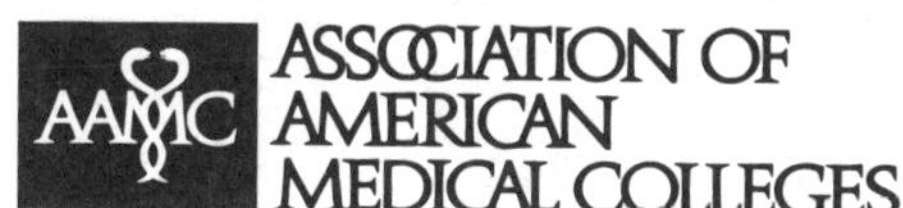

# Medical School
# ADMISSION REQUIREMENTS
## 1997-1998
### UNITED STATES AND CANADA

- Selection factors for each school
- Specific admission requirements
- Latest tuition figures
- Financial aid information and sources
- Current enrollment figures
- Combined-degree programs
- AMCAS-E and much more

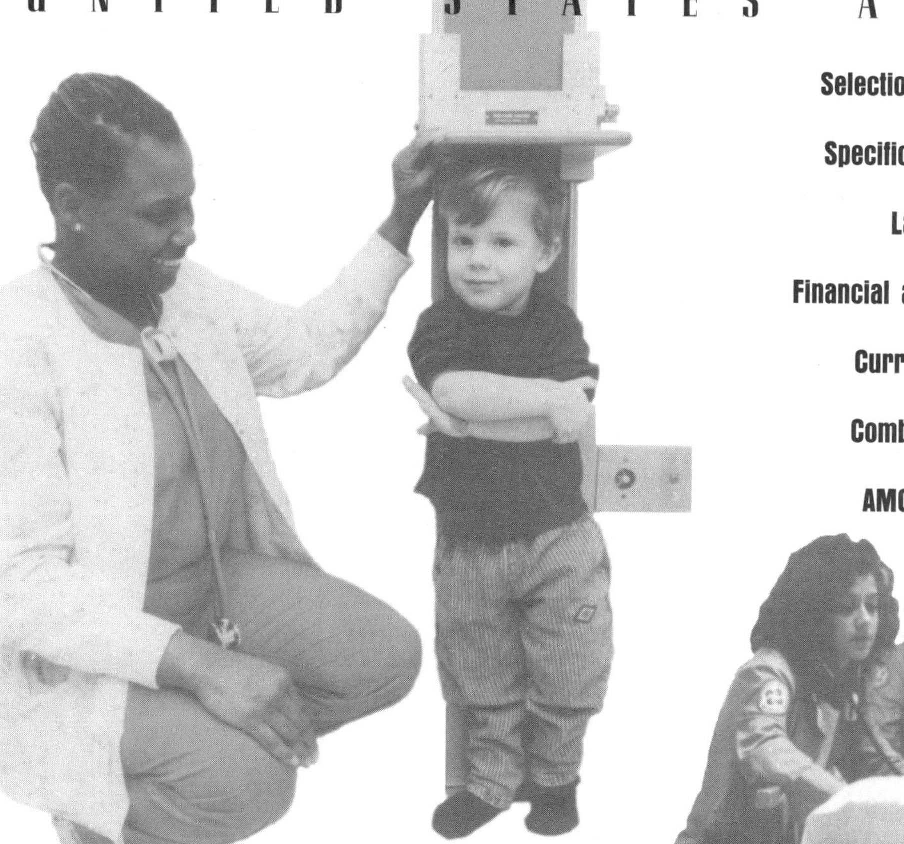

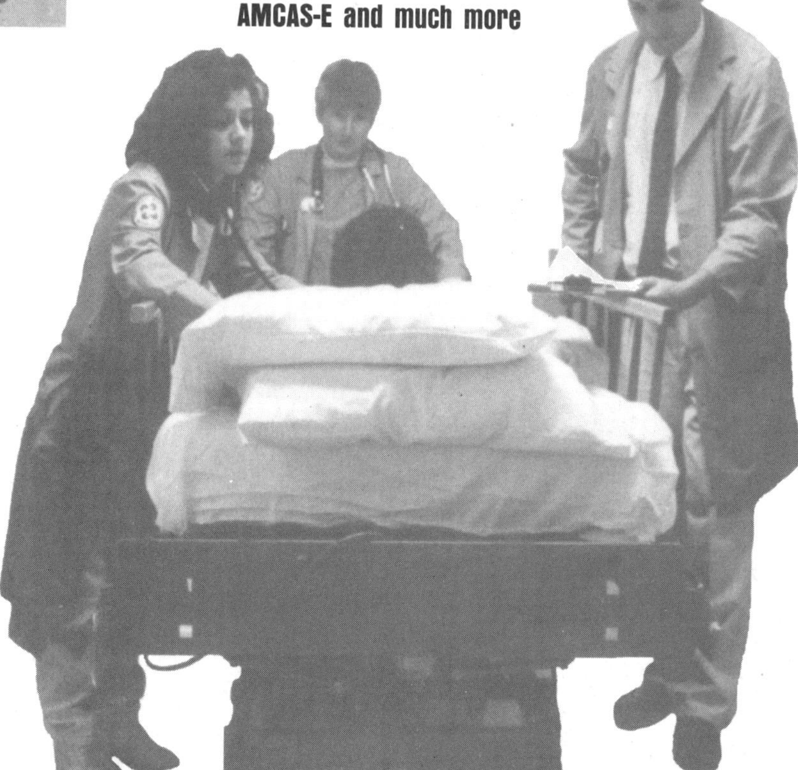

## 47TH Edition

Comprehensive admission information on every accredited medical school in the United States and Canada

The assistance of other AAMC staff members and the admission officers
and other representatives of the medical schools is noted with appreciation.


Revised annually; new edition available in April.


Address all inquiries to:
Cynthia T. Bennett, Editor
Coordinator of Special Publications
Association of American Medical Colleges
2450 N Street, NW
Washington, DC 20037
E-Mail: cbennett@aamc.org





ISBN 1-57754-000-X


Printed in the United States of America

**AAMC Staff for**
*Medical School Admission Requirements,*
*1997–98 United States and Canada*

Susan Neely, Vice President for Communications
Frances R. Hall, Director of Student Programs
Cynthia T. Bennett, Editor
M. LaVerne Alexander, Staff Associate
Kimberly S. Varner, Editorial Assistant

# ASSOCIATION OF AMERICAN MEDICAL COLLEGES

The Association of American Medical Colleges (AAMC) has as its purpose the advancement of medical education and the nation's health. In pursuing this purpose, the Association works with many national and international organizations, institutions, and individuals interested in strengthening the quality of medical education at all levels, the search for biomedical knowledge, and the application of these tools to providing effective health care.

As an educational association representative of members having similar purposes, the primary role of the AAMC is to assist those members by providing services at the national level which will facilitate the accomplishment of their mission. Such activities may include collecting data and conducting studies on issues of major concern, evaluating the quality of educational programs through the accreditation process, providing consultation and technical assistance to institutions as needs are identified, synthesizing the opinions of an informed membership for consideration at the national level, and improving communication among those concerned with medical education and the nation's health. Other activities of the Association reflect the expressed concerns and priorities of the officers and governing bodies.

The AAMC represents all 125 accredited U.S. medical schools; the 16 accredited Canadian medical schools; some 400 major teaching hospitals, including 74 Veterans Administration medical centers; 86 academic and professional societies representing 87,000 faculty members; and the nation's 67,000 medical students and 102,000 residents.

In addition to the types of activities listed above, the AAMC is responsible for the Medical College Admission Test (MCAT) and the American Medical College Application Service (AMCAS) and provides detailed admissions information to the medical schools and to undergraduate premedical advisers.

# Contents

# List of Tables

# Alphabetical Listing of Medical Schools

# Geographical Listing of Medical Schools

### Part 2 • Chapter 10 • U.S. Medical Schools

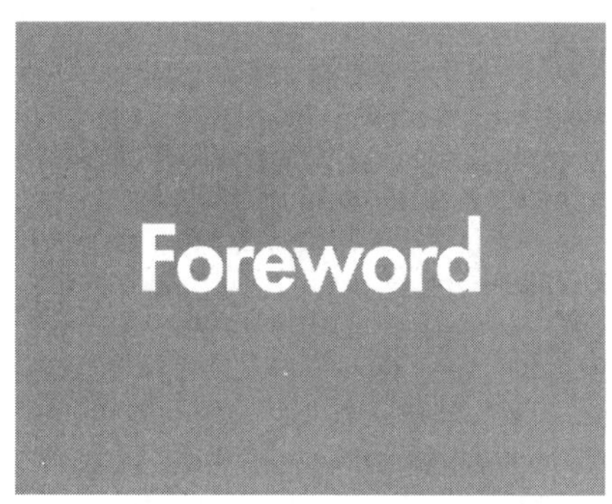


The medical profession offers a wide variety of career options that are exciting, challenging, and rewarding. Although the environment in which medical services are provided has been changing rapidly and will continue to change, the physician's role as diagnostician, healer, and patient advocate remains central to the provision of health care in our country.

The medical profession has, since World War II, assumed an enviable position in our society. The relief of suffering, the rehabilitation of injury, and the prevention of disease and premature death have always been regarded as worthy human endeavors. Modern science has enabled the pursuit of such objectives to become not only esteemed but also effective. The physician is no longer called upon primarily to comfort patients and alleviate suffering. The modern physician has the means to cure, control, and prevent many killing and crippling conditions.

This success has led to an increased demand for medical services. Unprecedented affluence and an egalitarian ethic have stimulated the growth of a societal commitment to provide access to quality medical services without regard to personal ability to pay for them. As a consequence, in the mid-1960s the nation greatly expanded its capacity to train health professionals.

The explosion of knowledge about biological processes and the consequent effectiveness of new clinical interventions have demanded longer and more specialized training of physicians. The rigor and discipline necessary to complete the training requires commitment and motivation. While society more and more recognizes the limits to its ability or at least its willingness to finance medical care, the intellectual challenges and the prospects for significant accomplishments attract large numbers to the profession.

The shortage of physicians perceived in the 1960s has not occurred. Indeed, some now describe an excess in some disciplines, while shortages of primary care specialists exist in all geographic areas, especially in rural and inner cities. The increased production of generalist physicians has become a priority for our medical schools and our nation. New forms of health care delivery are emerging as the health care environment becomes more price competitive. The expenditure for research, while increasing, has not matched the growth in science professionals and the increasing research opportunities. These stresses on the profession provide additional challenges and opportunities to an attractive and desirable career.

After a period of rapid growth in the 1960s and 1970s that saw the number of medical schools increase by 50 percent and total class size more than double, the national medical education enterprise plateaued in the 1980s. The size of the entering class has remained relatively stable, and the number of total enrollees dropped to reflect small decreases in class size at some institutions. With the dawn of this decade, the applicant pool has increased significantly. The number of applicants per medical school place dropped from 2.8 in the mid-1970s to 1.6 in 1988, but rose to nearly 3.0 in 1995. Women now comprise 42.5 percent of the applicant pool, compared with 11 percent in 1970. Minority applicants represented 11 percent of the 1995 applicant group. In 1975, 10 percent of all applicants were over age 27 compared with 17 percent in 1995.

This annually revised *Medical School Admission Requirements* book provides current and official information on premedical preparation and admission to medical school. It is designed to assist those who aspire to a medical career in approaching their goals realistically. It is also a source of assistance to premedical advisers in giving sound, informative, and practical advice to their students.

The prerequisites detailed in this volume by individual medical schools should not be the only guidance to those who seek a career in medicine. They reflect only the formal course work deemed necessary for admission to medical school. The preparation of an individual for a career in medicine must be much more extensive. In November 1984, the Association of American Medical Colleges (AAMC) published the final report of its Project Panel on the General Professional Education of the Physician and College Preparation for Medicine. The report states, "A broad and thorough baccalaureate education is an essential component of the general professional education of physicians." The report also stressed that the education of physicians includes teaching the following: values and attitudes that promote caring and concern for the individual and for society; concepts and principles derived from knowledge of the natural sciences, the social sciences, and the humanities; and skills in (a) the collection of information from and about patients, (b) the establishment of rapport with patients to facilitate both diagnosis and therapy, (c) the application of the scientific method to the analysis, synthesis, and management of clinical problems, (d) the identification and critical appraisal of the relevant literature in the assessment of clinical evidence, and (e) the continuation of effective learning.

The advancement of medical education, with all of the ramifications that affect the medical profession and the health sciences, has been the basic mission of the AAMC since its establishment in 1876. Through research, communications, and service, the AAMC seeks to serve both the medical schools and the public. It is active in student services; educational measurement and research; minority affairs; curriculum surveys; medical school, teaching hospital, and health care services. The Association's publications encompass newsletters, books, special reports, and the monthly journal *Academic Medicine*. The AAMC also sponsors conferences and workshops and national and regional meetings of the institutional membership as well as those of the student affairs faculties. Its fall Annual Meeting serves as a forum for discussion and action on matters of immediate and long-range interest to the nation, the AAMC, and its membership. Many of the activities of the AAMC involve cooperation with other professional organizations and a large number of private and governmental agencies.

The 47th edition of *Medical School Admission Requirements* contains current information from 122 medical schools in the United States, 3 in Puerto Rico, and 16 in Canada. It should be noted that all references made to U.S. medical schools are also applicable to the Puerto Rican medical schools listed in Chapter 10.

In making this information available, the AAMC hopes that individuals considering careers in medicine will be better informed of the opportunities available and more capable of realistically assessing their potential for admission.

JORDAN J. COHEN, M.D.
AAMC PRESIDENT

# Admission Information

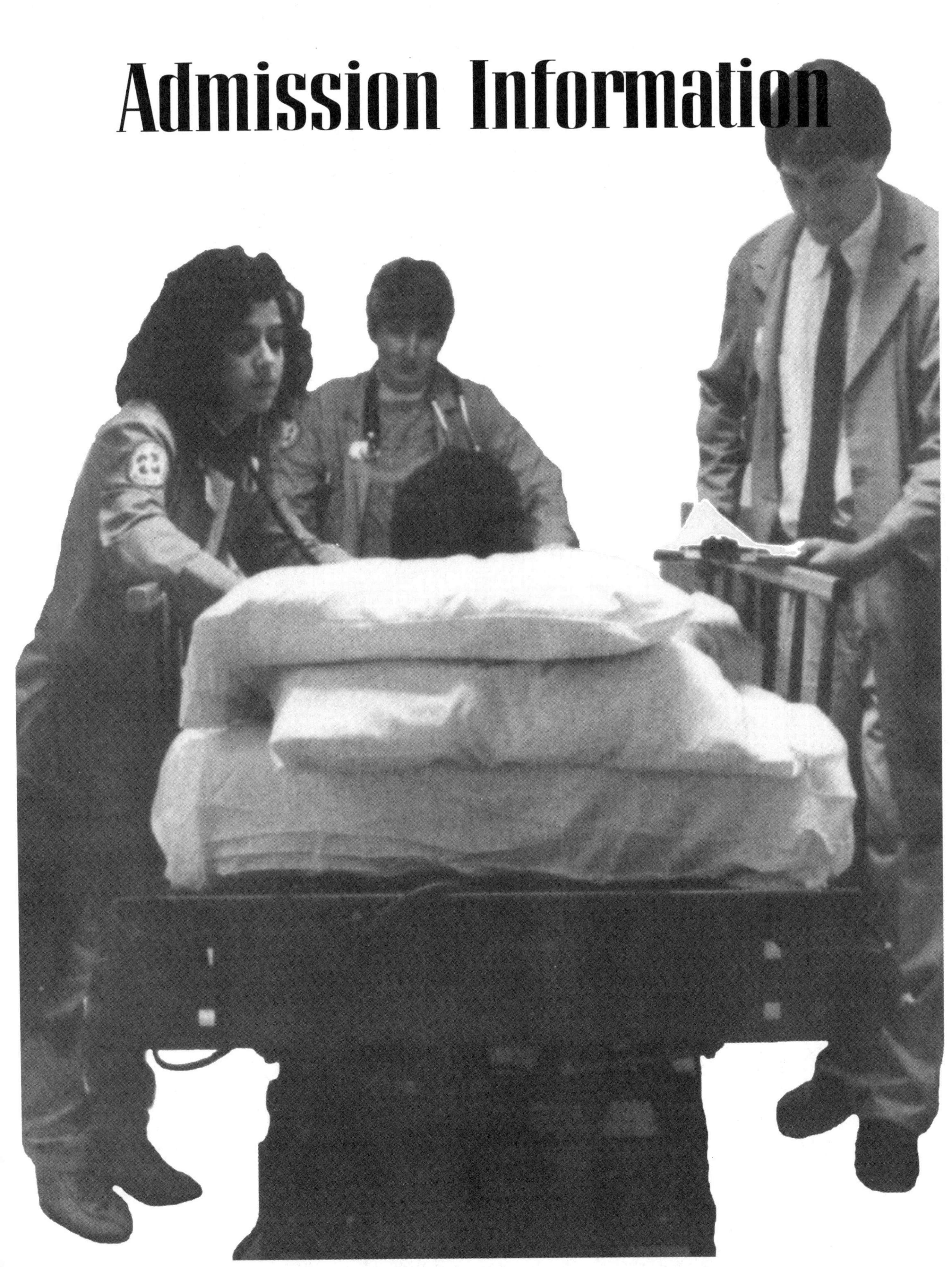

# The Nature of Medical Education

Programs of medical education that award the degree of doctor of medicine in the United States and Canada are accredited by the Liaison Committee on Medical Education (LCME). This voluntary accrediting agency is sponsored by the Association of American Medical Colleges and the American Medical Association. All state medical practice laws recognize the accreditation status conferred by the LCME on the medical schools. Holders of the M.D. degree awarded by the LCME-accredited schools are provided the opportunity for licensure subject to certain examinations and other requirements imposed by each state. The LCME has traditionally avoided narrowly dictating curriculum content and has encouraged institutions, while meeting national minimal standards of quality, to approach the education of physicians in a variety of ways. This philosophy has led to a significant diversity of educational approaches. The extent of this diversity may be observed in the annual *AAMC Curriculum Directory,* which provides details about the curriculum of each U.S. and Canadian medical school.

## THE M.D. CURRICULUM

Medical school curricula, although quite varied, have as their goal the preparation of students to enter a three- to seven-year period of graduate medical education. Many curricula are problem-based as contrasted to topical and discipline focused. The teaching methodologies include lecture, small group discussion, self-instruction, and laboratory experience. Instruction is provided in anatomy, biochemistry, physiology, microbiology, pharmacology, pathology, and behavioral sciences during the first several academic periods after matriculation. These basic sciences may be taught independently by departmental faculties or by interdisciplinary groups of faculty. The interdisciplinary approach often focuses on organ systems. In this approach, instruction in anatomy, biochemistry, physiology, pharmacology, and pathology of an organ system, such as the heart and blood vessels, is integrated with normal and abnormal functions of the system. Whether the basic sciences are taught by discipline or in an interdisciplinary fashion, there is a major emphasis in almost all medical schools on introducing contact with clinical problems early in the curriculum. In some schools students begin to learn in their first year how to interview and examine patients; in other schools the first clinical contact may be demonstrations of patients by faculty. In all schools, however, by the third semester or fifth quarter, students have begun to learn how to obtain historical data from patients and conduct physical and selected basic laboratory examinations. The teaching of bioethics, legal medicine, disease prevention, medical sociology, and characteristics of the health care delivery system occurs parallel to or interspersed within the basic and clinical sciences.

The last four semesters (six quarters) are usually devoted to education in the clinical setting. The immediate and specific aims of clinical education are to enable the student to establish desirable physician-patient relationships, to take a medical history, to conduct a physical examination, and to recognize the more familiar disease patterns. The overall aim, however, is to develop in the student both an understanding of the patient as a total human being and the sense of professional maturity that medicine demands.

The length and number of required clinical educational periods (clinical clerkships) vary  from school to school. Clinical clerkships are usually required in family medicine, internal medicine, obstetrics-gynecology, pediatrics, psychiatry, and surgery. Clerkships vary in length from 2 to 12 weeks. During clerkships, students are usually assigned to a hospital clinical service where they assume responsibility for "working-up," that is, collecting data and presenting to the faculty a specified number of patient studies each week. Students also participate with post-M.D. trainees (residents) and faculty in caring for patients admitted to the clinical service to which they are assigned. When feasible, students are provided the opportunity to follow their patients before and after discharge from the hospital in ambulatory care settings. In these first clerkships, basic science knowledge and fundamental clinical skills are applied to the solution of diagnostic and treatment problems. Lectures and seminars augment the bedside learning provided during patient visits, so-called "rounds," with teaching physicians.

As students progress through these early clinical experiences, the range of opportunity for career development becomes apparent. Elective courses in the basic, behavioral, and clinical sciences permit students to explore career options. In many institutions, courses taken in other colleges of the university may be applied for credit toward the M.D. degree. Depending upon individual interests and talent, students are provided the opportunity to arrange part of their programs. During the first four semesters, the opportunity to take electives varies greatly among the schools. In the last two semesters before graduation, many schools permit students to arrange their entire programs on an elective basis. Clinical electives include clerkships in the primary specialties and in their many subspecialties. Elective opportunities in clinical settings are often provided in other academic centers or in nonacademic settings. These may vary from a preceptorship with a practicing physician to a period of time spent in a research laboratory. Such settings allow students to become acquainted with the career possibilities of the medical specialties of their interest while enriching their education.

At present a major emphasis is placed on encouraging students to develop careers in the primary care specialties of family medicine, general internal medicine, and general pediatrics. This emphasis should not, however, deter students with interests in research and/or teaching from seeking the M.D. degree. There is also a need for well prepared physician-scientists to translate the rapid advances in biomedical knowledge into clinical applications.

## EVALUATION, PROMOTION, GRADUATION

Each medical school's faculty is responsible for establishing the criteria for evaluating student performance, promotion, and graduation. Many faculties have written learning objectives for the overall medical education program and for each course or segment of the curriculum. Determining whether students have met these objectives is accomplished by a combination of direct observation and written and/or oral assessments. The frequency and pattern of evaluation vary from institution to institution. Some form of year-end comprehensive exam is often required. Eighty-six schools report that they currently require students to pass Step 1 of the United States Medical Licensing Examination (USMLE) at the end of their basic science sequence or in order to graduate. Fifty-six schools report that they currently require students to pass Step 2 of the USMLE to graduate.

The USMLE is a single, three-step examination for medical licensure in the United States established by the Federation of State Medical Boards (FSMB) and the National Board of Medical Examiners (NBME). The USMLE provides a common evaluation system for all applicants for medical licensure. Each of the three steps consists of a written multiple-choice examination administered over two days. Step 1 assesses whether an examinee understands and can apply key concepts in biomedical sciences, with an emphasis on principles and mechanisms of health, disease, and modes of therapy. Step 2 assesses whether an examinee possesses the medical knowledge and understanding of clinical science considered essential for provision of patient care under supervision, including emphasis on health promotion and disease prevention. Step 3 is administered after graduation from medical school and assesses whether an examinee can apply the medical knowledge and understanding of biomedical and clinical science considered essential for the unsupervised practice of medicine with emphasis on patient management in ambulatory settings.

Currently, each step is administered twice during the year: Step 1 in June and October, Step 2 in March and August, and Step 3 in May and December. A plan to proceed with computer delivery of the step examinations by the end of the decade is under development.

Grading in less than half of the schools is pass/fail or honors/pass/fail. Regardless of the pattern or frequency of evaluation used, individual students' abilities are carefully scrutinized. This is particularly true in the clinical clerkships where one-to-one relationships between faculty and students permit close observation. Although student evaluation is rigorous, the rate of attrition in U.S. medical schools is low—slightly over 3 percent. Students with detected deficiencies in knowledge or skills are provided counseling and assistance. Students who are having difficulty may be offered the opportunity to repeat course work. However, all faculties reserve the right to drop students whose academic or personal characteristics are found to be incompatible with the professional responsibilities of a physician in this society.

## GRADUATE MEDICAL EDUCATION

Exposure to the various branches and aspects of medicine helps students to determine the course their education will take during the training period following medical school (residency). For students who have made a career decision to practice in a medical or surgical specialty, the requirements of the certifying board in that particular specialty will mold the choice of the first postgraduate year program. Specialties such as family medicine, internal medicine, pediatrics, and surgery encourage students to enter directly into first postgraduate year programs in that specialty and to continue in these programs until they have completed specialty board requirements. Satisfactory completion of three years of training in family medicine, internal medicine, or pediatrics generally qualifies an individual to take the examination(s) administered by the certifying boards of these specialties. General surgery requires five years of training while other surgical specialties require additional training.

Students seeking careers in other specialties will find they are encouraged or required to spend their first postgraduate year in a program offering a broad clinical experience. Examples of these specialties are anesthesiology, dermatology, psychiatry, and radiology. Usually these students will apply for a single year of internal medicine or for a diversified, transitional first postgraduate year with the expectation they will enter a program in the specialty of their choice in their second postgraduate year. In some cases a year of broad clinical experience may be located in the same institution where subsequent subspecialty training occurs. In other instances, specialty training must be completed elsewhere.

By the end of the third year of medical school, almost all students have made a career decision regarding the area of medicine in which they will specialize. Nearly all will eventually seek certification by one of the 24 specialty boards. Some will take one to two years of additional training in a subspecialty and will seek recognition through additional certification in that subspecialty. Descriptions of recognized specialties and subspecialties can be found in *Which Medical Specialist for You,* a brochure published by the American Board of Medical Specialties (ABMS). The ABMS also publishes a brochure entitled *Medical Specialty Certification and Related Matters* that provides information about the medical profession and specialty certification for the medical student, the resident and others, and lists sources of additional information. For more information, contact the ABMS at 1007 Church Street, Suite 404, Evanston, Illinois, 60201-5913.

## SPECIAL PROGRAMS

Individual medical schools offer a number of special programs. Many of these are listed in the *AAMC Curriculum Directory.* Specific details of the characteristics of a school's special programs may be obtained from that school. Several of the more common special programs are described below.

*B.A.- or B.S.-M.D. Degree Programs.* In 1995–96 a small number of U.S. medical schools provided limited programs beginning after high school that combined undergraduate college study and medical education. (These schools are listed in Table 2 in Chapter 2 and are fully described in Chapter 9.) Students are admitted provisionally to these programs based upon their high school credentials and, if their performance is satisfactory, are permitted to progress to the M.D. degree. This generally requires six or seven years. Students interested in this type of program should request information from the prospective medical school as early as possible.

*Accelerated Programs.* There are options for accelerating the standard four-year medical school curriculum. Since these options vary among schools, interested students should investigate the possibilities by consulting the dean's office at the institutions to which they intend to apply.

Several schools now offer programs that combine the undergraduate program and the first year of graduate medical education. These programs are especially designed to encourage careers in primary care through family practice or internal medicine. Students interested in these programs should inquire about their availability at the schools to which they apply.

*Research Training.* There is continuing need for physicians who have ability both to conduct research and interpret research findings. Students interested in research will find that most faculties are highly receptive to allowing them to engage in research projects. Depending upon the availability of resources and the student's willingness to invest time in research, programs ranging from a few months to a year or more can be arranged. These opportunities can be used by students to explore their creative talents for biomedical research. Such exploration can help students decide whether to pursue preparation for a career in academic medicine during graduate medical education.

*Medical Scientist Training Program (MSTP).* In recognition of a national need for medical scientists trained in both basic and clinical sciences, the National Institute of General Medical Sciences supports a combined M.D.-Ph.D. program, known as the Medical Scientist Training Program, at 33 schools. The goal of the MSTP is to provide combined scientific and medical training to highly motivated students with outstanding research and academic potential.

Medical scientists differ from most basic scientists in having had the medical training required to investigate human diseases. They differ from most clinicians in having had extensive research experience and training in the biological, chemical, physical, or behavioral sciences needed to bring the fundamental knowledge and insight of these disciplines into clinical investigation. The federal government supported approximately 841 MSTP students in 1995–96.

MSTP grants are made to universities and their medical schools, which are responsible for program operation and trainee selection. About 175 positions for new students are available each year. Therefore, selection for admission is highly competitive. For those selected, the program provides a maximum of six years of support, although an individual's course of study for the combined degree generally takes longer. Most institutions identify other sources of support for a trainee's additional years of study. The MSTP support provided includes a stipend of $10,008 a year plus a tuition allowance.

Continued support for an individual student is subject to annual renewal based on the trainee's satisfactory performance in the program and the institution's successful competition for funds at the time of grant renewal every three to five years. Since MSTP grants are a type of National Research Service Award (NRSA), trainees must be citizens or non-citizen nationals of the United States or have been lawfully admitted to permanent residence (i.e., possess an alien registration receipt card, I-151 or I-551). Effective with appointments made after June 10, 1993, newly appointed trainees now incur no payback obligation and existing trainees whose appointments are renewed incur no additional payback obligation.

Individuals who wish to enter the MSTP should contact the participating institution(s) of their choice for curriculum information and admission requirements.

The 33 schools offering the MSTP in 1995–96 are listed in Table 1-A. Other information about the MSTP may be obtained by contacting:

Program Administrator
Medical Scientist Training Program
National Institutes of Health
45 Center Drive, MSC 6200
Bethesda, Maryland 20892-6200
Telephone: (301) 594-3830

*M.D.-Ph.D. Degree Programs.* In 1995–96, 113 schools provided students the opportunity to earn both the M.D. and the Ph.D. in an area pertinent to medicine. These schools and some of the disciplines in which the Ph.D. is offered are listed in Table 1-B. This table does not include all disciplines and should only be used as a guide. See below for the names of the contact persons at each school.

*M.D.-J.D. Degree Programs.* In 1995–96, six schools (Duke, University of Illinois at Urbana-Champaign, Southern Illinois, University of North Carolina at Chapel Hill, West Virginia University, and Yale) offered programs that allowed the student the opportunity to earn both the M.D. and the J.D. degrees.

*Independent Study.* Several schools provide an option for students to pursue selected required courses of study at their own pace, using learning techniques of their own choosing. Characteristically, students engaged in independent study must meet periodically with faculty tutors to demonstrate their progress and must pass the comprehensive exams required of all students for promotion and graduation.

---

### TABLE 1-A

### U.S. Medical Schools Offering Medical Scientist Training Programs Supported by National Institutes of Health, 1995–96

| | |
|---|---|
| Alabama | Minnesota, Univeristy of |
| Albert Einstein | Mount Sinai |
| Baylor | New York University |
| California, Los Angeles (UCLA) | SUNY-Stony Brook |
| | Northwestern |
| California, San Diego | Pennsylvania, University of |
| California, San Francisco | Pittsburgh‡ |
| Case Western Reserve | Rochester |
| Chicago-Pritzker | Stanford |
| Colorado | Texas, Dallas |
| Columbia | (Southwestern) |
| Cornell* | Tufts |
| Duke | Vanderbilt |
| Emory | Virginia, University of |
| Harvard† | Washington University |
| Iowa | (St. Louis) |
| Johns Hopkins | Washington, University of |
| Michigan, University of | Yale |

*Conducted in cooperation with Rockefeller University—Sloan Kettering Institute.

†Conducted in cooperation with the Massachusetts Institute of Technology

‡Conducted in cooperation with Carnegie Mellon University.

# Contact Persons for M.D.-Ph.D. Programs at U.S. Medical Schools

**ALABAMA**

**University of Alabama
School of Medicine**
 Dr. Frank M. Griffin, Jr.
 Director, Medical Scientist Training
  Program

**University of South Alabama
College of Medicine**
 Dr. Mark Gillespie
 Director, Basic Medical Sciences
  Graduate Program

**ARIZONA**

**University of Arizona
College of Medicine**
 Dr. Raymond B. Nagle
 Professor of Pathology

**ARKANSAS**

**University of Arkansas for Medical
Sciences College of Medicine**
 Linda W. Williams
 Director, Student Admissions

**CALIFORNIA**

**University of California, Davis
School of Medicine**
 Edward D. Dagang
 Director of Admissions

**University of California, Irvine
College of Medicine**
 Patricia Terrell
 Medical Scientist Program
  Coordinator

**University of California, Los Angeles
UCLA School of Medicine**
 Alice del Rosario
 Program Administrator, Medical
  Scientist Training Program

**University of California, San Diego
School of Medicine**
 Kathleen Sexton
 Program Assistant

**University of California, San
Francisco, School of Medicine**
 Jana M. Toutolmin
 Program Administrator,
  Recruitment and Admissions
 Medical Scientist Training Program

**Loma Linda University
School of Medicine**
 Dr. W. Bart Rippon
 Dean, Graduate School

**University of Southern California
School of Medicine**
 Sandra M. Mosteller
 Administrative Director

**Stanford University
School of Medicine**
 Marjorie Weesner
 Administrative Assistant, Medical
  Scientist Training Program

**COLORADO**

**University of Colorado
School of Medicine**
 Dr. Arthur Gutierrez-Hartmann
 Assistant Professor and Director,
  Program MST

**CONNECTICUT**

**University of Connecticut
School of Medicine**
 Dr. Dominick L. Cinti
 Director, Combined M.D.-Ph.D.
  Degree Program

**Yale University School of Medicine**
 Dr. James D. Jamieson
 Director, M.D.-Ph.D. Program

**DISTRICT OF COLUMBIA**

**George Washington University
School of Medicine and Health
Sciences**
 Diane P. McQuail
 Director of Admissions

**Georgetown University
School of Medicine**
 W. Taylor Johnson
 Coordinator, Graduate Biomedical
  Education

**Howard University
College of Medicine**
 Dr. Verle Headings
 Assistant Dean for Student Affairs

**FLORIDA**

**University of Florida
College of Medicine**
 Dr. Alfred Lewin
 Director, Medical Scientist Training
  Program

**University of Miami
School of Medicine**
 Dr. Robert Hinkley
 Associate Dean for Admissions

**GEORGIA**

**Emory University
School of Medicine**
 Dr. Robert B. Gunn
 Director, M.D.-Ph.D. Program

**Medical College of Georgia
School of Medicine**
 Dr. James R. Goldenring
 Associate Director,
  M.D.-Ph.D. Program

**Morehouse University
School of Medicine**
 Dr. David E. Potter
 Chairman and Professor,
  Pharmacology/Toxicology

**HAWAII**

**University of Hawaii
John A. Burns School of Medicine**
 Marilyn M. Nishiki
 Admissions Officer/Registrar

## ILLINOIS

**University of Chicago**
**Pritzker School of Medicine**
Dr. Norma E. Wagoner
Dean of Students

**Finch University of Health Sciences**
**Chicago Medical School**
Dr. Yoon Berm Kim
Chairman, M.D.-Ph.D. Program

**University of Illinois**
**College of Medicine (Chicago)**
Dr. Edward P. Cohen
Director, M.D.-Ph.D. Training
Program

**University of Illinois**
**College of Medicine**
**at Urbana-Champaign**
Nora J. Few
Medical Scholars Program
Coordinator

**Loyola University Chicago**
**Stritch School of Medicine**
Paula Griffin-Arnold
Administrative Secretary

**Northwestern University**
**Medical School**
Charles A. Berry
Associate Dean for Admissions

**Rush Medical College of**
**Rush University**
Jan L. Schmidt
Director of Admissions

## INDIANA

**Indiana University School of Medicine**
Dr. William F. Bosron
Assistant Dean for Graduate Studies

## IOWA

**University of Iowa**
**College of Medicine**
Leslie Arnold
Program Associate

## KANSAS

**University of Kansas Medical Center**
**School of Medicine**
Dr. Joseph D. Bast
Associate Dean of Graduate Studies
and Research

## KENTUCKY

**University of Kentucky**
**College of Medicine**
Dr. Charles Snow
Director, M.D.-Ph.D. Program

## LOUISIANA

**Louisiana State University**
**School of Medicine in New Orleans**
Dr. Marilyn L. Zimny
Vice Chancellor for Academic Affairs
Dean, School of Graduate Studies

**Louisiana State University**
**School of Medicine in Shreveport**
Dr. Ronald J. Korthuis
Assistant Dean, Graduate Studies

**Tulane University School of Medicine**
Dr. Joseph C. Pisano
Associate Dean

## MARYLAND

**Johns Hopkins University**
**School of Medicine**
Dr. Stephen V. Desiderio
Director, M.D.-Ph.D. Program

**University of Maryland**
**School of Medicine**
Dr. Marshall L. Rennels
Professor of Anatomy
Director, M.D.-Ph.D. Program

## MASSACHUSETTS

**Boston University School of Medicine**
Sheila Welch
Coordinator, M.D.-Ph.D.

**Harvard Medical School**
Linda Burnley
Administrative Director

**University of Massachusetts Medical**
**School**
Dr. Michael R. Green
M.D.-Ph.D. Program

**Tufts University School of Medicine**
Cathenne Samson
Staff Assistant

## MICHIGAN

**Michigan State University**
**College of Human Medicine**
Dr. Jane M. Smith
Director of Admissions

**University of Michigan Medical**
**School**
Frances U. Simonds
Administrative Associate, Medical
Scientist
Training Program

**Wayne State University**
Dr. George E. Dambach
Associate Dean, Research and
Graduate Programs

## MINNESOTA

**Mayo Medical School**
Dr. Richard McGee
M.D.-Ph.D. Admissions Director

**University of Minnesota Medical**
**School–Minneapolis**
Dana Rechtzigel
Associate Administrator

## MISSISSIPPI

**University of Mississippi**
**School of Medicine**
Dr. Virginia H. Read
Chairman, Medical School
Admissions Committee

**MISSOURI**

**University of Missouri–Columbia**
**School of Medicine**
Dr. Herbert S. Goldberg
Associate Dean for Research and
Academic Affairs

**University of Missouri–Kansas City**
**School of Medicine**
Kim Huggett
Coordinator of Admissions

**Saint Louis University**
**Health Sciences Center**
Dr. Andrew J. Lechner
Chairman, M.D.-Ph.D. Program
Professor and Director of Medical
Physiology

**Washington University**
**School of Medicine**
Brian P. Sullivan
Program Administrator


**NEBRASKA**

**Creighton University**
**School of Medicine**
Dr. William L. Pancoe
Associate Dean for Student Affairs

**University of Nebraska**
**College of Medicine**
Dr. C. Kirk Phares
Associate Dean for Research and
Development


**NEVADA**

**University of Nevada**
**School of Medicine**
Dr. Gale Starich
Assistant Professor


**NEW HAMPSHIRE**

**Dartmouth Medical School**
Sheila M. Rembert
Assistant Director of Admissions


**NEW JERSEY**

**University of Medicine and Dentistry**
**of New Jersey**
**New Jersey Medical School**
Dr. George F. Heinrich
Assistant Dean for Admissions

**University of Medicine and Dentistry**
**of New Jersey**
**Robert Wood Johnson Medical School**
Dr. Michael J. Leibowitz
Associate Dean, Graduate School
of Biomedical Sciences


**NEW YORK**

**Albany Medical School**
Sara J. Kremer
Director of Admissions

**Albert Einstein College of Medicine**
**of Yeshiva University**
Cecile A. Brown
Assistant Director,
Sue Golding Graduate Division

**Columbia University**
**College of Physicians and Surgeons**
Joan R. Popovitch
Program Coordinator,
M.D.-Ph.D Program

**Cornell University Medical College**
Sheila Krauss
Program Coordinator, Tri-Institutional
M.D.-Ph.D. Program

**Mount Sinai School of Medicine**
**of the City University of New York**
Terry Ann Krulwich
Dean, Director of Medical Scientist
Training Program

**New York Medical College**
Dr. Mario A. Inchiosa, Jr.
Director, M.D.-Ph.D. Program

**New York University**
**School of Medicine**
Arlene Kohler
Administrative Assistant


**University of Rochester**
**School of Medicine and Dentistry**
Catherine Senecal-Rice
M.D.-Ph.D. Program Coordinator

**State University of New York**
**Health Science Center at Brooklyn**
**College of Medicine**
Liliana Montano
Director of Admissions

**State University of New York**
**at Buffalo**
**School of Medicine and**
**Biomedical Sciences**
Dr. Jerome A. Roth
Director, MSTP

**State University of New York**
**Health Science Center at Syracuse**
**College of Medicine**
Dr. Alexander Bortoff
M.D.-Ph.D. Chairperson

**SUNY Stony Brook**
**School of Medicine**
Dr. Paul A. Fisher, Director
Toni Douralo, Program Administrator


**NORTH CAROLINA**

**Duke University School of Medicine**
Pat Burks
Staff Specialist

**East Carolina University**
**School of Medicine**
Dr. Alvin Volkman
Associate Dean, Research and
Graduate Studies

**University of North Carolina at**
**Chapel Hill School of Medicine**
Kelly Collier
Administrative Coordinator


**NORTH DAKOTA**

**University of North Dakota**
**School of Medicine**
Dr. Thomas E. Norris
Executive Associate Dean

## OHIO

**Case Western Reserve University**
**School of Medicine**
Felicité Katz
MSTP Coordinator

**University of Cincinnati**
**College of Medicine**
Terri Berning
Administrative Secretary

**Medical College of Ohio**
Dr. Patricia J. Metting
Chairman, M.D.-Ph.D. Program

**Ohio State University**
**College of Medicine**
Priscilla K. North
Administrative Assistant

**Wright State University**
**School of Medicine**
Robert Fyffe
Director, Biomedical Sciences Ph.D.
Program


## OKLAHOMA

**University of Oklahoma**
**College of Medicine**
Dr. John B. Harley
Chair, M.D.-Ph.D. Advisory
Committee
Program Director


## OREGON

**Oregon Health Sciences University**
**School of Medicine**
Vicki Fields
Administrative Director


## PENNSYLVANIA

**Jefferson Medical College**
**of Thomas Jefferson University**
Dr. Benjamin Bacharach
Associate Dean for Admissions

**Medical College of Pennsylvania and**
**Hahnemann University**
**School of Medicine**
Office of Biomedical Graduate Stuies

**Penn State University**
**College of Medicine**
Dr. Judith S. Bond
Professor and Chair, Biochemistry
and Molecular Biology

**University of Pennsylvania**
**School of Medicine**
Dr. Glen N. Gaulton
Associate Dean

**University of Pittsburgh**
**School of Medicine**
Dr. Joseph M. Furman
Assistant Dean, M.D.-Ph.D. Program

**Temple University School of Medicine**
Dr. Peter N. Walsh
Director, M.D.-Ph.D. Program


## RHODE ISLAND

**Brown University Program**
**in Medicine**
Dr. Kim Baekelheide
Director, M.D.-Ph.D. Program


## SOUTH CAROLINA

**Medical University of South Carolina**
Dr. Perry V. Halushka
Director, Medical Scientist Training
Program
Professor of Pharmacology and
Medicine

**University of South Carolina**
**School of Medicine**
Dr. James Buggy
Assistant Dean for Graduate Studies


## SOUTH DAKOTA

**University of South Dakota**
**School of Medicine**
Dr. Gerald J. Yutrzenka
Director of Admissions

## TENNESSEE

**Meharry Medical College**
Dr. Fred Jones
Acting Dean, School of Graduate
Studies
Vice President for Research

**University of Tennessee, Memphis**
**College of Medicine**
Dr. David M. Mirvis
Associate Dean for VA Medical
Center

**Vanderbilt University**
**School of Medicine**
Dr. David Robertson
Director, Medical Scientist
Training Program


## TEXAS

**Baylor College of Medicine**
Leslie L. Walters
Senior Administrative Assistant

**Texas A&M University**
**Health Science Center**
**College of Medicine**
Dr. Gerald D. Frye
Professor, Pharmacology and
Toxicology

**Texas Tech University**
**Health Sciences Center**
**School of Medicine**
Dr. Kenneth L. Barker
Dean, Graduate School of
Biomedical Sciences

**University of Texas Southwestern**
**Medical Center at Dallas**
**Southwestern Medical School**
Dr. Rodney E. Ulane
Associate Dean

**University of Texas Medical**
**School at Galveston**
Jessica E. Thorp
M.D.-Ph.D. Combined Degree
Program Coordinator

**University of Texas—
Houston Medical School**
Doris Thornton
Education Coordinator, Special
Programs

**University of Texas
Medical School at San Antonio**
Dr. Terry Mikiten
Associate Dean, Graduate School of
Biomedical Sciences

## UTAH

**University of Utah School of Medicine**
Dr. Jerry Kaplan
Assistant Health Sciences Vice
President for Basic Science

## VERMONT

**University of Vermont
College of Medicine**
Dr. Paula B. Tracy
Associate Professor of Biochemistry

## VIRGINIA

**Eastern Virginia Medical School
of the Medical College of
Hampton Roads**
Dr. Gerald J. Pepe
Associate Dean for Research

**Virginia Commonwealth University
Medical College of Virginia
School of Medicine**
Dr. Jack L. Haar
Director, M.D.-Ph.D. Program

**University of Virginia
School of Medicine**
Susan Frasier
Director, Interdisciplinary Graduate
Studies

## WASHINGTON

**University of Washington
School of Medicine**
Maureen Levell
Program Coordinator

## WEST VIRGINIA

**Marshall University
School of Medicine**
Dr. L. Howard Aulick
Assistant Dean, Graduate and
Research Education

**West Virginia University
School of Medicine**
Dr. Diana S. Beattie
Professor and Chair, Director,
M.D.-Ph.D. Program

## WISCONSIN

**Medical College of Wisconsin**
Dr. Sidney E. Grossberg
Walter Schroeder Professor
Chair, Department of Microbiology

**University of Wisconsin Medical
School**
Dr. John F. Fallon
Director

## Combined M.D.-Ph.D. Program at U.S. Medical Schools, 1995–96

| Medical School | Anatomy | Biochemistry | Biomedical Engineering | Biophysics | Cell Biology | Genetics | Immunology | Microbiology | Molecular Biology | Neurosciences | Pathology | Pharmacology | Physiology | Other Disciplines |
|---|---|---|---|---|---|---|---|---|---|---|---|---|---|---|
| **Alabama** | | | | | | | | | | | | | | |
| Alabama | • | • | • | • | • | • | • | • | • | • | • | • | • | |
| South Alabama | • | • | | | • | • | • | • | • | • | | • | • | • |
| **Arizona** | | | | | | | | | | | | | | |
| Arizona | • | • | | | • | • | • | • | • | • | | • | • | • |
| **Arkansas** | | | | | | | | | | | | | | |
| Arkansas | • | • | | • | | | • | • | • | | | • | • | • |
| **California** | | | | | | | | | | | | | | |
| University of California | | | | | | | | | | | | | | |
| Davis | | • | • | | • | • | • | • | • | • | • | • | • | • |
| Irvine | • | • | | • | | | | • | • | | | • | • | • |
| Los Angeles | • | • | • | • | • | • | • | • | • | • | • | • | • | • |
| San Diego | | • | • | • | • | • | • | • | • | • | • | • | • | • |
| San Francisco | • | • | | • | • | • | • | • | • | • | • | • | • | |
| Loma Linda | • | • | | | | | • | | | | • | • | | |
| Southern California | • | • | • | • | • | • | • | • | • | • | • | • | • | |
| Stanford | | • | • | • | • | • | • | • | • | | • | | | • |
| **Colorado** | | | | | | | | | | | | | | |
| Colorado | | • | | • | • | | • | • | • | • | • | • | • | • |
| **Connecticut** | | | | | | | | | | | | | | |
| Connecticut | | • | | | • | | • | | | • | | • | | • |
| Yale | | • | | • | • | • | • | • | • | • | • | • | • | • |
| **District of Columbia** | | | | | | | | | | | | | | |
| George Washington | • | • | • | • | • | • | • | • | • | • | • | • | • | |
| Georgetown | | • | | • | • | | • | • | | • | • | • | • | • |
| Howard | • | • | | | | • | | • | | | • | • | • | |
| **Florida** | | | | | | | | | | | | | | |
| Florida | • | • | • | • | • | • | • | • | • | • | • | • | • | |
| Miami | • | • | | • | • | | • | • | • | | • | • | • | |
| **Georgia** | | | | | | | | | | | | | | |
| Emory | • | • | • | • | • | • | • | • | • | • | • | • | • | • |
| Medical College of Georgia | | • | | | | • | • | | | • | | • | | |
| Morehouse | | | | | | | | | | | | | | • |
| **Hawaii** | | | | | | | | | | | | | | |
| Hawaii | • | • | | • | • | • | • | • | • | | • | • | • | • |
| **Illinois** | | | | | | | | | | | | | | |
| Chicago Medical | • | • | | • | • | • | • | • | • | • | • | | • | |
| Chicago-Pritzker | • | • | | • | • | • | • | • | • | • | • | • | • | • |
| Illinois, Chicago | • | • | | • | • | • | • | • | | | • | • | • | |
| Illinois, Urbana-Champaign | | • | • | • | • | • | | • | | • | | | • | • |
| Loyola-Stritch | • | • | | | • | | • | • | • | • | | • | • | |

## Combined M.D.-Ph.D. Program at U.S. Medical Schools, 1995–96

| Medical School | Anatomy | Biochemistry | Biomedical Engineering | Biophysics | Cell Biology | Genetics | Immunology | Microbiology | Molecular Biology | Neurosciences | Pathology | Pharmacology | Physiology | Other Disciplines |
|---|---|---|---|---|---|---|---|---|---|---|---|---|---|---|
| **Illinois (Continued)** | | | | | | | | | | | | | | |
| Northwestern | | | | | | | | | | • | | | | • |
| Rush | • | • | | | | | • | • | | • | | • | • | • |
| **Indiana** | | | | | | | | | | | | | | |
| Indiana | • | • | | • | | • | • | • | • | • | • | • | • | |
| **Iowa** | | | | | | | | | | | | | | |
| Iowa | • | • | • | • | • | • | • | • | • | • | • | • | • | |
| **Kansas** | | | | | | | | | | | | | | |
| Kansas | | • | | | • | • | • | • | • | • | • | • | • | • |
| **Kentucky** | | | | | | | | | | | | | | |
| Kentucky | • | • | • | • | | | • | • | | | • | | • | |
| **Louisiana** | | | | | | | | | | | | | | |
| Louisiana State-New Orleans | • | • | | | • | • | • | • | • | • | • | • | • | |
| Louisiana State-Shreveport | • | • | | | • | | • | • | • | | | • | • | |
| Tulane | • | • | • | | • | • | • | • | • | • | | • | • | |
| **Maryland** | | | | | | | | | | | | | | |
| Johns Hopkins | • | • | • | • | • | • | • | • | • | • | • | | • | • |
| Maryland | • | • | • | • | • | • | • | • | • | • | • | • | • | • |
| **Massachusetts** | | | | | | | | | | | | | | |
| Boston | • | • | | • | • | • | • | • | • | • | • | • | • | |
| Harvard | | • | | • | • | • | • | • | • | • | • | • | | • |
| Massachusetts | • | • | • | • | • | • | • | • | • | • | • | • | • | • |
| Tufts | | • | | | • | • | • | • | • | • | | • | • | |
| **Michigan** | | | | | | | | | | | | | | |
| Michigan State | • | • | • | • | • | • | | • | • | • | • | • | • | • |
| University of Michigan | • | • | • | • | • | • | • | • | • | • | • | • | • | • |
| Wayne State | • | • | | • | • | • | • | • | • | • | • | • | • | • |
| **Minnesota** | | | | | | | | | | | | | | |
| Mayo | | • | | • | | | • | | | • | | • | • | |
| Minnesota-Minneapolis | | • | • | • | • | • | • | • | • | • | | • | • | • |
| **Mississippi** | | | | | | | | | | | | | | |
| Mississippi | • | • | | | | | | • | | | • | • | • | |
| **Missouri** | | | | | | | | | | | | | | |
| Missouri-Columbia | | • | | | | | • | • | | | • | • | | • |
| Missouri-Kansas City | | | | | | | | | | | | | | • |
| Saint Louis | • | • | | | • | • | • | • | • | • | • | • | • | |
| Washington University (Saint Louis) | | • | | | • | • | • | • | • | • | • | • | | • |
| **Nebraska** | | | | | | | | | | | | | | |
| Creighton | • | • | | | | | | • | | | | • | • | |
| Nebraska | • | • | | | • | • | • | • | • | • | • | • | • | • |
| **Nevada** | | | | | | | | | | | | | | |
| Nevada | | • | • | | • | | | • | • | | | • | • | • |

## Combined M.D.-Ph.D. Program at U.S. Medical Schools, 1995–96

| Medical School | Anatomy | Biochemistry | Biomedical Engineering | Biophysics | Cell Biology | Genetics | Immunology | Microbiology | Molecular Biology | Neurosciences | Pathology | Pharmacology | Physiology | Other Disciplines |
|---|---|---|---|---|---|---|---|---|---|---|---|---|---|---|
| **New Hampshire** | | | | | | | | | | | | | | |
| Dartmouth | | • | • | | • | • | • | • | • | | | • | • | • |
| **New Jersey** | | | | | | | | | | | | | | |
| New Jersey Medical | • | • | | | • | • | • | • | • | • | • | • | • | |
| Robert Wood Johnson | | • | • | | • | | | • | • | • | | • | • | • |
| **New York** | | | | | | | | | | | | | | |
| Albany | | • | | | • | | • | • | • | • | • | • | • | • |
| Albert Einstein | • | • | | • | • | | • | • | • | • | • | • | • | • |
| Columbia | • | • | | • | • | • | • | • | • | • | • | • | • | • |
| Cornell | | • | | • | • | • | • | • | • | • | | • | • | • |
| Mount Sinai | • | • | | • | • | • | • | • | • | • | • | • | • | • |
| New York Medical | • | • | | | • | • | • | • | • | • | • | • | • | |
| New York University | | • | | | • | • | • | • | • | • | • | • | • | • |
| Rochester | • | • | • | • | • | • | • | • | • | • | • | • | • | • |
| SUNY-Brooklyn | • | • | | • | • | | • | • | • | • | • | | • | |
| SUNY-Buffalo | • | • | | • | • | • | • | • | • | | • | • | • | |
| SUNY-Stony Brook | • | • | • | • | • | • | • | • | • | • | • | • | • | • |
| SUNY-Syracuse | • | • | | | • | | • | • | • | • | | • | • | |
| **North Carolina** | | | | | | | | | | | | | | |
| Duke | | • | • | • | • | • | • | • | • | • | • | • | • | |
| East Carolina | • | • | | | • | | • | • | | | • | • | • | |
| North Carolina | • | • | • | • | • | • | • | • | • | • | • | • | • | • |
| **North Dakota** | | | | | | | | | | | | | | |
| North Dakota | • | • | | | | | | | • | | | • | • | |
| **Ohio** | | | | | | | | | | | | | | |
| Case Western Reserve | | • | • | • | • | • | • | • | • | • | • | • | • | |
| Cincinnati | • | • | • | • | • | • | • | • | • | • | • | • | • | |
| Medical College of Ohio | • | • | | | | | | | • | | • | • | • | • |
| Ohio State | • | • | • | • | • | • | • | • | • | • | • | • | • | • |
| Wright State | • | • | | • | • | • | • | • | • | • | • | • | • | |
| **Oklahoma** | | | | | | | | | | | | | | |
| Oklahoma | • | • | | • | • | | • | • | • | • | • | • | • | • |
| **Oregon** | | | | | | | | | | | | | | |
| Oregon | | • | | • | • | • | • | • | • | • | • | • | • | |
| **Pennsylvania** | | | | | | | | | | | | | | |
| Jefferson | | • | | | • | • | • | • | • | • | • | • | • | • |
| Medical College of Pennsylvania and Hahnemann | • | • | | | • | | • | • | | • | • | • | • | • |
| Penn State | • | • | • | | | | • | • | • | • | • | | • | • |
| University of Pennsylvania | | • | • | • | • | • | • | • | • | • | • | • | • | • |
| Pittsburgh | • | • | • | • | • | • | • | • | • | • | • | • | • | • |
| Temple | • | • | | | | | • | • | • | • | • | • | • | |

## Combined M.D.-Ph.D. Program at U.S. Medical Schools, 1995–96

| Medical School | Anatomy | Biochemistry | Biomedical Engineering | Biophysics | Cell Biology | Genetics | Immunology | Microbiology | Molecular Biology | Neurosciences | Pathology | Pharmacology | Physiology | Other Disciplines |
|---|---|---|---|---|---|---|---|---|---|---|---|---|---|---|
| **Rhode Island** | | | | | | | | | | | | | | |
| Brown | | • | | | • | | | | • | • | | | | • |
| **South Carolina** | | | | | | | | | | | | | | |
| Medical University of South Carolina | • | • | | | • | | • | • | • | | • | • | • | • |
| University of South Carolina | • | | | | • | | • | • | | • | • | • | • | |
| **South Dakota** | | | | | | | | | | | | | | |
| South Dakota | • | • | | | | | | • | • | | | • | • | |
| **Tennessee** | | | | | | | | | | | | | | |
| Meharry | | • | | | • | | | • | • | • | | • | | |
| Tennessee-Memphis | • | • | | | • | | • | • | • | • | • | • | • | |
| Vanderbilt | | • | • | | • | | • | • | • | • | • | • | • | |
| **Texas** | | | | | | | | | | | | | | |
| Baylor | | • | | • | • | • | • | • | • | | | • | | • |
| Texas A&M | • | • | • | • | • | • | • | • | • | • | • | • | • | |
| Texas Tech | • | • | | | | | | • | | | | • | • | |
| University of Texas | | | | | | | | | | | | | | |
|   Southwestern, Dallas | | • | | • | • | • | • | • | • | • | • | • | • | |
|   Galveston | • | • | | • | • | • | • | • | • | • | • | • | • | • |
|   Houston Medical School | • | • | | • | • | • | • | • | • | • | • | • | • | |
|   San Antonio | | • | | | • | • | • | • | • | • | | • | • | • |
| **Utah** | | | | | | | | | | | | | | |
| Utah | • | • | | | • | • | • | | • | | • | | | |
| **Vermont** | | | | | | | | | | | | | | |
| Vermont | • | • | | • | • | | | • | • | | | • | • | • |
| **Virginia** | | | | | | | | | | | | | | |
| Eastern Virginia | • | • | | • | • | • | • | | • | • | • | • | • | |
| Medical College of Virginia | • | • | • | | • | • | • | • | • | • | • | • | • | |
| University of Virginia | | • | • | • | • | • | • | • | • | • | • | • | • | |
| **Washington** | | | | | | | | | | | | | | |
| University of Washington | • | • | • | • | • | • | • | • | • | • | • | • | • | • |
| **West Virginia** | | | | | | | | | | | | | | |
| Marshall | | | | | | | | | | | | | | • |
| West Virginia | • | • | • | | • | | • | • | • | | | • | • | |
| **Wisconsin** | | | | | | | | | | | | | | |
| Medical College of Wisconsin | • | • | | • | • | • | • | • | • | • | • | • | • | |
| University of Wisconsin | • | • | | • | • | • | • | • | • | • | • | • | • | • |

# Options for Individuals Considering a Career in Medicine

While it has been traditional for students to begin medical school immediately after graduation from college, in recent years several other options have become available. Some students have opted to enter a combined college/medical school program, others delay medical school for a number of years, and still others choose to prepare for medical school after a successful experience in another career. A wider range of options is now available. This chapter reviews these options.

## CAREERS IN MEDICINE

Medicine offers many careers. New opportunities emerge with each advance in medical knowledge and with each development in the organization of medical services. The physician's responsibilities cover a wide range of functions in health maintenance, including both acute care and preventive care approaches involving substantial patient education. These responsibilities include diagnosing disease, supervising the care of patients, prescribing treatment, and participating in improved delivery of health care. Although most physicians provide direct patient care, some concentrate on basic or applied research, others become teachers or administrators, still others combine various elements of these activities. Often students make these career decisions near completion of medical school.

Graduating students select an area of medicine for further training and eventual practice. Some physicians practice in the generalist specialties of general internal medicine, general pediatrics, or family practice. Other physicians choose from among the following specialties: allergy and immunology; anesthesiology; dermatology; emergency medicine; obstetrics and gynecology; pathology; psychiatry; radiology; and, surgery (general, neuro, orthopedic, plastic, urology, vascular).

The U.S. has a shortage of doctors in general internal medicine, general pediatrics, and family practice at the present time. These shortages are most acute in rural and center-city areas.

New patterns of practice are emerging. Physicians may be salaried, in partnership, or self-employed. A physician may choose from such varied settings as group practice, a managed care system, clinic, hospital, laboratory, industry, military, university, government, or various combinations of these.

The wide range of practice options, specialty choices, and availability of locations provides substantial diversity to individuals choosing a career in medicine. Benefits include the reward of caring for others, the intellectual challenge of medicine, and the social and economic rewards of providing services that are highly valued by society. The demands of a medical career are great in terms of the time, energy, and responsibility for other people's lives and a commitment to continuing service and education is essential.

## EDUCATIONAL PREPARATION

What does it take to be a physician? Briefly, it takes physical, emotional, and intellectual stamina; the desire to work with and for people; and, particularly, the ability to think logically and to use common sense. The educational pipeline involves four (occasionally three) years of college, four years of medical school, and three or more years of residency.

### Traditional Route

Most students apply to medical school during their senior year of undergraduate college. Admissions procedures are outlined in Chapter 6.

### Postbaccalaureate Programs

For those individuals who have completed college and perhaps embarked on another career before deciding to apply to medical school, a number of postbaccalaureate programs offer the opportunity to complete premedical courses and to participate in advising/counseling programs for premedical students. These programs are numerous and exist in every part of the country. Some provide a one- to two-year package of courses and health-related experiences for the individual who wishes to prepare on a half- or full-time schedule. Other programs are less structured and permit the individual to take premedical courses at their own pace while continuing their employment. Any U.S. medical school can provide the names of colleges and universities in their area that offer postbaccalaureate programs.

### Deferred Entry

An increasing number of medical schools will consider requests from accepted applicants for a one-year deferral of their matriculation to undertake a special opportunity or for specific personal reasons. Most schools require a specific request and review this request individually.

The remainder of this chapter provides special advice for (1) postbaccalaureate students who may be returning to college

**TABLE 2**

**U.S. Medical Schools Offering Combined College/M.D. Programs<br>Provisionally Admitting Students After Senior Year in High School, 1995–96**

| Schools offering programs of instruction combined with their undergraduate division: | Schools offering programs in collaboration with other undergraduate institutions: |
|---|---|
| South Alabama | Albany |
| Boston | Baylor |
| Brown | California, Los Angeles (UCLA) |
| Southern California | Chicago Medical |
| Case Western Reserve | Jefferson |
| Howard | Meharry Medical College |
| George Washington | UMDNJ—New Jersey Medical |
| Miami* | UMDNJ—Robert Wood Johnson† |
| Michigan State | SUNY Brooklyn |
| Michigan, University of | SUNY Syracuse |
| Missouri—Kansas City | Ohio, Northeastern |
| New York University | Pennsylvania, Medical College of and Hahnemann |
| Rochester | Pennsylvania State |
| Northwestern | Virginia, Eastern |
| East Tennessee State | |
| Wisconsin, University of | |

Source: Liaison Committee on Medical Education 1994–95 Questionnaire.

*Program acceptance limited to state residents.

†Students are selected at the end of their sophomore year in college.

after an absence of some years to complete premedical courses, and (2) high school students who may be considering an application to combined college/medical school programs.

## Combined College/Medical School Programs

There are a number of programs beginning after high school graduation that combine the undergraduate college and medical school curricula. Some of these programs result from special arrangements between a school of medicine and a particular undergraduate college and thus require enrollment in that respective undergraduate institution. For the 1995–96 academic year, those medical schools offering combined pro-

grams accepting high school seniors into the M.D. program on a provisional basis are indicated in Table 2. Several programs are limited to residents of the state where the medical school is located. See Chapter 9 for further information about specific programs.

## ADVICE FOR POSTBACCALAUREATE STUDENTS

Each year, an increasing number of individuals decide to enter medicine from other career fields or after several years of college in other areas. Such individuals bring maturity and life experience to medicine. Before applying, it is necessary to complete the premedical course requirements by taking or repeating the specific science and other course requirements that medical schools require of all applicants.

To complete premedical courses, postbaccalaureate students may choose between a structured program, which offers the opportunity to complete courses within one to two years, and a less structured approach, where courses are taken one at a time while the individual continues to work. Students are encouraged to investigate both types of programs, obtain information about the placement record of each, and weigh the pluses and minuses of each program with respect to their own personal needs. Prehealth advisers are available on most campuses and postbaccalaureate students are encouraged to consult these individuals and to make use of the services provided by their offices.

Postbaccalaureate students can expect their applications to be reviewed in competition with the entire applicant pool, with consideration given to both personal and academic qualifications, as discussed in Chapter 6. Admissions committees are interested in the process and experience that led to the applicant's choice of medicine as a career goal.

## ADVICE FOR HIGH SCHOOL STUDENTS

Choosing a medical career is a big decision and entry into the application process for a combined program should not be entered into lightly. It is important that high school students considering medicine weigh the relative advantages of combined undergraduate/medical school programs with those of the traditional route and consult carefully with high school advisers as well as appropriate college and medical school personnel in making a decision.

Medical schools accepting students in combined undergraduate college/medical school programs will be looking for a high level of academic achievement, maturity, well-developed communication skills, intellectual abilities, and social adjustment as well as a carefully thought-through career decision. Normally students applying for combined programs will have had some health-related experience while in high school.

## FINANCIAL PLANNING

In the U.S., much attention is currently directed at the rising costs of acquiring a higher education and the need for more financial assistance for students. Significant amounts of aid are available, but the award of aid to medical students is generally based on financial need. Parents of students of any age seeking assistance in medical school will almost certainly be asked to file a confidential report about their income, financial assets and liabilities.

It is important to start carefully estimating expenses for undergraduate college and medical school and analyzing the actual and potential income available from family resources, student earnings, and loans from a variety of national, regional, state, local, and institutional sources. Chapter 7 provides substantial detail regarding the types of financial aid (including loans and service commitment scholarships) available to medical students. In addition, readers are encouraged to consult *Financial Planning and Management Manual*, available through the AAMC Publications Office.

While substantial financial aid is available to medical students, much of this aid is in the form of loans. It is important to understand and plan for the accumulation of significant debt during medical school. In undergraduate college or during postbaccalaureate studies, it is wise to limit borrowing as much as possible. Undergraduate students may wish to work to defray expenses and reduce borrowing. Postbaccalaureate students who have accumulated financial assets during a prior career will find these assets invaluable in helping to finance both postbaccalaureate and medical studies. Since a medical career can be financially rewarding, medical schools expect all students to fully use liquid assets to pay for medical school expenses.

## Other Health Careers

Applicants considering other careers are encouraged to consult the following professional associations and references.

1. American Association of Colleges of Osteopathic Medicine, Suite 405, 6110 Executive Boulevard, Rockville, Maryland 20852-0000.

2. American Association of Colleges of Pharmacy, 1426 Prince Street, Alexandria, Virginia 22314-2841.

3. American Association of Colleges of Podiatric Medicine, Suite 322, 1350 Piccard Drive, Rockville, Maryland 20850-4307.

4. American Association of Dental Schools, Suite 502, 1625 Massachusetts Avenue, N.W., Washington, D.C. 20036-2212.

5. Association of American Veterinary Medical Colleges, Suite 710, 1101 Vermont Avenue, N.W., Washington, D.C. 20005-3521.

6. Association of Schools and Colleges of Optometry, Suite 690, 6110 Executive Boulevard, Rockville, Maryland 20852.

7. Association of Schools of Public Health, Suite 204, 1660 L Street, N.W., Washington, D.C. 20036.

8. *Allied Health Education and Rehabilitation Professions Directory.* 24th edition. 1996–1997. $54.95, plus $11.95 for handling and shipping. Order No. OP-417596. (American Medical Association, P.O. Box 109050, Chicago, Illinois 60610-9050; (1-800-621-8335); (312) 464-5600 (FAX).

9. *200 Ways To Put Your Talent To Work in the Health Field.* Single copy, $6.00. (National Health Council, 1730 M Street, N.W., Suite 500, Washington, D.C. 20036)

For further information on educational and financial planning, the following may be of interest.

1. M., and Cass-Liepmann, J., eds., *Cass & Birnbaum Guide to American Colleges,* 16th edition. $19.00 paperback, $40.00 hardcover. (Harper/Collins, Inc., Publications Department, Keystone Industrial Park, Scranton, Pennsylvania 18512)

2. *The College Board Guide to 150 Popular Majors.* $16.00. California residents add 7.25 percent sales tax and Pennsylvania residents add 6 percent sales tax. Revised annually each September. (College Board Publications, Box 886, New York, New York 10101–0886)

3. *The College Cost Book, 1992.* $15.00. Item #004817. California residents add 7.25 percent sales tax and Pennsylvania residents add 6 percent sales tax. Revised annually each September. (College Board Publications, Box 886, New York, New York 10101-0886)

4. *The College Handbook, 1994.* $20.00. Item #004795. California residents add 7.25 percent sales tax and Pennsylvania residents add 6 percent sales tax. Revised annually each September. (College Board Publications, Box 886, New York, New York 10101-0886)

5. *Dollars for College: The Quick Guide to Scholarships, Fellowships, Loans, and Other Financial Aid Programs for Medicine, Dentistry, and Related Fields.* $6.95 prepaid. Revised every 18 months. (Garrett Park Press, P.O. Box 190, Garrett Park, Maryland 20896) ISBN: 1-880774-15-1.

6. *Federal Student Aid Fact Sheet, 1990–91.* Department of Education. Free. (Federal Student Aid Information Center, P.O. Box 84, Washington, D.C. 20044 (1-800-333-INFO)

7. *Financial Planning and Management Manual for U.S. Medical Students, 1994.* $7.50 per copy. (Association of American Medical Colleges, 2450 N Street, N.W., Washington, D.C. 20037-1126)

8. *Index of Majors and Graduate Degrees, 1993.* $16.00. Item #004809. California residents add 7.25 percent sales tax and Pennsylvania residents add 6 percent sales tax. Revised annually each September. (College Board Publications, Box 886, New York, New York 10101–0886)

9. Keeslar, O. *Financial Aids for Higher Education.* 1995. 16th edition. $61.50, subject to change. (Brown & Benchmart Publishers, 2460 Kerper Boulevard, Dubuque, Iowa 52004–0539) ISBN: 0-697-22262-4.

10. *Meeting College Costs.* Revised annually in September. $10.00 per 50 copies. Available only in packages of 50 or from high school guidance offices. Item #236286. California residents add 7.25 percent sales tax and Pennsylvania residents add 6 percent sales tax. (College Board Publications, Box 886, New York, New York 10101-0886)

11. *Need a Lift? College Financial Aid Handbook.* $3.00 prepaid. (The American Legion, P.O. Box 1050, Indianapolis, Indiana 46206)

# Premedical Planning

This chapter presents general recommendations for the college student who is looking ahead to medical school and seeking information about criteria for admission in order to plan a program that satisfies academic requirements as well as enhances the student's own intellectual, personal, and social development. Supplementary information for students from minority groups traditionally underrepresented in medicine (black Americans, Native Americans, Mexican Americans, mainland Puerto Ricans) is presented in Chapter 8.

Although the process of selecting medical school applicants necessarily involves a variety of considerations (Chapter 4), in general, medical schools are concerned with academic, nonacademic, and personal characteristics of applicants. As medical schools respond to national social issues and problems in medical care, they are making efforts to select individuals whose personal and career goals appear to be compatible with the needs of society. Major curriculum revisions at some institutions have been designed to encourage students to pursue careers in primary care medicine and careers in underserved geographical areas. Some schools have designed curricula with a problem-based approach. Schools have broadened the socioeconomic diversity of entering medical school classes and expanded educational opportunities for men and women who are members of racial/ethnic groups that have been underrepresented in medicine. Prospective applicants should give careful attention to the selection factors and school characteristics presented for each medical school listed in Part 2.

## UNDERGRADUATE ACADEMIC PROGRAM

The medical profession needs individuals from diverse educational backgrounds who will bring to the profession a variety of talents and interests. Educational philosophies and goals, systems of education, and specific undergraduate course requirements and other qualifications for admission vary among the nation's medical schools. All, however, recognize the importance of a broad education—a strong foundation in the natural sciences (biology, chemistry, mathematics, and physics), highly developed communication skills, and a solid background in the social sciences and humanities.

An understanding of the principles of the sciences basic to medicine is required of entering medical students. A thorough understanding of modern concepts in biology, chemistry, and physics is necessary since the study and practice of medicine are based on these disciplines. In order to achieve the minimum level of understanding, medical schools generally require one year of biology, two years of chemistry (through organic chemistry), and one year of physics (Table 3-A). The courses should be rigorous and, in general, acceptable for students majoring in those areas. The courses should include adequate laboratory experience. Candidates for medical school must study in these areas in order to (1) confirm their interest in and capacity for proceeding further in these fields, (2) enable medical schools to estimate their achievement and potential in these areas, and (3) meet the requirements of state laws governing physician licensure.

Additional science courses are not required. Students may take upper level science courses out of educational interest or to fulfill the requirements of their undergraduate major course of study. The practice of taking additional science courses that cover material taught within the medical school curriculum in the belief that they will be useful in gaining admission to and succeeding in medical school is not recommended.

Although only a small number of medical schools demand a specific course sequence in mathematics, all value mathematical competence, and many require or strongly recommend mathematics and computer science courses. Mathematics courses provide a good basis for the student's understanding of rigorous courses in chemistry, physics, and modern biology. Increasing numbers of medical curricula also utilize computer theory and statistics.

Breadth of education is expected. The pursuit of some discipline in depth is encouraged. A successful medical student must effectively acquire, synthesize, apply, and communicate information. These are skills which can be developed through a great variety of academic disciplines. Studies in the humanities and in the social and behavioral sciences and opportunities for the development of effective writing skills are strongly suggested.

Honors courses and independent study or research are encouraged, because they permit the student to explore, in depth, an area of knowledge and provide a scholarly experience which will facilitate a lifelong habit of self-education.

Although most medical schools require a minimum of three years of undergraduate work before entrance to their regular M.D. programs, the majority of entering medical students have four years of college and a baccalaureate degree.

## UNDERGRADUATE MAJOR

The selection of an undergraduate major area of study should be a carefully considered decision. Students should select a major area of study that is of interest and that will provide a foundation of knowledge necessary for the pursuit of several career alternatives. Students who select a major area of study solely or primarily because of the perception that it will enhance the chance of acceptance to a school of medicine are not making a decision in their best interest.

A science major is not a prerequisite for medical school, and students should not major in science simply because they believe this will increase their chances for acceptance. Medical schools are most concerned with the overall quality and scope of undergraduate work. All students need to do well in the required premedical courses to ensure adequate preparation and favorable consideration by admission committees. For most physicians, however, the undergraduate years are the last available opportunity to pursue in depth a nonscience subject of interest, and all who hope to practice medicine should bear this in mind when selecting an undergraduate major.

Table 3-B indicates that, while there is some variation at the national level in the acceptance rates of applicants from different major fields of study in liberal arts programs, those majoring in certain areas of the humanities, for example, fared as well or better in gaining acceptance to the 1995–96 entering class as applicants majoring in certain scientific disciplines. These data also show, however, that students who concentrated in such professional fields as medical technology, nursing, and pharmacy were less successful in gaining admission to medical school that year.

## SELECTION FACTORS

Decisions about the undergraduate academic program can be made more realistically if the student is aware of the medical school selection process. Admission committees do not seek a stereotyped, ideal combination of characteristics in all applicants; diversity within an entering class is considered highly desirable. Chapter 4 discusses specific considerations for an applicant in choosing medical schools to which to apply.

Medical schools seek candidates with high levels of scholastic achievement and intellectual potential, as well as the motivation and humanistic concern necessary for success as a physician. These qualities are measured by college grades, particularly science grades; recommendations from undergraduate faculty, including premedical advisers; Medical College Admission Test (MCAT) scores; interview assessments; an applicant's personal statement and application; and occasionally the use of psychological tests of educational development, mental aptitude, and nonintellectual qualities.

College grades are perhaps the most important single predictor of medical school performance, although medical schools do recognize that grading policies may differ from one college to another or even within departments of the same institution. Most first-year medical students have achieved undergraduate averages of A or B, and in 1995–96, .8 percent of the applicants accepted to the first-year class had grade-point averages (GPAs) of equal to or less than 2.5. The mean undergraduate GPA of first-year entrants for the 1995–96 entering class was 3.52. In recent years those individuals admitted with less than a 3.00 GPA have either achieved strikingly improved performances in their later years of college or demonstrated other characteristics deemed desirable for medicine by the various medical school admission committees.

It is also important for students to demonstrate an understanding of course content in ways other than by grades achieved. For example, the student who undertakes special projects or independently investigates questions raised in course work may provide evidence of ability that is not reflected by grades alone.

Medicine demands superior personal attributes of its students and practitioners. Integrity and responsibility assume major importance in the classroom and research laboratory as well as in relationships with patients and colleagues. Medical schools also look for evidence of other traits such as leadership, social maturity, purpose, motivation, initiative, curiosity, common sense, perseverance, and breadth of interests.

---

### TABLE 3-A

#### Subjects Required by 10 or More U.S. Medical Schools, 1997–98 Entering Class

| Required Subject | No. of Schools (*n*=110) |
|---|---|
| Physics | 107 |
| Inorganic (general) chemistry | 105 |
| Organic chemistry | 104 |
| English | 74 |
| Biology or zoology | 55 |
| Biology | 53 |
| Calculus | 22 |
| College mathematics | 21 |
| Behavioral and/or social sciences | 16 |
| Humanities | 15 |

NOTE: Figures based on data provided fall 1995. Fifteen of the 125 medical schools (University of Arkansas, UCLA, Mercer, University of Illinois, Northwestern, Southern Illinois, Indiana, Michigan State, Wayne State, Duke, University of North Carolina, University of Pennsylvania, Medical Univesity of South Carolina, Meharry, and UT-Galveston) did not indicate specific course requirements and are not included in the tabulations.

Anyone considering a career as a physician must be able to relate to people effectively. The increasing emphasis on a team approach to medical care adds another dimension to the need for this skill.

Because of the demanding nature of both the training for and the practice of medicine, motivation is perhaps the most salient nonintellectual trait sought by most admission committees. It is assumed that a qualified applicant to medical school will have not only a general understanding of the profession but also a demonstrated interest in and knowledge of what the field of medicine encompasses. This could be accomplished, in part, by having experiences in health care settings (especially in a clinical setting), talking with health professionals, reading appropriate literature, and experiencing an exposure to research at the undergraduate level.

In all aspects of premedical planning, the prospective medical student is encouraged to consider not only the information and advice contained in this publication but also the resources and counseling available from undergraduate prehealth advisers. The prehealth adviser is an important source of information and guidance in the undergraduate institution on matters related to the application to medical school.

Another source of value to both applicants and advisers is the annual medical education issue of the *Journal of the American Medical Association*. The cost of the 1995 issue (Vol. 274, No. 9, September 6, 1995) is $5.00; copies are available from:

Customer Services
American Medical Association
515 North State Street
Chicago, Illinois 60610

**TABLE 3-B**

**Acceptance to Medical School by Undergraduate Major,
1995–96 Entering Class**

| Undergraduate Major | Total Applicants | | Accepted Applicants | |
|---|---|---|---|---|
| | No. | % of Total | No. | % of Major |
| **Biological Sciences** | | | | |
| Biology | 17,544 | 37.7 | 6,148 | 35.0 |
| Microbiology | 1,024 | 2.2 | 332 | 32.4 |
| Physiology | 597 | 1.3 | 178 | 29.8 |
| Science (other biology) | 1,069 | 2.3 | 471 | 44.1 |
| Zoology | 1,053 | 2.3 | 375 | 35.6 |
| Subtotal | 21,287 | 45.7 | 7,504 | 35.3 |
| **Physical Sciences** | | | | |
| Biochemistry | 2,549 | 5.5 | 1,050 | 41.2 |
| Biomedical Engineering | 534 | 1.1 | 238 | 44.6 |
| Chemical Engineering | 452 | 1.0 | 198 | 43.8 |
| Chemistry | 2,757 | 5.9 | 1,143 | 41.5 |
| Chemistry and Biology | 320 | 0.7 | 127 | 39.7 |
| Electrical Engineering | 567 | 1.2 | 208 | 36.7 |
| Mathematics | 347 | 0.7 | 151 | 43.5 |
| Natural Sciences | 260 | 0.6 | 102 | 39.2 |
| Physics | 310 | 0.7 | 145 | 46.8 |
| Science (General) | 200 | 0.4 | 62 | 31.0 |
| Subtotal | 8,296 | 17.8 | 3,424 | 41.3 |
| **Nonscience Subjects** | | | | |
| Anthropology | 310 | 0.7 | 155 | 50.0 |
| Economics | 556 | 1.2 | 240 | 43.2 |
| English | 671 | 1.4 | 334 | 49.8 |
| Foreign Language | 385 | 0.8 | 155 | 40.3 |
| History | 587 | 1.3 | 299 | 50.9 |
| Philosophy | 241 | 0.5 | 101 | 41.9 |
| Political Science | 399 | 0.9 | 164 | 41.1 |
| Psychobiology | 480 | 1.0 | 168 | 35.0 |
| Psychology | 2,612 | 5.6 | 892 | 34.2 |
| Sociology | 212 | 0.5 | 84 | 39.6 |
| Subtotal | 6,453 | 13.9 | 2,592 | 40.2 |
| **Other Health Professions** | | | | |
| Medical Technology | 282 | 0.6 | 48 | 17.0 |
| Nursing | 337 | 0.7 | 60 | 17.8 |
| Pharmacy | 309 | 0.7 | 85 | 27.5 |
| Subtotal | 928 | 2.0 | 193 | 20.8 |
| **Mixed Disciplines** | | | | |
| Double Major Science | 648 | 1.4 | 228 | 35.2 |
| Double Major Non-Science | 1,141 | 2.4 | 467 | 40.9 |
| Interdisciplinary Studies | 265 | 0.6 | 151 | 57.0 |
| Pre-Medical | 761 | 1.6 | 259 | 34.0 |
| Pre-Professional | 202 | 0.4 | 84 | 41.6 |
| Subtotal | 3,017 | 6.5 | 1,189 | 39.4 |
| **Other*** | | | | |
| Other | 6,610 | 14.2 | 2,455 | 37.1 |
| Subtotal | 6,610 | 14.2 | 2,455 | 37.1 |
| Grand Total | 46,591 | 100.0 | 17,357 | 37.3 |

*Those applicants not reporting an undergraduate major are included in "Other."

# Deciding Whether and Where To Apply to Medical School

The practice of medicine has never been more challenging and rewarding, offered more opportunities for accomplishing good, or provided more selection in styles of practice and practice patterns than it does today. Deciding whether to apply to medical school must be the outcome of serious personal reflection about one's motivations and aspirations as these relate to the realities of medical practice such as working with sick people, continuing study for 7 to 11 years after college, and commitment to lifelong learning. In this process of self-exploration, candid discussions with premedical advisers, knowledgeable faculty, and one's personal physician about the reasons for wanting to be a physician can be very helpful. Consulting books about medical education can provide an added perspective.

New scientific breakthroughs have extended the limits of treatment to the young and old and to individuals with serious, complex diseases. More and more medical care can be provided in the office, clinic, and home. Physicians are becoming more attuned to the promotion of health and the prevention of disease by risk screening and influencing healthier behaviors.

Medical schools have broadened the scientific foundation of medical training to include education in nutrition, geriatrics, epidemiology, environmental health and preventive medicine, medical humanities and bioethics, clinical decision-making, medical socioeconomics, and the systems and cost-effective application of health care.

The more complex therapies and the special opportunities for care present complicated ethical and social questions which demand the unique guidance of the health care team members and new interrelationships among the several health care professions. The trends named here are by no means all of the important changes that are occurring in the medical profession. Prospective medical students will want to seek more information by reading nationally distributed newspapers as well as medical periodicals, such as *The New England Journal of Medicine.*

If convinced that they genuinely want to study and practice medicine, students must decide whether they have a moderately good chance of being accepted to medical school, and, if so, where to apply.

## CHANCES FOR ACCEPTANCE

Over the past seven years, the applicant pool has been increasing, making it more competitive for applicants to gain admission to medical school. For the 1990 entering class, 54.7 percent of the 29,243 candidates who applied matriculated. For the 1995 entering class, 34.9 percent of 46,591 applicants matriculated. Although many factors other than college grades and test scores enter into the admission decision, it is unquestionably true that these two factors receive considerable attention in the preliminary review of each application. In 1995, 75.3 percent of matriculants had undergraduate grade-point averages (GPAs) of 3.26 or above. The majority of accepted applicants with GPAs below 3.26 achieved relatively high scores on the nationally standardized preadmission examination for medical school applicants, the Medical College Admission Test (MCAT). Only 7.6 percent of 1995 accepted applicants had GPAs lower than 3.0.

Admission committees understand that grades may not measure a student's true ability; extenuating circumstances, such as prolonged illness, unsettled family circumstances, or the need to work while in school, can affect academic performance.

The relationship between MCAT performance and performance in specific undergraduate courses can be evaluated through the examination of individual test scores. A low score in the Physical Sciences, for example, can be easily explained if a student has not completed introductory college level physics prior to taking the test. Admission committees will take such circumstances into consideration when evaluating an application.

It is important to recognize that medical schools consider not only grades and test scores but also such factors as personality, character, place of residence, career plans, motivation and interest in medicine, communication and interpersonal skills, leadership, critical thinking skills, maturity, integrity, empathy, level of difficulty of course work, and whether the applicant is from a minority and/or disadvantaged background. Again, students are encouraged to consult their premedical advisers, who ordinarily have access to pertinent data regarding the success of applicants from their institutions.

## CHARACTERISTICS OF SCHOOLS

All medical schools listed in this book maintain the high standards necessary for accreditation by the Liaison Committee on Medical Education. Most have similar basic undergraduate course requirements, and all seek to admit students with demonstrated learning, problem-solving, and communication skills and with the qualities of integrity, maturity, and caring.

The Association of American Medical Colleges (AAMC) and all its member schools strongly endorse the principle of equal opportunity for education and practice in the health professions without regard to sex, age, race, creed, national origin, disability, or sexual orientation. (See AAMC Position on Equal Opportunity.)

Medical schools differ, however, with respect to other factors, for example, policies and requirements regarding state or regional residence. They also vary considerably in such characteristics as size of student body, size of faculty, number and type of patients with whom medical students will have contact, general philosophy of education, geographic location, student services, sources of financial support, and opportunities for special activities such as research. Moreover, opportunities for postgraduate study and the aspects of medicine generally chosen as career paths by graduates differ among medical schools as well.

A number of schools have received funds from foundations to make major changes in their programs. The schools funded by the W.G. Kellogg Foundation will be developing programs in community-based health systems, while those funded by the Robert Wood Johnson Foundation will be making major curriculum changes to better integrate basic and clinical sciences. Other Robert Wood Johnson Foundation grants are directed at new initiatives to encourage students to become generalist physicians.

## STATE AND REGIONAL RESIDENCE POLICIES

The residence restrictions noted in the individual entries in chapters 9 and 10 are generally not subject to change. State-supported medical schools are required to give preference to state residents; some state-supported schools consider nonresidents only under the Early Decision Program discussed in Chapter 6. Some schools have quotas for counties or regions of the state. State residents pay a substantially lower tuition in publicly supported schools. In addition, there are private schools that give significant preference to residents of the state in which the schools are located, because the schools receive financial support from their state governments. Some states without medical schools within their boundaries participate in special interstate and regional agreements. These and similar arrangements are described later in this section.

Table 4-A shows the number of applicants, new entrants, and total enrollment for each medical school. Within each of these categories, percentages of in-state residents and women are also provided. For applicants and new entrants the in-state figure represents the percentage of individuals in that category who claim as their legal residence the state in which the medical school is located. (For example, of the 2,316 applicants to the University of Alabama, 25.0 percent were Alabama residents; and of the 165 new entrants, 86.1 percent were Alabama residents.) The total enrollment figure reflects total enrollment without regard to residency. Schools' practices regarding acceptance of in-state residents have been stable for the most part, and applicants can use these percentages as guides. Overall, 68.7 percent of 1995–96 first year students entered schools within their own states; 59.3 percent of public school entrants and 40.7 percent of private school entrants were in-state residents. Selection by a public school in another state is highly improbable unless the nonresident candidate has exceptionally strong credentials.

An applicant may be a resident of only one state at any given time. In view of the relationship between geographic residence and chances for admission, applicants are strongly

### AAMC Position on Equal Opportunity

The Association strongly reaffirms the principle of equal opportunity for individuals who are qualified for education and training in, and the practice of, the health professions, without regard to sex, race, creed, color, national origin, age, or handicap. In pursuit of this principle and policy, the AAMC:

1. Requests member institutions to continue to monitor their admission policies and practices to insure equal opportunity of admission to their educational and training programs.

2. Requests member institutions to continue to undertake and to reinforce programs of affirmative action to increase the numbers and proportions of students in the health professions from groups which are presently underrepresented in those professions.

Further, recognizing that the underrepresentation of some groups in health professions educational and training programs is but a symptom of broad social and economic problems, the AAMC:

1. Actively supports the organized study of the basic causes of underrepresentation and possible cures.

2. Actively supports the initiation of new programs, and the broadening of existing programs, which are designed to overcome these problems. These programs include, but are not limited to, those designed to permit women to fulfill their educational-professional goals and their cultural roles without sacrifice to either, programs designed to eliminate economic barriers to education in the health professions, and programs designed to develop increased interest in careers in the health professions on the part of members of underrepresented groups at the secondary school and college levels.

urged to clarify their official residency status, if it is uncertain, with the schools of their choice prior to making formal application. In most instances, the committee on admission will be responsible for official residency rulings regarding medical school applicants or will know what university office is responsible. University definitions of residency status may not always be identical with definitions of "legal residency" used for other purposes (for example, to determine liability for payment of state income taxes or voting registration).

The individual school entries in chapters 10 and 11 present nonresident statistics and note preference given to applicants on the basis of residence.

Three interstate agreements which provide special opportunities for residents of some states are:

*WICHE.* All accredited western medical schools except the University of Washington participate in the Western Interstate Commission for Higher Education (WICHE) Professional Student Exchange Program. After certification by their states, students from Alaska, Montana, and Wyoming can attend a participating school and pay the in-state tuition at a public institution or a reduced tuition at a private school. The student's home state then pays a support fee to the receiving school. In order to qualify for WICHE certification, a student must be a legal resident of the sending state and meet its eligibility requirements. Receiving WICHE certification does not guarantee admission to a participating school, however. Students must also apply directly to the participating schools of their choice, where they are considered on the basis of that school's admission criteria. Because funds available to the sending states for payment of support fees are limited, it is also possible that some students cannot be supported by their home states as exchange students, even though they are otherwise qualified for the exchange program. Further information is available from:

Professional Student Exchange Program
Western Interstate Commission for
    Higher Education
P.O. Drawer P
Boulder, Colorado 80301-9752

*WAMI.* In 1972 the WAMI Program was founded to meet the health needs of the states of Washington, Alaska, Montana, and Idaho. Under the supervision of the University of Washington School of Medicine, students from these northwest states take the first year of medical school at participating universities in their home states. Students spend their second year at the University of Washington School of Medicine. Clerkships are available for third- and fourth-year students in family medicine, internal medicine, pediatrics, obstetrics-gynecology, psychiatry, and surgery in communities in the four-state area. Through this program, students from Alaska, Idaho, and Montana are admitted to the University of Washington School of Medicine and pay in-state tuition and fees. By decentralizing medical education in this way, the University of Washington has been able to increase the number of students accepted from these states without medical schools and help correct the uneven distribution of physicians between urban and rural communities. Additional information about the program is available from:

Admissions Office
School of Medicine, Box 356340
University of Washington
Seattle, Washington 98195

*Southern Regional Education Board Program.* Certain students from the states of Alabama, Georgia, North Carolina, and Tennessee who are accepted at Meharry Medical College pay a reduced tuition under a program administered by the Southern Regional Education Board. Similar arrangements exist for a certain number of students from Alabama and Georgia who are accepted at Morehouse School of Medicine. Georgia residents also have this opportunity at Emory University and Mercer University School of Medicine. Further information is available from:

Southern Regional Education Board
592 Tenth Street, N.W.
Atlanta, Georgia 30318-5790

## Citizenship

In 1995–96, 118 foreign students entered the first-year class.

Prospective applicants from other countries should study carefully the application considerations and admission criteria discussed in this book, since they apply equally to both U.S. and non-U.S. citizens. Successful applicants from other countries will ordinarily have completed several years of their undergraduate college work in the United States. Proficiency in the English language is required, and medical schools may require proficiency certification either from the appropriate official agency in the applicant's own country or from the American undergraduate college the applicant has attended.

A majority of U.S. schools are required to give preference to applicants from their own states or regions.

Much of the financial aid available to U.S. medical schools comes from federal sources, which require U.S. citizenship or permanent residency. Since some countries impose severe restrictions on the exportation of currency, applicants should investigate the accessibility of financial resources before applying. In no case should foreign applicants assume that financial aid will be available in the United States. Foreign applicants should be prepared to present detailed plans for financing their medical education.

## Age

Medical schools review applications without regard to the candidate's age.

The numbers of older applicants have increased slightly in recent years. For the 1995–96 entering class, 23.5 percent of the 3,646 applicants who were 32 years or older were accepted; this represents about 5.3 percent of the total number

*(Text continued on page 32)*

## TABLE 4-A

### U.S. Medical School Applicants, New Entrants, and Total Enrollment by Residence and Sex, 1995–96

| Medical School[1] | Applicants | | | New Entrants | | | Total Enrollment | |
|---|---|---|---|---|---|---|---|---|
| | Total | Percent In-State | Percent Women | Total | Percent In-State | Percent Women | Total | Percent Women |
| Alabama | 2,316 | 25.0 | 37.8 | 165 | 86.1 | 40.0 | 702 | 36.0 |
| Alabama, South | 1,504 | 36.5 | 37.2 | 64 | 89.1 | 34.4 | 261 | 37.5 |
| Albany | 10,143 | 24.9 | 41.5 | 135 | 38.5 | 56.3 | 539 | 51.6 |
| Albert Einstein | 9,135 | 26.1 | 41.2 | 180 | 47.2 | 46.7 | 720 | 45.4 |
| Arizona | 1,142 | 47.2 | 39.8 | 100 | 98.0 | 49.0 | 404 | 53.7 |
| Arkansas | 905 | 43.4 | 39.1 | 143 | 97.2 | 39.9 | 566 | 39.6 |
| Baylor | 3,213 | 44.9 | 40.7 | 168 | 73.2 | 39.3 | 668 | 39.5 |
| Boston | 11,763 | 6.6 | 42.6 | 143 | 30.8 | 35.7 | 615 | 40.8 |
| Bowman Gray | 8,287 | 10.0 | 41.1 | 108 | 56.5 | 41.7 | 437 | 35.0 |
| Brown | 124 | 12.1 | 40.3 | 66 | 13.6 | 48.5 | 320 | 50.0 |
| California, Southern | 6,488 | 67.0 | 41.4 | 150 | 84.0 | 42.0 | 637 | 42.5 |
| California, University of | | | | | | | | |
|   Davis | 5,491 | 84.0 | 42.7 | 93 | 96.8 | 36.6 | 399 | 40.4 |
|   Irvine | 5,186 | 89.7 | 42.2 | 92 | 100.0 | 43.5 | 392 | 41.8 |
|   Los Angeles (UCLA) | 8,429 | 71.0 | 43.0 | 169 | 92.9 | 50.9 | 712 | 40.9 |
|     (and Drew program) | | | | | | | | |
|   San Diego | 5,564 | 75.1 | 41.9 | 122 | 95.9 | 45.1 | 498 | 44.6 |
|   San Francisco | 5,911 | 54.7 | 42.3 | 153 | 75.2 | 52.3 | 646 | 51.5 |
|     (and Berkeley program) | | | | | | | | |
| Caribe | 1,068 | 38.1 | 41.5 | 60 | 88.3 | 45.0 | 256 | 43.8 |
| Case Western Reserve | 7,702 | 15.1 | 42.4 | 138 | 59.4 | 44.2 | 579 | 44.6 |
| Chicago Medical | 12,798 | 10.5 | 39.6 | 168 | 29.2 | 38.7 | 723 | 37.1 |
| Chicago-Pritzker | 8,407 | 13.9 | 39.7 | 104 | 40.4 | 41.4 | 421 | 44.4 |
| Cincinnati | 5,219 | 28.6 | 40.0 | 160 | 83.1 | 36.9 | 651 | 36.3 |
| Colorado | 3,075 | 24.7 | 38.7 | 129 | 82.2 | 42.6 | 508 | 42.5 |
| Columbia | 4,120 | 24.3 | 43.5 | 150 | 24.7 | 41.3 | 602 | 41.4 |
| Connecticut | 3,336 | 13.4 | 42.9 | 83 | 86.8 | 49.4 | 335 | 51.6 |
| Cornell | 7,429 | 23.5 | 40.6 | 101 | 39.6 | 49.5 | 395 | 49.1 |
| Creighton | 9,072 | 3.0 | 36.3 | 112 | 16.1 | 31.3 | 463 | 33.5 |
| Dartmouth | 8,048 | 1.0 | 39.9 | 91 | 13.2 | 37.4 | 313 | 39.0 |
| Duke | 7,493 | 6.4 | 39.0 | 100 | 33.0 | 45.0 | 405 | 40.7 |
| East Carolina | 1,972 | 49.9 | 42.0 | 72 | 100.0 | 48.6 | 294 | 49.7 |
| Emory | 8,612 | 8.3 | 42.6 | 114 | 53.5 | 44.7 | 449 | 43.2 |
| Florida | | | | | | | | |
|   (and FSU/FAMU/UWF program) | 3,642 | 61.9 | 39.7 | 115 | 95.7 | 50.4 | 468 | 44.4 |
| Florida, South | 1,993 | 71.8 | 40.6 | 96 | 99.0 | 34.4 | 377 | 34.5 |
| George Washington | 12,371 | 0.7 | 43.4 | 158 | 12.0 | 54.4 | 640 | 48.6 |

## TABLE 4-A (continued)

## U.S. Medical School Applicants, New Entrants, and Total Enrollment by Residence and Sex, 1995–96

| Medical School[1] | Applicants | | | New Entrants | | | Total Enrollment | |
| --- | --- | --- | --- | --- | --- | --- | --- | --- |
| | Total | Percent In-State | Percent Women | Total | Percent In-State | Percent Women | Total | Percent Women |
| *Georgetown* | 12,448 | 0.5 | 40.5 | 165 | 1.2 | 41.8 | 736 | 36.5 |
| Georgia, Medical College of | 1,911 | 51.1 | 40.5 | 180 | 97.8 | 35.6 | 731 | 33.9 |
| *Hahnemann*[2] | n/a | n/a | n/a | n/a | n/a | n/a | 531 | 37.9 |
| *Harvard* | 3,913 | 8.5 | 40.4 | 165 | 9.7 | 50.9 | 735 | 46.0 |
| Hawaii | 1,631 | 13.1 | 39.8 | 56 | 78.6 | 48.2 | 229 | 48.9 |
| *Howard* | 6,163 | 1.1 | 46.6 | 111 | 3.6 | 52.2 | 455 | 51.6 |
| Illinois, Southern | 2,103 | 68.5 | 41.5 | 72 | 98.6 | 47.2 | 287 | 46.3 |
| Illinois, University of | 6,646 | 31.9 | 40.9 | 317 | 95.9 | 29.3 | 1,321 | 34.3 |
| Indiana | 3,124 | 23.4 | 38.8 | 280 | 92.1 | 34.6 | 1,103 | 38.1 |
| Iowa | 3,513 | 10.2 | 39.0 | 175 | 85.1 | 49.7 | 698 | 42.8 |
| *Jefferson* | 11,694 | 12.0 | 40.8 | 223 | 40.4 | 43.1 | 918 | 35.5 |
| *Johns Hopkins* | 3,714 | 8.9 | 43.0 | 119 | 15.1 | 45.4 | 477 | 45.3 |
| Kansas | 2,474 | 18.3 | 36.5 | 175 | 92.0 | 38.9 | 724 | 37.8 |
| Kentucky | 2,294 | 24.2 | 37.5 | 95 | 88.4 | 37.9 | 379 | 33.8 |
| *Loma Linda* | 5,052 | 50.9 | 37.6 | 159 | 52.8 | 36.5 | 649 | 35.7 |
| Louisiana State—New Orleans | 1,412 | 63.1 | 39.6 | 175 | 99.4 | 38.3 | 711 | 42.9 |
| Louisiana State—Shreveport | 1,078 | 71.7 | 39.9 | 101 | 100.0 | 35.6 | 408 | 32.4 |
| Louisville | 1,967 | 27.8 | 40.8 | 136 | 89.7 | 48.5 | 553 | 46.1 |
| *Loyola-Stritch* | 10,346 | 16.2 | 40.9 | 130 | 50.0 | 46.2 | 521 | 45.7 |
| Marshall | 1,464 | 20.8 | 38.9 | 49 | 91.8 | 24.5 | 199 | 33.2 |
| Maryland | 4,645 | 23.1 | 44.6 | 146 | 82.9 | 49.3 | 628 | 49.8 |
| *Massachusetts* | 1,527 | 60.8 | 46.4 | 100 | 100.0 | 53.0 | 409 | 49.6 |
| *Mayo* | 3,905 | 10.8 | 39.0 | 42 | 23.8 | 47.6 | 161 | 44.1 |
| *Medical Col. of PA/Hahnemann*[3] | 13,602 | 10.6 | 43.5 | 240 | 55.8 | 48.3 | 652[3] | 51.2 |
| *Meharry* | 5,871 | 5.1 | 44.4 | 80 | 11.3 | 47.5 | 380 | 52.4 |
| *Mercer* | 1,471 | 49.8 | 39.1 | 55 | 100.0 | 36.4 | 206 | 37.4 |
| *Miami* | 3,271 | 42.8 | 39.1 | 138 | 98.6 | 51.5 | 605 | 44.8 |
| Michigan State | 3,728 | 34.1 | 44.2 | 104 | 76.0 | 51.0 | 490 | 49.8 |
| Michigan, University of | 5,909 | 19.6 | 40.2 | 165 | 64.2 | 41.8 | 704 | 40.2 |
| Minnesota—Duluth[4] | 1,605 | 37.9 | 39.3 | 52 | 88.5 | 46.2 | 107 | 46.7 |
| Minnesota—Minneapolis | 2,917 | 27.9 | 42.1 | 185 | 91.9 | 48.1 | 887 | 46.8 |
| Mississippi | 630 | 49.1 | 37.1 | 100 | 100.0 | 34.0 | 383 | 31.3 |
| Missouri—Columbia | 1,333 | 42.9 | 39.9 | 92 | 98.9 | 48.9 | 385 | 48.8 |
| Missouri—Kansas City | 95 | 74.7 | 48.4 | 95 | 74.7 | 48.4 | 382 | 57.3 |
| *Morehouse* | 2,930 | 13.7 | 48.9 | 34 | 76.5 | 52.9 | 152 | 57.2 |
| *Mount Sinai* | 8,455 | 29.4 | 42.5 | 116 | 61.2 | 50.9 | 496 | 47.2 |
| Nebraska | 1,654 | 23.0 | 37.6 | 119 | 97.5 | 44.5 | 492 | 42.1 |

# TABLE 4-A (continued)

## U.S. Medical School Applicants, New Entrants, and Total Enrollment by Residence and Sex, 1995–96

| Medical School[1] | Applicants | | | New Entrants | | | Total Enrollment | |
|---|---|---|---|---|---|---|---|---|
| | Total | Percent In-State | Percent Women | Total | Percent In-State | Percent Women | Total | Percent Women |
| Mount Sinai | 8,455 | 29.4 | 42.5 | 116 | 61.2 | 50.9 | 496 | 47.2 |
| Nebraska | 1,654 | 23.0 | 37.6 | 119 | 97.5 | 44.5 | 492 | 42.1 |
| Nevada | 1,222 | 16.0 | 38.0 | 52 | 73.1 | 40.4 | 210 | 39.0 |
| New Jersey: | | | | | | | | |
| UMDNJ—New Jersey Medical | 4,321 | 32.6 | 43.0 | 170 | 90.6 | 30.0 | 687 | 37.8 |
| UMDNJ—Robert Wood Johnson | 4,636 | 31.4 | 43.0 | 138 | 91.3 | 44.2 | 624 | 41.3 |
| New Mexico | 1,283 | 27.4 | 45.4 | 73 | 90.4 | 63.0 | 306 | 55.9 |
| New York Medical | 12,289 | 21.0 | 40.3 | 188 | 22.9 | 39.9 | 777 | 32.2 |
| New York University | 4,445 | 30.0 | 43.6 | 159 | 42.8 | 37.7 | 655 | 37.6 |
| New York: | | | | | | | | |
| SUNY—Brooklyn | 6,141 | 46.1 | 42.3 | 186 | 97.3 | 41.4 | 816 | 38.4 |
| SUNY—Buffalo | 3,778 | 74.3 | 42.6 | 139 | 98.6 | 46.0 | 578 | 41.0 |
| SUNY—Stony Brook | 3,982 | 72.5 | 42.6 | 100 | 92.0 | 43.0 | 427 | 43.1 |
| SUNY—Syracuse | 4,085 | 70.8 | 42.4 | 146 | 95.2 | 40.4 | 607 | 47.0 |
| North Carolina | 3,420 | 30.4 | 43.3 | 160 | 89.4 | 43.1 | 670 | 43.6 |
| North Dakota | 326 | 40.8 | 45.1 | 57 | 71.9 | 42.1 | 237 | 41.4 |
| Northwestern | 9,522 | 14.4 | 40.8 | 174 | 47.6 | 48.9 | 706 | 50.3 |
| Ohio, Medical College of | 4,818 | 28.0 | 38.7 | 140 | 85.7 | 37.9 | 567 | 38.3 |
| Ohio, Northeastern | 1,479 | 58.3 | 39.5 | 105 | 94.3 | 41.9 | 421 | 43.9 |
| Ohio State | 5,911 | 24.2 | 39.7 | 210 | 79.5 | 37.6 | 845 | 34.0 |
| Oklahoma | 1,701 | 28.0 | 39.6 | 149 | 88.6 | 42.3 | 592 | 38.7 |
| Oregon | 2,083 | 18.9 | 42.6 | 96 | 75.0 | 43.8 | 399 | 44.9 |
| Pennsylvania State | 7,285 | 19.0 | 41.5 | 119 | 49.6 | 45.4 | 448 | 47.3 |
| Pennsylvania, University of | 8,927 | 11.3 | 41.4 | 151 | 27.2 | 39.1 | 689 | 41.8 |
| Pittsburgh | 6,693 | 18.4 | 41.8 | 141 | 61.0 | 48.9 | 560 | 46.3 |
| Ponce | 974 | 37.8 | 39.1 | 60 | 71.7 | 43.3 | 257 | 42.8 |
| Puerto Rico | 984 | 36.2 | 41.0 | 115 | 96.5 | 47.8 | 438 | 50.9 |
| Rochester | 3,958 | 27.8 | 44.9 | 99 | 35.4 | 56.6 | 387 | 46.0 |
| Rush | 5,627 | 30.9 | 42.0 | 120 | 86.7 | 40.8 | 498 | 47.0 |
| Saint Louis | 8,632 | 5.9 | 36.5 | 152 | 28.3 | 35.5 | 606 | 32.5 |
| South Carolina, Medical University of | 3,402 | 14.3 | 41.0 | 140 | 90.7 | 41.4 | 570 | 38.9 |
| South Carolina, University of | 1,878 | 21.2 | 38.8 | 72 | 88.9 | 43.1 | 285 | 38.9 |
| South Dakota | 1,231 | 9.3 | 34.9 | 51 | 82.4 | 43.1 | 205 | 48.3 |
| Stanford | 7,015 | 40.7 | 40.0 | 86 | 55.8 | 47.7 | 452 | 41.6 |
| Temple | 8,784 | 16.1 | 42.5 | 187 | 57.2 | 42.8 | 715 | 36.4 |
| Tennessee State, East | 2,089 | 30.1 | 36.8 | 60 | 85.0 | 50.0 | 245 | 44.9 |
| Tennessee, University of | 2,334 | 30.5 | 37.0 | 165 | 91.5 | 35.8 | 683 | 35.4 |

**TABLE 4-A (continued)**

## U.S. Medical School Applicants, New Entrants, and Total Enrollment by Residence and Sex, 1995–96

| Medical School[1] | Applicants | | | New Entrants | | | Total Enrollment | |
|---|---|---|---|---|---|---|---|---|
| | Total | Percent In-State | Percent Women | Total | Percent In-State | Percent Women | Total | Percent Women |
| Texas A & M | 1,519 | 90.1 | 39.4 | 64 | 100.0 | 37.5 | 211 | 39.8 |
| Texas Tech | 1,600 | 95.7 | 36.8 | 120 | 96.7 | 24.2 | 443 | 26.9 |
| Texas, University of | | | | | | | | |
|    Dallas (Southwestern) | 3,365 | 73.1 | 39.4 | 199 | 87.4 | 32.7 | 811 | 35.4 |
|    Galveston | 3,218 | 78.6 | 39.6 | 200 | 94.0 | 38.0 | 841 | 43.2 |
|    Houston | 3,363 | 75.8 | 39.6 | 200 | 91.5 | 54.5 | 806 | 47.1 |
|    San Antonio | 3,272 | 77.1 | 39.6 | 201 | 90.1 | 42.3 | 826 | 37.5 |
| *Tufts* | 11,534 | 6.8 | 42.9 | 176 | 29.6 | 47.7 | 679 | 44.2 |
| *Tulane* | 11,147 | 5.5 | 40.3 | 148 | 22.3 | 47.3 | 587 | 41.9 |
| Uniformed Services University | 3,238 | n/a | 29.1 | 166 | n/a | 29.5 | 666 | 26.3 |
| Utah | 1,409 | 30.9 | 29.0 | 100 | 75.0 | 39.0 | 399 | 29.1 |
| *Vanderbilt* | 6,888 | 4.8 | 38.1 | 103 | 9.7 | 30.1 | 396 | 33.3 |
| Vermont | 8,656 | 1.2 | 40.2 | 93 | 33.3 | 40.9 | 378 | 48.9 |
| *Virginia, Eastern* | 7,354 | 14.6 | 42.3 | 101 | 75.3 | 49.5 | 412 | 47.8 |
| Virginia, Medical College of | 5,297 | 22.3 | 42.8 | 174 | 71.3 | 42.5 | 681 | 40.1 |
| Virginia, University of | 5,435 | 19.1[5] | 42.9 | 139 | 70.5[5] | 41.7 | 553 | 44.8 |
| *Washington University (St. Louis)* | 7,013 | 4.3 | 40.1 | 122 | 9.8 | 50.8 | 481 | 45.3 |
| Washington, University of | 3,923 | 24.8 | 42.7 | 166 | 94.6 | 49.4 | 693 | 48.1 |
| Wayne State | 4,409 | 32.2 | 41.0 | 247 | 93.5 | 35.2 | 1,051 | 40.8 |
| West Virginia | 1,794 | 16.5 | 37.2 | 88 | 96.6 | 36.4 | 354 | 43.2 |
| *Wisconsin, Medical College of* | 7,772 | 6.7 | 38.3 | 204 | 45.1 | 34.8 | 805 | 38.5 |
| Wisconsin, University of | 3,034 | 18.8 | 40.0 | 143 | 80.4 | 51.1 | 595 | 46.6 |
| Wright State | 3,672 | 36.5 | 42.3 | 90 | 86.7 | 61.1 | 371 | 53.1 |
| *Yale* | 3,355[5] | 4.0 | 40.5 | 101 | 12.9 | 46.5 | 490 | 45.1 |
| Total | 46,591[6] | n/a | 42.5 | 16,253 | n/a | 42.7 | 66,970 | 41.9 |

Sources: Final Admission Action Summary, Geographic Source of Entering Students, Geographic Source of Applicants, and 1995 Fall Enrollment Questionnaire.

Notes:
[1] Italics indicate privately supported schools.
[2] Applicant and New Entrant data is not applicable due to the consolidation of Hahnemann and the Medical College of Pennsylvania. Total enrollment data reflects students who matriculated at Hahnemann prior to the 1995 Entering Class.
[3] Total enrollment data reflects the consolidated Medical College of PA/Hahnemann new entrants and students who matriculated at the Medical College of PA prior to the 1995 Entering Class.
[4] Two-year school of basic medical sciences.
[5] In-state residents include residents of Alaska, Idaho, and Montana.
[6] These applicants submitted a total of 595,975 applications.

of accepted applicants. Additional information will be found in Chapter 2.

## Disabled Applicants

Medical school graduates must have the knowledge and skills to function in a broad variety of clinical situations and to render a wide spectrum of patient care. Thus, schools may ask applicants to respond to a statement of technical standards, describing the standards expected of students who will be candidates for the M.D. degree. Applicants may be questioned on their ability to meet these standards and may be asked to provide documentation to support their statement.

The LCME standards for accreditation of medical schools state: "While physical disability should not preclude a student from consideration for admission, each school should develop and publish technical standards for the admission of handicapped applicants, in accordance with legal requirements." The AAMC has distributed information regarding the development of technical standards by institutions to ensure that their admission policies are in compliance with the Americans with Disabilities Act (ADA).

## Special Information for Women

The AAMC continues to assist medical schools in creating an educational environment as conducive to the professional development of women as it is to men. Currently, about 20 percent of U.S. physicians are women, up from less than 8 percent in 1970. The proportion of women in the applicant pool did not rise last year but appears to have at least temporarily plateaued at about 42 percent (Table 4-C). In 1970–71, 2,734 women and 22,253 men applied to medical school. The corresponding figures for 1995–96 were 19,779 and 26,812 (Table 4-D). In 1995–96 the acceptance rates of both men and women were virtually the same, 37.0) percent and 37.6 percent, respectively. Data for 1993–94 were essentially the same as well. Table 4-B demonstrates that for the 1995–96 entering class, as in previous years, the acceptance rate of women 35 years and older is generally slightly higher than that of men. Many of these individuals have acquired experience in another health career or in community service.

Table 4-A shows the proportion of new entrants into each U.S. medical school who are women. Large school-to-school variations are apparent, from a low of 24.3 percent to a high of 63.0 percent. At 13 schools, women make up over 50 percent of new entrants. In recent years the proportion of underrepresented minorities who are women has been increasing; in 1995–96, 53.5 percent of those minorities accepted were women.

Women considering medicine as a career often have questions about the medical school environment, future career options, and combining a medical career with parenting responsibilities. Changes in the health care system are creating opportunities in primary care and team building that women physicians are particularly well positioned to lead. Likewise, with increasing attention being focused on women's health needs, there has never been a more exciting time for women to enter the medical field.

Overall, women currently in practice report a high level of satisfaction with both their professional and personal lives. Approximately two-thirds of practicing physicians have children, and medical students are increasingly likely to meet female residents and faculty members who are also mothers. For applicants with questions along these lines, student chapters of the American Medical Women's Association (AMWA), present at many of the medical schools, can be good resources. Some of the local AMWA chapters offer housing arrangements for women applicants interviewing at their institution. At schools without such chapters, the admission office may be able to provide names of local women physicians who could talk with applicants about their experiences in the practice of medicine.

Women students are finding more women faculty members at medical schools each year. Since 1968 the percentage of women faculty in U.S. medical schools has grown from 13.3 percent to 25 percent. However, women are far from being proportionately represented in leadership positions in academic medicine. Only 10 percent of women faculty are full professors, compared to 32 percent of men faculty. The low number of women reaching this rank partially explains the low number of women who chair academic departments; there are currently fewer than 120 women chairs.

The AAMC's Women in Medicine Coordinating Committee works on programs and avenues to address this paucity of women leaders. This includes annual Women in Medicine professional development seminars for junior and senior faculty desiring to increase their leadership skills. All U.S. medical schools and many teaching hospitals have designated an individual to serve as the Women Liaison Officer (WLO) to the AAMC and with others outside their medical centers on matters of special interest and concern to women in academic medicine. WLOs are periodically surveyed regarding the activities they have initiated to improve the environment for women students and faculty at their institutions; their responses are compiled into a handbook and distributed among the WLOs. The name and address of the WLO at any institution and data about women in medical education are available from:

Staff, Women Liaison Officers
Division of Institutional Planning
   and Development
Association of American Medical Colleges
2450 N Street, N.W.
Washington, D.C. 20037-1126

## RESOURCES FOR AND REFERENCES ABOUT WOMEN IN MEDICINE

Women with questions that pertain more to the practice of medicine than to medical education are encouraged to contact the AMA Department of Women in Medicine (515 N. State St.,

Chicago, Illinois 60610; (312) 464-4392), or AMWA (801 North Fairfax Street, Alexandria, Virginia 22314; (703) 838-0500). The American Medical Students Association (1890 Preston White Drive, Reston, Virginia 22091; (703) 620-6600) has a Standing Committe on Women in Medicine that can connect female students to sources of support and information. As noted above, many medical schools have student AMWA chapters. Moreover, AMWA publishes the *Journal of the American Medical Women's Association,* which includes diverse articles of interest to women physicians and medical students.

The books and articles included in the following bibliography are also valuable resources. Familiarity with information included in any of the following may be of great advantage in responding to interviewers' questions, especially inquiries related to combining family and career, and to gender-related issues in medicine.

1. American Medical Association, *Women in Medicine Services. Women in Medicine in America: In the Mainstream.* $12.00 for AMA members, $15.00 for non-members. (American Medical Association, 515 North State Street, Chicago, Illinois 60610; 1-800-621-8335).

2. Association of Women Surgeons. *Pocket Mentor: A Manual for Surgical Residents.* Westmont, Illinois: AWS, 1993 (708/655-0394).

3. Bickel, J. Scenarios for Success—Enhancing Women Physician's Professional Advancement. *Western Journal of Medicine,* 162:165-9, 1995.

4. Bickel, J., Povar, G. Women as Health Professionals: Contemporary Issues. *Encyclopedia of Bioethics,* ed. W. Reich, New York: Simon and Schuster, 1995.

5. Bickel, J. and Quinnie, R. *Building a Stronger Women's Program: Enhancing the Educational and Professional Environment.* Washington, D.C.: AAMC, 1993 (Call 202/828-0416 to order).

6. Bickel, J., Ruffin, A. Gender-associated Differences in Matriculating and Graduating Medical Students. *Academic Medicine,* 70:552-559, June 1994.

7. Bongiovi, M., et al. Maternity Leave Experiences of Resident Physicians. *Journal of the American Medical Women's Association,* 48 (6): 185–93, 1993.

8. Carr, P., et. al., Comparing the Status of Women and Men in Academic Medicine. *Annals of Internal Medicine,* 119:908-13, 1993.

9. Conley, F. Toward a More Perfect World—Eliminating Sexual Discrimination in Academic Medicine. *New England Journal of Medicine,* 328–351-2, 1993.

10. Crandall, S.J., et al., Medical Students' Attitudes Toward Providing Care for the Underserved: Are We Training Socially Responsible Physicians? *Journal of the American Medical Association,* 269: 2519–23, 1993.

11. Jamieson, K. *Beyond the Double Bind: Women and Leadership.* New York: Oxford University Press, 1995.

12. Jeruchim, J. and Shapiro, P. *Women, Mentors, and Success.* New York: Ballantine Books, 1992.

13. Klebanoff, M.A., et. al. Outcomes of Pregnancy in a National Sample of Resident Physicians. *New England Journal of Medicine,* 323:1040–45, 1990.

14. Lenhart, S., Evans C. Sexual harassment of gender discrimination: A primer for women physicians. *Journal of American Medical Womens' Association,* 46:77–82, May/June 1991.

15. Levinson, W., Tolle, S. W., and Lewis, C. Women in Academic Medicine: Combining Career and Family. *New England Journal of Medicine,* 321:1511–7, 1989.

16. Lillemoe, K., et. al. Surgery—Still An "Old Boys" Club? *Surgery,* 116:255–61, 1994.

17. Mendelsohn, K., et. al. Sex and Gender Bias in Anatomy and Physical Diagnosis Text Illustrations. *Journal of the American Medical Association,* 272:1267–70, 1994.

18. Morantz-Sanchez, R. *Sympathy & Science: Women Physicians in American Medicine.* 1987. $12.95. ISBN: 0195049853. (Oxford University Press, (800) 451-7556).

19. Sandrick, J. The residency experience: The woman's perspective. *American College of Surgeons Bulletin,* 77:10–17, August 1992.

20. Stobo, J., et al. Understanding and Eradicating Bias Against Women in Medicine. *Academic Medicine,* 68:249, 1993.

21. Tannen, D. *Talking from 9 to 5: Language, Sex and Power.* New York: Ballantine Books, 1990.

22. Tesch, B., et. al. Promotion of Women Physicians: Glass Ceiling or Sticky Floor? *Journal of the American Medical Association,* 273:1022-5, 1995.

23. Walters, B., et al. *The Annotated Bibliography of Women in Medicine,* 1993. $40.00. (Ontario Medical Association, 525 University Avenue, Suite 300, Toronto, Ontario M5G 2K7; 416/599-2580).

24. Wear, D. and Nixon, L.L. *Literary Anatomies: Women's Bodies and Health in Literature.* Ithaca: SUNY Press, 1994. $15.00 (607/277-2211).

## INFORMATION ABOUT FINANCIAL AID AND SPECIAL PROGRAMS

Because of the strong national movement encouraging women to pursue professional careers, a number of informational resources have been designed specifically for women.

The following list of published resources was developed from a publication prepared by the Project on the Status and Education of Women (Association of American Colleges, 1818 R Street, N.W., Washington, D.C. 20009).

1. American Fellowships and Selected Professions Fellowships, American Association of University Women (AAUW) Educational Foundation, 1111 16th

Street, N.W., Washington, D.C. 20036; (202) 728-7603. Awarded to American women to conduct research or study in the final year at the following levels: dissertation and postdoctoral in any field of study and selected professions (including medicine and osteopathic medicine underrepresented for minorities). Request announcement flier and applications from August through November only. Applications must be postmarked for dissertation/postdoctoral by November 15 and for selected professions by December 15.

2. American Medical Women's Association (AMWA), Medical Education Loan Program, 801 North Fairfax Street, Suite 400, Alexandria, Virginia 22314. Women in their first, second, or third year of medical school are eligible to apply. Loans of $1,000 and $2,000 at 10 percent interest are granted. Applicants must be U.S. citizens or permanent residents attending a U.S. institution full-time and be student members of AMWA.

   American Medical Women's Association Wilhelm-Frankowski Medical Education Scholarship of approximately $4,000 to women in their first, second, or third year of medical school. Applicants must be U.S. citizens or permanent residents attending a U.S. institution full-time and be student members of AMWA. Criteria include community service, AMWA activities, and women's health.

3. Business and Professional Women's Foundation Scholarship Program, 2012 Massachusetts Avenue, N.W., Washington, D.C. 20036. This program awards scholarships to nontraditional female students with critical financial need who are seeking the education necessary for entry into, re-entry into, or advancement within the work force. Applicants must be 30 years of age or older, have U.S. citizenship, and be within 24 months of completing an accredited program at a U.S. institution. Applicants may be full- or part-time students in the fields of computer science, teacher education, paralegal studies, engineering, science, or professional (J.D., M.D., D.D.S.) degrees. Applications are only available from November 1 to April 1. The deadline is April 15. To receive additional information, submit a business-size, self-addressed, double-stamped envelope to the above address.

4. *Financial Aid for Minorities in Health Fields.* 1994. $4.95. ISBN 0-912048-96-4. (Garrett Park Press, P.O. Box 190, Garrett Park, Maryland 20896)

5. Schlachter, G. A. *Directory of Financial Aids for Women* (7th Edition). 1995–97 (revised biennially). $45. (Reference Service Press, 1100 Industrial Road, Suite 9, San Carlos, California 94070.) A list of over 1,700 scholarships, fellowships, loans, grants, internships, awards, and prizes are available to women. Also included is a list of state sources of educational benefits and a bibliography of financial aid directories.

Information about other sources of medical student financing is presented in Chapter 7.

## Marital Status

Medical school admission decisions are made without regard to marital status.

## Minority Status

Efforts continue to be made to encourage better representation in medical schools of students from racial/ethnic groups underrepresented in medicine and students from nontraditional or economically disadvantaged backgrounds. Medical schools focus their affirmative action recruitment on ethnic minority groups that have been traditionally underrepresented among the physician workforce in the United States. These groups are black Americans, mainland Puerto Ricans, Mexican Americans, and Native Americans.

Many schools have programs directed at the preparation of the prospective minority medical school applicant; recruitment and retention programs; programs that offer funds for scholarships to minority undergraduate and medical students; establishment of more direct relationships between the medical schools and the predominantly minority colleges; and special projects, such as summer study programs, for minority undergraduate students.

Table 4-E shows the national application and acceptance rate for underrepresented minorities from 1991–92 through 1995–96. Table 4-F shows first-year new entrants and total enrollments, by racial/ethnic categories, for 1995–96. Chapter 8 provides more detailed information and a list of information sources for minority group students.

**TABLE 4-B**

## Acceptance Rates of Applicants by Age and Sex, 1995–96 First-Year Class

| | All Applicants | | | Men | | | Women | | |
|---|---|---|---|---|---|---|---|---|---|
| Age* | Number | Percent | Percent Accepted | No. of Applicants | Percent | Percent Accepted | No. of Applicants | Percent | Percent Accepted |
| 20 and Under | 792 | 1.7 | 65.0 | 398 | 1.5 | 66.6 | 394 | 2.0 | 63.5 |
| 21–23 | 24,328 | 52.2 | 44.1 | 13,531 | 50.5 | 44.6 | 10,797 | 54.6 | 43.5 |
| 24–27 | 13,682 | 29.4 | 29.8 | 8,306 | 31.0 | 29.4 | 5,376 | 27.2 | 30.5 |
| 28–31 | 4,143 | 8.9 | 28.2 | 2,543 | 9.5 | 27.3 | 1,600 | 8.1 | 29.6 |
| 32–34 | 1,526 | 3.3 | 25.4 | 877 | 3.3 | 26.0 | 649 | 3.3 | 24.5 |
| 35–37 | 1,008 | 2.2 | 25.2 | 590 | 2.2 | 23.7 | 418 | 2.1 | 27.3 |
| 38 and Over | 1,112 | 2.4 | 19.5 | 567 | 2.1 | 20.1 | 545 | 2.8 | 18.9 |
| Total | 46,591 | 100.0 | 37.3 | 26,812 | 100.0 | 37.0 | 19,779 | 100.0 | 37.6 |

*In 1995 the mean ages for these applicant groups were as follows: 24.7 (all applicants), 23.9 (applicants accepted), 24.7 (men applicants), 24.0 (men accepted), 24.7 (women applicants), 23.8 (women accepted).

**TABLE 4-C**

## Women Applicants and First-Year Women New Entrants to U.S. Medical Schools, 1991–92 Through 1995–96

| First-Year Class | Total Applicants | Women Applicants | % of Total Applicants | Total First-Year New Entrants* | Women First-Year New Entrants | % of Total First-Year New Entrants* |
|---|---|---|---|---|---|---|
| 1991–92 | 33,301 | 13,700 | 41.1 | 16,211 | 6,433 | 39.7 |
| 1992–93 | 37,410 | 15,619 | 41.8 | 16,289 | 6,772 | 41.6 |
| 1993–94 | 42,808 | 17,957 | 42.0 | 16,307 | 6,851 | 42.0 |
| 1994–95 | 45,365 | 18,968 | 41.8 | 16,287 | 6,819 | 41.9 |
| 1995–96 | 46,591 | 19,779 | 42.5 | 16,253 | 6,941 | 42.7 |

Source: AAMC Section for Student Services (Final Admission Action Summary Reports)
*First-year new entrants are students entering medical school of the first time.

**TABLE 4-D**

**Comparative Acceptance Data for Men and Women Applicants,
1991–92 Through 1995–96**

| First-Year | No. of Applicants | | No. Accepted | | % Accepted | |
|---|---|---|---|---|---|---|
| Class | Men | Women | Men | Women | Men | Women |
| 1991–92 | 19,601 | 13,700 | 10,493 | 6,943 | 53.5 | 50.7 |
| 1992–93 | 21,791 | 15,619 | 10,207 | 7,257 | 46.8 | 46.5 |
| 1993–94 | 24,851 | 17,957 | 10,074 | 7,288 | 40.5 | 40.6 |
| 1994–95 | 26,397 | 18,968 | 10,062 | 7,255 | 38.1 | 38.2 |
| 1995–96 | 26,812 | 19,779 | 9,920 | 7,437 | 37.0 | 37.6 |

Source: AAMC Section for Student Services (Final Admission Action Summary Reports)

**TABLE 4-E**

**Application and Acceptance Rate of Selected Minority Group Applicants to
First-Year Classes in U.S. Medical Schools, 1991–92 Through 1995–96**

| | Black American | | | | American Indian | | | |
|---|---|---|---|---|---|---|---|---|
| | Applicants | | Acceptees | | Applicants | | Acceptees | |
| First-Year Class | No. | % of All Applicants | No. | % Accepted | No. | % of All Applicants | No. | % Accepted |
| 1991–92 | 2,659 | 8.0 | 1,193 | 44.9 | 161 | 0.5 | 93 | 57.8 |
| 1992–93 | 2,917 | 7.8 | 1,291 | 44.3 | 194 | 0.5 | 103 | 53.1 |
| 1993–94 | 3,489 | 8.2 | 1,381 | 39.6 | 238 | 0.6 | 120 | 50.4 |
| 1994–95 | 3,659 | 8.1 | 1,427 | 39.0 | 261 | 0.6 | 116 | 44.4 |
| 1995–96 | 3,595 | 7.7 | 1,407 | 39.1 | 305 | 0.7 | 138 | 45.2 |

| | Mexican American/Chicano | | | | Mainland Puerto Rico | | | |
|---|---|---|---|---|---|---|---|---|
| | Applicants | | Acceptees | | Applicants | | Acceptees | |
| First-Year Class | No. | % of All Applicants | No. | % Accepted | No. | % of All Applicants | No. | % Accepted |
| 1991–92 | 568 | 1.7 | 327 | 57.6 | 217 | 0.7 | 125 | 57.6 |
| 1992–93 | 699 | 1.9 | 418 | 59.8 | 224 | 0.16 | 127 | 56.7 |
| 1993–94 | 747 | 1.8 | 399 | 53.4 | 241 | 0.6 | 115 | 47.7 |
| 1994–95 | 861 | 1.9 | 478 | 55.5 | 279 | 0.6 | 152 | 54.5 |
| 1995–96 | 917 | 2.0 | 497 | 54.2 | 329 | 0.7 | 137 | 41.6 |

Source: AAMC Section for Student Services (Final Admission Action Summary Reports).

**TABLE 4-F**

## U.S. Medical School Enrollments, 1995–96

| Racial/Ethnic Category | First-Year Entrants* | | Total Enrollments | |
|---|---|---|---|---|
| | Total | % of Grand Total | Total | % of Grand Total |
| **U.S. Citizens** | | | | |
| White | 10,552 | 64.9 | 44,594 | 66.6 |
| Underrepresented Minorities | | | | |
|   Black | 1,290 | 7.9 | 5,337 | 8.0 |
|   American Indian or Alaskan Native | 137 | 0.8 | 501 | 0.7 |
|   Mexican American/Chicano | 476 | 2.9 | 1,769 | 2.6 |
|   Puerto Rican (Mainland) | 107 | 0.7 | 455 | 0.7 |
|   **Subtotal** | **2,010** | **12.4** | **8,062** | **12.0** |
| **Other U.S. Students** | | | | |
| Asian or Pacific Islander | 2,964 | 18.2 | 11,352 | 17.0 |
| Puerto Rican (Commonwealth) | 207 | 1.3 | 878 | 1.3 |
| Other Hispanic | 312 | 1.9 | 1,247 | 1.9 |
| **Subtotal** | **3,483** | **21.4** | **13,477** | **20.1** |
| **Foreign Student** | | | | |
| Black | 39 | 0.2 | 154 | 0.2 |
| Other | 79 | 0.5 | 397 | 0.6 |
| **Subtotal** | **118** | **0.7** | **551** | **0.8** |
| Unidentified | 90 | 0.6 | 286 | 0.4 |
| **Grand Total** | **16,253** | **100.0** | **66,970** | **100.0** |

Source: AAMC Section for Student Services (Fall Enrollment Questionnaire). Reflects enrollments as of October 13, 1995 at 125 U.S. medical schools.

*First-year new entrants are students entering medical school for the first time.

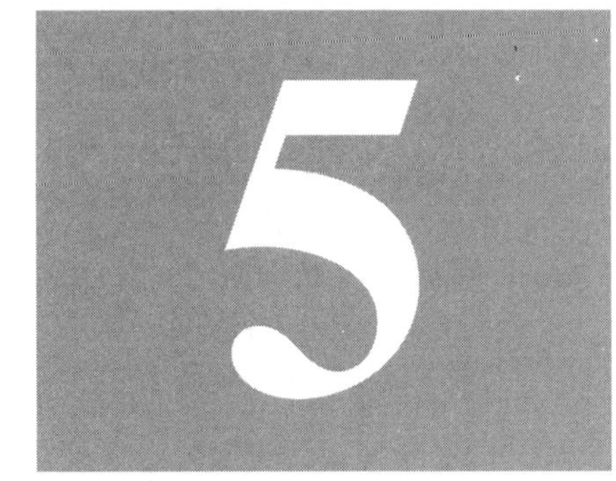

# MCAT and AMCAS

This chapter provides information on the Medical College Admission Test (MCAT) and the American Medical College Application Service (AMCAS). Details concerning application and selection procedures are presented in Chapter 6.

## MEDICAL COLLEGE ADMISSION TEST (MCAT)

The MCAT is a standardized, multiple-choice examination designed to help admission committees predict which of their applicants will perform adequately in the medical school curriculum. It provides these committees with a standardized measure of academic performance for all examinees under equivalent conditions. The battery is developed by medical school admission officers, premedical instructors, medical educators, practicing physicians, the Association of American Medical Colleges (AAMC), and a group of testing experts under contract to the AAMC.

In response to the rapid changes occurring in medical education and medical practice, an intensive review of the content and format of the MCAT was conducted by an MCAT Evaluation Panel comprised of medical school faculty, students, deans, practicing physicians, and undergraduate advisers. In accordance with revisions suggested by the Evaluation Panel, a substantially different MCAT was introduced in 1991.

Although the goal of the MCAT has not changed, the revised test is also designed to encourage students interested in medicine to pursue broad undergraduate study in the natural and social sciences and in the humanities. The updated MCAT assesses facility with scientific problem solving, critical thinking, and writing skills, as well as understanding of science concepts and principles identified as prerequisite to the study of medicine. The four parts of the revised MCAT are as follows: Verbal Reasoning, Physical Sciences, Writing Sample, and Biological Sciences.

Verbal Reasoning is designed to assess students' abilities to comprehend, reason, and think critically. It draws upon materials from the humanities, social sciences, and natural sciences. Subject matter knowledge is not tested; content information necessary to answer test questions is presented in each passage. In preparation for this section of the MCAT, examinees are encouraged to familiarize themselves with the practice of critical thinking and the use of reasoning skills in these disciplines.

The Biological Sciences and Physical Sciences sections are constructed to test material covered in first-year, introductory undergraduate courses in general biology; general chemistry, including both organic and inorganic chemistry; and general, noncalculus physics. Both sections consist entirely of science problems and may include data presented in graphs, tables, and charts. Each section is designed to assess knowledge of basic concepts and facility with scientific problem solving as well as the ability to interpret data presented in a tabular or graphic format.

The essay topics which constitute the Writing Sample section are designed to provide examinees with an opportunity to demonstrate their writing and analytical skills. Examinees receive 60 minutes for the writing of two essays at the beginning of the afternoon session. Each essay question will provide a specific topic that will require an expository response. Essay topics will not pertain to the technical content of biology, chemistry, physics, or mathematics; the medical school application process or reasons for the choice of medicine as a career; social or cultural issues not in the general experience of MCAT examinees; or religious or other emotionally charged issues.

The test-day schedule is as follows:

| Section | Number of Questions | Time in Minutes |
|---|---|---|
| Verbal Reasoning | 65 | 85 |
| Physical Sciences | 77 | 100 |
| Writing Sample | 2 | 60 |
| Biological Sciences | 77 | 100 |

*Total testing time: 5-3/4 hours*

Four scores are reported, one for each section. Verbal Reasoning, Physical Sciences, and Biological Sciences are presented on a scale ranging from 1 (lowest) to 15 (highest). The Writing Sample is presented on a scale ranging from J (lowest) to T (highest).

Information about the specific content of the examination, its organization, and scoring scheme appears in the MCAT Student Manual available at some college and university bookstores. The manual includes detailed descriptions of the content and cognitive skills assessed and a full-length practice test with a scoring key.

### Test Dates and Registration

The MCAT is administered twice a year—on a Saturday in April and August. It is recommended that students take it about 18 months before they expect to enter medical school. Testing dates for the MCAT in 1996 are April 20 and August 17. All students, especially those taking the test in August, should bear in mind that there is no provision for makeup examinations. Where possible, special Sunday testings are arranged for applicants presenting, in advance, satisfactory evidence that (1) their religious convictions prevent them from taking the examination on Saturday or (2) unavoidable conflicts prevent them from taking the examination on one of the regularly scheduled dates. An additional $10 fee is charged for these special testing arrangements. Only those persons who plan to apply to a school of allopathic, osteopathic, podiatric, and/or veterinary medicine will be permitted to take the MCAT without special permission.

Most medical schools prefer that the test be taken in April because of the short period of time between the availability of the August test scores and application deadlines. Taking the April test decreases the possibility that procedural problems will prevent the completion of an applicant's file and its timely review. Furthermore, in most cases, very little content that would be helpful to a student for the test is covered between the April and the August administrations, except for those students who complete introductory science courses during the intervening summer months. For these students, the August testing date may be preferable.

The MCAT is administered and scored by the MCAT Program Office at the direction of the AAMC. The examination fee is $155 for the 1996 administrations. A registration packet that contains an announcement, registration card, and all up-to-date information about the MCAT (including test dates, testing locations, distribution of scores, and deadlines) is available in February through premedical advisory offices and at major university testing centers. It may also be obtained by writing directly to:

MCAT Program
P.O. Box 4056
Iowa City, Iowa 52243
Telephone: (319) 337-1357

It is essential that students apprise themselves of the information provided in this packet.

## Fee Reduction

The Fee Reduction Program makes the MCAT accessible to financially disadvantaged individuals by lowering the MCAT testing fee for eligible individuals to $55. The MCAT Fee Reduction Program is operated according to eligibility policies and processing procedures established by the Association of American Medical Colleges. Information on criteria for financial eligibility and the administrative processes for the program are published in the MCAT Fee Reduction Request Form. Fee Reduction Request Forms are contained in the MCAT registration packet. You may also request that materials be sent to you by calling the Section for Student Services, AAMC, at (202) 828-0600.

## Score Reporting

Payment of the examination fee will entitle the candidate to have test scores sent to six medical schools, **provided the scores are released by the examinee at the time of the examination.** Students need to direct these six free reports only to medical schools not participating in AMCAS, since AMCAS automatically provides official reports of MCAT scores released by the candidate to the participating schools to which the candidate applies. MCAT examinees are encouraged to request at the time the test is taken that their scores be sent, at no added cost, directly to their current pre-medical advisers. MCAT examinees may not cancel or delete their scores.

Additional non-AMCAS score reports beyond the six included in the MCAT examination fee, score reports from previous MCAT administrations to non-AMCAS destinations, or reports of pre-1991 MCAT scores to any institution can be arranged by submitting a completed MCAT Additional Score Report form and fees to the address below. Further information is provided in the *1996 MCAT Announcement* and is also available from:

Additional Score Reports
Section for Student Services
Association of American Medical Colleges
2450 N Street, N.W.
Washington, D.C. 20037-1130

AAMC policy does not permit the waiver of fees for additional score reports. This policy applies to all examinees.

## Publications

To help students prepare for the MCAT, the AAMC publishes three sets of materials. The first set includes the *MCAT Student Manual* and the full-length *MCAT Practice Test I*. The *MCAT Student Manual* describes the four sections of the test and the content and reasoning skills covered by each of the sections; it also offers suggestions for preparing to take the test.

A second set of publications includes *MCAT Practice Items: Verbal Reasoning and Writing Sample, MCAT Practice Items: Physical Science* and *Biological Science,* and *MCAT Practice Test II. MCAT Practice Test II* is a released operational test form from the April 1991 administration. Items in the *Practice Item* booklets are similar to test materials used in an actual MCAT. They have not, however, received the same level of review and testing as the materials that appear on the MCAT examination; they are intended to provide examinees with additional practice with MCAT item formats and do not constitute a sample test.

The *MCAT Practice Test III* is the most recently released operational test form. Included with this publication is a set of tables that allows individuals to conduct an in-depth analysis of their strengths and weaknesses. *Practice Test III* became available in February 1995.

The AAMC also produces a videocassette, *Preparing for the MCAT.* Designed to be used in conjunction with the *MCAT Student Manual,* this tape provides information about the knowledge and skills tested by the MCAT and discusses preparation strategies for each of the four sections of the test.

For information about purchasing publications from the AAMC, call the AAMC's Section for Membership and Publication Orders at (202) 828-0416, or write to them at the following address:

Membership and Publication Orders
Association of American Medical Colleges
2450 N Street, N.W.
Washington, D.C. 20037-1129

## Retaking the Test

If an applicant's MCAT scores are low, the advisability of retaking the test may be discussed with a premedical adviser. Legitimate reasons for retaking the test include: unusual discrepancy between college grades and MCAT scores; having taken the MCAT prematurely, that is, before completing the introductory science courses that provide the necessary background for the science areas of the test; serious illness at the time of the test; and recommendation by a member of a medical school admission committee that the test be retaken. Application procedures for retaking the test are identical to those for initial testing.

## THE AMERICAN MEDICAL COLLEGE APPLICATION SERVICE (AMCAS)

### General Information

AMCAS is a nonprofit, centralized service developed by medical school admission officers to facilitate the process of applying to participating U.S. medical schools.

AMCAS does not render any admission decisions or advise applicants where to submit applications. Each participating school is completely autonomous in its admission decisions. AMCAS only provides the processing service.

AMCAS benefits both the applicant and the participating medical schools by efficiently collecting, coordinating, and processing data, which frequently reduces the time and expense of application. The total operation neither alters nor depersonalizes the principles of traditional application procedures.

AMCAS further assists admissions committees by providing rosters and statistical reports relative to the individual medical school and the national applicant pools. For example, a list of accepted applicants is forwarded to all medical schools beginning in April and continuing through October of the matriculation year. This list identifies each applicant holding an acceptance and the schools where those acceptances are being held. AMCAS also enables the AAMC to initiate research projects focusing on the medical school admission process.

For the 1995–96 entering class 43,958 or 94.3 percent of all applicants applied to at least one AMCAS-participating school. One hundred and nine medical schools and two programs are participating in AMCAS for the 1996 entering class. AMCAS participation is indicated in individual school entries in Chapter 10.

### The AMCAS Application

All individuals applying to medical schools participating in the American Medical College Application Service (AMCAS) for the first-year entering class must apply through AMCAS.

**For the first time, applicants to the 1997 entering class can complete their AMCAS application using a personal computer and software developed by the Association of American Medical Colleges.**

This software, **AMCAS-E,** significantly reduces the time needed to supply data required by AMCAS, while preserving the final product forwarded by AMCAS to designated medical schools—the standard verified AMCAS application.

The process is simple. Applicants using AMCAS-E software (in either the Windows or Macintosh formats) supply required information in response to prompts, making use of pull down tables for common data elements such as colleges attended, state and county of legal residence, etc. In addition, the process of standardizing course work grades and credit hours is automated. These prompts, supporting data tables, automation of grade/credit hour conversion, and an audit of all required data fields ensure that all required information is provided to AMCAS, speeding the processing of your application. In addition, AMCAS-E software also includes the AMCAS Fee Waiver Request Form and other forms, such as the Additional Designation Form used by applicants to apply to other medical schools after their initial application has been submitted, and the Post Submission Change Form which applicants may use to change information after they have submitted their initial application. Applicants will also be able to print a "replica" copy of the AMCAS application or text only copies of other forms for their personal records.

Applicants without access to a personal computer will be able to complete the traditional AMCAS paper application.

### How to get the AMCAS Application

The AMCAS application, electronic version (AMCAS-E) or paper, is available in April and can be obtained from a number of sources: pre-professional health advisers, participating medical schools, or by contacting AMCAS at the following address:

AMCAS
Section for Student Services
Association of American Medical Colleges
2450 N Street NW, Suite 201
Washington, DC 20037-1130
(202) 828-0600

In addition to written and telephone requests, applicants may also order materials from the AAMC World Wide Web site at **http://www.aamc.org** or by sending an e-mail to **amcas@aamc.org.**

AMCAS-E software, when released for distribution in April 1996, will also be available as a downloadable file from the AAMC's Web Site.

## Transcript Requirements and Deadlines

Before submitting application materials, the applicant should request that one set of official transcripts be forwarded directly to AMCAS by the registrar of every school at which he or she has registered. Official transcripts are required from each junior college, community college, college, university, graduate school, U.S. medical school, trade school, or professional school within the United States, Canada, or U.S. Territories, regardless of whether credit was earned. The applicant is also encouraged to simultaneously request a personal copy of each transcript in order to properly complete his or her AMCAS application materials.

*Transcripts submitted to AMCAS in prior years cannot be reactivated and will not be used.*

AMCAS begins accepting official transcripts on March 15. Except for the Early Decision Program for which application materials and official transcripts must be received by August 1, all official transcripts must be received no later than two weeks following the deadline for application materials. Refer to the AMCAS instructions for detailed information on official transcript requirements and deadlines.

## Application Processing

Applicants submit only one set of application materials (**paper or data diskette**) and have one set of official transcripts forwarded to AMCAS regardless of the number of AMCAS participating medical schools they are applying to. The service fee is based on the number of schools an applicant designates and can be paid by check, money order, or credit card.

The AMCAS Fee Waiver Program is provided by the AAMC for applicants whose inability to pay the AMCAS service fee would absolutely prohibit them from applying to medical school. Applicants must complete and forward to AMCAS the Fee Waiver Request Form found in both the paper AMCAS application packet and in the AMCAS-E software to determine eligibility prior to submitting their application materials.

AMCAS will not accept completed applications (paper or diskette) until June 1, 1996. Materials received prior to June will be returned to the applicant. The deadline for submitting applications to AMCAS for each medical school is listed in Chapter 10.

The processing of an application is contingent upon receipt by AMCAS of both the completed application and all required official transcripts by the published deadlines.

Upon receiving the completed application, AMCAS verifies the applicant's academic record against the required transcripts to ensure accuracy. After verification, grade point averages and credit hour totals are computed. These data, as well as other information extracted from the application (paper or diskette), are forwarded to the applicant's designated medical schools with a copy of the application form.

After receiving application materials from AMCAS, medical schools will notify the applicant directly of any supplemental items that may be required, such as additional fees, letters of recommendation, or updated transcripts. These items should be forwarded by the applicant directly to the medical schools upon request.

The fee listed in Chapter 10 under each school entry is the supplemental fee to be paid directly to that school upon request, not the AMCAS service fee. Applicants should contact individual schools regarding the waiver of supplemental fees.

## Sample Screen from the AMCAS-E Application

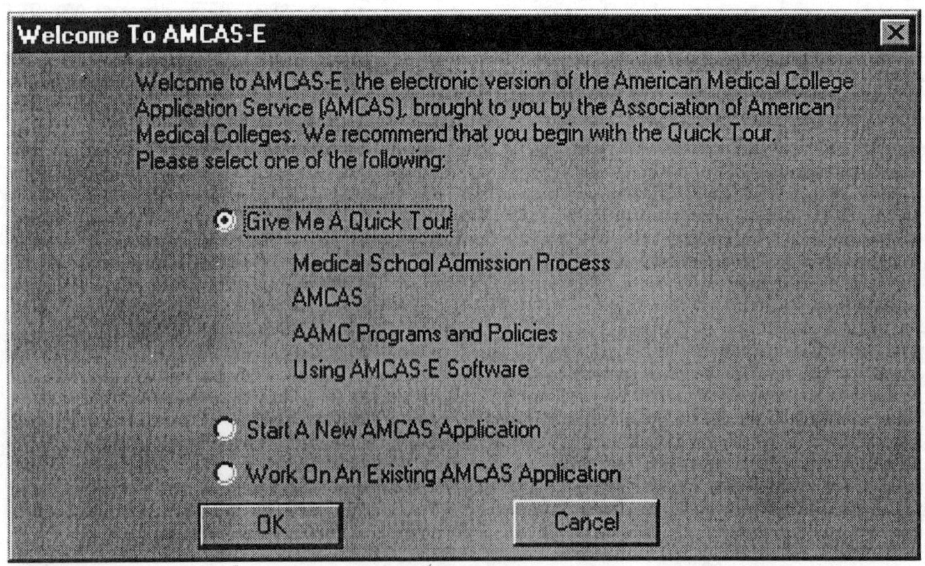

# Sample AMCAS Application (Paper Format)

## Page 1 — AMCAS Application for the 1997 Entering Class

**1. SSN:** 028-26-2288

**AMCAS® APPLICATION FOR THE 1997 ENTERING CLASS** — AMCAS USE ONLY

- **2A. Last Name:** ZYLER
- **2B. First Name:** Richard
- **2C. Middle Name:** Ross
- **2D. Suffix:** III
- **3A. Permanent Address - Street:** 434 Columbus Avenue, Apt. 2
- **3B. City and Province:** New Haven
- **3C. St:** CT
- **3D. Zip/Postal Code:** 06519 - 1234
- **3E. County (if in U.S.A.):** New Haven
- **3F. Country (if not U.S.A.):**
- **4. Telephone:** (203) 555-5125

**5. Parents or Guardian**

| Name | Living? Yes | No | Occupation | Legal Residence | Education/College (highest level) |
|---|---|---|---|---|---|
| **Father** Ralph E. Zyler | x | | Teacher | Mass. | M.A., Boston Univ. |
| **Mother** Edwina Alexander | x | | Economist | Calif. | Ph.D., Harvard |
| **Guardian** | | | | | |

**6A. Ages of your Brothers:** 9  
**6B. Ages of your Sisters:**  
**7A. Secondary School — Name:** William Penn H. S.  
**7B. Location:** Davis, CA  
**7C. Grad Yr.:** 1987

**8. All Colleges, Graduate and Professional Schools Attended (list in chronological order)**

| Name | Location | Dates of Attendance MM/YY to MM/YY | Check if summer only | Check if Jr/Comm College | Major | Degree Granted or Expected (with date) |
|---|---|---|---|---|---|---|
| Sorbonne | Paris, France | 6/87 to 8/87 | x | | French | None |
| Bennett College | Millbrook, NY | 9/87 to 8/88 | | x | Science | None |
| Nassau Cmty. Col. | Garden City, NY | 9/88 to 6/89 | | x | Biology | None |
| Michigan State U. | East Lansing, MI | 9/89 to 8/90 | | | Biology | None |
| Bowdoin College | Brunswick, Maine | 9/90 to 6/91 | | | Biology | B.S. 6/91 |
| St. Mercy Hospital | Duncannon, PA | 1/91 to 6/91 | | | Med Tech | None |
| Penn State Univ. | Univ. Park, PA | 9/91 to 6/95 | | | Psych | M.A. 6/95 |
| Abcd University | Washington, DC | 9/95 to 6/96 | | | Microbiol | None |
| | | to | | | | |
| | | to | | | | |

**9. Post-Secondary Honors/Awards:**
Phi Beta Kappa; Dean's List for three semesters; National Biology Honor Society; National Psychology Honor Society; Biology Student of the Year (Bowdoin College); Varsity Lacrosse Player (Michigan State); Outstanding Volunteer Award from St. Mercy Hospital (continued)

**10. Extracurricular, Community, and Avocational Activities:**
Community activities: Sickle Cell Anemia screening, Penn State Univ.

**11. Chronological Post-Secondary History, including Volunteer, Part-Time and Full-Time Employment**

Summer 1989 - Lab Technician, Allstate Labs.

1989-90 - Junior Year - Waiter/Cook, Pizza Restaurant - 20 hrs/wk

1995-96 Academic Year - Lab Assistant, Hematology - 15 hrs/wk

*See AMCAS instructions before completing this form.*

## Page 2 — Personal Comments

**PERSONAL COMMENTS** (Your comments must not exceed the space provided. Use a font at least 10 points in size.) — NAME (LAST NAME FIRST)

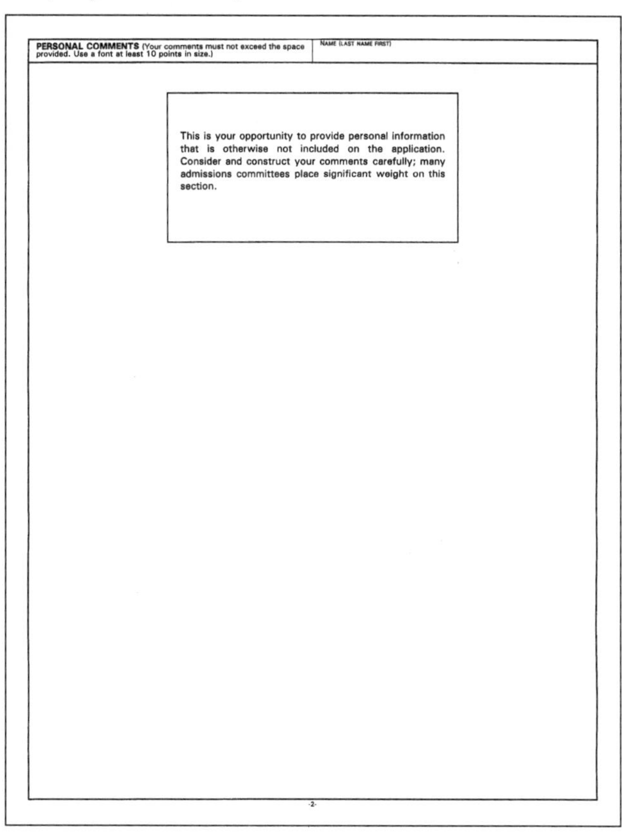


-2-

## Page 3 — Academic Record

**SSN:** 028-26-2288 — **ACADEMIC RECORD** — AMCAS USE ONLY

**Last Name:** ZYLER  **First Name:** Richard  **Middle Name:** Ross  **Suffix:** III

| College Name / Location | Academic Status | BCPM/A | Academic Year | Term | Course Name | Number | Type | Transcript Grade | Semester Hours Attempted | AMCAS Grade | AMCAS Use |
|---|---|---|---|---|---|---|---|---|---|---|---|
| Bennett College, | FR | A | 87 | SS | Credit (French) | | PF | S | 6 | P | |
| Transfer Credit | | A | | | Adv. French Convers | | | B+ | | | |
| (Sorbonne/Paris) | | A | | | French Civiliz.(Art) | | | A | | | |
| Bennett College | | A | | S1 | Elementary French | | AP | | 6 | G | |
| Millbrook, N.Y. | | A | | | Intermed French I | | AP | B | 3 | B | |
| | | A | | | American History | | CL | | 6 | L | |
| | | C | | S1 | Gen Chemistry I+Lab | 115 | | A- | 4 | A- | |
| | | A | | | Volleyball | 118 | | A+ | 1 | A | |
| | | A | | | Philosophy | 101 | | A+ | 3 | A | |
| | | A | | | Fresh. English Comp | 180 | H | A- | 3 | A- | |
| | | P | | | General Physics I | 125 | | B | 4 | B | |
| | | M | | SM | Calculus I | 125 | | B- | 4 | B- | |
| | | A | | S2 | English Literature | 109 | | A | 3 | A | |
| | | C | | | Gen Chemistry II+Lab | 116 | | B | 4 | B | |
| | | A | | | First Aid & Safety | 116 | | B | 2 | B | |
| | | A | | | European History | 104 | | B | 3 | B | |
| | | M | | | Calculus II | 126 | | B | 4 | B | |
| | SO | P | 88 | SS | Electromagnetism | 103 | | B | 4.5 | B | |
| | | A | | | Literature | 131 | | A- | 3 | A- | |
| Nassau Cmty. Col | | A | | S1 | French Literature | 001 | EX | | | | |
| Garden City, NY | | B | | | General Biology | 201 | | B+ | 4 | AB | |
| | | C | | | Organic Chemistry | 223 | | B | 3 | B | |
| | | A | | | Medical Ethics | 225 | AU | NG | | | |
| | | C | | | Organic Chem Lab | 223 | | C | 1 | C | |
| | | B | | S2 | General Biology | 202 | | B | 3 | B | |
| | | C | | | Organic Chemistry | 224 | PF | S | 3 | P | |
| | | C | | | Organic Chem Lab | 224 | PF | U | 1 | N | |
| | | A | | | Social Psychology | 227 | | A | 3 | A | |
| | | P | | | General Physics II | 222 | | C+ | 3 | BC | |
| Michigan State U. | JR | A | 89 | Q1 | Political Science | 241 | | 3.5 | 2.7 | AB | |
| E. Lansing, MI | | A | | | Revolution and War | 243 | H/I | 2.0 | 2.7 | C | |
| [Narrative | | C | | | Basic Biochemistry | 401 | | 3.5 | 3.3 | AB | |
| Evaluations | | B | | | Comp Vertebrate Anat | 314 | R | 1.0 | 3.3 | D | |
| Enclosed] | | A | | | Military Drill | 259 | | 4.0 | 0.7 | A | |
| | | B | | Q2 | Comp Vertebrate Anat | 314 | R | 4.0 | 3.3 | A | |
| | | A | | | Mythology | 250 | | 2.0 | 2.7 | C | |
| | | M | | | Statistics I | 201 | | 2.5 | 2.7 | BC | |
| | | A | | | Modern Ideologies | 242 | | 1.5 | 2.7 | CD | |
| | | A | | Q3 | Anthropology | 171 | | 2.0 | 2.7 | C | |
| | | B | | | Zoology | 331 | | 3.0 | 2.0 | B | |
| | | A | | | Humanities | 251 | | 0.0 | 2.7 | F | |
| Michigan State U. | | M | 90 | QS | Linear Functions | 302 | | 3.0 | 2.7 | B | |
| Study Abroad Prog | | A | | | History of England I | 307 | | 4.0 | 2.7 | A | |
| (Oxfrd/Londn, Eng) | | A | | | Hist of England II | 308 | | 2.0 | 2.7 | A | |
| Bowdoin College, | SR | M | | Q1 | Statistics II | 91 | | P | 3 | C | |
| Brunswick, ME | | B | | | Cell & Molec Biol | 122 | | HP | 3 | B | |
| | | B | | | Physiology | 163 | | HH | 4 | A | |
| | | M | | | Scientific Analysis | 22 | | HH | 4 | A | |
| | | A | | | Economics (micro) | 2 | | P | 4 | C | |

-3-  
*Be sure to complete and sign page 4. >>*

## Page 4 — Academic Record (continued)

| College Name / Location | Academic Status | BCPM/A | Academic Year | Term | Course Name | Number | Type | Transcript Grade | Semester Hours Attempted | AMCAS Grade | AMCAS Use |
|---|---|---|---|---|---|---|---|---|---|---|---|
| Bowdoin College, | SR | B | 90 | Q2 | Med Tech Internship: | | PF | CR | 16 | P | |
| Brunswick, ME | | B | | | Hematology | 101 | | 86 | | | |
| Transfer Credit | | B | | | Serology | 107 | | 91 | | | |
| (St. Mercy Hsp, PA) | | B | | | Lab Techniques | 111 | | 96 | | | |
| | | B | | | Virology | 113 | | 92 | | | |
| Penn State Univ. | PB | A | 91 | T1 | Occult Literature | 120 | W | WF | | | |
| Univ. Park, PA | | A | | | Tolstoy | 220 | | A | 3 | A | |
| | | A | | | Modern Novel | 224 | | A | 3 | A | |
| | | A | 92 | T1 | Physio. Psychology | 301 | | A | 3 | A | |
| | | A | | | Psych. of Learning | 304 | W | WN | | | |
| | | A | | T2 | Research Psychology | 340 | | A | 2 | A | |
| | | A | | T3 | Semantics | 307 | NR | NG | 3 | | |
| | GR | A | 93 | T1 | Child Psychology | 435 | | A | 4 | A | |
| | | A | | | Educ. Psychology | 441 | | B | 4 | B | |
| | | A | | T2 | Social Psychology | 415 | | A | 4 | A | |
| | | A | | | Abnormal Psychology | 460 | | A | 4 | A | |
| | | A | | | Psych. Field Work | 490 | I | INC | 4 | | |
| | | A | 94 | T1 | Advanced Research | 477 | PF | PS | 4 | P | |
| | | A | | T2 | Death and Dying | 503 | DG | DF | 4 | | |
| | | A | | | Advanced Research | 477 | PF | PS | 4 | P | |
| | | A | | T3 | Death and Dying | 503 | | A | 4 | A | |
| Abcd University, | GR | M | 95 | S1 | Quantitative Data | 668 | | H | 3 | A | |
| Washington, DC | | B | | | Epidemiology | 635 | | HP | 4 | A- | |
| | | B | | S2 | Microbiology | 665 | | P | 3 | B | |
| | | B | 96 | S1 | Biology of Tumors | 230 | CC | | 2 | | |
| | | B | | | Microbiology | 665 | CC | | 3 | | |
| | | B | | S2 | Virus Infections | 668 | CC | | 1 | | |

**14. MCAT Testing Status**
Number of MCATs taken since April 1991: **3**
Have you taken, or do you plan to take, the August 1996 MCAT? YES [x]  NO [ ]

**15. Medical School — You must answer this Question**
Have you ever matriculated at or attended any medical school as a candidate for the M.D. degree? YES [ ]  NO [x]

**16. Institutional Action — You must answer this Question**
[Refer to AMCAS instructions before answering.] Were you ever the recipient of any action (e.g., dismissal, disqualification, suspension, etc.) by any college or medical school for: (1) unacceptable academic performance or (2) conduct violations? If "YES," explain fully in the "Personal Comments" section (page 2). YES [ ]  NO [x]

**Certification Statement**
I have read and understand the AMCAS instructions. I certify that the information submitted in this application and associated materials is current, complete, and accurate to the best of my knowledge.

Signature (Black Ink Only) or Certification  
Date: June 15, 1996

NO. E-6 REV. 2/96    DCIC No. 008-96    -4-    COPYRIGHT 1996 BY THE ASSOCIATION OF AMERICAN MEDICAL COLLEGES

# The Medical School Application and Selection Process

Each medical school faculty has the responsibility and authority to select the individuals who will be admitted to the school. Responsibility for the admission process is delegated to an admission officer who, with the assistance of an office staff, organizes and conducts the procedures for the receipt and processing of applications. Through this process, candidates' credentials are reviewed, and decisions to admit or reject a candidate are made by a faculty admission committee. The composition of admission committees and the selection process vary from school to school, but each school follows the general principles discussed below.

## COMPOSITION OF COMMITTEES

Admission committees are composed principally of faculty members from both basic science and clinical departments. Frequently one or more medical student members are included. At a few schools, committees include faculty members from other colleges in the university and/or individuals from the community.

## PROCESSING OF APPLICATIONS

Applications are screened and placed in priority categories according to policies established by the faculty. Supplementary application materials may be requested from all applicants or from only those in specified categories. A general discussion of the criteria and approach used by admissions committees in the evaluation of applicants is found in chapters 3 and 4.

Applicants in the highest priority are contacted by the admission office to arrange an interview appointment. As the process continues, applicants in successively lower categories are contacted.

The admission committee schedules interviews regularly throughout the fall, winter, and spring. Applicants are interviewed by one or more committee members, either sequentially or by several committee members together Subsequently, the full committee reviews the complete file of all interviewed candidates.

Interviewed applicants are informed of the committee's decision sometime after the interview. The exact schedule will vary from school to school.

The decision will be to offer an acceptance, reject the applicant, or place the applicant on an alternate list.

### Investigation Policies and Procedures

One significant responsibility of the Association of American Medical Colleges (AAMC) is to promote integrity and high ethical standards in the processes associated with admission to and enrollment in medical school. Applicants are expected to provide complete, current, and accurate information at the time application materials are submitted and during all phases of this process. Registrants for the MCAT are also obligated to present accurate and current information at the time registration materials are submitted and to adhere to all Test Center Regulations and Procedures as outlined in the *MCAT Announcement*.

Any falsification, omission, or discrepancy in application materials, including incomplete or invalid financial transactions, as well as any irregular behavior exhibited during the administration of the MCAT will prompt an inquiry by the AAMC. An investigation is conducted in accordance with procedures established by the AAMC's Executive Council as outlined in *AAMC Policies and Procedures for Investigating Reported Violations of Admission and Enrollment Standards*.

If the investigation confirms that such an action has occurred, a report thereof will be issued to all current and future medical schools to which the individual has applied or matriculated and all MCAT score recipients. In addition, it is the position of the AAMC to cooperate with report requests from duly constituted agencies, because reports may contain information relevant to academic or disciplinary proceedings, criminal investigations, graduate medical education, and/or professional licensure.

As the process continues through the admission cycle, acceptances are offered until the requisite number of acceptees is achieved to fill all the positions in the entering class for that year.

## NUMBER IN ENTERING CLASSES

Each medical school predetermines the number of students to be matriculated each year. (An estimate of the expected size of the entering class is provided in each school entry in

**TABLE 6**

**Trends Related to Medical School Applications for First-Year Centering Classes,
1991–92 Through 1995–96**

| Entering Year | Individuals Filing Applications | Applications Filed | Number of New Entrants* | Percent of Applicants Enrolled |
|---|---|---|---|---|
| 1991–92 | 33,301 | 354,017 | 16,211 | 49 |
| 1992–93 | 37,410 | 405,720 | 16,289 | 44 |
| 1993–94 | 42,808 | 482,788 | 16,307 | 38 |
| 1994–95 | 45,365 | 561,593 | 16,287 | 36 |
| 1995–96 | 46,591 | 595,975 | 16,253 | 35 |

Source: AAMC Section for Student Services (Final Action Summary Reports)
*New entrants are those students entering medical school for the very first time.

Chapter 10.) Budgetary and other policies may modify this number in any given year, so it is wise to check directly with the school. There were 16,253 new entrants in 1995 (Table 6).

## NUMBER OF APPLICANTS

Nationwide, 46,591 individuals applied for the 1995 entering class, a 2.7 percent increase over the number of applicants for the entering class of 1994. In other words, there were 2.9 applicants for each place. It is estimated that there will be approximately 47,000 applicants for the entering class of 1996, and the ratio of applicants to entering students may stay the same as 1995.

## PROPORTION OF APPLICANTS ACCEPTED

Overall, 37.3 percent of the candidates applying in 1995 were accepted. This is a decrease from 1994. Among first-time applicants, who numbered 32,176, the acceptance rate was 40.6 percent. Those 8,165 candidates who had applied for the second time after not being admitted in 1994 had a 29.4 percent acceptance rate.

## TIMING OF APPLICATIONS

Applicants are encouraged to submit their application as early as feasible in the admission cycle. For schools participating in the American Medical College Application Service (AMCAS), applications received beginning June 1 will be processed and forwarded to the schools designated by each applicant. (Applications received prior to June 1 will be returned to the applicant.) The 16 schools not participating in AMCAS have varying dates for the earliest receipt of applications (see school entries in Chapter 10).

All schools (whether using or not using AMCAS) determine the closing date for applications. For AMCAS-participating schools, the deadline date shown in the school's Chapter 10 entry is the date when the application must be received at AMCAS.

## EARLY DECISION PROGRAM (EDP)

The Early Decision Program (EDP) provides the well-qualified applicant who has a strong preference for a particular school with the opportunity to secure an acceptance by October 1. By applying as an EDP candidate, the individual agrees not to apply to any other U.S. medical school (AMCAS or non-AMCAS) until any of the following occurs: (1) receipt of an EDP rejection; (2) receipt of a formal release from the EDP commitment; or, (3) the October 1 notification deadline has passed. In addition, the applicant also agrees to attend the school if offered an EDP acceptance. Any violation of these conditions will be investigated and, if confirmed, reported to legitimately interested parties.

For the 1995 entering class, 90 medical schools offered admission through EDP. The EDP deadline for the receipt of application materials and official transcripts for AMCAS-participating schools is August 1. The EDP deadlines for non-AMCAS schools are listed in Chapter 10. If an EDP applicant is not accepted by the school, the applicant still has sufficient time to apply to other schools.

## NUMBER OF APPLICATIONS

Early Decision Program applicants initially file only one application. In 1995, there were 2,990 EDP candidates, and 1,076 (36 percent) were offered acceptances under the EDP. An additional 2,780 non-EDP candidates filed only one appli-



CHAPTER 6   APPLICATION AND SELECTION

cation to AMCAS-participating schools, and 70 percent were accepted at these institutions. For the 1995 entering class, AMCAS applicants applied to an average of 12.8 AMCAS-participating schools. AMCAS applicants who applied to from 7 to 19 AMCAS-participating schools for the 1995 entering class had an average acceptance rate of 37.5 percent at these institutions. AMCAS applicants who applied to 20 or more AMCAS-participating schools for the 1995 entering class had an average acceptance rate of 37.9 percent at these institutions.

The number of applications an applicant should file depends upon the qualifications of the individual relative to the overall level of competition of the schools to which the individual is applying. The decision of how many schools and to which schools to apply to is an important decision that should be made only after careful consultation with the pre-medical adviser. The considerations detailed in Chapter 4 should be used as guides.

## SELECTION FACTORS

Decisions to admit candidates are based upon multiple factors that are to a degree unique for each school. In general, however, all schools are looking for (1) evidence of an ability to accomplish the academic work necessary to progress through the school's curriculum and (2) evidence of possession of the personal qualities and attributes of physicians.

### Academic Ability

An admission committee seeks students who have acquired the knowledge and study skills needed to progress through the medical curriculum and to be active learners throughout their medical careers. To evaluate this, committees rely on candidates' college records and on the scores achieved on the MCAT. College transcripts are carefully reviewed from the standpoint of the grades earned, the credit hours carried during successive academic periods, and the distribution of courses among the biological, physical, and social sciences and the humanities. Although each school sets its own scale of preferences, in general, schools prefer candidates who have accomplished their college work on a normal schedule, who have a balanced distribution of credits among the sciences and humanities, and who have consistently earned grades in the 3.0 to 4.0 range.

In analyzing candidates' transcripts, the characteristics of the colleges they have attended are also considered. Thus, work accomplished and grades earned at colleges known by admission committees to have rigorous standards will be accorded greater weight than those from colleges considered to have lesser standards. The acceptability of advanced placement (AP) credits earned in high school varies from school to school. The individual school entries in Chapter 10 should be reviewed regarding their policies. If a school's policies for AP are unclear, the school's admission office should be consulted.

Scores on the MCAT provide ancillary information on candidates' academic ability. The method by which the scores achieved on the MCAT tests are factored into determining whether candidates can reasonably be expected to accomplish the academic work necessary to progress through a school's curriculum is established by each school. The range of acceptable MCAT scores varies among schools. MCAT scores are given greater attention when evaluating the academic records of candidates from colleges that are unfamiliar to an admission committee. Comparing MCAT scores with grades earned provides an estimation of such candidates' academic accomplishments in relationship to candidates from colleges that are familiar to the committee.

In summary, academic ability is an important selection factor, but judgments of academic ability vary among schools. Assessments of the academic ability of older candidates will include additionally their achievement in postbaccalaureate courses. The academic abilities of socioeconomically disadvantaged and underrepresented minority candidates require special assessments (see Chapter 8 and the AAMC publication, *Minority Student Opportunities in United States Medical Schools*).

### Personal Qualities and Attributes

Candidates' personal qualities are important factors in selection decisions. Evidence of maturity, character and integrity, self-discipline, concern with helping others, and leadership is sought through information obtained from the personal statement on applications, evaluations by premedical advisers and college faculty members, and interviews.

In writing a personal statement, the applicant should record not only the reasons for desiring a career in medicine but also extracurricular and work accomplishments. The activities deemed particularly significant should be described clearly and succinctly.

All medical schools will ask the applicant to designate persons from whom letters of evaluation should be requested. Generally, a letter from the premedical committee at the applicant's undergraduate college or university where premedical courses are taken is required. Evaluations from premedical advisers and college faculty members who know the applicant are given much greater weight by admission committees than letters of recommendation from friends, family members, clergymen, or political figures. If the applicant has worked extensively during college or is applying several years after college, letters from employers and supervisors are helpful.

Character, integrity, and maturity are important factors to medical schools. Applicants who have experienced disciplinary action in college for infractions of citizenship codes of conduct are expected to disclose this information in their application and to discuss the incident on their personal growth in a personal statement. Failure to disclose such official college action will prompt an investigation.

### Interviews

Policies regarding scheduling of interviews vary from school to school. Some will grant interviews to all candidates requesting one. Others invite candidates for an interview only after initial screening and priority categorization. In almost all cases, acceptances are offered only after candidates have been interviewed. Usually, the applicant will be asked to come to the school for the interview. Some schools have designated interviewers in various regions of the country to reduce the financial and time expenditures for candidates. However, the interview trip is also a good opportunity for the applicant to see the medical school.

Information about a school's interview policies and procedures is generally provided to candidates in the initial stage of the school's selection process. If these are not clear, applicants should ask for clarification from the admission office. At the interview, applicants should be prepared to discuss their personal histories and motivation for medicine candidly.

## NOTIFICATION OF ACCEPTANCE

Since 1961, the constituent medical schools of the AAMC have agreed to observe a new set of recommendations concerning medical school acceptance procedures for first-year entering students, commonly referred to as the "traffic rules." The recommendations for the 1997 entering class are noted on page 55. The purpose of these recommendations is to complete the admissions cycle in as timely a fashion as possible so that both students and schools will know who is entering the first year prior to the summer months.

The earliest and latest dates for notification and the time allowed for the applicant's response to an acceptance are shown in each school's entry in Chapter 10. Some schools permit accepted students to defer their entrance for one or more years. Applicants desiring to defer entrance to medical school should request deferment no later than when responding to a school's offer of acceptance.

The AAMC recommends that deposits required of accepted students not exceed $100 and that they be refundable until May 15. The amount of the deposit and the refund policy for each school are shown in the school entries in Chapter 10.

## APPLICANT RESPONSIBILITIES

In order for medical school admission committees to fully consider an application, the applicant must assume certain responsibilities in the application process. The observance of the responsibilities in the box below will ensure both applicants and admission committees of an orderly and timely process of student selection.

## CANDIDATES OFFERED MULTIPLE ACCEPTANCES

In 1995, 36.1 percent of accepted candidates were accepted by two or more medical schools. To provide an orderly and fair admission process, candidates are obligated to hold no more than one acceptance at a time. An applicant receiving acceptances from two or more schools simultaneously is expected to accept the offer of the most preferred school and notify the others that their offers are not accepted. If subsequent offers are received from other schools, the applicant may withdraw from the school originally accepted and accept the offer of a more preferred school. The schools are expected not to offer acceptances to students who have already arrived at another medical school for orientation and matriculation.

---

### Responsibilities of Medical School Applicants

1. Applicants are expected to become familiar with and observe the application procedures at each school to which they apply. All application documents including primary and secondary application forms, transcript(s), letters of evaluation, fees, etc., must be submitted in a timely manner.
2. Applicants must promptly notify AMCAS and medical schools not participating in AMCAS of any change of address.
3. Applicants must respond promptly to all invitations for a medical school interview. In those instances when an applicant cannot appear for a previously scheduled interview, the applicant is responsible for promptly notifying the school of the cancellation of the appointment. The cancellation should be undertaken by telephone, followed by a letter.
4. Applicants in need of financial aid must initiate the steps necessary to determine their eligibility as early as possible. This includes filing the appropriate need analysis forms in January or February and encouraging their parents (if required) to file their income tax forms early.
5. Applicants who remain under consideration for admission should keep the medical schools informed of the address and telephone number where they can be reached. Applicants who are unavailable (e.g. foreign travel) should instruct and grant authority to a parent or other individual to act on their behalf.
6. Applicants who have made a final decision on the medical school they plan to attend have the obligation to promptly withdraw their applications from all other schools.

## AAMC Recommendations Concerning
## Medical School Acceptance Procedures for
## First-Year Entering Students

*For the information of prospective medical students and their advisers, the recommended procedures for offering acceptance to medical school and for student responses to those offers are as follows:*

1. Each school of medicine should prepare and distribute to applicants and college advisers a detailed schedule of its application and acceptance procedures and should adhere to this schedule unless it is publicly amended.

2. Each school of medicine should agree not to notify its applicants (except for those applying via Early Decision Program [EDP]) of acceptance prior to October 15 of each admission cycle.

3. By March 15 of the year of matriculation, each school of medicine should have issued a number of acceptances at least equal to the size of its first-year entering class.

4. Only after May 15 are schools free to apply appropriate rules for dealing with accepted applicants who, without adequate explanation, hold one or more places in other schools. These rules should recognize the problems of the applicant who has multiple offers and also of those applicants who have not yet been accepted. Only schools whose first official day of classes begins prior to August 1 may start to request decisions from accepted applicants prior to May 15 but not earlier than April 15.

5. By May 15 of the year of matriculation, an applicant who has received offers of admission from more than one school should choose the one school that he or she prefers and withdraw from all other schools to which he or she has been accepted.

*6. Prior to May 15 of the year of matriculation, an applicant should be given at least two weeks to reply to an offer of admission. After May 15, schools may require applicants to respond to acceptance offers in less than two weeks. An applicant may be required to file a statement of intent, or a deposit, or both. The statement of intent should provide freedom to withdraw if the applicant is later accepted by a school that he or she prefers.

*7. It is recommended that the acceptance deposit not exceed $100 and be refundable until May 15. After that date, a school may retain the deposit as a late withdrawal fee. If the applicant matriculates at the school, the school is encouraged to credit the deposit toward tuition.

8. Subsequent to June 1, a school of medicine seeking to admit an applicant already known to be accepted by another school for that entering class should advise that school of its intent. Because of the administrative problems involved in filling a place vacated just prior to the commencement of the academic year, schools should communicate fully with each other with respect to anticipated late roster changes in order to keep misunderstandings at a minimum.

9. After an applicant has enrolled in a U.S. school of medicine or begun a brief orientation program contiguous to enrollment, no further acceptances should be offered to that individual. Once enrolled in a school, students have an obligation to withdraw their applications promptly from all other schools. Enrollment is defined as being officially registered as a member of the first-year entering class at a school.

*Most of what is stated in these two procedures does not pertain to students accepted through the Early Decision Program (EDP), because such students agree in advance to attend a given medical school if offered a place during the "early decision" segment of the application year.

# Financial Information for Medical Students

This chapter, which is designed for individuals seeking to finance their medical education, includes general information on financial planning and debt management, financial aid application procedures, distribution of aid, and common sources of student funding. Medical school applicants who need to supplement their resources to pay for the cost of a medical education need not feel intimidated by the profusion of financial aid programs, the amount of paperwork involved, or the variety of requirements. However, the following points should be kept in mind:

1. The primary responsibility for financing a medical education rests with the student and/or the student's family.
2. Borrowing is the most common form of assistance.
3. Applicants who are in default on federal educational loans or who owe refunds to federal grant programs are prohibited from obtaining additional support from a number of federal programs.
4. The amount of assistance available and how it is awarded to students differs from one medical school to another.
5. Funding and eligibility requirements for federal programs may change at any time.
6. The financial aid officer is responsible for coordinating all sources of financial assistance for each enrolled student.

## FINANCIAL PLANNING

The cost of attaining a medical education has increased markedly in the last decade. Individual school entries in Chapter 10 provide information on the cost of attendance for the 1995–96 academic year. Table 7-A provides tuition and student fees for 1995–96 first-year medical students at U.S. medical schools. For the 1995 graduating class, the average indebtedness of all medical students with debt was $69,059. The primary source of financial aid is in the form of loans (79 percent). For students who must depend extensively on loans to pay for medical school, two fundamental concepts are critical.

First, borrowing is defined as obligating future income. It is income yet to be earned that is obligated today for some benefit such as buying a car or paying for tuition to acquire an M.D. degree. When that income is finally earned, the amount that has been obligated cannot be used for any purpose other than the repayment of the past debt.

The second concept is a corollary to the first—an individual who decides to borrow to obtain an M.D. degree has also decided implicitly that the degree is equal in value to the amount of future income that has been obligated in order to attend medical school. Borrowing, therefore, has a direct effect on future professional and personal lifestyle; it is also an investment in one's own future. In deciding whether to pursue a medical education, the individual assesses whether the return is worth the investment.

Even if a student must borrow, it is possible to acquire a sense of fiscal awareness and responsibility that will permit significant control over the amount of future income obligated. Following the guidelines described below—and these are guidelines that will serve a lifetime—has the two-fold benefit of setting limits on the level of indebtedness while the student is in school and of successfully dealing with repayments after graduation.

## DEBT MANAGEMENT

Formulating a budget and living within its limits are essential. It requires delaying gratification in terms of purchases and lifestyle decisions while the individual is enrolled in school. Doing so can mean borrowing less and having more money in the future. To assist students, each medical school prepares a standard student budget, which can serve as a guideline for creating an individual budget. It is possible to live on less than the amount budgeted—by having roommates, sharing transportation, and preparing meals at home, for example. Participating in seemingly small economies can free literally thousands of dollars of future income for purposes other than repaying educational debts.

### Meeting Deadlines

Meeting deadlines for assistance is fundamental to receiving both sufficient and the least expensive funding while in school. Students are urged to maintain personal calendars in which due dates for applications, other documents, and tuition payments can be recorded. Meeting all deadlines will prevent late fees on tuition bills and, later on, defaults on educational loans while enhancing a good credit rating.

### Debt Reduction Methods

Limiting undergraduate borrowing, working (as long as academic standing is not jeopardized), and aggressively seek-

## TABLE 7-A

### Tuition and Student Fees for 1995–96 First-Year Students in U.S. Medical Schools (In Dollars)

| Categories of Students | Private Schools | | | Public Schools | | |
|---|---|---|---|---|---|---|
| | Range | Median | Average | Range | Median | Average |
| Resident | 8,879–30,973 | 23,695 | 22,509 | 2,685–18,490 | 8,715 | 9,447 |
| Nonresident | 15,188–30,973 | 24,495 | 24,131 | 7,983–49,577 | 20,133 | 20,681 |

Figures based on data provided summer 1995. Uniformed Services University of the Health Sciences, a public institution, does not charge tuition or student fees; books and equipment are also furnished without charge.

ing private sources of assistance are very effective methods for reducing debt and increasing future disposable earnings. For more information on private organizations and agencies—medical societies, state programs, brotherhoods, sisterhoods, and church groups—applicants are urged to explore their college libraries, contact their state departments of education, and review the material offered by their medical school's financial aid office. Although the search for private assistance requires considerable effort, the prospect of meeting the cost of education and decreasing the level of indebtedness makes the effort worthwhile.

### Record Maintenance

Maintaining good records is the responsibility of the borrower and is indispensable to the financial health of that borrower. Students should not expect others to maintain their records. The maintenance of precise records, including copies of application forms and signed promissory notes, enables the borrower to verify any errors and potentially save money that may be inappropriately assigned. Further, lenders often sell their loans to other lenders. A borrower with poor records may inadvertently default because deferment forms or payments are forwarded to the wrong financial institution.

### Borrower Responsibility

*The onus for keeping in touch with the lender/holder of the loan is on the borrower.* It is very important that lenders are notified of any change of permanent address. Default is inevitable if the lender is unable to communicate with the borrower or the borrower does not provide deferment forms or payments to the lender. **Default results in long-term negative effects on the borrower's credit rating.**

## SOURCES OF ASSISTANCE AND APPLICATION PROCEDURES

This chapter describes the rudiments of financial aid; each medical school has its own policies and procedures for distributing funds to students. Applicants must, therefore, maintain close contact with the financial aid offices at the schools to which they have been accepted.

Despite the variations of policies, procedures, application forms, and deadlines among institutions, a calendar showing general deadlines and dates of procedures is included here to help applicants with their plans for financing a medical education (Table 7-C); individual schools may deviate somewhat from the schedule in the table.

In addition to understanding the financial aid award cycle and the need to meet program deadlines, applicants should be aware that there are some general eligibility requirements and some specific requirements based on particular programs.

### General Eligibility Criteria

Most programs—federal and private, need- and cost-based—will normally require that the applicant be a U.S. citizen or permanent resident of the United States, make satisfactory academic progress, and comply with Selective Service registration requirements. Further, the student may not be in default on other loans. Applicants who have defaulted on prior educational debts will be unable to obtain loans from most federal programs. An individual in this circumstance may be prevented from attending medical school because of being barred from a substantial source of aid—the federal government. It is critical, therefore, to remain in good standing with all loan and scholarship programs. Some programs also may require a commitment of service as a condition for receiving financial assistance.

*(Text continued on page 55)*

## TABLE 7-B

### Federal Loan Programs for Students

| Characteristic | Primary Care Loan | Perkins* | Subsidized Stafford* | Unsubsidized Stafford* | HEAL* |
|---|---|---|---|---|---|
| Lender | Medical school financial aid office | Medical school financial aid office | Financial or credit institution, or eligible school | Financial or credit institution, or eligible school | Financial or credit institution, or eligible school |
| Based on need | Note[1] | Yes | Yes | No | No |
| Citizenship Requirement | U.S. citizen, U.S. National, or U.S. permanent resident | U.S. citizen, U.S. National, or U.S. permanent resident | U.S. citizen, U.S. National, or U.S. permanent resident | U.S. citizen, U.S. National, or U.S. permanent resident | U.S. citizen, U.S. National, or U.S. permanent resident |
| Borrowing limits | Tuition plus $2,500 | $5,000/year $30,000 aggregate undergraduate and graduate | $18,500 aggregate undergraduate and graduate | $138,500 aggregate undergraduate and graduate less the subsidized amount | $20,000/year $80,000 aggregate |
| Interest rate | Note[2] | 5% | Variable (91-Treasury Bill + 2.5%) adjusted annually, capped at 8.25% | Variable (91-Treasury Bill + 2.5%) adjusted annually, capped at 8.25% | Variable, no more than 91-day Treasury Bill + 3% (discounted by all lenders) |
| Interest accrues during: | | | | | |
| School | No | No | No | Yes | Yes |
| Deferments | No | No | No | Yes | Yes |
| Grace Period | No | No | No | Yes | Yes |

[1]Yes; in addition, borrower must agree upon signing loan agreement to enter and complete primary care residency and practice in a primary care field until the loan is repaid in full.

[2]Five percent, if borrower fails to meet primary care requirement at any time before the completion of repayment, the unpaid balance is recomputed from date of issuance at 12%, and the recomputed balance must be repaid not later than 3 years after borrower fails to comply with the agreement.

**TABLE 7-B (Continued)**

**Federal Loan Programs for Students**

| Characteristic | Primary Care Loan | Perkins* | Subsidized Stafford* | Unsubsidized Stafford* | HEAL* |
|---|---|---|---|---|---|
| Grace Period | 1 year after graduation | 9 months after graduation | 6 months after graduation | 6 months after graduation | 9 months after graduation or 9 months after approved internship or residency completion |
| Deferments | Allowable. Check with lending institution for current deferment categories | Allowable. Check with lending institution for current deferment categories | Allowable. Check with lending institution for current deferment categories | Allowable. Check with lending institution for current deferment categories | Note[3] |
| Repayment requirements | Minimum: $15/month including interest; maximum 10 years to repay | Minimum: $40/month including interest; maximum 10 years to repay; eligible for loan consolidation | Minimum: $50/month maximum 10 years to repay; eligible for loan consolidation | Minimum: $50/month maximum 10 years to repay; eligible for loan consolidation | Minimum amount negotiable with lender; maximum 10–25 years to repay; eligible for loan consolidation |
| Prepayment penalties | n/a | None | None | None | None |
| Allowable cancellations | n/a | Death, totally and permanently disabled | Death, totally and permanently disabled; up to 70% cancellation for service as a Peace Corps or VISTA volunteer | Death, totally and permanently disabled; up to 70% cancellation for service as a Peace Corps or VISTA volunteer | Death, totally and permanently disabled |

[3]Up to 4 years for internship and residency; up to 3 years for active military duty. Public Health Service Corps, ACTION/Peace Corps service and National Health Service Corps; up to 2 years fellowship and full-time educational activity; up to 3 years for a borrower who has completed an internship or residency in family medicine, general internal medicine, preventive medicine or general pediatrics, and is practicing primary care.

*Perkins = Federal Perkins Loan; Subsidized and Unsubsidized Stafford = Federal Stafford Loan; HEAL = Health Education Assistance Loan

---

**TABLE 7-C**

**Calendar of Deadlines and Procedures for Financial Aid
for Incoming Students**

| Event | Dates |
| --- | --- |
| Need analysis forms sent to student | November–March |
| Financial aid information sent to students | January–March |
| School-based aid application sent to students | January–March |
| Deadline for submission of state scholarship applications by students | February–March |
| Deeadline for submission of need analysis forms by students | March–May |
| Processing of applications to federal loan programs begins | March–June |
| Deadline for submission of institutional aid forms by students | March–June |
| Notification to students of estimated award of school-based aid | April–August |
| Notification to students of complete award package | April–August |

*NOTE: This schedule is approximate. Contact individual schools for specific dates.*

---

## Need-Based Funds

Financial need is determined by subtracting the student's family resources from the school's standard student budget. The family contribution is usually calculated by using a national need analysis service. Supporting materials such as tax returns are also required. Most medical schools expect full disclosure of parents' financial information—even for independent, older, or married students—to be considered for certain types of aid. It is important for applicants to ask their parents to file their income tax forms as early in the year as possible. Applicants should submit the required need analysis form(s) in March, April, or May of the year they expect to be accepted to medical school. Medical school financial aid officers can assist accepted students in determining their financial assistance requirements in a timely manner *only if applicants submit the necessary forms early.*

Examples of federal need-based funds are listed in Table 7-B. School-administered programs and a number of private sources are also need-based. Individual medical schools, state departments of education, and college libraries are the best sources of information for these programs.

## Cost-Based Funds

Some programs are cost-based, which means a formal need analysis of family contribution is not necessarily required. The student's resources must still be taken into account and subtracted from the budget established by the school in order to determine the amount that may be obtained. Two federally insured loans are not associated with need—the Federal Unsubsidized Stafford Loan and the HEAL. Detailed information about these two cost-based loan programs can be found in Table 7-B. The Alternative Loan Program (ALP), a component of the Association of American Medical Colleges' MEDLOANS Program, is an instance of private, non-need-based financial assistance. A description of the AAMC MEDLOANS Program and the ALP loan is presented below.

## AAMC MEDLOANS℠ PROGRAM

MEDLOANS is a comprehensive loan program for allopathic medical students sponsored by the Association of American Medical Colleges. MEDLOANS can provide all the loan assistance a student will need for medical school through access to the Federal Stafford Loan (both subsidized and unsubsidized), the Alternative Loan Program (ALP), and the MEDEX loan.

Now entering its second decade, MEDLOANS offers numerous benefits to borrowers who finance their education through MEDLOANS. Some of these benefits are immediate, and others carry on throughout the life of the loan. These benefits include:

- borrower benefits which result in reduced repayment amounts for MEDLOANS borrowers over the life of the loan;
- reduced guarantee fees on the Federal Stafford Loan;
- state of the art processing of applications and delivery of loan proceeds;
- superior customer assistance and loan servicing;
- competitive interest rates on the ALP and MEDEX loans;

- favorable capitalization terms on the ALP and MEDEX loans;
- loan forgiveness in the event of death prior to repayment for the ALP and MEDEX; and
- the combined expertise of leaders in the student loan industry.

In order to borrow the Federal Stafford Loan through MEDLOANS, the borrower must meet the eligibility criteria as described in the previous section. However, in order to borrow through either the ALP or MEDEX programs, an applicant must be a U.S. citizen, be enrolled full-time in a U.S. accredited allopathic medical school, be making satisfactory progress, not be in default on any loans, and be deemed credit worthy.

The ALP is used to help supplement other borrowing, including borrowing through the Federal Stafford Loan program and other federal, state, and institutional loan programs. In this regard, it should always be considered a loan of last resort, and the borrower should always contact the financial aid office prior to applying for the ALP. The maximum annual amount a student may borrow through the ALP is the cost of attendance less other aid received during the year, with the total aggregate educational indebtedness of the student from all loan sources not to exceed $175,000.

The ALP is a variable interest rate loan, with a rate of 2.5% plus the 91-Day T-Bill during school, and 2.85% plus the 91-Day T-Bill following graduation. The ALP is currently capitalized once at graduation and annually thereafter until repayment begins. Repayment on the ALP can be delayed up to four years following graduation. However, once repayment begins, the loan must be repaid within 20 years. The ALP may be administratively consolidated with other loans in the MEDLOANS program.

The MEDLOANS program also offers senior medical students access to the MEDEX loan, a loan designed to provide funding for both interview and relocation expenses, expenses not allowed through regular financial aid programs. Terms of the MEDEX loan are similar to those of the ALP.

The MEDLOANS program continues to provide dependable, low cost, affordable, state of the art financing for medical students, and does so with a program that always compares favorably with other loan programs designed for medical students.

Additional information on MEDLOANS can be obtained by either calling MEDLOANS Customer Assistance at 1-800-858-5050 or by contacting the financial aid office at your medical school. In addition, you can contact the AAMC's Division of Student Affairs and Education Services at:

AAMC MEDLOANS Program
Division of Student Affairs and Education Services
Association of American Medical Colleges
2450 N Street, N.W.
Washington, D.C. 20037

## SERVICE COMMITMENT PROGRAMS

The commitment service scholarship programs—military awards available through the Army, Navy, and Air Force are not need-based or cost-based, nor are they, strictly speaking, financial aid.

The Armed Forces Health Professions Scholarship Program essentially offers full support to the medical student while in school in exchange for service in the funding organization once the scholarship recipient has received the M.D. degree. Participation in a postgraduate training program conducted at a military facility does not count toward the service commitment. Applications are very competitive and are handled by military recruiters. Addresses and further information are outlined in Table 7-D.

Medical students have the opportunity to enlist in the National Health Service Corps (NHSC) Scholarship Program upon matriculation to medical school. The NHSC is administered by the Bureau of Health Care Delivery and Assistance in the Health Resources and Services Administration, an agency of the U.S. Public Health Service. Among the goals of the NHSC is the improvement of the delivery of primary care health services in health professional shortage areas (HPSA). The NHSC offers two major types of financial support in exchange for professional services: competitive scholarships and loan repayment. Awards are made in various amounts and service obligations range from two to four years.

### The Federal Scholarship Program

This program awards tuition and fees; payment towards books, supplies, and equipment; and a monthly stipend. In return, awardees commit to service in a federally designated HPSA one year for each year the scholarship is awarded with a minimum two-year obligation.

### The Federal Loan Repayment Program

This program provides payment towards both government and commercial education loans—up to $25,000 per year for the first two years and up to $35,000 for every year thereafter with a minimum two-year commitment. The program also provides funds for increased income taxes resulting from loan repayment. This is in addition to full salary and benefits.

The NHSC also provides a State Loan Repayment Program and Community Scholarship Program in selected states. For more information:

National Health Service Corps
　Scholarship Program
U.S. Public Health Recruitment
8201 Greensboro Drive
Suite 600
McLean, Virginia 22102

Students may also want to inquire about whether the state in which they intend to eventually practice has a loan forgiveness or repayment program in return for a commitment to serve in that state's areas of need. These programs are often aimed at residents and practicing physicians, though some are available to medical students who are still in school. Financial aid officers in the medical schools are a good source of information in this area. Inquire about the reference handbook, *State and Other Loan Repayment/Forgiveness and Scholarship Programs,* when you are gathering other information from the medical school financial aid office.

## Loan Consolidation

Under the federal consolidation loan program, lenders, student loan guarantee agencies, and the Student Loan Marketing Association (Sallie Mae) now have the authority to consolidate the following loans: Federal Stafford Loan (subsidized and unsubsidized), Federal Perkins Loan, and Health Professions Student Loans (HPSL). (See Table 7-B, "Repayment Requirements.")

Depending on the size of the total educational indebtedness, an individual could have up to 30 years to repay. The interest rate charged on consolidated loans is the weighted average of the underlying loans, rounded upward to the nearest whole percentage point. In addition, an "administrative" consolidation of loans made under the Health Education Assistance Loan (HEAL) program is also possible. This enables a borrower to write one repayment check each month for loans under all of the federal programs.

More information on personal financial planning and debt management can be found in the publications listed below.

## INFORMATION SOURCES

The following books, articles, brochures, and newsletters should be readily available in libraries, university counseling offices, and medical school student affairs and financial aid offices, or they may be ordered directly from the publishers. Study of these materials may help students in their financial planning and lead them to further sources of financial aid.

1. *The Student Guide, 1995–96.* Department of Education. Free. (Federal Student Aid Information Center, P.O. Box 84, Washington, D.C. 20044; 1-800-4-FED AID (1-800-433-3243).

2. *Dollars for College: The Quick Guide to Scholarships, Fellowships, Loans, and Other Financial Aid Programs for Medicine, Dentistry, and Related Fields.* $6.95 prepaid. Revised every 18 months. (Garrett Park Press, P.O. Box 190, Garrett Park, Maryland 20896) ISBN: 1-880774-15-1.

3. *Financial Planning and Management Manual for U.S. Medical Students, 1994.* Association of American Medical Colleges. $7.50 plus shipping and handling. (Association of American Medical Colleges, Department 66, Washington, D.C. 20055; (202) 828-0416.)

4. *Informed Decision-Making: Part I, Financial Planning and Management for Medical Students; Part II, Sources of Financial Assistance for Medical School.* National Medical Fellowships, Inc. 1993. $15.00 per set. (Scholarship Department, National Medical Fellowships, Inc., 110 West 32nd Street, 8th Floor, New York, New York 10001)

## TABLE 7-D

## Federal Loan Programs for Students

| Characteristic | Source of Grant | | | | |
| --- | --- | --- | --- | --- | --- |
| | Air Force | Army | Navy | EFN Program* | FADHPS Program† |
| Provider | Medical Recruiting Division HQ USAFRS/RSOHM 550 D Street West, Suite 1 Randolph AFB, TX 78150-4527 | US Army Health Professions Support Agency SGPS-PD 5109 Leesburg Pike Falls Church, VA 22041-3258 | Commander, Navy Recruiting Command (Code 32) 801 North Randolph St. Arlington, VA 22203-1991 | Medical school financial aid office | Medical school financial aid office |
| Based on need | No | No | No | Yes—family contribution not to exceed the lesser of $5,000 or one-half cost of education | Yes—family contribution not to exceed the lesser of $5,000 or one-half cost of education plus student must be from disadvantaged background |
| Citizenship requirement | U.S. citizen only | U.S. citizen only | U.S. citizen only | U.S. citizen, U.S national, or U.S. permanent resident | U.S. citizen, U.S. national, or U.S. permanent resident |
| Service commitment | Yes | Yes | Yes | None | None |
| Nature of commitment | One year of service for each year of support | One year of service for each year of support | One year of service for each year of support | Not applicable | Not applicable |
| Level of support | Full tuition, monthly living stipend, book and supply allowance | Full tuition, monthly living stipend, book and supply allowance | Full tuition, monthly living stipend, book and supply allowance | Tuition and other educational expenses | Up to $10,000 per year |

*Scholarship Program for Students of Exceptional Financial Need.
†Financial Assistance for Disadvantaged Health Professions Students.

# Information for Minority Group Students

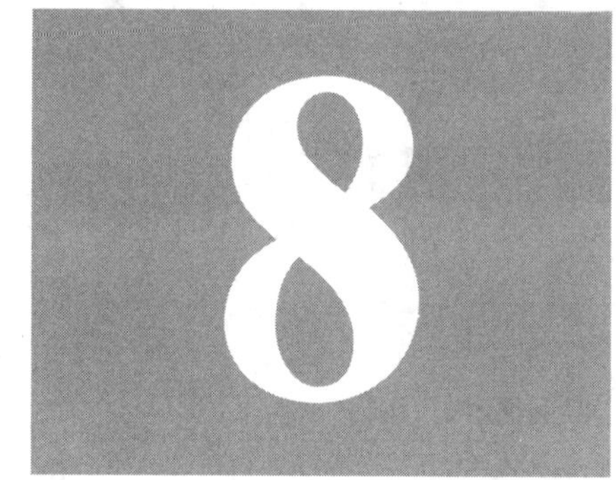

This chapter provides information for students interested in applying to medical school who are from minority groups underrepresented in medicine—blacks, Native Americans (American Indian, Alaskan Natives or Native Hawaiian), Mexican Americans, and mainland Puerto Ricans. These four groups were designated as underrepresented in medicine more than 20 years ago by the Association of American Medical Colleges (AAMC). They continue to be underrepresented in medical school enrollment—underrepresented minorities constitute 19.4 percent of the U.S. population (1990 U.S. Census), but only 12.4 percent of 1995 medical school matriculants. Designation as underrepresented not only reflects these groups' numerical score underrepresentation but also a history of discrimination and exclusion in the United States.

Increasing the number of physicians from racial and ethnic groups underrepresented in medicine has been a priority of medical schools for many years. The Executive Council of the AAMC issued a policy statement in 1970 on the medical education of minority group students. The AAMC reaffirmed this commitment in 1987 by issuing the "AAMC Statement on Medical Education of Minority Group Students" (page 69). In 1991 AAMC officially launched *Project 3000 by 2000*. The goal of this project is to increase the number of underrepresented minority students entering medical school each year to 3,000 by the Year 2000. The project emphasizes the development of partnerships linking medical school systems with undergraduate colleges and local school systems.

Most medical schools have programs and resources specifically designed to assist in the recruitment and enrollment of underrepresented minority students. Premedical advisers at undergraduate colleges can also provide pertinent information on medical school admissions or refer students to appropriate contact persons or offices.

The number of applicants to medical school has increased dramatically (42,808 in 1993, 45,355 in 1994, and 46,591 in 1995). The number of underrepresented minority applicants to medical school has also increased. There were 5,164 underrepresented minority applicants to medical school in 1995 (5,060 in 1994). Underrepresented minority new entrants to the 1995 entering class was 2,010, comprising 12.4 percent of all new entrants (Table 4-F). However, the disparity continues to exist. Tables 8-A and 8-B show the trend in minority first year and total enrollment from 1986–87 to 1995–96. Table 4-E in Chapter 4 presents additional information pertaining to the number of underrepresented minorities enrolled in medical school in 1995–96.

Once enrolled in medical school, academic and personal support programs are available to students. These support systems promote the successful completion of medical studies by minority students to help achieve the ultimate goal: increasing the numbers of minority physicians entering careers in patient care, teaching, and research.

Table 8-C identifies the individual primarily responsible for minority affairs at each U.S. medical school who can provide more detailed information on each school's programs and admissions procedures. Enrollment data on new entrants, first year, and total number of underrepresented minority students for each medical school is also included in the table.

Additional information concerning programs at medical schools for minority students can be obtained from the medical school contact persons or offices listed in Table 8-C and from premedical advisers at the undergraduate colleges.

## MEDICAL MINORITY APPLICANT REGISTRY (MED-MAR)

One of the services initiated by the AAMC for students from underrepresented minority groups is the Medical Minority Applicant Registry (Med-MAR). This program provides the opportunity for any medical school applicant belonging to a minority group traditionally underrepresented in medicine to have basic biographical information and MCAT scores circulated, at no cost, to the minority affairs and admissions offices of all U.S. medical schools as well as to other health services institutions and organizations that request the Med-MAR lists. At the time students take the MCAT, they indicate on the MCAT form their interest in being included on the Med-MAR. The lists are circulated twice a year (usually in July and November) following the administration of the MCAT. Medical schools correspond directly with students and may request more detailed information.

Waiver of medical school application fees is determined by each school on an individual basis. Similarly, fees for the American Medical College Application Service (AMCAS) are waived on an individual basis. MCAT fees are not waived, but a fee reduction program is in place (see Chapter 5).

For information about matters related to minority students, the applicant should write to:

Minority Student Information Clearinghouse
Division of Community and Minority Programs
Association of American Medical Colleges
2450 N Street, N.W.
Washington, D.C. 20037-1126

## SUMMER AND ENRICHMENT PROGRAMS

To encourage and prepare underrepresented minority students for a career in medicine, a variety of academic enrichment programs are available. There are programs designed for almost every stage in the educational continuum. These are programs for middle school and high school students, college programs, and postbaccalaureate programs, as well as research opportunities. There are also laboratory research internships available for high school and college students.

## FINANCIAL AID

Because of the variety and scope of financial assistance plans, applicants to both public and private medical schools should not think that they are unqualified for admission solely because of financial status. Generally, medical schools have been successful in providing adequate funding to meet the needs of their students, regardless of financial means. However, it is the responsibility of applicants to devote careful and thorough attention to all aspects of their educational financing. Before enrolling, applicants should obtain specific information from the medical schools about possibilities of financial assistance. (See Chapter 7.)

Financial assistance is usually made available to medical students in the form of loans or a combination of grants, scholarships, and loans. The amount awarded is determined by most schools on the basis of economic need rather than on the basis of academic performance. Financial need is usually determined by a need analysis system belonging to one of the national organizations established specifically for this purpose. Student aid comes from a variety of sources, some of which are listed below:

1. Directly from the medical school, usually from endowments or grants made to the school for use in the support of students.
2. The federally supported Scholarship Program for Students of Exceptional Financial Need (EFN).
3. The federally supported National Health Service Corps Scholarship Program and the Armed Forces Health Professions Scholarship Program, which may include payment of tuition and other reasonable expenses plus a monthly stipend in return for specific periods of service following graduation from medical school. (Places in the National Health Service Corps Scholarship Program will be limited, if available at all.)
4. The Federal Stafford Loan Program (subsidized and unsubsidized) and the Health Education Assistance Loan Program (HEAL)—the student borrows money from a bank or other private lender, a state, or a medical school, and the federal government guarantees to repay a major portion of the loan should the student default. In some cases the federal government pays the interest on the loan while the student is in school. The student should be aware of whether or not the government will pay the interest.
5. The federally sponsored Health Professions Student Loan Program, which is limited to applicants who are committed to primary care.
6. The federally administered Perkins Loan Program, which provides loans at 5 percent interest through the medical schools.
7. National Medical Fellowships, Inc., which provides grants to aid minority group students to reduce the amount of loan indebtedness incurred by the students.
8. Loans or scholarship funds available in certain states to residents to enable them to study medicine. The amounts awarded and the programs themselves differ widely among the states that offer them.
9. Loans and scholarship funds available to medical students directly from various philanthropic organizations.

The federal financial assistance programs described in the preceding list are subject to change due to congressional and executive review. Students should obtain up-to-date information on each of these programs from the school's financial aid office either when interviewed or accepted.

Further information about these sources and about financial aid programs in general is provided in Chapter 7. Information on admission procedures for individual medical schools is given in Chapter 10.

## INFORMATION SOURCES

Students may find the following articles, books, and brochures helpful in planning their medical careers.

1. *Career Choices: Health Professions Opportunities for Minorities.* Free. (Office of Statewide Health Planning and Development, Health Professions Career Opportunity Program, 1600 Ninth Street, Room 441, Sacramento, California 95814)
2. *Choosing a Health Professional Career: A Reference Guide.* National Medical Fellowships, Inc. 1993. $15.00 per set. (National Medical Fellowships, Inc., 110 West 32nd Street, Eighth Floor, New York, New York 10001; (212) 714-1007)
3. *Educational Survival Skills Reading Package.* Free. (Office of Statewide Health Planning and Development, Health Professions Career Opportunity Program, 1600 Ninth Street, Room 441, Sacramento, California 95814)
4. Epps, A. C., and Pisano, J. C. *MEdREP at Tulane: Effectiveness of a Medical Education Reinforcement and Enrichment Program for Minorities in the Health Professions.* 1985. $12.00. (Futura Publishing Com-

## AAMC Statement on Medical Education of Minority Group Students

The findings and recommendations of the 1970 AAMC Task Force on Minority Student Opportunities in Medical Education, combined with federal and private philanthropy support, provided the first impetus for the academic medical community to address the issue of access to the profession of medicine for individuals of underrepresented minority groups in our society.

The following decade witnessed significant progress as total enrollment of underrepresented minorities surged from 3.12 percent in 1969 to 8.0 percent in 1979. Whereas in 1969 Howard and Meharry accounted for 75 percent of all black medical students, by 1979 they accounted for only 20 percent.

Minority enrollments in U.S. medical schools reached their peak in 1975, when minorities represented 8.1 percent of the total student body. Since then, however, a leveling-off effect has dominated, and no significant increase in the number of underrepresented minorities entering medical school has occurred.

This long-term plateau indicates that if the progress achieved in providing access for more minorities to pursue careers in medicine is to continue, educational institutions, the federal government, and philanthropic organizations must reaffirm their commitment to the education of underrepresented minorities for careers in medicine as a national goal.

The AAMC and its constituent members are directing an earnest effort toward the goal of increasing opportunities for underrepresented minorities who wish to pursue careers in medical service, teaching, and research. These goals are described in detail in the 1970 "Report of the AAMC Task Force to the Inter-Association Committee on Expanding Educational Opportunities in Medicine for Blacks and Other Minority Students." These goals were also reaffirmed in the 1978 "Report of the AAMC Task Force on Minority Student Opportunities in Medicine."

Medical schools, working with cooperating undergraduate institutions, the AAMC, other agencies, and interested entities, are urged to help increase minority student awareness of the opportunities for professional education and specific preparation necessary for medical school. Minority students, thus motivated, prepared, and recruited, should be provided with the necessary encouragement and support to ensure their retention in and graduation from medical schools. To strengthen these efforts, medical schools are encouraged to continue to identify a faculty member or administrator who can be specifically charged with responsibility for minority student affairs. The person designated for this role should be a member of a minority group and should work closely with the AAMC Group on Student Affairs to represent the medical school in the activities of the Group on Student Affairs' Minority Affairs Section.

Medical schools are encouraged to pursue actively the expansion of minority student support funds from local, state, and federal levels. The AAMC is making known to the American public and to the federal government these needs to increase financial aid for minority students and for all students.

The AAMC-AMA Liaison Committee on Medical Education (LCME) is strongly encouraged to review critically the degree of individual opportunity provided to minority students. The LCME should continue to include in its membership and accreditation teams representatives from minority group members who have experience and knowledge in the education of minority group students.

The AAMC and its constituent members reaffirm their commitment to these efforts. Many current trends point to the urgency and timeliness of this affirmation: a perceived physician surplus in the face of an underrepresentation of minority physicians, the continuing physician maldistribution vis-a-vis minority and other underserved areas, the lack of opportunity for minorities in graduate medical programs, the underrepresentation of both minority medical students and faculty members in medical education, and the increasing cost of medical education to minorities and other low-income individuals. The AAMC and its member schools urge that, in any deliberations regarding physician manpower, the recruitment and graduation of individuals from underrepresented minorities in medical education be considered with particular care.

Approved by the AAMC Executive Council
June 1987

pany, Inc., 2 Bedford Ridge Road, Mount Kisco, New York 10549)

5. *Financial Advice and Health Careers Resources Directory for Minority Students.* Free. (Office of Statewide Health Planning and Development, Health Professions Career Opportunity Program, 1600 Ninth Street, Room 441, Sacramento, California 95814)

6. *Financial Aid for Minorities in Health Fields.* 1993. $4.95. ISBN 0-912048-96-4. (Garrett Park Press, P.O. Box 190, Garrett Park, Maryland 20896)

7. *Financing Medical Education, 1995–1996.* $6.00 (includes shipping and handling) Checks made payable to NAMME (Charles Terrell, Associate Dean for Student Affairs, Boston University School of Medicine, 80 East Concord Street, Boston, Massachusetts 02118)

8. *Financing Your Health Professions Education and Financial Planning and Debt Management for Health Professions Students.* National Medical Fellowships, Inc. 1993. $15.00 per set. (National Medical Fellowships, Inc., 110 West 32nd Street, Eighth Floor, New York, New York 10001; (212) 714-1007)

9. *Getting In: A Guide for Pre-Med Students.* Written by students who have recently gone through or are currently going through the process of applying to medical school. From the Premedical Education Task Force. 1993. (American Medical Student Association, 1902 Association Drive, Reston, Virginia 22091. $5.00 for AMSA members; $8.00 for non-members. Call (703) 620-6600 to order.)

10. Haller, E. H., and Myers, R. A. (Eds.). *Searching, Teaching, Healing: American Indians and Alaskan Natives in Biomedical Research Careers.* 1986. $9.95. (Futura Publishing Company, Inc., 2 Bedford Ridge Road, Mount Kisco, New York 10549)

11. Health Pathways. Free. (Office of Statewide Health Planning and Development, Health Professions Career Opportunity Program, 1600 Ninth Street, Room 441, Sacramento, California 95814)

12. *Informed Decision-Making: Part I, Financial Planning and Management for Medical Students; Part II, Sources of Financial Assistance for Medical School.* National Medical Fellowships, Inc. 1993. $15.00 per set. (National Medical Fellowships, Inc., 110 West 32nd Street, New York, New York 10001; (212) 714-1007)

13. *Minorities in Medicine: A Guide for Premedical Students.* Free. (Office of Statewide Health Planning and Development, Health Professions Career Opportunity Program, 1600 Ninth Street, Room 441, Sacramento, California 95814)

14. *Minority Student Opportunities in United States Medical Schools, 1995–96.* 13th edition. Association of American Medical Colleges. (Membership and Publication Orders, Association of American Medical Colleges, 2450 N Street, N.W., Washington, D.C. 20037-1126)

15. Schlachter, G. A., and Weber, D. *Directory of Financial Aids for Minorities, 1995–96.* $47.50 plus $4.00 shipping. Includes over 2,200 scholarships, fellowships, loans, grants, awards, and internships for black, Hispanic, Asian, and Native Americans. (Reference Service Press, 1100 Industrial Road, Suite 9, San Carlos, California 94070)

16. *Time Management for Students.* Free. (Office of Statewide Health Planning and Development, Health Professions Career Opportunity Program, 1600 Ninth Street, Room 441, Sacramento, California 95814)

## TABLE 8-A

### Selected Minority Group Enrollment in First-Year Classes in U.S. Medical Schools, 1986–87 Through 1995–96*

| | Black American | | American Indian | | Mexican American/Chicano | | Mainland Puerto Rican | | |
|---|---|---|---|---|---|---|---|---|---|
| Year | Number Enrolled* | % of Total First-Year Enrollment | Number Enrolled | % of Total First-Year Enrollment | Number Enrolled | % of Total First-Year Enrollment | Number Enrolled | % of Total First-Year Enrollment | Total First-Year Enrollment |
| 1986–87 | 1,174 | 7.0 | 61 | 0.4 | 331 | 2.0 | 111 | 0.7 | 16,819 |
| 1987–88 | 1,221 | 7.3 | 68 | 0.4 | 308 | 1.8 | 116 | 0.7 | 16,713 |
| 1988–89 | 1,210 | 7.2 | 76 | 0.5 | 295 | 1.7 | 127 | 0.8 | 16,868 |
| 1989–90 | 1,221 | 7.3 | 82 | 0.5 | 307 | 1.8 | 139 | 0.8 | 16,756 |
| 1990–91 | 1,263 | 7.5 | 76 | 0.5 | 285 | 1.7 | 120 | 0.7 | 16,876 |
| 1991–92 | 1,304 | 7.6 | 93 | 0.5 | 351 | 2.1 | 128 | 0.7 | 17,071 |
| 1992–93 | 1,425 | 8.3 | 123 | 0.7 | 447 | 2.6 | 126 | 0.7 | 17,079 |
| 1993–94 | 1,489 | 8.7 | 129 | 0.8 | 437 | 2.6 | 106 | 0.6 | 17,121 |
| 1994–95 | 1,519 | 8.9 | 131 | 0.8 | 501 | 2.9 | 137 | 0.8 | 17,085 |
| 1995–96 | 1,528 | 9.0 | 150 | 0.9 | 535 | 3.1 | 127 | 0.7 | 17,058 |

NOTE: First-year class enrollment figures include new entrants and those students repeating, reentering, or continuing the initial year.

*These figures include Black Americans enrolled at predominantly black schools. In 1995, a total of 186 were enrolled at Howard, Meharry, and Morehouse medical schools.

## TABLE 8-B

### Selected Minority Group Total Enrollment in U.S. Medical Schools, 1986–87 Through 1995–96*

| | Black American | | American Indian | | Mexican American/Chicano | | Mainland Puerto Rican | | |
|---|---|---|---|---|---|---|---|---|---|
| Year | Number Enrolled* | % of Total First-Year Enrollment | Number Enrolled | % of Total First-Year Enrollment | Number Enrolled | % of Total First-Year Enrollment | Number Enrolled | % of Total First-Year Enrollment | Total First-Year Enrollment |
| 1986–87 | 3,892 | 5.9 | 242 | 0.4 | 1,153 | 1.7 | 435 | 0.7 | 66,125 |
| 1987–88 | 3,968 | 6.0 | 233 | 0.4 | 1,144 | 1.7 | 467 | 0.7 | 65,735 |
| 1988–89 | 3,995 | 6.1 | 237 | 0.4 | 1,128 | 1.7 | 438 | 0.7 | 65,300 |
| 1989–90 | 4,145 | 6.4 | 258 | 0.4 | 1,087 | 1.7 | 452 | 0.7 | 65,016 |
| 1990–91 | 4,241 | 6.5 | 277 | 0.4 | 1,109 | 1.7 | 457 | 0.7 | 65,163 |
| 1991–92 | 4,334 | 6.6 | 301 | 0.5 | 1,205 | 1.8 | 485 | 0.7 | 65,602 |
| 1992–93 | 4,638 | 7.0 | 333 | 0.5 | 1,332 | 2.0 | 484 | 0.7 | 66,142 |
| 1993–94 | 4,900 | 7.4 | 364 | 0.5 | 1,450 | 2.2 | 444 | 0.7 | 66,629 |
| 1994–95 | 5,117 | 7.6 | 430 | 0.6 | 1,623 | 2.4 | 445 | 0.7 | 67,072 |
| 1995–96 | 5,337 | 8.0 | 501 | 0.7 | 1,769 | 2.6 | 455 | 0.7 | 66,970 |

*These figures include Black Americans enrolled at predominantly black schools. In 1995, a total of 720 were enrolled at Howard, Meharry, and Morehouse medical schools.

Source: AAMC Section for Student Services (Fall Enrollment Questionnaires).

## TABLE 8-C

## Minority Student Information by Individual Medical School

| Medical School | Contact Person or Office | Minority Enrollment, Fall 1995 (New Entrant/First Year/Total)* | | | |
|---|---|---|---|---|---|
| | | Black American | American Indian | Mexican-American | Mainland Puerto Rican |
| Alabama | Sylvia Strothers<br>Coordinator, Minority<br>  Enhancement Program<br>(205) 934-2330 | 16/18/60 | 2/ 2/ 5 | 0/ 0/ 0 | 0/ 0/ 1 |
| Alabama, South | Dr Hattie M. Myles<br>Assistant Dean, Office of<br>  Special Programs and<br>  Student Affairs<br>(334) 460-7313 | 4/ 5/22 | 1/ 1/ 2 | 0/ 0/ 1 | 0/ 0/ 0 |
| Albany† | Assie Bishop<br>Director of Minority Affairs<br>(518) 262-5824 | 4/ 4/19 | 1/ 1/ 1 | 2/ 2/ 5 | 0/ 0/ 4 |
| Albert Einstein† | Dr. Milton Gumbs<br>Vice President,<br>  Medical Director<br>(718) 901-8712 | 10/12/38 | 0/ 0/ 2 | 3/ 4/ 5 | 2/ 2/ 8 |
| Arizona | Linda K. Don<br>Program Coordinator<br>(602) 626-7146 | 4/ 5/10 | 2/ 2/10 | 13/15/44 | 2/ 2/ 2 |
| Arkansas | Dr. Phillip L. Rayford<br>Associate Dean for Minority<br>  Affairs<br>(501) 686-5123 | 12/15/52 | 4/ 4/ 5 | 0/ 0/ 2 | 0/ 0/ 1 |
| Baylor† | Dr. James L. Phillips<br>Senior Associate Dean<br>(713) 746-6457 | 12/15/32 | 1/ 1/ 4 | 18/18/36 | 2/ 3/ 6 |
| Boston† | Dr. Kenneth Edelin<br>Associate Dean for Student<br>  and Minority Affairs<br>(617) 638-4163 | 9/15/37 | 3/ 3/ 3 | 1/ 2/10 | 0/ 1/ 2 |
| Bowman Gray† | Dr. Velma G. Watts<br>Director of Minority Affairs<br>(910) 716-4201 | 8/12/48 | 0/ 0/ 0 | 0/ 0/ 2 | 0/ 0/ 0 |
| Brown† | Dr. Alicia D. Monroe<br>Associate Dean<br>(401) 863-3335 | 5/ 7/24 | 0/ 0/ 1 | 1/ 1/ 1 | 0/ 1/ 2 |

## Minority Student Information by Individual Medical School

|  |  | Minority Enrollment, Fall 1995 (New Entrant/First Year/Total)* | | | |
| **Medical School** | **Contact Person or Office** | Black American | American Indian | Mexican- American | Mainland Puerto Rican |
|---|---|---|---|---|---|
| California, University of Davis | Dr. Lindy Kumagai Assistant Dean for Minority Affairs (916) 752-8119 | 3/ 3/30 | 0/ 0/ 4 | 4/ 5/46 | 0/ 0/ 1 |
| Irvine | Assistant Dean, Outreach Student Affairs (714) 856-4771 | 2/ 3/17 | 0/ 0/ 1 | 3/ 4/32 | 0/ 0/ 0 |
| Los Angeles (Drew and Riverside) | Dr. Patricia Pratt (UCLA) Office of Student Support Services (310) 825-3575<br><br>Dr. Theodore Miller (Drew) Associate Dean for Student Affairs (213) 563-4960 | 23/26/93 | 0/ 0/ 2 | 25/25/89 | 2/ 2/ 5 |
| San Diego | Dr. Percy J. Russell Associate Dean, Student Outreach (619) 534-4184 | 5/ 6/25 | 0/ 0/ 1 | 7/11/48 | 0/ 0/ 2 |
| San Francisco (and Berkeley) | Dr. Michael V. Drake Associate Dean, Admissions (415) 476-4044 | 16/16/63 | 2/ 2/10 | 22/22/71 | 3/ 3/ 6 |
| California, Southern† | Althea Alexander Assistant Dean for Minority Affairs (213) 342-1050 | 8/ 9/43 | 0/ 0/ 8 | 20/23/69 | 1/ 1/ 3 |
| Caribe† | Dr. Luis Marti Dean for Admissions and Student Affairs (809) 740-1600 | 0/ 0/ 0 | 1/ 1/ 1 | 0/ 0/ 1 | 7/ 7/14 § |
| Case Western Reserve† | Dr. Ruben Pamies Associate Dean | 19/21/78 | 0/ 0/ 0 | 3/ 3/ 6 | 0/ 2/ 3 |
| Chicago Medical† | Dr. Timothy Hansen Associate Dean, Ancillary Programs (708) 578-3314 | 14/19/61 | 0/ 0/ 3 | 3/ 4/ 6 | 0/ 0/ 0 |

**TABLE 8-C (continued)**

**Minority Student Information by Individual Medical School**

|  |  | Minority Enrollment, Fall 1995 (New Entrant/First Year/Total)* | | | |
|---|---|---|---|---|---|
| **Medical School** | **Contact Person or Office** | Black American | American Indian | Mexican-American | Mainland Puerto Rican |
| Chicago-Pritzker† | Rosita Ragin<br>Director of Student Programs<br>(312) 702-1939 | 5/ 5/27 | 1/ 1/ 2 | 0/ 0/ 4 | 2/ 2/ 4 |
| Cincinnati | Clarice Fooks<br>Assistant Dean for Admissions<br>  and Student Affairs<br>(513) 558-7314 | 12/12/62 | 1/ 1/ 2 | 0/ 0/ 1 | 0/ 0/ 2 |
| Colorado | Marguerite Childs<br>Acting Director,<br>  Center for<br>  Multicultural Enrichment<br>(303) 270-7278 | 6/ 7/12 | 2/ 2/ 5 | 10/10/35 | 0/ 0/ 0 |
| Columbia† | Dr. Gerald E. Thomson<br>Associate Dean for Minority<br>  Affairs and Assistant Vice<br>  President for Health Science<br>(212) 305-4158 | 7/ 8/37 | 0/ 0/ 0 | 1/ 1/ 5 | 3/ 4/13 |
| Connecticut | Dr. Marja Hurley<br>Associate Dean, Minority<br>  Student Affairs | 8/ 9/34 | 0/ 0/ 0 | 0/ 0/ 1 | 0/ 0/ 4 |
| Cornell† | Dr. Bruce L. Ballard<br>Associate Dean for Student<br>  Affairs and Equal Opportunity<br>  Programs<br>(212) 746-1058 | 9/ 9/29 | 2/ 2/ 4 | 7/ 7/13 | 6/ 7/16 |
| Creighton† | Jacqueline R. Harris<br>Director, Minority Affairs for<br>  Health Sciences<br>(402) 480-2981 | 0/ 1/13 | 0/ 0/ 2 | 8/11/20 | 0/ 0/ 3 |
| Dartmouth† | Dr. Martha Regan-Smith<br>Associate Dean for Education<br>  and Assistant Dean,<br>  Minority Affairs<br>(603) 650-1156 | 4/ 5/19 | 2/ 2/ 5 | 3/ 3/ 9 | 0/ 0/ 2 |
| Duke† | Dr. Brenda E. Armstrong<br>Associate Professor of Pediatrics<br>(919) 681-2916 | 10/10/34 | 1/ 1/ 3 | 0/ 0/ 0 | 0/ 0/ 0 |

## Minority Student Information by Individual Medical School

| Medical School | Contact Person or Office | Minority Enrollment, Fall 1995 (New Entrant/First Year/Total)* | | | |
| --- | --- | --- | --- | --- | --- |
| | | Black American | American Indian | Mexican-American | Mainland Puerto Rican |
| East Carolina | Dr. Julius J. Mallette<br>Assistant Dean for<br>Student Affairs<br>(919) 816-2870 | 11/12/45 | 1/ 1/ 5 | 0/ 0/ 2 | 0/ 0/ 0 |
| Emory† | Dr. Robert Lee<br>Associate Dean/Director of<br>Minority Affairs<br>(404) 727-0016 | 15/15/46 | 0/ 0/ 1 | 0/ 0/ 0 | 0/ 0/ 1 |
| Florida<br>(and FSU/FAMU<br>program) | Dr. Cheryl Debose<br>Interim Assistant Dean<br>for Minority Relations<br>(904) 392-3015 | 12/13/35 | 2/ 2/ 3 | 0/ 0/ 0 | 1/ 1/ 2 |
| Florida, South | Dr. Marvin T. Williams<br>Coordinator of Minority<br>Affairs<br>(813) 974-3393 | 10/11/22 | 2/ 3/ 8 | 1/ 1/ 4 | 0/ 0/ 5 |
| George Washington† | Dr. John F. Williams, Jr.<br>Associate Vice President for<br>Graduate Medical Education<br>(202) 994-3506 | 23/28/57 | 2/ 2/ 3 | 2/ 3/ 5 | 1/ 1/ 3 |
| Georgetown† | Dr. Arthur H. Hoyte<br>Director, Office of Minority<br>Affairs<br>(202) 687-1602 | 8/ 8/45 | 2/ 2/ 5 | 3/ 3/ 8 | 2/ 2/ 7 |
| Georgia, Medical<br>College of | Dr. Rosie Allen-Noble<br>Associate Dean,<br>Special Academic Programs | 13/14/44 | 0/ 0/ 1 | 0/ 0/ 2 | 1/ 1/ 3 |
| Harvard | Dr. Alvin F. Poussaint<br>Associate Dean for Student<br>Affairs<br>(617) 232-8390 | 11/11/77 | 2/ 2/10 | 7/ 7/32 | 2/ 2/ 6 |
| Hawaii | Dr. Maurice A. Hitchcock<br>Professor and Director,<br>Native Hawaiian Center<br>for Excellence<br>(808) 956-5826 | 0/ 0/ 1 | 0/ 0/ 1 | 1/ 1/ 2 | 0/ 0/ 0 |

**Minority Student Information by Individual Medical School**

| Medical School | Contact Person or Office | Minority Enrollment, Fall 1995 (New Entrant/First Year/Total)* | | | |
|---|---|---|---|---|---|
| | | Black American | American Indian | Mexican-American | Mainland Puerto Rican |
| Howard† | Sterling M. Lloyd, Jr. Assistant Dean for Student Affairs (202) 806-7679 | 69/81/282 | 0/ 0/ 1 | 1/ 1/ 3 | 0/ 0/ 0 |
| Illinois | Dr. Jorge A. Girotti Associate Dean and Director of Urban Health Program (312) 996-3500 | 30/54/175 | 1/ 1/ 5 | 14/21/61 | 3/ 3/13 |
| Illinois, Southern | Dr. Harold R. Bardo Director, MEDPREP (618) 536-5513 | 4/ 4/23 | 1/ 1/ 2 | 4/ 4/ 6 | 1/ 1/ 2 |
| Indiana | Associate Director of Admissions (317) 274-3772 | 5/ 7/38 | 0/ 0/ 2 | 0/ 0/ 7 | 0/ 0/ 1 |
| Iowa | Barbara Barlow Program Associate for Equal Opportunity Programs (319) 335-8056 | 6/ 7/33 | 2/ 2/ 4 | 6/ 6/25 | 2/ 2/ 3 |
| Jefferson† | Dr. Edward Christian Assistant Dean for Student Affairs and Special Projects (215) 955-6763 | 5/ 6/25 | 1/ 1/ 1 | 2/ 2/ 7 | 0/ 0/ 2 |
| Johns Hopkins† | Dr. Roland T. Smoot Assistant Dean for Student Affairs (410) 955-3419 | 13/13/48 | 0/ 0/ 0 | 1/ 1/ 2 | 0/ 0/ 1 |
| Kansas | Dr. Shadrach Smith Associate Dean for Minority Affairs (913) 588-7285 | 12/14/42 | 1/ 1/15 | 7/ 7/18 | 2/ 2/ 3 |
| Kentucky | Dr. Carol Elam Assistant Dean for Admissions (606) 328-6161 | 8/11/29 | 0/ 0/ 0 | 0/ 0/ 0 | 0/ 0/ 0 |
| Loma Linda† | Dr. Abel Torres Assistant Dean for Clinical Affairs (909) 824-4466 | 4/ 6/30 | 0/ 0/ 1 | 2/ 3/10 | 2/ 2/ 2 |

## Minority Student Information by Individual Medical School

| Medical School | Contact Person or Office | Minority Enrollment, Fall 1995 (New Entrant/First Year/Total)* | | | |
|---|---|---|---|---|---|
| | | Black American | American Indian | Mexican-American | Mainland Puerto Rican |
| Louisiana State—New Orleans | Dr. Edward Helm<br>Assistant Dean, Minority Affairs<br>(504) 568-8501 | 24/30/71 | 3/ 3/ 5 | 1/ 1/ 2 | 1/ 1/ 3 |
| Louisiana State—Shreveport | Shirley Roberson<br>Director, Multicultural Affairs<br>(318) 675-5190 | 8/ 9/22 | 1/ 1/ 1 | 0/ 0/ 1 | 0/ 0/ 0 |
| Louisville | Michael Byrne<br>Director of Special Programs<br>(502) 852-7182 | 10/14/38 | 1/ 1/ 2 | 0/ 0/ 0 | 0/ 0/ 2 |
| Loyola-Stritch† | Dr. Michael L. Rainey<br>Associate Dean for Student Affairs<br>(702) 216-3220 | 4/ 4/15 | 1/ 1/ 2 | 2/ 2/12 | 0/ 0/ 2 |
| Marshall | Dr. Patrick I. Brown<br>Associate Dean, Student Affairs and Academic Affairs<br>(304) 696-7229 | 0/ 1/ 2 | 1/ 2/ 2 | 1/ 1/ 1 | 0/ 0/ 0 |
| Maryland | Dr. Robert L. Harrell<br>Assistant Dean of Student Affairs<br>(410) 706-7689 | 30/30/92 | 1/ 1/ 3 | 1/ 1/ 1 | 0/ 0/ 3 |
| Massachusetts | Dr. Deborah Harmon Hines<br>Associate Provost<br>(508) 856-2444 | 6/ 6/23 | 0/ 0/ 2 | 1/ 1/ 3 | 0/ 0/ 3 |
| Mayo† | Dr. Richard McGee, Jr.<br>Associate Dean for Student Affairs<br>(507) 284-0339 | 2/ 2/12 | 2/ 2/ 7 | 1/ 1/ 9 | 1/ 1/ 2 |
| Meharry† | Dr. Thomas W. Johnson, Sr.<br>Associate Dean for Student/Academic Affairs<br>(615) 327-6413 | 60/72/309 | 0/ 0/ 0 | 0/ 0/ 0 | 0/ 0/ 0 |
| Mercer† | Dr. Roger Comeau<br>Associate Dean for Admissions/Student Affairs<br>(912) 752-2547 | 1/ 1/ 7 | 0/ 0/ 0 | 0/ 0/ 0 | 0/ 0/ 0 |

## Minority Student Information by Individual Medical School

| Medical School | Contact Person or Office | Minority Enrollment, Fall 1995 (New Entrant/First Year/Total)* | | | |
|---|---|---|---|---|---|
| | | Black American | American Indian | Mexican-American | Mainland Puerto Rican |
| Miami† | Dr. Astrid Mack<br>Associate Dean for Minority<br>Affairs<br>(305) 547-6965 | 10/10/48 | 0/ 0/ 0 | 0/ 0/ 0 | 1/ 1/ 1 |
| Michigan State | Dr. Carrie B. Jackson<br>Assistant Dean for<br>Student Affairs<br>(517) 353-7140 | 22/22/67 | 2/ 2/ 8 | 8/ 8/27 | 1/ 1/ 7 |
| Michigan, University of | Dr. Joyce M. Mitchell<br>Assistant Dean for Student<br>and Minority Affairs<br>(313) 764-8185 | 14/14/71 | 0 0/ 2 | 8/ 8/30 | 2/ 3/ 4 |
| Minnesota—Duluth‡ | Dr. Gerald L. Hill<br>Director, CAIMH<br>(218) 726-7235 | 0/ 0/ 0 | 5/ 5/15 | 0/ 0/ 0 | 0/ 0/ 0 |
| Minnesota—Minneapolis | Dr. Cassius Ellis III<br>Assistant to the Dean for<br>Student Affairs<br>(612) 624-1188 | 4/ 4/20 | 4/ 6/24 | 3/ 3/ 7 | 0/ 0/ 0 |
| Mississippi | Dr. Leon Anderson, Jr.<br>Director of Minority Affairs<br>(601) 984-1340 | 14/15/42 | 0/ 0/ 0 | 0/ 0/ 2 | 0/ 0/ 0 |
| Missouri—Columbia | Dr. Michael Hosokawa<br>Assistant Dean for Curriculum<br>and Minority Affairs<br>(314) 882-1566 | 1/ 1/14 | 1/ 1/ 1 | 0/ 0/ 5 | 0/ 0/ 1 |
| Missouri—Kansas City | Dr. Reaner Shannon<br>Director, Office of Minority Affairs<br>(816) 235-1780 | 3/ 3/12 | 0/ 0/ 0 | 2/ 2/ 7 | 0/ 0/ 0 |
| Morehouse† | Dr. Angela Franklin<br>Associate Dean for Student<br>Affairs and Curriculum<br>(404) 752-1651 | 28/33/129 | 0/ 0/ 0 | 0/ 0/ 1 | 0/ 0/ 0 |
| Mount Sinai† | Dr. Marta Rico<br>Assistant Dean, Student Affairs<br>(212) 241-8276 | 14/16/46 | 1/ 1/ 2 | 0/ 0/ 2 | 4/ 5/15 |

## Minority Student Information by Individual Medical School

|  |  | Minority Enrollment, Fall 1995 (New Entrant/First Year/Total)* | | | |
| --- | --- | --- | --- | --- | --- |
| **Medical School** | **Contact Person or Office** | Black American | American Indian | Mexican-American | Mainland Puerto Rican |
| Nebraska | Alfonso Lopez<br>Director, Multicultural<br>Affairs Office<br>(402) 559-7260 | 2/ 3/ 7 | 1/ 1/ 4 | 1/ 1/11 | 0/ 0/ 1 |
| Nevada—Reno | Ann Diggins<br>Director of Recruitment<br>(702) 784-1317 | 2/ 2/ 5 | 0/ 0/ 2 | 1/ 1/ 7 | 0/ 0/ 1 |
| UMDNJ-New Jersey Medical | James Foster<br>Assistant Dean for Minority<br>Affairs<br>(201) 456-5431 | 13/16/70 | 0/ 0/ 0 | 4/ 5/ 8 | 5/ 6/27 |
| UMDNJ-Robert Wood Johnson | Dr. Florence Kimball<br>Assistant Dean for Special<br>Academic Programs<br>(908) 235-4510 | 26/31/99 | 0/ 0/ 2 | 1/ 1/ 6 | 2/ 4/23 |
| New Mexico | Dr. Roberto Gomez<br>Associate Dean<br>(505) 277-2728 | 2/ 2/ 3 | 2/ 2/13 | 15/15/55 | 0/ 0/ 0 |
| New York Medical College† | Dr. Anthony Clemendor<br>Associate Dean for Student Affairs<br>(914) 993-4623 | 7/10/38 | 1/ 1/ 3 | 2/ 2/ 9 | 0/ 0/ 5 |
| New York University† | Dr. Margaret Haynes<br>Associate Dean, Office of<br>Minority Student Services<br>and Recruitment<br>(212) 263-8948 | 6/ 7/24 | 0/ 0/ 0 | 0/ 0/ 2 | 0/ 0/ 2 |
| SUNY—Buffalo | Dr. Maggie S. Wright<br>Director of Minority Affairs<br>(716) 831-2811 | 6/ 6/40 | 0/ 0/ 0 | 0/ 0/ 1 | 2/ 2/ 7 |
| SUNY—Brooklyn | Dr. Constance Hill<br>Associate Dean for Minority<br>Affairs<br>(718) 270-3765 | 21/25/66 | 0/ 0/ 0 | 0/ 0/ 0 | 1/ 1/12 |
| SUNY—Stony Brook | Dr. Aldustus E. Jordan<br>Associate Dean for Student and<br>Minority Affairs<br>(516) 444-2341 | 8/11/30 | 0/ 0/ 0 | 0/ 0/ 0 | 1/ 2/ 9 |

## Minority Student Information by Individual Medical School

| | | Minority Enrollment, Fall 1995 (New Entrant/First Year/Total)* | | | |
|---|---|---|---|---|---|
| **Medical School** | **Contact Person or Office** | Black American | American Indian | Mexican-American | Mainland Puerto Rican |
| SUNY—Syracuse (Binghamton Campus) | Georgette Cowans<br>Director, Office of Minority Affairs<br>(315) 464-5433 | 6/14/35 | 0/ 0/ 1 | 0/ 0/ 0 | 1/ 1/ 5 |
| North Carolina | Dr. Marion Phillips<br>Associate Dean<br>(919) 962-8331 | 31/33/87 | 3/ 3/13 | 1/ 1/ 1 | 2/ 2/ 3 |
| North Dakota | Barbara Anderson<br>Administrative Officer, INMED Program<br>(701) 777-3037 | 0/ 0/ 0 | 7/ 8/29 | 0/ 0/ 0 | 0/ 0/ 0 |
| Northwestern† | Dr. Tacoma A. McKnight<br>Assistant Dean for Minority Affairs<br>(312) 503-0461 | 10/10/25 | 0/ 0/ 1 | 4/ 4/ 8 | 2/ 2/ 4 |
| Ohio, Medical College of | Dr. Barry L. Richardson<br>Associate Dean for Admissions and MinorityAffairs<br>(419) 381-3438 | 12/23/63 | 0/ 0/ 2 | 1/ 1/ 4 | 0/ 1/ 2 |
| Ohio, Northeastern | Dr. Kenneth B. Durgans<br>Special Assistant to the President for Minority Affairs and Affirmative Action<br>(216) 325-2511 | 5/ 6/17 | 0/ 0/ 1 | 1/ 1/ 2 | 0/ 0/ 0 |
| Ohio State | Associate Dean for Admissions and Minority Affairs<br>(614) 292-7755 | 13/15/63 | 0/ 0/ 0 | 4/ 4/19 | 1/ 1/ 7 |
| Oklahoma | Susan Massara<br>Assistant Director of Student Affairs<br>(405) 271-2331 | 5/ 6/16 | 11/14/50 | 1/ 1/ 2 | 0/ 0/ 2 |
| Oregon | Alfonso Lopez Vasquez<br>Director, Multicultural Affairs<br>(503) 494-7574 | 3/ 3/ 8 | 0/ 0/ 2 | 2/ 2/13 | 0/ 0/ 0 |

## Minority Student Information by Individual Medical School

Minority Enrollment, Fall 1995
(New Entrant/First Year/Total)*

| Medical School | Contact Person or Office | Black American | American Indian | Mexican-American | Mainland Puerto Rican |
|---|---|---|---|---|---|
| Pennsylvania, Medical College of and Hahnemann† | Ann Hill<br>Director of Minority Affairs<br>(215) 991-8215 | 35/40/76 | 0/ 1/ 4 | 8/ 9/16 | 1/ 1/ 5 |
| Pennsylvania State† | Dr. Alphonse E. Leure-duPree<br>Associate Dean for Student Affairs<br>(717) 531-8651 | 15/15/46 | 0/ 0/ 0 | 0/ 0/ 2 | 1/ 1/ 1 |
| Pennsylvania,† University of | Dr. Karen Hamilton<br>Assistant Dean for Student Affairs and Director, Minority Affairs<br>(215) 898-4409 | 13/14/62 | 0/ 0/ 1 | 7/ 8/22 | 4/ 4/18 |
| Pittsburgh† | Paula K. Davis<br>Director, Minority Programs | 11/11/52 | 1/ 1/ 1 | 1/ 1/ 2 | 3/ 4/ 5 |
| Ponce† | Dr. Wanda Velez<br>Department of Physiology<br>Assistant Professor<br>(809) 840-2511 | 0/ 0/ 0 | 0/ 0/ 0 | 0/ 0/ 0 | 4/ 6/14 § |
| Puerto Rico | Dr. America Facunds<br>Associate Director, Hispanic Center of Excellence<br>(809) 758-2525 Ext. 1810 | 1/ 1/ 1 | 0/ 0/ 0 | 0/ 0/ 0 | 6/ 7/19 § |
| Rochester† | José M. Bayona<br>Associate Dean, Ethnic and Multicultural Affairs<br>(716) 275-2842 | 12/13/35 | 1/ 1/ 4 | 1/ 1/ 4 | 1/ 1/ 2 |
| Rush† | Dr. Fred Richardson<br>Assistant Dean, Minority Affairs<br>(312) 942-6913 | 6/ 9/40 | 0/ 0/ 1 | 3/ 3/ 5 | 0/ 0/ 0 |
| Saint Louis | Dr. Manuel R. Comas<br>Associate Dean, Admissions and Student Affairs<br>(314) 577-8205 | 7/ 9/13 | 0/ 0/ 1 | 0/ 0/ 0 | 0/ 0/ 0 |

## Minority Student Information by Individual Medical School

| Medical School | Contact Person or Office | Minority Enrollment, Fall 1995 (New Entrant/First Year/Total)* | | | |
|---|---|---|---|---|---|
| | | Black American | American Indian | Mexican-American | Mainland Puerto Rican |
| South Carolina, Medical University of | Dr. Thaddeus J. Bell<br>Assistant Dean, Minority<br>Students<br>(803) 792-2081 | 21/22/62 | 1/ 1/ 2 | 0/ 0/ 0 | 0/ 0/ 0 |
| South Carolina, University of | Dr. Robert F. Sabalis<br>Associate Dean,<br>Student Programs<br>(803) 733-3135 | 5/ 5/16 | 0/ 0/ 0 | 0/ 0/ 1 | 0/ 0/ 2 |
| South Dakota | Minority Affairs Officer | 0/ 0/ 0 | 3/ 3/ 9 | 0/ 0/ 0 | 0/ 0/ 0 |
| Stanford† | Dr. Fernando S. Mendoza<br>Associate Dean for<br>Student Affairs<br>(415) 725-4727 | 7/ 7/30 | 1/ 1/ 7 | 11/11/44 | 0/ 0/ 1 |
| Temple† | Charles S. Ireland, Jr.<br>Assistant Dean<br>(215) 707-3653 | 15/18/84 | 1/ 1/ 2 | 5/ 6/15 | 1/ 1/ 9 |
| Tennessee State, East | Dr. Dorothy Dobbins<br>Associate Dean, Student Affairs<br>(615) 929-6269 | 7/ 7/24 | 0/ 0/ 2 | 1/ 1/ 1 | 0/ 0/ 0 |
| Tennessee, University of | Dr. Kenneth Robinson<br>Assistant Dean, Admissions<br>and Students<br>(901) 448-7228 | 20/22/71 | 0/ 0/ 0 | 0/ 0/ 0 | 0/ 0/ 0 |
| Texas A&M | Tommy Boquez<br>Coordinator, Minority<br>Access to Medical Careers<br>(409) 845-7743 | 1/ 1/ 2 | 0/ 0/ 0 | 5/ 5/16 | 0/ 0/ 0 |
| Texas Tech | Dr. J.E. Mendez<br>Assistant Dean for<br>Minority Affairs<br>(806) 743-2890 | 1/ 1/ 2 | 0/ 0/ 0 | 10/13/31 | 0/ 1/ 1 |
| Texas—Dallas (Southwestern) | Dr. Drew Alexander<br>Assistant Dean for Minority<br>Student Affairs<br>(214) 648-2168 | 3/ 4/28 | 6/ 6/ 8 | 9/ 9/70 | 0/ 0/ 0 |

## Minority Student Information by Individual Medical School

Minority Enrollment, Fall 1995
(New Entrant/First Year/Total)*

| Medical School | Contact Person or Office | Black American | American Indian | Mexican-American | Mainland Puerto Rican |
|---|---|---|---|---|---|
| Texas—Galveston | Dr. Billy Ray Ballard<br>Associate Dean for Student Affairs<br>Director, Medical School<br>Admissions<br>(409) 772-1442 | 21/30/81 | 4/ 4/10 | 31/40/144 | 2/ 2/ 4 |
| Texas—Houston | Dr. Patricia Butler<br>Associate Dean for<br>Educational Programs<br>(713) 792-5518 | 13/14/34 | 1/ 1/ 2 | 41/50/110 | 0/ 0/ 1 |
| Texas—San Antonio | Dr. Leonard E. Lawrence<br>Associate Dean for Student<br>Affairs<br>(210) 567-4429 | 10/11/36 | 1/ 1/ 5 | 35/37/114 | 1/ 1/ 4 |
| Tufts† | Colleen Romain<br>Assistant Director of<br>Student Services<br>(617) 636-6576 | 6/ 9/38 | 0/ 0/ 5 | 0/ 0/ 6 | 0/ 0/ 2 |
| Tulane† | Dr. Anna Cherrie Epps<br>Associate Dean for Student<br>Services<br>(504) 588-5327 | 3/ 6/29 | 2/ 2/ 7 | 2/ 2/ 4 | 0/ 0/14 |
| Uniformed Services University | Dr. Jeannette South-Paul<br>Associate Professor,<br>Family Practice<br>(301) 295-3965 | 3/ 3/20 | 1/ 1/ 5 | 2/ 2/14 | 1/ 1/ 3 |
| Utah | Jessie M. Soriano<br>Director, Health Sciences<br>Minority Affairs<br>(801) 585-7012 | 2/ 2/ 3 | 4/ 5/ 9 | 3/ 4/12 | 0/ 0/ 0 |
| Vanderbilt† | Dr. Deborah German<br>Associate Dean for<br>Student Affairs<br>(615) 322-6109 | 2/ 2/10 | 4/ 4/ 5 | 1/ 1/ 4 | 0/ 0/ 0 |
| Vermont | Dr. Marga S. Sproul<br>Associate Dean for Student<br>Affairs and Admissions<br>(802) 656-2150 | 0/ 1/ 3 | 0/ 0/ 3 | 1/ 2/ 7 | 0/ 0/ 2 |

## Minority Student Information by Individual Medical School

Minority Enrollment, Fall 1995
(New Entrant/First Year/Total)*

| Medical School | Contact Person or Office | Black American | American Indian | Mexican-American | Mainland Puerto Rican |
|---|---|---|---|---|---|
| Virginia, Eastern† | Gail C. Williams<br>Assistant Dean for Student<br>Affairs and Director of<br>Minority Affairs<br>(804) 446-5869 | 4/ 4/33 | 1/ 1/ 1 | 0/ 0/ 0 | 0/ 0/ 2 |
| Virginia, Medical College of | Aileen Edwards<br>Assistant Director,<br>Admissions | 15/15/66 | 0/ 0/ 0 | 1/ 1/ 1 | 0/ 0/ 1 |
| Virginia, University of | Dr. Maurice Apprey<br>Associate Dean<br>(804) 924-1867 | 18/22/75 | 1/ 1/ 3 | 1/ 1/ 2 | 1/ 1/ 2 |
| Washington University† (St. Louis) | Dr. Helen E. Nash<br>Acting Director,<br>Minority Admissions<br>(314) 362-6844 | 9/10/37 | 1/ 1/ 1 | 0/ 0/ 0 | 0/ 0/ 0 |
| Washington, University of | Charles Garcia<br>Director, Minority<br>Affairs Program<br>(206) 685-2489 | 2/ 2/19 | 5/ 8/22 | 5/ 6/24 | 1/ 1/ 3 |
| Wayne State | Dr. Jane Thomas<br>Assistant Dean for<br>Student Affairs<br>(313) 577-1463 | 32/48/132 | 0/ 0/ 4 | 3/ 3/ 6 | 0/ 0/ 2 |
| West Virginia | Dr. John W. Traubert<br>Associate Dean for<br>Student Affairs<br>(304) 293-2408 | 1/ 1/ 6 | 0/ 0/ 1 | 0/ 0/ 0 | 0/ 0/ 0 |
| Wisconsin,† Medical College of | Dr. Lauree Thomas<br>Associate Dean for Minority<br>Student Affairs<br>(414) 456-8734 | 8/ 9/27 | 2/ 2/ 4 | 10/12/28 | 2/ 3/ 5 |
| Wisconsin, University of | Dr. Gloria V. Hawkins<br>Assistant Dean for<br>Minority Affairs<br>(608) 263-3713 | 8/ 8/41 | 3/ 3/14 | 6/ 7/28 | 1/ 1/ 7 |

## Minority Student Information by Individual Medical School

| | | Minority Enrollment, Fall 1995 (New Entrant/First Year/Total)* | | | |
|---|---|---|---|---|---|
| **Medical School** | **Contact Person or Office** | Black American | American Indian | Mexican-American | Mainland Puerto Rican |
| Wright State | Jacqueline McMillan<br>Director of Recruitment<br>(513) 873-2934 | 14/18/62 | 0/ 0/ 0 | 0/ 0/ 2 | 0/ 0/ 1 |
| Yale† | Dr. Forrester A. Lee<br>Assistant Dean of<br>    Multicultural Affairs<br>(203) 785-7545 | 12/12/49 | 2/ 2/ 4 | 2/ 2/10 | 3/ 3/ 7 |
| Grand Total | | 1,290/1,528/5,337 | 137/150/501 | 476/535/1,769 | 107/127/455 |

* The first figure under each minority category is the number of these students who are new entrants for 1995; the second figure is the number of these students who are in the first year class; and the third is the total number of these students enrolled in the medical school.

† Privately supported medical schools.

‡ Two year school of basic medical sciences.

§ These figures represent students who are mainland Puerto Rican residents only and do not include residents of commonwealth of Puerto Rico.

Source: 1995 Fall Enrollment Survey. Reflects enrollments as of October 13, 1995, at 125 medical schools. First-year new entrants are students entering medical school for the first time.

# Information on Medical Schools Offering Combined College/M.D. Program for High School Students

Many of the medical schools providing programs of undergraduate college and medical education for high school students offer an accelerated course of study. These programs take a minimum of six to eight years to complete. The first two to four years of the curriculum consist of undergraduate courses and include the necessary premedical requirements. At various stages, a graduate receives a bachelor's degree from the university and then the M.D. degree from the medical school on completion of the program. There are several schools which offer an integrated curriculum and are primarily designed for students entering from high school.

Admission is open to highly qualified high school seniors with a strong desire to pursue medicine as a career. State-supported schools generally do not admit many out-of-state applicants into their programs. Prospective applicants seeking admission to state-supported schools will have a better chance of acceptance at institutions located in their own state of residence. Private schools are, for the most part, more flexible; enrollment is generally not limited to state residents.

Academic prerequisites for admission vary among the schools conducting these programs but usually include the following subjects: introductory calculus, biology, physics, chemistry, English, and social studies. Any high school student who has an early aspiration to become a physician should consult with a guidance counselor to be certain that the curriculum incorporates those specific courses required for the program(s) in which the student would like to enroll.

The following program descriptions were compiled from responses to a questionnaire sent to all medical schools with programs of interest to high school students. For medical school tuitions for the 1995–96 entering class, refer to the school entries in Part 2. For further information, please contact the schools directly.

## ABBREVIATIONS

Listed below are the abbreviations used in the school entries in this chapter.

ACT Assessment—American College Testing Program Assessment

CEEB—College Entrance Examination Board

GPA—Grade-point average

MCAT—Medical College Admission Test

SAT—Scholastic Aptitude Test

USMLE—United States Medical Licensing Examination

### List of Medical Schools Offering Combined College/
### M.D. Programs for High School Students

**Alabama**
University of South Alabama College of Medicine

**California**
University of California, Riverside and University of California, Los Angeles,
UCLA School of Medicine
University of Southern California College of Letters, Arts, and Sciences and School of Medicine

**District of Columbia**
The George Washington University School of Medicine and Columbian College
Howard University

**Florida**
University of Miami

**Illinois**
Finch University of Health Sciences/Chicago Medical School
and Illinois Institute of Technology
Northwestern University

**Massachusetts**
Boston University

**Michigan**
Michigan State University College of Human Medicine
University of Michigan

**Missouri**
University of Missouri—Kansas City School of Medicine

**New Jersey**
University of Medicine and Dentistry of New Jersey/New Jersey Medical School
Rutgers University and University of Medicine and Dentistry of New Jersey
Robert Wood Johnson Medical School

**New York**
Binghamton University and State University of New York Health Science Center at Syracuse
Brooklyn College and State University of New York Health Science Center at Brooklyn College of Medicine
New York University
Rensselaer Polytechnic Institute and Albany Medical College
University of Rochester School of Medicine and Dentistry
Siena College and Albany Medical College
Sophie Davis School of Biomedical Education/City University of New York
Union College and Albany Medical College

**Ohio**
Case Western Reserve University
Northeastern Ohio Universities College of Medicine

**Pennsylvania**
Lehigh University and Medical College of Pennsylvania and
  Hahnemann University School of Medicine
Penn State University and Jefferson Medical College of Thomas Jefferson University
Villanova University and Medical College of Pennsylvania and Hahnemann University School of Medicine

**Rhode Island**
Brown University

**Tennessee**
East Tennessee State University
Fisk University and Meharry Medical College

**Texas**
Rice University and Baylor College of Medicine

**Virginia**
Eastern Virginia Medical School

**Wisconsin**
University of Wisconsin—Madison Medical School

# University of South Alabama
# College of Medicine

Mobile, Alabama

## ADDRESS INQUIRIES TO:

Office of Admissions
University of South Alabama
Administrative Building
Room 182
Mobile, Alabama 36688-0002
(334) 460-6141 or (800) 872-5247

## PURPOSE

Candidates selected for the program will receive early acceptance from the University of South Alabama and College of Medicine. Students participating in the program are expected to enter the University of South Alabama College of Medicine following the fall after completion of the baccalaureate degree.

## REQUIREMENTS FOR ENTRANCE

Students in the senior year of high school or recently graduated individuals who have not yet entered college will be eligible to apply for the program. Both residents and nonresidents of Alabama may apply.

## SELECTION FACTORS

Candidates must have a minimum high school GPA of 3.5 as computed by the University of South Alabama and must present a minimum enhanced composite ACT score of 28 (or comparable SAT). Candidates must also have demonstrated leadership qualities and motivation toward the study of medicine.

## CURRICULUM

The curriculum will include core requirements for the selected baccalaureate program and prerequisites for matriculation in medical school. Students in the program must maintain a minimum overall GPA of 3.5 and a minimum GPA of 3.4 in the sciences (biology, chemistry, physics) and mathematics. All required courses must be taken at the University of South Alabama unless otherwise approved in advance by their undergraduate program director and the associate dean of the College of Medicine.

Students will be required to participate in CP-200 (Career Planning; Clinical Observation) for a minimum of four quarters. Students will be given the opportunity to participate in a special summer premedical clerkship. The activities will be planned to give the participant a broad exposure to medical education.

Students will be required to take the MCAT for admission to the College of Medicine and will be required to score above the national average. A formal assessment, including an interview, will be conducted after the student has completed 96 quarter hours of work. At this time, the student's academic performance and continued interest in a medical career will be assessed.

## EXPENSES

The 1995–96 annual tuition for students at the University of South Alabama was $2,382 for residents; $3,807 for non-residents.

## FINANCIAL AID

Information can be obtained from Office of Financial Aid, Administration Building, Room 260, University of South Alabama, Mobile, AL 36688-0002; or phone (334) 460-6231.

## APPLICATION AND ACCEPTANCE POLICIES

Filing of application:
   Latest date: March 1
Application fee: $25
Acceptance notice:
   Earliest date: April 15
   Latest date: July 1
Applicant's response to acceptance offer:
   Maximum time: 30 days
Deposit to hold place in class: None
Starting date: End of September

## INFORMATION ON 1995–96 ENTERING CLASS

| Number of | In-State | Out-of-State | Total |
|---|---|---|---|
| Applicants | 90 | 45 | 135 |
| Applicants Interviewed | 25 | 10 | 35 |
| New Entrants | 10 | 5 | 15 |

# University of California, Riverside, and University of California, Los Angeles UCLA School of Medicine

Riverside, California

## ADDRESS INQUIRIES TO:

Student Affairs Officer
Division of Biomedical Sciences
University of California, Riverside
Riverside, California 92521-0121
(909) 787-4333

## PURPOSE

This program offers an accelerated curriculum which allows receipt of a B.S. degree after four years of college work and the M.D. degree seven years after matriculation as an undergraduate freshman.

## REQUIREMENTS FOR ENTRANCE

Admission to this combined-degree program occurs in two phases: first, admission from high school to the University of California, Riverside, as a freshman; and second, admission to UCLA School of Medicine after completion of three undergraduate years at Riverside. Residents of California as well as out-of-state students are eligible to apply. For admission to Riverside, students are required to take the SAT I and three scholastic assessment tests. One test must be in writing, and one must be in mathematics. In addition, applicants are required to complete six semesters of laboratory science courses in chemistry, physics, or biology and qualify for placement in calculus.

## SELECTION FACTORS

To gain admission as a freshman in the combined-degree program at Riverside, an applicant must meet the selection criteria for the University of California, as mentioned above. Subsequent admission to UCLA School of Medicine depends on the student's undergraduate science GPA at Riverside, non-science and overall GPA, results of the MCAT taken in the summer before the third year at Riverside, letters of recommendation including one from the student faculty adviser at Riverside, and three required interviews. In the 1995–96 class entering UCLA School of Medicine from Riverside's combined-degree program, the 24 students had an average undergraduate GPA of 3.82, an average MCAT score of 10.2, and an average combined SAT score of 1151.

## CURRICULUM

This program leads to a baccalaureate degree granted by the University of California, Riverside, and the M.D. degree awarded by the University of California, Los Angeles, UCLA School of Medicine.

Students must complete work for a bachelor's degree in biomedical sciences. Requirements for that degree include three courses in the humanities, three courses in the social sciences, and five courses in the natural and physical sciences.

The curriculum for both degrees takes seven years to complete. Students benefit from having medical faculty serve as their advisers during the undergraduate phase. Students are expected to take steps 1 and 2 of the USMLE examinations while at UCLA, but passing these examinations is not a graduation requirement.

## EXPENSES

For California residents, there is no tuition for undergraduate work, but there are fees amounting to $4,092 per year. For out-of-state students, tuition was $7,698 per year for undergraduate work as well as fees of $4,092 per year.

## FINANCIAL AID

Sources of aid are scholarships, grants, work-study, and student loans. Applicants can receive more information from the Financial Aid Office, University of California, Riverside, Riverside, CA 92521.

---

### APPLICATION AND ACCEPTANCE POLICIES FOR UNDERGRADUATE PORTION AT RIVERSIDE

Filing of application:
  Earliest date: Nov. 1
  Latest date: Nov. 30
Application fee: $40
Acceptance notice:
  Earliest date: March 1
  Latest date: March 15
Applicant's response to acceptance offer:
  Maximum time: May 1
Deposit to hold place in class: $100; nonrefundable
Starting date: September 25

### INFORMATION ON 1995–96 ENTERING CLASS UCLA SCHOOL OF MEDICINE FROM THE COMBINED-DEGREE PROGRAM AT RIVERSIDE

| Number of | In-State | Out-of-State | Total |
|---|---|---|---|
| Applicants | 50 | 0 | 50 |
| Applicants Interviewed | 50 | 0 | 50 |
| New Entrants | 24 | 0 | 24 |

# University of Southern California
# College of Letters, Arts, and Sciences
# School of Medicine

**Los Angeles, California**

## ADDRESS INQUIRIES TO:

Office of College Academic Services
College of Letters, Arts, and Sciences
University of Southern California
Los Angeles, California 90089-0152
(213) 740-5930

## PURPOSE

The goal of this program, initiated in 1993, is to encourage bright and highly motivated students to expand the breadth of their education through a diverse liberal arts education. Students accepted into this program have the opportunity to study a wide variety of disciplines beyond the course of the standard premedical curriculum. It is the hope of the University to graduate physicians who are educated in medical science, art, and the humanities.

## REQUIREMENTS FOR ENTRANCE

Students are selected for this program in the senior year of high school. Both residents and nonresidents of California are eligible to apply. There are no specific high school course requirements, but applicants are required to take either the SAT or ACT Assessment.

## SELECTION FACTORS

Academic factors considered include grades and standardized test scores. Additionally, participation in extracurricular activities and demonstrated leadership and community service are highly valued. In the 1995–96 entering class, the high school GPA averaged 4.18, and the average mean SAT score was 1416. An interview is required.

## CURRICULUM

This program leads to a baccalaureate degree awarded by the University of Southern California, and the M.D. degree granted by the University of Southern California School of Medicine.

This is not an accelerated program; all students must complete four years of undergraduate education and four years of medical school.

Students must complete requirements for the bachelor's degree and may pursue any major offered in the university that is compatible with the requirements of the program. There are specific requirements for the bachelor's degree, which include the humanities, social, natural, and physical sciences.

Advancement to the medical school phase of the program is based on acceptable academic performance and MCAT scores as defined by the program. The MCAT is required and must be taken by the spring of junior year. Students must take steps 1 and 2, and pass Step 1 of the USMLE examinations in order to graduate.

## EXPENSES

In 1995–96, undergraduate tuition for residents and nonresidents was $18,246 plus annual fees of $278.

## FINANCIAL AID

Sources of aid include scholarships, grants, work-study programs, and loans. Contact the Office of Financial Aid, University of Southern California, Los Angeles, California 90089-0912; or call (213) 740-5466 for additional information.

## APPLICATION AND ACCEPTANCE POLICIES

Filing of application:
  Latest date: Dec. 15
Application fee: None
Acceptance notice:
  Latest date: April 1
Applicant's response to acceptance offer:
  Maximum time: May 1
Deposit to hold place in class: $200; refundable
Starting date: August 28

## INFORMATION ON 1995–96 ENTERING CLASS

| Number of | Total |
| --- | --- |
| Applicants | 400 |
| Applicants Interviewed | 100 |
| New Entrants | 35 |

# Howard University

**Washington, D.C.**

## ADDRESS INQUIRIES TO:

Dr. G. Aboko-Cole, *Director*
Center for Preprofessional Education
P.O. Box 473
Administration Building
Howard University
Washington, D.C. 20059
(202) 806-7231

## PURPOSE

The aims of this combined-degree program are to encourage bright young students to choose medicine as a career and to enter the Howard University College of Medicine for their medical education.

## REQUIREMENTS FOR ENTRANCE

Students can be selected for this program during the senior year of high school or during the first year of college. There are no state residence requirements. Applicants are expected to have completed the following courses by the time they graduate from high school: at least two years of a foreign language; at least one year each of biology, chemistry, and physics; two years of mathematics; and four years of English, including literature. They must take either the SAT or the ACT Assessment.

## SELECTION FACTORS

The academic factors considered in offering admission to an applicant are rank in high school class, GPA, and test scores. Applicants are expected to be in the top five percent of their high school class. In the 1995–96 entering class, the average GPA was 3.7, and the average SAT combined score was 1300. ACT Assessment cumulative scores ranged from 25 to 29. Personal qualities considered include self-esteem, realistic self-appraisal, a realistic assessment of the medical profession, leadership, and superior writing skills. An interview is required.

## CURRICULUM

This program leads to a bachelor's degree awarded by the College of Liberal Arts at Howard University and the M.D. degree granted by the College of Medicine, also at Howard.

Students must complete work for a baccalaureate degree. They are expected to complete at least 40 semester hours of humanities and social sciences to fulfill general education requirements and at least 46 semester hours of natural and physical science. Students meet with the director of the Center for Preprofessional Education to design a curriculum tailored to individual needs, and the specific course selection must have the adviser's approval. Students are encouraged to select a major of personal interest.

The curricula for both degrees are completed in six years. In the first two years the curriculum focuses on work toward the bachelor's degree and premedical requirements, and in the last four years the focus is on studies related to medicine. Students in this program must take the MCAT in April of the second year. Results of this test are a factor in gaining admission to the medical school phase of the combined-degree program. Students are also expected to take steps 1 and 2 of the USMLE examinations while at Howard University College of Medicine, and they must pass these examinations for graduation from that school.

## EXPENSES

In 1995–96 the annual tuition for students in the College of Liberal Arts was $7,005. There are also student fees, which are subject to change.

## FINANCIAL AID

Information can be obtained from the Office of Financial Aid, Howard University, Johnson Administration Building, 2400 – 6th Street, N.W., Washington, D.C. 20059.

---

## APPLICATION AND ACCEPTANCE POLICIES

Filing of application:
    Latest date: Rolling admission
Application fee: $25
Deposit to hold place in class: $100; nonrefundable
Starting date: Late Aug.

## INFORMATION ON 1995–96 ENTERING CLASS

| Number of | Total |
|---|---|
| Applicants | 25 |
| Applicants Interviewed | 15 |
| New Entrants | 10 |

# George Washington University School of Medicine and Columbian College

Washington, D.C.

## ADDRESS INQUIRIES TO:

Office of Admissions
George Washington University
2121 "I" Street, N.W.
Washington, D.C. 20052
1 (800) 447-3765

## PURPOSE

The undergraduate program includes basic training in the hard sciences with the opportunity to explore another field of interest. The baccalaureate degree is awarded after year four (first year of medical school).

## REQUIREMENTS FOR ENTRANCE

Students are selected in their senior year of high school. Both residents of the District of Columbia and nonresidents may apply. There are no specific high school course requirements. Applicants are required to take the SAT II Subject Tests in writing, mathematics, and science.

## SELECTION FACTORS

Applicants should be in the top five percent of their class. The average GPA for the 1995–96 entering class was 3.70. The average test score for the ACT was 32, and the average scores were 650 for the SAT Mathematics and 710 for the SAT Verbal. In addition to academic factors, extracurricular, health related activities, and letters of recommendation are reviewed. An interview is required.

## CURRICULUM

This seven-year program leads to the baccalaureate degree granted by The George Washington University and the M.D. degree granted by the School of Medicine. The course requirements for the baccalaureate degree in the humanities and social sciences varies, but students must complete 32 semester hours in the natural and physical sciences. Passing the MCAT examination is not a factor in the admission or promotion phase to the medical school program. Students are required to take Step 1 of the USMLE at the end of year 2 of medical school. Passing Step 1 is a requirement for promotion and graduation. Students must take Step 2 of the USMLE, but are not required to pass in order to graduate.

## EXPENSES

In 1995–96, tuition was $29,125 per year for seven years. This includes a $10,000 per year scholarship.

## FINANCIAL AID

Information may be obtained from the George Washington University, Office of Student Financial Assistance, 2121 "I" Street, N.W., Rice Hall, Washington, D.C. 20037.

## APPLICATION AND ACCEPTANCE POLICIES

Filing of application:
   Earliest date: Sept.
   Latest date: Dec. 1 (Part I)
Application fee: $50
Acceptance notice:
   Earliest date: mid-March
Applicant's response to acceptance offer:
   Maximum time: 6 weeks
Deposit to hold place in class: $650; nonrefundable

## INFORMATION ON 1995–96 ENTERING CLASS

| Number of | Total |
|---|---|
| Applicants | 648 |
| Applicants Interviewed | 55 |
| New Entrants | 8 |

# University of Miami

## Coral Gables, Florida

## ADDRESS INQUIRIES TO:

Office of Admissions
University of Miami
P.O. Box 248025
Coral Gables, Florida 33124
(305) 284-4323

## PURPOSE

The Honors Program in Medicine (HPM) offers exceptionally motivated and talented students the opportunity to earn the B.S. and M.D. degrees in either six or seven years, at the students' option.

## REQUIREMENTS FOR ENTRANCE

Students are selected for this program only during their senior year of high school. To be eligible to apply, students must have a minimum combined score of 1360 on the SAT or a composite score of 31 on the ACT Assessment and take the SAT II Subject Tests in English, mathematics, and science. Only residents of Florida are eligible to apply. Applicants are expected to have completed eight semesters of English and mathematics and two semesters each of biology and chemistry by the time they graduate from high school.

## SELECTION FACTORS

Academic factors taken into account in offering admission to an applicant are scores on the standardized admissions tests; the quality of the high school curriculum, including the number and nature of advanced placement courses; the amount of university-level work already completed; as well as research awards and other distinctions won at the national level. In the 1995–96 class entering the HPM Program as college freshmen, the average combined SAT score was 1388. The average score of students in this class for the CEEB Achievement Tests were: English composition, 613; mathematics II, 727; and science, 646. An interview at the university campus is required.

## CURRICULUM

The HPM Program leads to a baccalaureate degree granted by the College of Arts and Sciences at the University of Miami and to the M.D. degree awarded by the University of Miami School of Medicine.

Students are required to complete a bachelor's degree. Minimum requirements for this degree include two semester courses in humanities and four semester courses in natural and physical sciences. HPM students major in biology most frequently, followed by chemistry and physics. An important educational innovation in the HPM Program is the Undergraduate Research Institute, which provides continuing research opportunities with stipends for students throughout the undergraduate years.

At the student's option, the HPM curriculum can take either six or seven years to complete. In years 1 and 2 of the six-year option, the curriculum focuses exclusively on work related to the bachelor's degree. In years 3 through 6, the curriculum is devoted to medical school courses.

HPM students must take the MCAT examination. However, the results do not factor into subsequent promotion to the medical school at Miami. While at the medical school, students must take steps 1 and 2 of the USMLE examinations. Passing the examinations is currently not a graduation requirement.

## EXPENSES

The 1995–96 tuition for the undergraduate portion of these programs was $17,700 per year.

## FINANCIAL AID

Scholarships, work-study, loans, and state tuition vouchers are sources of financial assistance. Information on undergraduate financial aid is available from the Office of Financial Assistance Services at (305) 284-5212. At the medical school, contact the Office of Financial Assistance at (305) 547-6211.

## APPLICATION AND ACCEPTANCE POLICIES

Filing of application:
   Earliest date: Oct. 15
Latest date for receipt of all materials: Jan. 15
Application fee: $35
Acceptance notice:
   Earliest date: April 1
   Latest date: May 20
Applicant's response to acceptance offer:
   Maximum time: May 1 or 14 days
Deposit to hold place in class (applied to tuition):
   $300; nonrefundable

## INFORMATION ON 1995–96 ENTERING CLASS

| Number of | Total |
| --- | --- |
| Applicants | 150 |
| Applicants Interviewed | 80 |
| New Entrants | 19 |

# Finch University of Health Sciences/ Chicago Medical School and Illinois Institute of Technology

Chicago, Illinois

## ADDRESS INQUIRIES TO:

Director of Admissions
B.S./M.D. Program
10 West 33rd Street
Chicago, Illinois 60616
(312) 567-3025
outside Chicago, 1-800-448-2329

## PURPOSE

The honors program allows superior students to earn both an Accreditation Board for Engineering and Technology (ABET) accredited Bachelor of Science degree in chemical, electrical, or mechanical engineering or computer science and an M.D. degree in eight years. The goal is to produce graduates who understand the intricacies of technology applied to medicine who will be the future innovators in improving medical diagnoses and treatment for their patients.

## REQUIREMENTS FOR ENTRANCE

Students are selected for this program during their senior year of high school. The program is open to U.S. citizens and permanent residents. Both residents and nonresidents of Illinois are eligible to apply. Applicants are expected to have completed the following courses by the time they graduate from high school: four years of mathematics (through calculus) and three years of life sciences (chemistry, biology, and physics). Applicants must take either the SAT or the ACT Assessment.

## SELECTION FACTORS

Academic factors considered in offering admission to an applicant include high school class rank, GPA, and curriculum. In the 1995–96 entering class, the average score on the ACT was 30 and the SAT was 1375; the average high school grade point average was 3.9/4.0. An interview is required.

## CURRICULUM

This program leads to a baccalaureate degree granted by the Illinois Institute of Technology (IIT) and to an M.D. degree granted by the Finch University of Health Sciences/Chicago Medical School. The most frequent major for a baccalaureate degree is chemical engineering. The curriculum focuses on studies for the bachelor's degree in the first four years. Continuation on to medical school is contingent upon maintaining a 3.3 GPA, no course grade below a "C," and displaying ethical behavior appropriate for a future physician. Students enter medical school in the fifth year. Students are required to pass Step 1 and Step 2 of the USMLE before graduation.

## EXPENSES

In 1995–96, the undergraduate tuition was $15,280. The medical school tuition was $29,106, plus $100 in yearly fees. Tuition is subject to change at both institutions.

## FINANCIAL AID

Applicants can receive more information by calling the Illinois Institute of Technology Admissions Office at the numbers above, or Chicago Medical School, Office of Financial Aid, at (847) 578-3216.

## APPLICATION AND ACCEPTANCE POLICIES

Filing of application:
  Latest date: January 1
Application fee: $30
Acceptance notice:
  Latest date: April 1
Applicant's response to acceptance offer:
  Maximum time: May 1
Deposit to hold place in class: $100; nonrefundable
Starting date: August 26

## INFORMATION ON 1995–96 ENTERING CLASS

| Number of | In-State | Out-of-State | Total |
| --- | --- | --- | --- |
| Applicants | 57 | 155 | 212 |
| Applicants Interviewed | 6 | 28 | 34 |
| New Entrants | 3 | 5 | 8 |

# Northwestern University

Evanston, Illinois



Office of Admission and Financial Aid
Northwestern University
1801 Hinman Avenue
Evanston, Illinois 60204-3060
(847) 491-7271

## PURPOSE

The Honors Program in Medical Education (HPME), one of the oldest in the nation, provides highly motivated and gifted students an individualized undergraduate curriculum that shortens the premedical preparation and assures entry to medical school.

## REQUIREMENTS FOR ENTRANCE

Students are selected for this program during the senior year of high school. Both residents and nonresidents of Illinois are eligible to apply. Applicants must meet the following high school course requirements: English, eight semesters; mathematics including differential and integral calculus, eight semesters; chemistry, two semesters; physics, two semesters; biology, two semesters; foreign language, four semesters. They must take either the SAT or the ACT Assessment plus the SAT II Subject Tests in mathematics IIC, chemistry, and writing.

## SELECTION FACTOR

Academic factors considered in selecting applicants include class rank, grades in high school, and scores on college entrance tests. Average test scores of students in the 1995–96 entering class were: SAT Verbal, 673; SAT Mathematics, 764; CEEB Achievement Tests—English, 669; Mathematics II, 780; Chemistry, 725. Nonacademic factors considered are motivation, concern for others, maturity, and involvement in extracurricular activities. An interview is required.

## CURRICULUM

The degrees offered in the Honors Program are a baccalaureate degree (B.S. in medicine, B.S. in biomedical engineering, B.S. in Speech, or B.A.) and the M.D., all from Northwestern University.

Students must complete requirements for a baccalaureate degree. Most students major in the biological sciences followed by psychology. Course requirements include the following: 11 quarters of natural and physical sciences and courses in the humanities and social sciences. The engineering curriculum also includes courses in basic and advanced engineering and mathematics. The third option is in Communication Sciences and Disorders—Human Communication Sciences. It includes courses in that department in addition to the HPME requirements.

The curriculum normally takes seven years to complete. In years 1 through 3, the curriculum consists entirely of courses in the liberal arts and sciences, engineering or speech. In years 4 through 7, the curriculum focuses on medicine. By the spring of year 2, students must take the MCAT, but it is not a factor in admission to the medical school or in promotion. Students must also take Step 1 of the USMLE examinations, but passing that examination is not a requirement for graduation from the medical school.

## EXPENSES

In 1995–96 tuition for the B.S. degree was $16,404 per year.

## FINANCIAL AID

Sources of aid include Northwestern University and federal, state, and private programs. Applicants can receive more information from the Office of Admission and Financial Aid, 1801 Hinman Avenue, Evanston, IL 60204; or phone: (847) 491-7271.

## APPLICATION AND ACCEPTANCE POLICIES

Filing of application:
  Latest date: Jan. 1
    of applicant's senior year of high school
Application fee: $50
Acceptance notice:
  Earliest date: April 1
Applicant's response to acceptance offer:
  Maximum time: May 1
Deposit to hold place in class: $200; nonrefundable
Starting date: Sept. 16

## INFORMATION ON 1995–96 ENTERING CLASS

| Number of | Total |
|---|---|
| Applicants | 792 |
| Applicants Interviewed | 707 |
| New Entrants | 70 |

# Boston University

**Boston, Massachusetts**

## ADDRESS INQUIRIES TO:

Assistant Director, Admissions
Boston University
121 Bay State Road
Boston, Massachusetts 02215
(617) 353-2300

## PURPOSE

This combined-degree program, one of the oldest in the nation, provides an  undergraduate premedical preparation which emphasizes the humanities and social sciences and affords a quality medical education even though the overall period of study is shortened.

## REQUIREMENTS FOR ENTRANCE

Students are selected for the program at Boston University during the senior year of high school or after high school if they have not been enrolled in any other degree-granting program. Since Boston University is a private institution, there are no state residence requirements. Applicants are expected to have completed the following courses by the time they graduate from high school: four years each of English and mathematics (including calculus), three years of foreign language, and one year each of biology, chemistry, and physics. They must take either the ACT Assessment or the SAT II Subject Exams in English composition with writing sample, mathematics I or II, and chemistry. The CEEB Achievement Test in foreign language is recommended.

## SELECTION FACTORS

The academic factors taken into account in offering admission to an applicant include the following: the high school GPA, the SAT or ACT score, scores on the CEEB Achievement Tests, rank in high school class, and the nature of the applicant's high school curriculum. In the 1995–96 entering class, the average high school GPA was 4.0; the average SAT Verbal was 670, SAT Mathematics was 750. SAT II Subject Exam scores were greater than 650, and rank in class was in the top 4 percent. Personal characteristics sought in applicants are motivation, maturity, and understanding of a career in medicine. An interview is required.

## CURRICULUM

This program leads to a baccalaureate degree granted by the College of Liberal Arts in Boston University and to the M.D. degree awarded by Boston University School of Medicine.

Students must complete work for the baccalaureate degree with a major in medical sciences. Requirements for this degree include four semester courses in the humanities, four courses in the social sciences, and nine courses in the natural and physical sciences. The program is seven years in length with an eight-year option. The program integrates the undergraduate and medical curricula in Year 3 and provides students with an early exposure to research opportunities and M.D.-Ph.D. programs.

Students must take the MCAT by the third year, but it is not a factor in admission to the medical school or in promotion. They are also required to take steps 1 and 2 of the USMLE examinations during the medical school portion of the program. Passing Step 2 of the USMLE examination is not a requirement for graduation.

## EXPENSES

In 1995–96 undergraduate tuition was $19,420 per year for residents and nonresidents, plus $280 for student fees.

## FINANCIAL AID

The usual sources of financial aid are available to students during the undergraduate portion of this program. Once into the medical school, students can qualify for need-based, low-interest, and government-sponsored loans. More information about aid can be obtained from the Office of Financial Assistance, Boston University, 881 Commonwealth Avenue, Boston, MA 02215; or phone (617) 353-9695.

## APPLICATION AND ACCEPTANCE POLICIES

Filing of application:
  Earliest date: Sept. 1
  Latest date: Dec. 15
Application fee: $50
Acceptance notice:
  Earliest date: March 15
  Latest date: April 15
Applicant's response to acceptance offer:
  Maximum time: May 1
Deposit to hold place in class: $400; nonrefundable

## INFORMATION ON 1995–96 ENTERING CLASS

| Number of | In-State | Out-of-State | Total |
| --- | --- | --- | --- |
| Applicants | 71 | 841 | 912 |
| Applicants Interviewed | 9 | 100 | 109 |
| New Entrants | 3 | 17 | 20 |

# Michigan State University
# College of Human Medicine

**East Lansing, Michigan**

## ADDRESS INQUIRIES TO:

College of Human Medicine
Office of Admissions
A-239 Life Sciences
Michigan State University
East Lansing, Michigan 48824
(517) 353-9620

## PURPOSE

The goal of the program is to educate excellent primary care physicians who will establish caring relationships with patients, who will practice in Michigan, especially in under-served rural and inner-city areas, and who will commit to a lifetime of learning and ethical practices.

## REQUIREMENTS FOR ENTRANCE

Students are selected for this program in the senior year of high school. Both residents and nonresidents of Michigan are eligible to apply. There are no specific high school course requirements, but applicants are required to have an ACT composite score in the range of 29 or higher, or an SAT composite score in the range of 1200 or higher.

## SELECTION FACTORS

Academic factors considered in selecting applicants include consistently high grades or a strong upward trend, class rank in the top 10 percent, and a GPA of at least 3.6. An interview is required.

In the 1995–96 entering class, the high school GPA averaged 3.93, and the average mean ACT score was 31; the SAT score averaged 1323.

## CURRICULUM

This program leads to a baccalaureate degree awarded by the Michigan State University, and the M.D. degree granted by the Michigan State University College of Human Medicine. It is not an accelerated program; all students must complete four years of undergraduate education and four years of medical school.

The most frequent major for the baccalaureate degree is physiology followed by biology. Course requirements include eight semesters each of humanities, social sciences, and natural and physical sciences. These credit requirements are minimums and are dependent on the academic major.

Medical Scholars are encouraged to complete a specialization in health and humanities and to participate in a research project under the direction of a medical school faculty, as well as participate in a year-long service commitment to a community service agency.

Students in this program are not required to take the MCAT for promotion or admission to the medical school. The student must pass steps 1 and 2 of the USMLE examinations in order to graduate. The USMLE Step 1 examination is administered at the completion of Year 2.

## EXPENSES

In 1995–96, undergraduate tuition was $4,268 for residents and $11,084 for nonresidents. Student fees averaged $573 for the year. Medical school tuition for residents was $13,699.50 (three semesters); nonresidents, $30,097.50 (three semesters). The average cost for student fees was $854.25.

## FINANCIAL AID

A number of options are available for aid. These include college work study, Pell grants, student aid grants, Supplemental Educational Opportunities Grant, Subsidized and Unsubsidized Stafford loans, Perkins loan, and private loans. Applicants can receive more information from Michigan State University, Office of Financial Aid, 252 Student Services Building, East Lansing, Michigan 48824.

## APPLICATION AND ACCEPTANCE POLICIES

Filing of application:
   Earliest date: Aug. 15
   Latest date: Nov. 1
Application fee: $50
Acceptance notice: March 15
Applicant's response to acceptance offer:
   Maximum time: 2 weeks
Deposit to hold place in class: $50; nonrefundable
Starting date: Aug. 26

## INFORMATION ON 1995–96 ENTERING CLASS

| Number of | Total |
| --- | --- |
| Applicants | 307 |
| Applicants Interviewed | 60 |
| New Entrants | 10 |

# University of Michigan

Ann Arbor, Michigan

## ADDRESS INQUIRIES TO:

Inteflex Program
5113 Medical Science I Building, Wing "C"
University of Michigan
Ann Arbor, Michigan 48109-0611
(313) 764-9534
(313) 936-3510 (FAX)

## PURPOSE

The primary goal of the Integrated Premedical/Medical (Inteflex) Program is to educate physicians who are scientifically competent, compassionate, and socially conscious and who can apply the insights gained in the study of the humanities and social sciences in addressing the challenges of medicine in the 21st century.

## REQUIREMENTS FOR ENTRANCE

Students are selected for this program during the senior year of high school. Both residents and nonresidents of Michigan are eligible to apply. Students must first apply to and be admitted to the College of Literature, Science, and Arts. In general, applicants are expected to have a solid background in mathematics and science. To be considered, they must take either the SAT or the ACT Assessment and achieve a minimum score of 1320 total on the SAT or 30 cumulative on the ACT Assessment.

## SELECTION FACTORS

Academic factors considered in selecting applicants include the high school GPA, scores on college entrance tests, and type of high school courses completed. Personal factors such as extracurricular activities, honors and awards, letters of recommendation, and motivation to study medicine are evaluated. Students interested in a career as a generalist physician and students from minority groups underrepresented in medicine are encouraged to apply. In 1995, the average SAT score for incoming Michigan resident students was 1376; the average for nonresidents was 1392. The average high school GPA for both groups was 3.9. An interview is required for admission.

## CURRICULUM

Degrees offered in the Inteflex Program are a baccalaureate degree from the College of Literature, Science, and Arts at the University of Michigan and a M.D. degree from the University of Michigan Medical School.

Students may elect from a variety of liberal arts majors and must complete all requirements for the baccalaureate degree prior to advancement to the medical four years of the program. Most students major in the biomedical sciences. Some course requirements for the baccalaureate degree include three semesters of humanities, three semesters of social science, three semesters of natural and physical sciences, four semesters of a foreign language, and two semesters of writing.

The curriculum normally takes eight years to complete. The study of medicine is integrated with the study of liberal arts beginning with the first year of the program. Advancement to the medical school phase is based on the overall undergraduate record *and* a successful performance on the required MCAT examination. Students must complete all requirements of the standard four-year medical curriculum (including steps 1 and 2 of the USMLE) to complete the program and receive the M.D. degree.

## EXPENSES

Students are responsible for tuition and fees set by the university for four years of both undergraduate and medical school. For the 1995–96 entering class, the in-state annual tuition (including spring term) was $6,713; out-of-state tuition was $21,118. For reference, medical school annual tuition was $16,040 for in-state and $25,140 for out-of-state. University fees are approximately $175 per year. Costs for room and board are additional.

## FINANCIAL AID

Sources of aid include grants, loans, work-study through the undergraduate Financial Aid Office (undergraduates in Inteflex), 2011 Student Activities Building, University of Michigan, Ann Arbor, MI 48109-1316.

## APPLICATION AND ACCEPTANCE POLICIES

Filing of application:
   Latest date—University: Jan. 10
      of applicant's senior year of high school
   Latest date—Inteflex Application: Feb. 15
Application fee: $40
Acceptance notice: Mailed by April 15
Applicant's response to acceptance offer:
   Maximum time: 1 month
Deposit to hold place in class: $200; nonrefundable
Starting date: Early Sept.

## INFORMATION ON 1995–96 ENTERING CLASS

| *Number of* | *In-State* | *Out-of-State* | *Total* |
|---|---|---|---|
| Applicants | 242 | 464 | 706 |
| Applicants Interviewed | 97 | 52 | 149 |
| New Entrants | 25 | 10 | 35 |

# University of Missouri—Kansas City School of Medicine

**Kansas City, Missouri**

## ADDRESS INQUIRIES TO:

Council on Selection
University of Missouri—Kansas City
School of Medicine
2411 Holmes
Kansas City, Missouri 64108
(816) 235-1870

## PURPOSE

This combined baccalaureate-M.D. degree program integrates the humanities, basic sciences, and clinical medicine throughout the curriculum so graduates will have the background for lifelong learning in order to meet the needs of their patients. It is one of the few U.S. programs in which the vast majority of students are pursuing a combined-degree.

## REQUIREMENTS FOR ENTRANCE

The program is primarily designed for high school graduates who are entering college. Residents and nonresidents of Missouri are eligible to apply. An applicant's high school curriculum must include at a minimum the following: eight semesters of English; eight semesters of mathematics; six semesters of science, including two semesters of biology and two semesters of chemistry; six semesters of social studies; two semesters of fine arts; four semesters of foreign language; and one semester of computer science. Applicants must meet a minimum academic screen based on the ACT composite score and rank in high school class.

## SELECTION FACTORS

Applicants' academic potential is judged by the quality of high school courses, rank in high school class, and scores on the ACT. In the 1995–96 entering class, the average ACT score was at the 93rd percentile, and the average rank in class was at the 93rd percentile. Personal qualities include maturity, leadership, stamina, reliability, motivation for medicine, range of interests, interpersonal skills, compassion, and job experience. Qualified applicants are invited for a required interview.

## CURRICULUM

The six-year curriculum leads to a baccalaureate degree granted by the School of Biological Sciences or the College of Arts and Sciences and the doctor of medicine degree granted by the School of Medicine.

Students must complete requirements for the bachelor's degree. Students may pursue any major offered in the college, but most major in liberal arts or biology. Course requirements for the bachelor's degree in liberal arts include 21 semester hours of humanities, 21 semester hours of social sciences, and 50 semester hours of natural and physical sciences.

The curriculum normally takes six years to complete. During the first two years of the curriculum, students spend 75 percent of their time in course work related to the bachelor's degree. Conversely, in the last four years students spend 75 percent of their time in courses, clerkships, and electives related to the M.D. degree. Thus, the study of liberal arts, basic sciences, and clinical medicine is integrated throughout the entire curriculum. Beginning in Year 1, students are involved with patients and the health care delivery system. Problem-solving plus learning and teaching in small groups are emphasized. Students are assigned a faculty adviser (docent), and younger students are paired with older students. During the last four years of the curriculum students attend a general medicine outpatient clinic for a half-day each week.

Students in this program do not take the MCAT. They must pass steps 1 and 2 of the USMLE examinations for graduation.

An alternative path is available for extended study, and a combined eight-year baccalaureate/M.D./Ph.D. degree program is open to a small number of highly qualified individuals.

## EXPENSES

In 1995–96 estimated tuition and fees for years 1 and 2 were $12,460 in-state per year and $25,654 out-of-state.

## FINANCIAL AID

Contact the UMKC Financial Aid Office, 4825 Troost Avenue, Kansas City, MO 64110; or phone (816) 235-1154.

## APPLICATION AND ACCEPTANCE POLICIES

Filing of application:
  Earliest date: Aug. 1
  Latest date: Nov. 15
Application fee: $25 in-state; $50 out-of-state
Acceptance notice:
  Earliest date: April 1
Applicant's response to acceptance offer:
  Maximum time: No later than May 1
Deposit to hold place in class: $100; refundable before
  May 15
Starting date: August

## INFORMATION ON 1995–96 ENTERING CLASS

| Number of | In-State | Out-of-State | Total |
|---|---|---|---|
| Applicants | 419 | 348 | 767 |
| Applicants Interviewed | 276 | 89 | 365 |
| New Entrants | 87 | 17 | 104 |

# University of Medicine and Dentistry of New Jersey/New Jersey Medical School

Newark, New Jersey

## ADDRESS INQUIRIES TO:

Office of Admissions
C653 MSB
UMDNJ—New Jersey Medical School
185 South Orange Avenue
Newark, New Jersey 07103-2714
(201) 982-4631

## PURPOSE

New Jersey Medical School has established accelerated baccalaureate-M.D. degree programs in collaboration with seven undergraduate institutions. The goal of these programs is to give highly qualified high school students an opportunity to broaden their premedical preparation without having to compete for admission for medical school.

## REQUIREMENTS FOR ENTRANCE

The programs are open to all high school seniors who are either U.S. citizens or permanent residents. Application procedures vary slightly among the programs, but SATs are required.

## SELECTION FACTORS

Applicants should be in the top 5 to 10 percent of their high school class and have a minimum combined SAT score of 1400 (1350 if in top 3 percent of their high school class). Applicants are screened on the basis of academic credentials, letters of recommendation, and an essay; those who meet screening criteria are invited for an interview at the undergraduate school and at the medical school. The deadline for applications to the undergraduate college is January 7. However, the earliest applicants have an advantage.

## CURRICULUM

The course of study consists of three years at the undergraduate school, followed by the regular four year medical program. Students must take the MCAT in their junior year, but scores are not a factor for promotion or admission to the medical school phase. Promotion to the medical school is contingent upon achieving grades of B or better in all premedical courses and maintaining an overall grade point average of at least 3.2 each semester. The baccalaureate degree is awarded by the undergraduate institution upon completion of the first year of medical school. The M.D. degree is awarded by New Jersey Medical School.

Students are required to pass Step 1 of the USMLE in order to be graduated. Students must also take Step 2 of the USMLE, but passing is not a requirement for graduation.

Seven programs are currently available:

*Boston University* provides an undergraduate emphasis in liberal arts or humanities. This program is open only to residents of New Jersey. Mailing address: Jessica Marinaccio, Assistant Director of Admissions, Boston University, Commonwealth Avenue, Boston, MA 02215.

*Drew University* offers premedical preparation in all sciences and liberal arts subjects. Mailing address: Dr. Harold Rohrs, Department of Biology, Drew University, Madison, NJ 07940; (201) 408-3802; E-mail: HRohrs@Daniel.Drew. EDU.

*Montclair State University* offers premedical preparation in biology, chemistry, biochemistry, molecular biology, computer science, mathematics, psychology, and anthropology. The mailing address is Dr. Judith Shillcock, Health Professions Committee, Department of Biology, Montclair State University, Upper Montclair, NJ 07043.

*New Jersey Institute of Technology* offers undergraduate study in the Honors Premedical Curriculum within the Engineering Science Program. Mailing address: Dr. David Kristol, Director, Center for Biomedical Engineering, New Jersey Institute of Technology, University Heights, Newark, NJ 07102; phone: (201) 596-3584.

*Stevens Institute of Technology* offers premedical preparation in chemical biology. Mailing address: Edwina W. Fleming, Director of Honors Admissions Programs, Stevens Institute of Technology, Castle Point on the Hudson, Hoboken, NJ 07030.

*The Richard Stockton College of New Jersey* offers preparation in chemistry, biology, physics and liberal arts. Mailing address: Judith Hain, Associate Vice President for Academic Affairs, Stockton State College, Pomona, NJ 08240-9988; phone: (609) 652-4514.

*Trenton State College* offers preparation in biology, chemistry, history, philosophy and psychology. Mailing address: Dr. Dennis Shevlin, Co-chairman, Biology Department, Trenton State College CN 4700, Trenton, NJ 08650-4700; phone: (609) 771-2021.

Application is made through the undergraduate institutions listed above.

# Rutgers University and University of Medicine and Dentistry of New Jersey Robert Wood Johnson Medical School

Piscataway, New Jersey

## ADDRESS INQUIRIES TO:

Bachelor/Medical Degree Program
Nelson Biological Laboratory
Rutgers University
P.O. Box 1059
Piscataway, New Jersey 08855-1059
(908) 445-5270

## PURPOSE

The program permits the early identification and admission of high quality medical students. It also integrates medical studies with liberal arts study.

## REQUIREMENTS FOR ENTRANCE

Applicants must be students at Rutgers University and are selected for this program at the end of their sophomore year. Residents and nonresidents of New Jersey are considered.

## SELECTION FACTORS

An applicant's high school and college transcripts plus faculty recommendations are taken into account in offering admission. In the 1995–96 entering class, matriculants had achieved a 3.84 GPA at the end of two years of college. They had an average score of 596 on the SAT Verbal section and 735 on the Mathematics section. Maturity, motivation, and broad interests are personal characteristics sought in applicants. An interview is required. The MCAT is not used.

## CURRICULUM

This program leads to the baccalaureate degree awarded by Rutgers University and to the M.D. degree granted by the University of Medicine and Dentistry of New Jersey Robert Wood Johnson Medical School. Students must complete requirements for a baccalaureate degree. The most frequent majors for that degree are biological sciences, followed by biochemistry.

The program is eight years in duration. As indicated in the curriculum chart below, the basic sciences and the liberal arts are studied together during a four-year period.

While in medical school, students must take and pass steps 1 and 2 of the USMLE examinations.

| Year | Percent Liberal Arts | Percent Basic Sciences |
|---|---|---|
| 1 | 100 | 0 |
| 2 | 100 | 0 |
| 3 | 50 | 50 |
| 4 | 50 | 50 |
| 5 | 20 | 80 |
| 6 | 0 | 100 |
| 7 | 0 | 100 |
| 8 | 0 | 100 |

## EXPENSES

In 1995–96 residents of New Jersey paid $3,786 per year in undergraduate tuition and $13,295 per year in medical school tuition. In the same year, nonresidents paid $7,707 per year in undergraduate tuition and $17,445 annually in medical school tuition. Fees averaged $1,050 for undergraduates each year and $1,187 for medical students per year.

## FINANCIAL AID

Undergraduates should contact the Office of Financial Aid, Records Hall, College Avenue, Rutgers University, New Brunswick, NJ 08901.

## APPLICATION AND ACCEPTANCE POLICIES

Filing of application:
  Latest date: June 1
    of sophomore year
    at Rutgers University
Application fee: None
Acceptance notice:
  Latest date: July 1
Applicant's response to acceptance offer:
  Maximum time: 2 weeks
Deposit to hold place in class: $50; refundable
Starting date: Aug.

## INFORMATION ON 1995–96 ENTERING CLASS

| Number of | In-State | Out-of-State | Total |
|---|---|---|---|
| Applicants | 39 | 3 | 42 |
| Applicants Interviewed | 33 | 2 | 35 |
| New Entrants | 12 | 0 | 12 |

# Binghamton University and State University of New York Health Science Center at Syracuse

Binghamton, New York

## ADDRESS INQUIRIES TO:

Rural Primary Care Recruitment Programs
College of Medicine
State University of New York
Health Science Center at Syracuse
P.O. Box 1000
Binghamton, New York 13902
(607) 770-8515

## PURPOSE

The scholars program will offer a unique pathway for exceptionally able students who possess both academic and personal attributes which will lead to primary care practice in rural areas.

## REQUIREMENTS FOR ENTRANCE

Students are selected for this program during their senior year of high school. Only residents of New York are eligible to apply. Applicants must meet the entrance requirements of Binghamton University and take the SAT.

## SELECTION FACTORS

To be considered for this program, applicants must have a grade point average of 92 or above, a combined SAT of 1200 or higher, and must be a U.S. citizen or permanent resident. An interview is required.

## CURRICULUM

This eight-year program leads to a baccalaureate degree granted by Binghamton University, and to the M.D. degree awarded by the State University of New York Health Science Center at Syracuse.

Students are expected to complete work for the bachelor's degree. Requirements for that degree vary according to the major chosen, but all include course work in the humanities and two semesters each of social sciences, and natural and physical sciences. They are not required to take the MCAT to advance to the medical school.

Educational innovations include: (a) a primary care mentor in college; (b) health care-related classes; (c) participation in hospital and private practice settings; (d) and community-based clinical medical education in a primary care setting.

Students are required to take Step 1 of the USMLE, and passing this exam is required for promotion and graduation. Students also must take Step 2 of the USMLE.

## EXPENSES

Annual tuition for undergraduates is $3,200, and $10,840 for the medical school.

## FINANCIAL AID

For more information, applicants can contact the Office of Rural Primary Care Recruitment Programs, College of Medicine, State University of New York, Health Science Center at Syracuse, P.O. Box 1000, Binghamton University, New York 13902; or phone (607) 770-8515.

## APPLICATION AND ACCEPTANCE POLICIES

Filing of application:
   Earliest date: Sept. 1
   Latest date: Jan. 1
Application fee: None
Applicant's response to acceptance offer:
   Maximum time: May 1
Starting date: Aug. 1997

## INFORMATION ON 1995–96 ENTERING CLASS

More information may be obtained from the Office of Rural Primary Care Recruitment Programs, College of Medicine, State University of New York, Health Science Center at Syracuse, P.O. Box 1000, Binghamton University, New York 13902; or phone (607) 770-8515.

# Brooklyn College and State University at New York Health Science Center at Brooklyn College of Medicine

Brooklyn, New York

## ADDRESS INQUIRIES TO:

Director of Admissions
1602 James Hall
Brooklyn College
Brooklyn, New York 11210
(718) 951-5044

## PURPOSE

The aims of this program are to produce physicians who are humanists and to offer an economically sound path to medicine.

## REQUIREMENTS FOR ENTRANCE

Students are selected in their senior year of high school. Residents and nonresidents of New York are considered. Applicants are expected to have completed the following high school courses: a full year of biology, chemistry, and physics plus mathematics through trigonometry. They usually have a high school average of at least 90 and SAT combined scores of at least 1200.

## SELECTION FACTORS

The academic factors taken into account in offering admission to an applicant include: the high school GPA, SAT scores, New York State Regents Examination scores, Advanced Placement courses, and CEEB Achievement Tests scores. In the 1995–96 entering class, most students had a high school average of at least 94, and the median SAT combined score was 1320. Maturity and motivation are personal characteristics sought among applicants. An interview is required.

## CURRICULUM

This program leads to a baccalaureate degree awarded by Brooklyn College and to the M.D. degree granted by the State University of New York Health Science Center at Brooklyn College of Medicine.

The baccalaureate program includes eight required semester courses in the natural and physical sciences, seven semester courses in humanities, and three semester courses in the social sciences. Several of these classes are honors sections specifically for students in the B.A.-M.D. program. The most frequent major is biology. The next most frequent majors are chemistry and psychology. Students may major in any subject, but nonscience majors are encouraged. Students must maintain a 3.4 overall, and 3.2 science undergraduate GPA to progress to the medical school.

The program is eight years in length with a seven-year option. Students are encouraged to do an internship at the medical school during the summer after their second college year. The four-year medical school program focuses on the M.D. degree exclusively.

During medical school, students must take and pass steps 1 and 2 of the USMLE examinations.

## EXPENSES

In 1995–96 the undergraduate tuition for state residents was $3,200 per year and for nonresidents $6,800. The 1995–96 medical school tuition was $10,840 for state residents and $21,940 for nonresidents. Student fees cost an additional $160 per year at Brooklyn College and $220 per year at the Medical College.

Brooklyn College has no dormitory facilities, so students must commute or find lodging in the community. Dormitory space is available during the medical school portion of the program.

## FINANCIAL AID

Pell grants, Stafford Student Loans, work-study, Hearst Scholarships for minority female students, and institutional scholarships are available. Applicants can receive more information from the Director of Financial Aid, 1203 James Hall, Brooklyn College, Brooklyn, NY 11210.

## APPLICATION AND ACCEPTANCE POLICIES

Filing of application:
  Earliest date: Nov. 1
  Latest date: Dec. 29
Application fee: None
Acceptance notice: April 1
Applicant's response to acceptance offer:
  Maximum time: May 1
Deposit to hold place in class: None
Starting date: Aug. 29

## INFORMATION ON 1995–96 ENTERING CLASS

| Number of | In-State | Out-of-State | Total |
|---|---|---|---|
| Applicants | 291 | 24 | 315 |
| Applicants Interviewed | 54 | 7 | 61 |
| New Entrants | 21 | 1 | 22 |

# New York University

New York, New York

## ADDRESS INQUIRIES TO:

Admissions Office
New York University
College of Arts and Science
22 Washington Square North
Room 904 Main Building
New York, New York 10003
(212) 998-4500

## PURPOSE

The goal of the B.A.-M.D. program is to train broadly educated doctors who are interested in people and their place in society and who are excited about the science of medicine.

## REQUIREMENTS FOR ENTRANCE

Students are selected for this program only during the senior year of high school. There are no state residency requirements. No specific courses are required. Applicants must take the ACT Assessment or SAT and either three CEEB Achievement Tests or three Advanced Placement Tests (one of which must be English in either case).

## SELECTION FACTORS

Academic factors considered in offering admission include high school GPA, rank in high school class, and honors or advanced placement course work. The admissions committee looks very closely at each applicant's extracurricular and/or service activities, writing skills, knowledge of and enthusiasm for the medical profession, and general intellectual curiosity. Students with broad interests are sought. Minority applicants are encouraged to apply. Interviews at the College of Arts and Science and the School of Medicine are required. Four students were admitted to the 1995–96 entering class. The average high school GPAs of previous classes have been 3.9/4.0.

## CURRICULUM

The B.A.-M.D. program is not accelerated. All students must complete four years of undergraduate education and four years of medical school.

Students earn a bachelor's degree, which includes completion of a major and the college's Liberal Education Program. Students in the combined-degree program are encouraged to pursue any liberal arts major they wish. Additionally, they are required to complete an independent interdisciplinary research project over a period of several semesters. Students are expected to maintain good progress and a satisfactory GPA while in college. They are not required to take the MCAT to advance to the medical school.

## EXPENSES

The annual tuition and fees for the undergraduate portion of the combined-degree program totaled $19,748 in 1995–96. The medical school portion was $24,620.

## FINANCIAL AID

Special merit scholarships are available. These awards include participation in a scholarship group which pays for cultural events and two study trips per year: one to a domestic point and one to an international destination. The usual loans, grants, and work-study programs are available. Applicants can receive more information from the Office of Financial Aid, 23 West 4th Street, New York, NY 10003.

---

### APPLICATION AND ACCEPTANCE POLICIES

Filing of application:
   Latest date: Jan. 15
Application fee: $45
Acceptance notice:
   Earliest date: April 3
Applicant's response to acceptance offer:
   Maximum time: until May 1
Deposit to hold place in class: $200; nonrefundable
Starting date: Sept.

### INFORMATION ON 1995–96 ENTERING CLASS

| Number of | Total |
| --- | --- |
| Applicants | 200 |
| Applicants Interviewed | 11 |
| New Entrants | 4 |

# Rensselaer Polytechnic Institute and Albany Medical College

Troy, New York

## ADDRESS INQUIRIES TO:

Admissions Counselor
Rensselaer Polytechnic Institute
Troy, New York 12180
(518) 276-6216

## PURPOSE

The Six-Year Biomedical Program, begun in the early 1960s, offers qualified individuals the opportunity to earn the B.S. and M.D. degrees in six calendar years. Participants receive a strong science-based education in a technological university before entering Albany Medical College.

## REQUIREMENTS FOR ENTRANCE

Students are selected for this program during the senior year of high school. Residents of New York as well as nonresidents of the state are eligible to apply. Applicants are expected to have completed the following courses by the time they graduate from high school: four years of English; one year each of biology, chemistry, and physics; and three years of mathematics (through trigonometry). They must take the SAT plus CEEB Achievement Tests in Mathematics I or II, English composition, and a science. In lieu of these tests, ACT Assessment scores may be submitted.

## SELECTION FACTORS

Academic factors considered in offering admission to an applicant include the quality and nature of course work in high school, performance in those courses, rank in high school class, and test scores. The 1995–96 entering class had an average score of 652 on the SAT Verbal and 730 on the SAT Math (tests administered prior to April 1995). Personal qualities sought in applicants are motivation, maturity, and personal development. An interview is required.

## CURRICULUM

This program leads to a B.S. degree awarded by Rensselaer Polytechnic Institute and the M.D. degree granted by Albany Medical College.

Students must complete work for a bachelor's degree. Requirements for that degree include 18 courses in the natural and physical sciences and eight elective courses in the humanities and social sciences.

The curriculum for both degrees normally requires six years to complete. During the first two years of the program spent at Rensselaer, the curriculum involves 70 percent pre-medical science courses and 30 percent liberal arts courses. The medical college has replaced the traditional two years of basic science and two years of clinical science with an integrated four-year curriculum. Emphasis is placed on the pivotal role of primary care.

Students admitted to the program are not required to take the MCAT for admission to Albany Medical College. Students are expected to take steps 1 and 2 of the USMLE examinations while at Albany Medical College, but passing these examinations is not a graduation requirement.

## EXPENSES

The tuition and fees for 1995–96 were $17,995 at Rensselaer, and $24,074 for residents and $25,346 for nonresidents at Albany Medical College.

## FINANCIAL AID

Sources of financial aid are restricted and endowed scholarships based on need, merit scholarships, work-study, and student loans through federal and institutional programs. Applicants can receive more information by contacting the Financial Aid Office of Rensselaer Polytechnic Institute at (518) 276-6813 or Albany Medical College at (518) 262-5435.

## APPLICATION AND ACCEPTANCE POLICIES

Filing of application:
   Earliest date: Sept. 1
   Latest date: Dec. 1
Application fee: $35 (RPI);
   $75 (Albany Medical College)
Acceptance notice:
   Earliest date: Jan.
   Latest date: until class is filled
Applicant's response to acceptance offer:
   Maximum time: May 1
Deposit to hold place in class: $250; nonrefundable
Starting date: Sept.

## INFORMATION ON 1995–96 ENTERING CLASS

| Number of | In-State | Out-of-State | Total |
| --- | --- | --- | --- |
| Applicants | 131 | 324 | 455 |
| Applicants Interviewed | 28 | 72 | 100 |
| New Entrants | 6 | 14 | 20 |

# Siena College and Albany Medical College

Loudonville, New York

## ADDRESS INQUIRIES TO:

Siena College
Office of Admissions
Route 9
Loudonville, New York 12211
(518) 783-2423

## PURPOSE

This program offers an eight-year continuum of education which has a special emphasis on the humanities and on community service while providing a sound understanding of both the natural and social sciences.

## REQUIREMENTS FOR ENTRANCE

Students are selected for this program during the senior year of high school. Both residents and nonresidents of New York are eligible to apply. There are no specific high school course requirements, but applicants are required to take the SAT.

## SELECTION FACTORS

Academic factors considered in offering admission to an applicant include the following: required and elective courses taken, grades earned, class standing, SAT scores, honors received, letters of recommendation, and unique academic experiences. Of great importance to the admission committee are such factors as extracurricular activities, evidence of intellectual curiosity, and interest in the humanities and in the sciences. Students generally rank among the top 10 percent of their high school class. The 1995–96 entering class had an average score of 590 on the SAT Verbal and 680 on the SAT Math (tests administered prior to April 1995). An interview is required.

## CURRICULUM

This program offers a coordinated eight-year curriculum of premedical and medical education. The undergraduate phase offers an equal distribution of science and nonscience courses. Students graduate in four years with a bachelor of arts degree in biology with a minor in the humanities. The undergraduate phase of the program also includes a required summer of human service in a health related agency, usually in an urban ghetto or developing nation. Passage from the undergraduate to the medical school requires achievement of a 3.20 GPA and

a continued interest in the human service dimension of the program. The medical college has replaced the traditional two years of basic science and two years of clinical science with an integrated four-year curriculum. Emphasis is placed on the pivotal role of primary care. The summer between the sophomore and junior year is dedicated to medically related volunteer service, usually in a rural or inner city clinic.

Students are not required to take the MCAT for admission to Albany Medical College. Students are expected to take Step 1 and Step 2 of the USMLE, but passing these examinations is not a requirement for graduation.

## EXPENSES

In 1995–96 tuition and fees were $11,340 at Siena College, and $24,074 for residents and $25,346 for nonresidents at Albany Medical College.

## FINANCIAL AID

Applicants can receive more information by contacting Siena College, Financial Aid Office, Route 9, Loudonville, NY 12211, (phone: (518) 783-2427); or Albany Medical College, Financial Aid Office, Albany, NY 12208 (phone: (518) 262-5435).

## APPLICATION AND ACCEPTANCE POLICIES

Filing of application:
  Earliest date: Sept. 1
  Latest date: Dec. 15
Application fee: $40 (Siena);
  $75 (Albany Medical College)
Acceptance notice:
  Earliest date: March 15
  Latest date: until classes are filled
Applicant's response to acceptance offer:
  Maximum time: May 1
Deposit to hold place in class: $200; nonrefundable
Starting date: Sept.

## INFORMATION ON 1995–96 ENTERING CLASS

| Number of | In-State | Out-of-State | Total |
| --- | --- | --- | --- |
| Applicants | 154 | 159 | 313 |
| Applicants Interviewed | 24 | 12 | 36 |
| New Entrants | 8 | 3 | 11 |

# Sophie Davis School of Biomedical Education/ City University of New York

New York, New York

## ADDRESS INQUIRIES TO:

Sophie Davis School of Biomedical Education
City University of New York
Office of Admissions
Y Building, Room 205N
138th Street and Convent Avenue
New York, New York 10031
(212) 650-7707/7712

## PURPOSE

The purposes of this combined-degree program are to train primary care physicians who will work in medically under-served urban areas and to increase the number of minority physicians.

## REQUIREMENTS FOR ENTRANCE

Students are selected for this program in the senior year of high school. Only residents of New York are eligible to apply. Applicants are expected to have completed the following courses by the time they graduate from high school: two semesters each of chemistry and biology and six to eight semesters of mathematics. They must take the ACT Assessment and a local mathematics placement test.

## SELECTION FACTORS

Academic factors taken into account in offering admission to an applicant are: the high school GPA, scores on the ACT Assessment, and scores on the New York State Regents Examinations. In the 1995–96 entering class, the high school grades averaged 93.0, and the subscore on the Mathematics ACT Assessment averaged 28. The SAT Mathematics average was 630 and the SAT Verbal average was 610. Personal qualities sought in applicants include interest in people, concern for others, initiative, and leadership. An interview is required.

## CURRICULUM

This seven-year program leads to a baccalaureate degree granted by the City College of New York and to the M.D. degree awarded by one of seven New York medical schools.

During the first five years of the program, students fulfill all requirements for the B.S. degree and study the preclinical portion of the medical school curriculum. After successfully com-pleting the five-year sequence and passing Step 1 of the USMLE examinations, students transfer to one of the partici-pating medical schools in New York for their final two years of clinical training. Students are expected to pass steps 1 and 2 of the USMLE examinations to graduate.

There is a strong emphasis on humanities and social sciences courses. The introduction of community medicine courses with field work and medical biochemistry and anatomy during the undergraduate phase is an innovative feature of this program. Students also benefit from counseling and academic support services.

## EXPENSES

In 1995–96, resident undergraduate tuition per year was $1,600. Student fees were $95. Tuition for the final two years of the program varies according to the medical school attended.

## FINANCIAL AID

Pell grants, New York State tuition assistance, and the City College of New York biomedical stipend are sources of financial aid. More information about aid is available from the Office of Student Affairs.

---

### APPLICATION AND ACCEPTANCE POLICIES

Filing of application:
   Earliest date   Oct. 15
   Latest date: Jan. 15
Application fee: None
Acceptance notice: April 1
Applicant's response to acceptance offer:
   Maximum time: 1 month
Deposit to hold place in class: None
Starting date: Sept.

### INFORMATION ON 1995–96 ENTERING CLASS

| Number of | Total |
|---|---|
| Applicants | 500 |
| Applicants Interviewed | 182 |
| New Entrants | 70 |

# Union College
# and Albany Medical College

Schenectady, New York

## ADDRESS INQUIRIES TO:

Associate Dean of Admissions
Union College
Schenectady, New York 12308
(518) 388-6112

## PURPOSE

Stressing both the sciences and humanities, the Medical Education Program offers students the opportunity to earn the B.S. degree and the M.D. degree in seven years.

## REQUIREMENTS FOR ENTRANCE

Students are selected for this program during the senior year of high school. Residents of New York as well as nonresidents of the state are eligible to apply. Applicants are expected to have completed the following courses by the time they graduate from high school: four years of English, one year of biology, one year of chemistry, and three years of mathematics (at least through trigonometry). They must take either the ACT Assessment or the SAT and three CEEB Achievement Tests, specifically in Mathematics I or II, English composition, and a science.

## SELECTION FACTORS

Academic factors considered in offering admission to an applicant include the quality and nature of course work in high school, performance in those courses, rank in high school class, and standardized test scores. In the 1995–96 entering class, the average SAT score was 646 for SAT Verbal and 720 for SAT Mathematics (tests administered prior to April 1995). Personal qualities sought in applicants include motivation, maturity, and personal development. An interview is required.

## CURRICULUM

This program leads to a bachelor's degree awarded by Union College and an M.D. degree granted by Albany Medical College.

Students must complete work for a bachelor's degree. Minimum requirements for this degree include 11 courses in the humanities and social sciences plus 18 courses in natural and physical sciences. Students take an interdepartmental major which combines work in two fields, one in the field of science and the other in a nonscience area. This requirement to major in both a science and in a nonscience is an important educational innovation offered at Union College.

The curriculum for both degrees requires seven years to complete. During the first three years of the program spent at Union College, students devote 45 percent of their curricular time to the humanities and social sciences and remainder to premedical sciences. Students take a course in health and human values during the summer before matriculation in the medical school. The medical college has replaced the traditional two years of basic science and two years of clinical science with an integrated four-year curriculum. Emphasis is placed on the pivotal role of primary care.

Students admitted to the program are not required to take the MCAT for admission to Albany Medical College. Students are expected to take steps 1 and 2 of the USMLE examinations while at Albany Medical College, but passing these examinations is not a graduation requirement.

## EXPENSES

The 1995–96 tuition was $19,782 for study at Union College and $24,074 for residents and $25,346 for nonresidents at Albany Medical College.

## FINANCIAL AID

Sources of financial aid include various programs based on need, student loans through federal and state assistance, work-study, and merit scholarships. Applicants can receive more information by contacting the Financial Aid Office of Union College at (518) 388-6123 or Albany Medical College at (518) 262-5435.

## APPLICATION AND ACCEPTANCE POLICIES

Filing of application:
    Earliest date: Sept. 1
    Latest date: Jan. 1
Application fee: $50 (Union College);
    $75 (Albany Medical College)
Acceptance notice:
    Earliest date: Feb.
    Latest date: until class is filled
Applicant's response to acceptance offer:
    Maximum time: May 1
Deposit to hold place in class: $400; nonrefundable
Starting date: Sept.

## INFORMATION ON 1995–96 ENTERING CLASS

| Number of | In-State | Out-of-State | Total |
| --- | --- | --- | --- |
| Applicants | 213 | 318 | 531 |
| Applicants Interviewed | 44 | 51 | 95 |
| New Entrants | 14 | 6 | 20 |

# University of Rochester
# School of Medicine and Dentistry

Rochester, New York

## ADDRESS INQUIRIES TO:

Stephen Robson
Rochester Early Medical Scholars
University of Rochester
Undergraduate Admissions—Meliora Hall
Rochester, New York 14627
(716) 275-3221

## PURPOSE

The Rochester Early Medical Scholars Program (REMS) provides conditional acceptance to the University of Rochester School of Medicine and Dentistry to a group of exceptionally talented and motivated students. REMS allows undergraduates the utmost flexibility in degree programs, mentoring relationships with medical school staff, and early exposure to medical school curriculum through a series of lectures and seminars.

## REQUIREMENTS FOR ENTRANCE

Students are selected for this program during their senior year of high school from a national pool. A recommended high school curriculum includes two years of foreign language and four years each of English, social studies, mathematics, and science. A transcript which includes Honors or AP courses is preferable. Applicants are expected to take the SAT or ACT Assessment.

## SELECTION FACTORS

Outstanding achievement in a challenging high school curriculum, character, interests, maturity and motivation necessary for a career in medicine as well as a required interview for finalists are the academic and personal characteristics considered for entry into the REMS program. Interviews are required. In the 1995–96 entering class, REMS students had an average SAT verbal score of 640 and a math score of 707. In order to take their place in the first year medical school class, students must maintain a 3.0 overall grade point average and a 3.3 grade point average in their premedical course requirements.

## CURRICULUM

The eight-year program leads to a baccalaureate degree and the M.D. degree, both granted by the University of Rochester. Students must complete the baccalaureate degree. The most popular major is biology. Undergraduates are encouraged to pursue a variety of academic disciplines in addition to completing their premedical course requirements.

## EXPENSES

Undergraduate tuition in 1995–96 was $18,730 per year and annual fees total $445.

## FINANCIAL AID

University of Rochester scholarships and loans plus governmental loans are available. For more information, write the Office of Financial Aid, University of Rochester, Meliora Hall, Rochester, NY 14627; or phone (716) 275-3226.

## APPLICATION AND ACCEPTANCE POLICIES

Filing of application:
  Earliest date: Oct. 15
  Latest date: Dec. 20
Application fee: $50
Acceptance notice:
  Earliest date: April 1
  Latest date: April 15
Applicant's response to acceptance offer: May 1
Deposit to hold place in class: $400; nonrefundable
Starting date: Sept.

## INFORMATION ON 1995–96 ENTERING CLASS

| Number of | In-State | Out-of-State | Total |
|---|---|---|---|
| Applicants | 205 | 299 | 504 |
| Applicants Interviewed | 14 | 26 | 40 |
| New Entrants | 3 | 7 | 10 |

# Case Western Reserve University

## Cleveland, Ohio

### ADDRESS INQUIRIES TO:

John D. Cameron, *Assistant Director of Admissions*
Office of Undergraduate Admission
Case Western Reserve University
10900 Euclid Avenue
Cleveland, Ohio 44106-7055
(216) 368-4450

### PURPOSE

This program is intended to provide college students with a greater sense of freedom and choice in the pursuit of a premedical baccalaureate degree.

### REQUIREMENTS FOR ENTRANCE

Students are selected for this program during the senior year of high school. Both residents and nonresidents of Ohio are considered for admission. Applicants are expected to have completed the following courses by the time they graduate from high school: one year each of biology, chemistry, and physics and four years of mathematics. They must take either the ACT Assessment or the SAT I and three SAT II Tests.

### SELECTION FACTORS

The high school academic record, standardized test reports, the applicant's history of interests and activities, and a required interview are factors taken into account in offering admission to an applicant. Evidence of strong interpersonal and leadership skills is also sought. In the 1995–96 entering class, the average combined SAT scores were 1480. The average combined ACT score was 33, and the average high school GPA was 4.35.

### CURRICULUM

This eight-year program leads to the baccalaureate and M.D. degrees granted by Case Western Reserve University. Students are expected to complete the requirements for any of the baccalaureate degrees awarded by the colleges of the university. They are expected to satisfy all requirements of and earn a baccalaureate prior to matriculating in the School of Medicine. The work taken for the baccalaureate must include the studies specifically required of applicants by the School of Medicine: one year of biology, two years of chemistry includ-ing organic chemistry, one year of physics, and freshman expository writing. No specific major concentration is required for the premedical undergraduate phase. To date, the majors most commonly taken have been chemistry and biochemistry. Biology has been the next most popular major.

The first four years of the program are devoted to study for the baccalaureate and the last four years to the curriculum for medicine. Students in the medical phase are required to pass Step 1 of the USMLE examinations for promotion within the program and are required to pass Step 2 of the USMLE examination in order to graduate.

### EXPENSES

In 1995–96 the tuition for the undergraduate phase of the program was $16,300 per year.

### FINANCIAL AID

Sources of aid for the undergraduate phase include student loans, work-study, and university grants and scholarships. For information about aid in the undergraduate phase, write the Office of Financial Aid, Case Western Reserve University, 10900 Euclid Avenue, Cleveland, OH 44106-7049. For information about financial aid during medical school, contact Financial Aid Officer, Room T303, School of Medicine, Case Western Reserve University, Cleveland, OH 44106-4920.

### APPLICATION AND ACCEPTANCE POLICIES

Filing of application:
   Latest date: Jan. 1
Application fee: None
Acceptance notice:
   Latest date: April 15
Applicant's response to acceptance offer:
   Maximum time: 2 weeks
Deposit to hold place in class: $200; nonrefundable
Starting date: Last week in Aug.

### INFORMATION ON 1995–96 ENTERING CLASS

| Number of | Total |
|---|---|
| Applicants | 750 |
| Applicants Interviewed | 60 |
| New Entrants | 19 |

# Northeastern Ohio Universities College of Medicine

Rootstown, Ohio

## ADDRESS INQUIRIES TO:

Karen Berger, *Associate Director of Admissions*
Northeastern Ohio Universities
College of Medicine
4209 State Route 44, P.O. Box 95
Rootstown, Ohio 44272-0095
(216) 325-2511

## PURPOSE

The mission of the Northeastern Ohio Universities College of Medicine (NEOUCOM) is to graduate qualified physicians oriented to the practice of medicine at the community level, with an emphasis on primary care: family medicine, internal medicine, pediatrics, and obstetrics-gynecology.

## REQUIREMENTS FOR ENTRANCE

Students are selected for this program during the senior year of high school. Both residents and nonresidents of Ohio are eligible to apply; however, strong preference is given to in-state applicants. Applicants are expected to have pursued a solid college preparatory curriculum, including four years of mathematics and four years of science. They must take either the ACT or the SAT.

## SELECTION FACTORS

High school grades and test scores are some of the academic factors taken into account in offering admission to applicants. In 1995–96, the mean high school GPA of Ohio resident matriculants was 3.87 and 3.99 for nonresidents. The average test score for Ohio residents who took the ACT was 29 and 30 for nonresidents. Ohio residents taking the SAT scored an average of 1275 while nonresidents scored an average of 1293. Career maturity and emotional maturity are among the personal qualities weighed by the admissions committee. An interview is required by invitation only.

## CURRICULUM

Students in this combined-degree program study for a baccalaureate degree granted by Youngstown State University, Kent State University, or the University of Akron and for the M.D. degree granted by NEOUCOM.

Students must complete requirements for a bachelor's degree with a major in integrated life sciences. The curriculum takes six or seven years to complete. Some of the educational innovations offered include an introduction to clinical medicine course taught at area family practice centers in the sophomore medical school year and a one-month primary care preceptorship course in the junior medical school year. Further, most of the basic science courses are taught in just one year (M 1) in contrast to the more traditional two-year sequence.

Students are expected to pass both Step 1 and Step 2 of the USMLE examinations for graduation from Northeastern Ohio Universities College of Medicine.

## EXPENSES

Tuition and fees for years 1 and 2 for 1995–96 were determined by each undergraduate university.

## FINANCIAL AID

Sources of aid are scholarships, grants, loans, and work. For more information on financial aid, contact Northeastern Ohio Universities College of Medicine, Financial Aid Office at (216) 325-2511 (x508/509); University of Akron, Financial Aid Office, (216) 972-7032; Kent State University, Financial Aid Office, (216) 672-2972; or Youngstown State University, Financial Aid Office; or phone (216) 742-3505.

## APPLICATION AND ACCEPTANCE POLICIES

Filing of application*:
  Earliest date: Sept. 1
  Latest date: Dec. 31
Application fee: $25
Acceptance notice:
  Earliest date: April 1
  Latest date: July 20
Applicant's response to acceptance offer:
  Maximum time: 1 to 2 weeks
Deposit to hold place in class: None
Starting date: June or July
*Beginning with the 1995 entering class, applicants apply directly to NEOUCOM, not the individual undergraduate universities.

## INFORMATION ON 1995–96 ENTERING CLASS

| Number of | In-State | Out-of-State | Total |
| --- | --- | --- | --- |
| Applicants | 455 | 345 | 800 |
| Applicants Interviewed | 217 | 33 | 250 |
| New Entrants | 99 | 6 | 105 |

# Lehigh University and Medical College of Pennsylvania and Hahnemann University School of Medicine

Bethlehem, Pennsylvania

## ADDRESS INQUIRIES TO:

Office of Admissions
27 Memorial Drive West
Lehigh University
Bethlehem, Pennsylvania 18105
(610) 758-3100

## PURPOSE

This program gives gifted high school students who are certain that they want to become physicians the opportunity to obtain a liberal arts education and to reduce their total educational cost.

## REQUIREMENTS FOR ENTRANCE

Students are selected for this program during the senior year of high school. Residents and nonresidents of Pennsylvania are considered for this program. Applicants are expected to have completed the following courses by the time they finish high school: four years each of English and mathematics and two years each of history, science, and foreign language. Applicants are expected to take the SAT. SAT II tests are not required but are recommended (i.e., math, English composition, and chemistry).

## SELECTION FACTORS

Generally, a combined SAT score of 1360 (recentered) and rank in the top 10 percent of the high school class are necessary for entrance in this program. In 1995–96, matriculants had a high school GPA of 3.9, a SAT Verbal score of 650 (original), and an SAT Math score of 750 (original). Maturity, stability, scholarship, flexibility, independence, and service to others are personal characteristics sought among applicants. An interview is required. Once admitted to the program, students are expected to maintain an overall grade-point average of 3.45 or better with no grade less than a C in any course. Candidates are required to take the MCAT. It is required that the three numbered scores equal or exceed 9 on a 1–15 scale.

## CURRICULUM

This program, six years in duration, allows students to obtain a bachelor's degree from Lehigh University and an M.D. degree from the medical college. Students do have the flexibility of remaining three years rather than two at Lehigh, however, to pursue additional coursework or study abroad.

Students are not required to complete work for the bachelor's degree; however, specific course requirements for the degree include eight semesters of English, eight semesters of math, nine semesters of natural and physical sciences, three semesters each of humanities and social sciences, a freshman seminar, a writing intensive, and four semesters of electives.

All students must pass USMLE Step 1 in order to graduate from medical school and post a score for Step 2.

## EXPENSES

In 1995–96 tuition at Lehigh University was $19,650 per year.

## FINANCIAL AID

Institutional scholarships and loans are available, as well as federal loan programs and armed services scholarships. More financial aid information can be obtained from the Financial Aid Office, Lehigh University, 218 W. Packer Avenue, Bethlehem, PA 18015.

## APPLICATION AND ACCEPTANCE POLICIES

Filing of application:
  Earliest date: Sept. 1
  Latest date: Dec. 1
Application fee: $40
Acceptance notice:
  Earliest date: April 1
  Latest date: April 15
Applicant's response to acceptance offer:
  Maximum time: May 1
Deposit to hold place in class: $300; nonrefundable
Starting date: August

## INFORMATION ON 1995–96 ENTERING CLASS

| Number of | Total |
| --- | --- |
| Applicants | 284 |
| Applicants Interviewed | 76 |
| New Entrants | 14 |

# Penn State University and Jefferson Medical College of Thomas Jefferson University

University Park, Pennsylvania

## ADDRESS INQUIRIES TO:

Undergraduate Admissions Office
201 Shields Building
Box 3000
Penn State University
University Park, Pennsylvania 16802
(814) 865-5471

## PURPOSE

This program, which began in 1963, is a cooperative effort between Pennsylvania State University and Jefferson Medical College of Thomas Jefferson University in Philadelphia. Students can earn both the B.S. and M.D. degrees in six calendar years after graduation from high school.

## REQUIREMENTS FOR ENTRANCE

Students are selected for this program only during the senior year of high school. Both residents and nonresidents of Pennsylvania are considered for admission, but preference is given to qualified applicants from Pennsylvania. Applicants are expected to have completed the following courses by the time they graduate from high school: four units of English, one and one-half units of algebra, one unit of plane geometry, one-half unit of trigonometry, three units of science, and five units from social studies, humanities, and/or arts.

## SELECTION FACTORS

To be considered for this program, applicants must be in the top 10 percent of their high school class and offer a combined SAT score of 1380 or higher and 1440 (recentered). In the 1995–96 entering class, the average combined score on the SAT was 1410. Motivation, compassion, integrity, dedication, and performance in nonacademic areas are among the personal characteristics sought in applicants. An interview is required.

Special attention is given to the student's progress during each semester while at Penn State University. Students must take a full course load and maintain a minimum GPA of 3.5 in both science and nonscience courses. For subsequent admission to Jefferson Medical College, students in this combined-degree program must take the MCAT prior to matriculation into medical school.

## CURRICULUM

This six-year program leads to a baccalaureate degree granted by Penn State University and to the M.D. degree awarded by Jefferson Medical College.

Students begin this program in June immediately after high school graduation. They spend two full years on the Penn State, University Park campus and then proceed to Jefferson Medical College for their regular four-year curriculum. The B.S. degree from Penn State University is awarded after successful completion of the sophomore year at Jefferson Medical College, and the M.D. degree is awarded after successful completion of the senior year at Jefferson. While at Jefferson students must take and pass steps 1 and 2 of the USMLE examinations.

## EXPENSES

Undergraduate tuition at Penn State in 1995–96 for residents of Pennsylvania was $4,548 per semester and for nonresidents $9,574 per semester. Tuition for 1995–96 at Jefferson Medical College was $24,500 for residents and nonresidents.

## FINANCIAL AID

Scholarships, loans, and grants are the sources of financial assistance available. For more information write the Office of Student Financial Aid, Penn State University, University Park, PA 16802.

## APPLICATION AND ACCEPTANCE POLICIES

Filing of application:
  Earliest date: Sept. 1
  Latest date: Nov. 30
Application fee: $40
Acceptance notice:
  Earliest date: March 1
Applicant's response to acceptance offer:
  Maximum time: May 1
Deposit to hold place in class: $225;
  all but $75 refundable
Starting date: June

## INFORMATION ON 1995–96 ENTERING CLASS

| Number of | Total |
|---|---|
| Applicants | 476 |
| Applicants Interviewed | 139 |
| New Entrants | 61 |

# Villanova University and Medical College of Pennsylvania and Hahnemann University School of Medicine

Villanova, Pennsylvania

## ADDRESS INQUIRIES TO:

Office of Undergraduate Admissions
Villanova University
800 Lancaster Avenue
Villanova, Pennsylvania 19085-1699
1-800-338-7927

## PURPOSE

This combined-degree program provides outstanding high school seniors who are highly motivated toward a medical profession an opportunity to complete a strong liberal arts undergraduate program and medical school in six or seven years.

## REQUIREMENTS FOR ENTRANCE

Students are selected for this program during the senior year of high school. Residents and nonresidents of Pennsylvania are considered for the program. Applicants are expected to have completed the following courses by the time they finish high school: four years each of English and mathematics; two years each of history, and modern language; and one year each of biology, chemistry and physics. Applicants are expected to take the SAT.

## SELECTION FACTORS

Generally, a combined SAT score of 1300 and rank in the top 10 percent of the high school class are necessary for entrance in this program. In 1995–96 matriculants had a high school GPA of 3.9, an SAT Verbal score of 661, and an SAT Mathematics score of 709. Maturity, stability, scholarship, flexibility, independence, and service to others are personal characteristics sought among applicants. An interview is required. Once admitted to the program, students are required to take the MCAT in the spring of their second or third year. A score of 9 or better and a 3.45 GPA are required for medical school admission.

## CURRICULUM

This program, six or seven years in duration, allows students to obtain a bachelor's degree from Villanova University and an M.D. degree from the medical school.

Students may elect a six- or seven-year program majoring in biology and general science comprehensive. The following chart shows the emphasis of the curriculum:

| Year | Percent Liberal Arts | Percent Medicine |
|---|---|---|
| 1 | 30 | 70 |
| 2 | 30 | 70 |
| 3 | 70 | 30 |
| 4 | 0 | 100 |
| 5 | 0 | 100 |
| 6 | 0 | 100 |
| 7 | 0 | 100 |

All students must post a passing score on Step 1 and post a score on Step 2 of USMLE in order to graduate from medical school.

## EXPENSES

In 1995–96, tuition at Villanova University was $16,100 per year plus student fees.

## FINANCIAL AID

Institutional scholarships and loans are available as well as federal loan programs. More information about financial aid can be obtained from the Office of Financial Aid, Villanova University, Villanova, PA 19085; phone: (610) 519-4010.

## APPLICATION AND ACCEPTANCE POLICIES

Filing of application:
    Earliest date: Sept. 1
    Latest date: Dec. 15
Application fee: $40
Acceptance notice:
    Earliest date: March 1
    Latest date: April 1
Applicant's response to acceptance offer:
    Maximum time: May 1
Deposit to hold place in class: $400; nonrefundable
Starting date: Aug.

## INFORMATION ON 1995–96 ENTERING CLASS

| Number of | In-State | Out-of-State | Total |
|---|---|---|---|
| Applicants | 84 | 275 | 359 |
| Applicants Interviewed | 9 | 48 | 57 |
| New Entrants | 8 | 1 | 9 |

# Brown University

## Providence, Rhode Island

### ADDRESS INQUIRIES TO:

College Admission Office
Brown University
Box 1876
Providence, Rhode Island 02912
(401) 863-2378

### PURPOSE

The Program in Liberal Medical Education (PLME) offers a unique experience in medical education. Designed as an eight-year continuum, the program combines liberal arts and professional education to enable each student to develop advanced level competence in a chosen field of scholarship. Great flexibility is built into the program. Each student develops an individualized educational plan in close collaboration with PLME faculty advisers. The PLME is the primary route of admission to Brown University's medical school.

### REQUIREMENTS FOR ENTRANCE

Students are selected for the PLME in the senior year of high school. The Brown Admission Office recommends that applicants should have pursued the following: four years of English, with significant emphasis on writing; three years of college preparatory mathematics; three years of foreign language; two years of laboratory science above the freshman level; two years of history, including American history; at least one year of course work in the arts; and at least one year of elective academic subjects. Prospective science or engineering majors should have taken physics, chemistry, and advanced mathematics. Familiarity with computers is recommended for all applicants. Applicants must take the SAT (SAT I) and three CEEB Achievement Tests (SAT II), or the ACT.

### SELECTION FACTORS

Students are selected on the basis of scholarship, accomplishment and promise, and intellectual curiosity. Those applicants who indicate an interest in pursuing an academic area to an advanced degree of scholarship are particularly sought. In addition, emotional maturity, character, motivation, sensitivity, and caring are personal characteristics considered in offering admission to an applicant. In the 1995–96 entering class, students on average were in the top 2 percent of their high school class and had achieved on the average a score of 640 on the SAT Verbal and 710 on the SAT Mathematics. An interview is not required.

### CURRICULUM

The PLME leads to a baccalaureate degree and to the M.D. degree granted by Brown University. Students must complete a baccalaureate degree in the field of their choice. Each student's educational plan is highly individualized. The PLME has introduced several innovations in medical education, including a competency-based curriculum that defines nine abilities and a core knowledge base expected of all graduates in the M.D. class of 2000 and beyond. All students must post a passing score on Step 2 of USMLE in order to graduate from medical school.

### EXPENSES

In 1995–96 the undergraduate tuition at Brown University was $20,608 per year plus $640 in yearly fees.

### FINANCIAL AID

For undergraduates in the first four years of the PLME, financial aid is awarded by the Financial Aid Office at Brown University as a package. Students are awarded monies via scholarships, work-study, and loans. During the last four years of the PLME, financial aid is administered by the Office of Admissions and Financial Aid of the school of medicine. Both loans and scholarships are available, although loans are the most common form of assistance.

### APPLICATION AND ACCEPTANCE POLICIES

Filing of application:
   Earliest date: Nov. 1
   Latest date: Jan. 1
Application fee: $55
Acceptance notice:
   Earliest date: Dec. 15
   Latest date: April 3
Applicant's response to acceptance offer:
   Maximum time: May 1
Deposit to hold place in class: None
Starting date: Early Sept.

### INFORMATION ON 1995–96 ENTERING CLASS

| Number of | In-State | Out-of-State | Total |
|---|---|---|---|
| Applicants | 56 | 2,146 | 2,202 |
| New Entrants | 5 | 58 | 63 |

# East Tennessee State University

**Johnson City, Tennessee**

## ADDRESS INQUIRIES TO:

Dr. Lattie F. Collins
*Director, Premedical-Medical Program*
Office of Medical Professions Advisement
East Tennessee State University
P.O. Box 70,592
Johnson City, Tennessee 37614-0592
(423) 439-5602; 439-6905 (FAX)

## PURPOSE

The Premedical-Medical (PMMD) Program at East Tennessee State University integrates the undergraduate premedical and medical education curricula and establishes a continuum of medical education from college entry through the awarding of the M.D. degree. This is not an accelerated program; eight full years are required from college entry until completion of the M.D. degree.

## REQUIREMENTS FOR ENTRANCE

Students are selected for the PMMD Program at the end of their freshman year on the East Tennessee State University (ETSU) campus, during which they enroll in a prescribed group of courses. This is not a transfer program; students who have earned more than 14 semester hours credit before entering ETSU are not eligible for selection. There are no state residency requirements, but residents of Tennessee may be given preference in the selection process. There are no specific high school course requirements. Applicants must have taken the ACT and/or SAT assessments.

## SELECTION FACTORS

Applicants must have graduated in the top 20 percent of their high school classes, and must have scored at or above the 80th percentile for college-bound high school seniors on the ACT and/or SAT. Students must maintain a GPA of 3.3/4.0 or better during their freshman year in order to qualify for selection. The average high school GPA for the 1995–96 entering student was 3.7/4.0. The average GPA for the freshman year was 3.5/4.0. The average composite ACT assessment was 28. Two or more interviews are required. Students are not required to take the MCAT for selection, but are required to take the MCAT and to perform at a satisfactory level prior to beginning the medical school component of the program.

## CURRICULUM

The Premedical-Medical Program leads to a baccalaureate degree in the College of Arts and Sciences and the M.D. degree awarded by the James H. Quillen College of Medicine. All students in this program must complete a major or minor in an approved humanities discipline and must participate in a special non-credit seminar on topics of current interest in medicine.

Students are required to pass Step 1 of the USMLE before entering the final year of clerkship studies. Students must pass Step 2 of the USMLE in order to graduate.

## EXPENSES

In 1995–96, the undergraduate tuition rate was $1,880 per year and the medical school tuition rate was $8,910 per year for Tennessee residents. The corresponding out-of-state tuition rates were $6,010 and $15,890.

Premedical-medical students pay undergraduate tuition for the first four years and medical school tuition for the remaining four years.

## FINANCIAL AID

For more information, contact the Office of Financial Aid, East Tennessee State University, P.O. Box 70,772, Johnson City, TN 37614 (undergraduate); and the Office of Financial Aid, James H. Quillen College of Medicine, East Tennessee State University, P.O. Box 70,580, Johnson City, TN 37614 (medical school).

## APPLICATION AND ACCEPTANCE POLICIES

Filing of application (end freshman year):
   Earliest date (typical): March 15
   Latest date (typical): April 1
Application fee: None
Acceptance notice:
   Earliest date: July 1
   Latest date: August 1
Applicant's response to acceptance offer:
   Maximum time: 2 weeks
Deposit to hold place in class: None
Starting date: Aug. 15

## INFORMATION ON 1995–96 ENTERING CLASS

| Number of | In-State | Out-of-State | Total |
|---|---|---|---|
| Applicants | 12 | 2 | 14 |
| Applicants Interviewed | 12 | 2 | 14 |
| New Entrants | 9 | 2 | 11 |

# Fisk University
# Meharry Medical College

**Nashville, Tennessee**

## ADDRESS INQUIRIES TO:

Henry A. Moses, Ph.D., *Associate Vice President for College Relations and Lifelong Learning*
1005 D.B. Todd, Jr. Boulevard
Nashville, TN 37208
(615) 327-6425

## PURPOSE

The Joint Program in Biomedical Sciences is designed to address America's need to train bright young minorities who are dedicated to find solutions to biomedical problems through research, and who will be future health care providers.

## REQUIREMENTS FOR ENTRANCE

Students are selected at the end of their first semester of undergraduate course work on the Fisk University campus. There are no specific high school course requirements. Applicants must have taken the ACT and/or SAT assessments.

## SELECTION FACTORS

The courses taken and grades earned at Fisk University, plus ACT and/or SAT scores are considerations for eligibility for this program. Applicants must rank in the top 20 percent of their high school class. Students must take the MCAT prior to admission into the clinical phase of the program, and a satisfactory score is required for medical school admission.

## CURRICULUM

The Joint Program in Biomedical Sciences, seven years in duration, allows students to obtain a baccalaureate degree from Fisk University and an M.D. degree from Meharry Medical College.

Course requirements for the baccalaureate degree include 8 semesters of natural and physical sciences and 12 semesters each in the humanities and social sciences. Students are required to spend two summers in structured academic enrichment.

Students must take steps 1 and 2 of the USMLE during the medical school portion of the program. Passing these examinations is a factor in promotion and graduation from medical school.

The most frequent major chosen by students is biology, followed by chemistry. The following chart shows the emphasis of the curriculum:

| *Year* | *Percent Liberal Arts* | *Percent Medicine* |
|---|---|---|
| 1 | 100 | 0 |
| 2 | 100 | 0 |
| 3 | 100 | 0 |
| 4 | 0 | 100 |
| 5 | 0 | 100 |
| 6 | 0 | 100 |
| 7 | 0 | 100 |

## EXPENSES

Undergraduate tuition is $6,740 for residents and nonresidents, plus $250 in annual fees. Tuition for medical school is $16,500, plus $1,865 in annual fees.

## FINANCIAL AID

Sources of financial aid include college scholarships, need-based grants, and federal and private loans. Applicants can receive more information from the Office of Student Financial Aid, Meharry Medical College, 1005 D.B. Todd Boulevard, Nashville, TN 37208.

---

### APPLICATION AND ACCEPTANCE POLICIES

Filing of application:
  Earliest date: Feb. 1
  Latest date: Feb. 15
Application fee: None
Acceptance notice:
  Earliest date: Feb. 21
  Latest date: March 1
Applicant's response to acceptance offer:
  Maximum time: one week
Deposit to hold place in class: None
Starting date: Retroactive second semester, undergraduate year 1

### INFORMATION ON 1995–96 ENTERING CLASS

More information may be obtained from the Office of Student Financial Aid at the above address.

---

# Rice University
# Baylor College of Medicine

Houston, Texas

## ADDRESS INQUIRIES TO:

Office of Admissions
One Baylor Plaza
Room 106A
Houston, Texas 77030
(713) 798-4841

## PURPOSE

To promote the education of future physicians who are sci-entifically competent, compassionate, and socially conscious in order to apply insight from extensive study of liberal arts and other disciplines to the study of modern medical science.

## REQUIREMENTS FOR ENTRANCE

Students are selected for this program during their senior year of high school. Both residents and nonresidents of Texas are considered for admission. Applicants are expected to have had a varied and rigorous high school program with high aca-demic achievement. They must take the SAT I or ACT plus three SAT II subject tests.

## SELECTION FACTORS

The high school academic record, standardized test scores, course selection, and school recommendation are factors taken into account in offering admission to an applicant. In the 1995–96 entering class, students averaged above the top five percent.

## CURRICULUM

This is is not an accelerated program; all students must complete four years of undergraduate education and four years of medical school.

Students earn a baccalaureate degree from Rice University, and are awarded an M.D. degree from Baylor College of Medicine. Minimum course requirements for this program include at least two semesters each in the humanities and social sciences, and eight semesters in the natural and physical sciences.

The medicine portion of the curriculum devotes roughly 1½ years to the basic sciences with clinical experience, and 2½ years to clinical science with some basic sciences.

The MCAT is not required for promotion or admission to the medical school. Students are required to take Step 1 of the USMLE in their sophomore or junior year. They are also required to take Step 2 of the USMLE, but passing these examinations is not a graduation requirement.

## EXPENSES

In 1995–96 the undergraduate tuition for all students was $11,650 per year plus $375 in student fees. The medical school tuition for residents was $6,550; for nonresidents it was $19,650 annually plus $1,559 in student fees.

## FINANCIAL AID

Sources of aid include academic and athletic scholarships, and need-based loans. Applicants can receive more informa-tion from the Rice Admission Office, M.S. 17, 6100 Main Street, Houston, Texas 77035.

## APPLICATION AND ACCEPTANCE POLICIES

Filing of application:
   Earliest date: Nov. 1
   Latest date: Dec. 1
Application fee: $25
Acceptance notice:
   Latest date: Mid-April
Applicant's response to acceptance offer:
   Maximum time: two weeks
Deposit to hold place in class: $100; nonrefundable
Starting date: Aug 20

## INFORMATION ON 1995–96 ENTERING CLASS

Total number of applicants: 748

| Number of | In-State | Out-of-State | Total |
| --- | --- | --- | --- |
| Applicants Interviewed | 18 | 21 | 39 |
| New Entrants | 10 | 4 | 14 |

# Eastern Virginia Medical School

## Norfolk, Virginia

## ADDRESS INQUIRIES TO:

Office of Admissions
Eastern Virginia Medical School
721 Fairfax Avenue
Norfolk ,Virginia 23507-2000
(804) 446-5812

## PURPOSE

We currently have combined programs with four universities—The College of William and Mary, Old Dominion University, Hampton University, and Norfolk State University. The purpose of these programs is to enlist outstanding high school and undergraduate students into a track which provides great freedom and choice in the pursuit of a baccalaureate degree.

## REQUIREMENTS FOR ENTRANCE

Depending on the undergraduate institution, students are selected during their senior year of high school or their freshman year of college. Both residents and nonresidents of Virginia are eligible to apply. There are no specific high school course requirements, but students must take the SAT.

## SELECTION FACTORS

Although the criteria for consideration into the program differs at each of the undergraduate institutions, all applicants are screened on the basis of their academic qualifications. Selected applicants are invited for an interview.

## CURRICULUM

The eight-year curriculum leads to a baccalaureate degree awarded by the College of William and Mary, Old Dominion University, Hampton University, or Norfolk State University. The M.D. degree is granted by Eastern Virginia Medical School. The course requirements for the baccalaureate degree vary at each undergraduate institution, but the most frequent major is biology.

Hampton University and Norfolk State University require students to take the MCAT in April of the year that they apply to AMCAS; it is not a factor in promotion to the medical school. The College of William and Mary, and Old Dominion University do not require students to take the MCAT. Step 1 of the USMLE must be taken at the completion of the second year of medical school. Students must pass steps 1 and 2 of the USMLE to complete the program and receive the M.D. degree.

## EXPENSES

In 1995–96 the annual tuition for medical school for residents was $13,000 and for nonresidents it was $23,000. The student fees were $1,283 per year.

## FINANCIAL AID

For information about financial aid during the undergraduate phase, contact the Office of Financial Aid at the institutions outlined. Four programs are available: The College of William and Mary, Randolph A. Coleman, Ph.D., (804) 221-2476; Old Dominion University, Christopher Osgood, Ph.D., (804) 683-3595; Hampton University, Alfred McQueen, Ph.D., (804) 727-5282; and Norfolk State University, Larry Mattix, Ph.D., (804) 683-2511. For information about financial aid during the medical school phase contact the Office of Financial Aid at (804) 446-5813.

## APPLICATION AND ACCEPTANCE POLICIES

Information varies at each undergraduate institution.

## INFORMATION ON 1995–96 ENTERING CLASS

Total number of applicants: 119

| Number of | In-State | Out-of-State | Total |
| --- | --- | --- | --- |
| Applicants Interviewed | 24 | 17 | 41 |
| New Entrants | 9 | 0 | 9 |

# University of Wisconsin— Madison Medical School

Madison, Wisconsin

## ADDRESS INQUIRIES TO:

Medical Scholars Program
University of Wisconsin—Madison Medical School
1300 University Avenue, Room 1250
Madison, Wisconsin 53706
(608) 263-7561

## PURPOSE

The Medical Scholars Program provides conditional admission to the University of Wisconsin—Madison Medical School for 50 highly qualified Wisconsin high school seniors. Medical scholars are a part of the medical school community and may participate in specially designed basic science and clinical experiences.

## REQUIREMENTS FOR ENTRANCE

Students are selected for this program during the senior year of high school. Only residents of Wisconsin are eligible to apply. Applicants are expected to have completed the following courses by the time they graduate from high school: eight semesters of mathematics, eight semesters of English, six semesters of science (at least one semester each of biology, chemistry, and physics), six semesters of social studies, and four semesters of foreign language. They must take either the SAT or the ACT Assessment.

## SELECTION FACTORS

To be eligible for application, a student must have attained a minimum academic GPA of 3.8 (includes English, mathematics, science, social studies, and foreign language in grades 9 through 11) and be ranked in the top five percent of their high school class or have a minimum combined SAT score of 1300 or a minimum composite score of 30 on the ACT Assessment. In the 1995–96 entering class, the average GPA was 3.96, the average SAT Verbal score was 700, and the average composite score on the ACT Assessment was 31. An interview is not required.

## CURRICULUM

This program, normally seven to nine years in duration, allows students to obtain a bachelor's degree from the University of Wisconsin—Madison and an M.D. degree from the University of Wisconsin Medical School.

Students are expected to complete work for the bachelor's degree. Requirements for that degree vary according to the major chosen, but all include course work in the humanities, social sciences, and natural and physical sciences. The most frequent major chosen by students in this program is molecular biology, followed by zoology.

Educational innovations offered include the following: (a) a wide range of experiences in medical science research and exposure to clinical medicine allowing students to integrate undergraduate and medical education; (b) the opportunity to major in any subject; (c) completion of the undergraduate program in three to five years; and (d) a semester or year studying in a foreign country.

Students are expected to take Step 1 of the USMLE examinations at the end of the second year of medical school, with a passing score required in order to begin clinical work. Passing both steps 1 and 2 is a graduation requirement.

## EXPENSE

In 1995–96, residents of Wisconsin paid $2,880.50 per year to attend the University of Wisconsin—Madison and $13,041.50 per year at the University of Wisconsin Medical School.

## FINANCIAL AID

Scholarships and loans are available to students according to their need. More information can be obtained from the University of Wisconsin—Madison Financial Aid Office, 432 North Murray Street, Madison, WI 53706.

## APPLICATION AND ACCEPTANCE POLICIES

Filing of application:
    Earliest date: Sept. 30
    Latest date: Jan. 1
Application fee: None
Acceptance notice:
    Earliest date: April 1
    Latest date: April 1
Applicant's response to acceptance offer:
    Maximum time: May 1
Deposit to hold place in class: None

## INFORMATION ON 1995–96 ENTERING CLASS

| Number of | Total |
| --- | --- |
| Applicants | 275 |
| New Entrants | 52 |

# School Entries

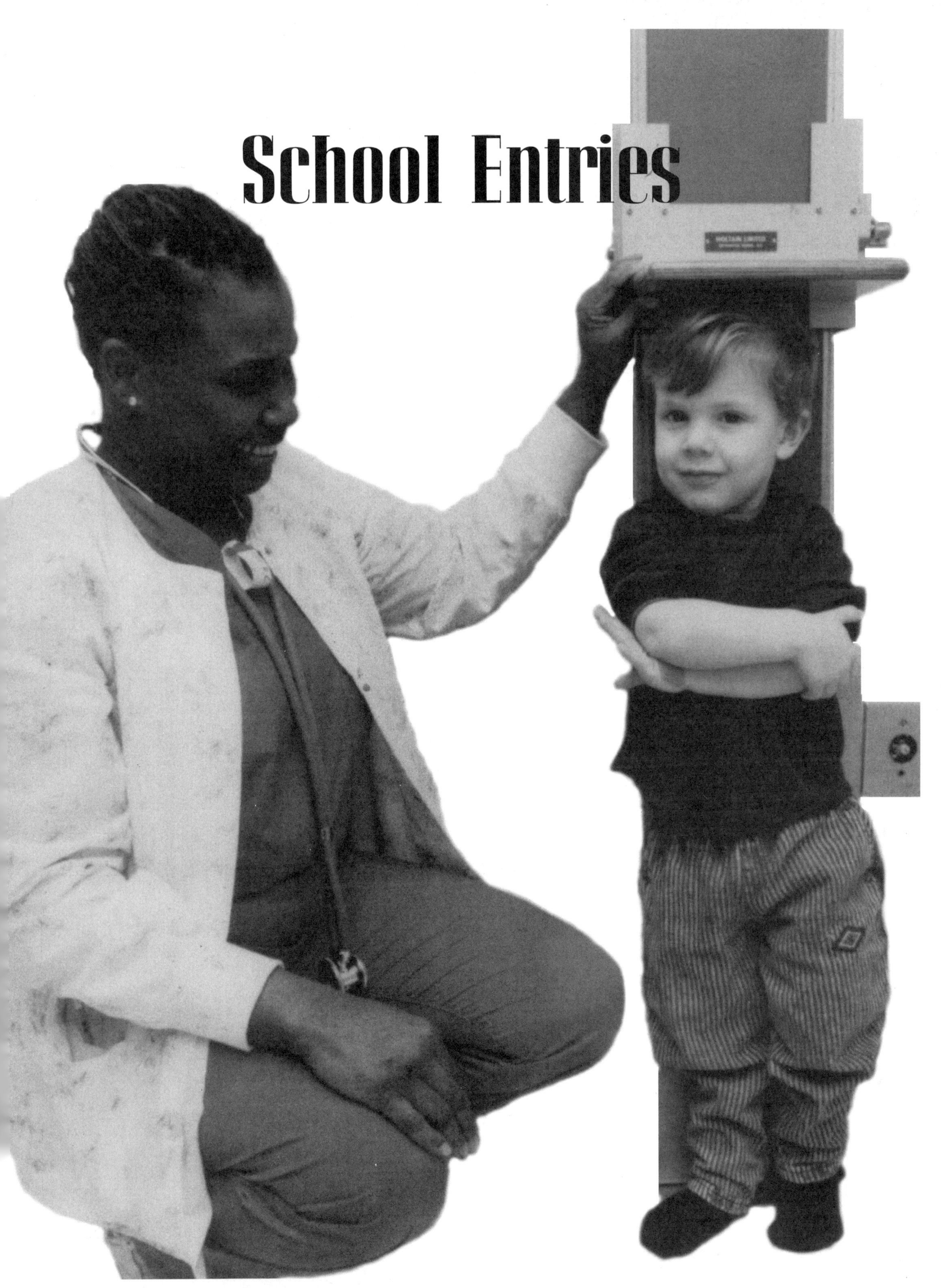

# Information About U.S. Medical Schools
## Accredited by the LCME

Information about individual medical schools is given in the following two-page entries for 122 schools in the United States and 3 schools in Puerto Rico that will be considering applications for fall 1997 entering classes. The schools presented here are fully accredited as of fall 1995 by the Liaison Committee on Medical Education (LCME), which is sponsored by the Association of American Medical Colleges (AAMC) and the American Medical Association (AMA).

The University of Minnesota—Duluth School of Medicine has a two-year basic medical science program; students transfer to the University of Minnesota Medical School—Minneapolis to complete their training. Individual school entries provide the tuition and student fees for a 1995–96 first-year student.

Each school entry provides statistics on the number of applicants, interviewed applicants, and new entrants (students entering medical school for the first time, excluding repeaters and reentrants) to the 1995–96 first-year class. These statistics are presented by residence status—in-state and out-of-state. Foreign nationals who do not have permanent resident status in the United States are included in the out-of-state figures.

## ABBREVIATIONS

Listed below are the abbreviations used in the school entries in this chapter.

AMCAS—American Medical College Application Service

CLEP—College Level Examination Program

FAF—Financial Aid Form

FAFSA—Free Application for Federal Student Aid

GAPSFAS—Graduate and Professional School Financial Aid Service

GPA—Grade-point average

MCAT—Medical College Admission Test

VR—Verbal Reasoning

PS—Physical Sciences

WS—Writing Sample

BS—Biological Sciences

USMLE—United States Medical Licensing Examination

WICHE—Western Interstate Commission for Higher Education

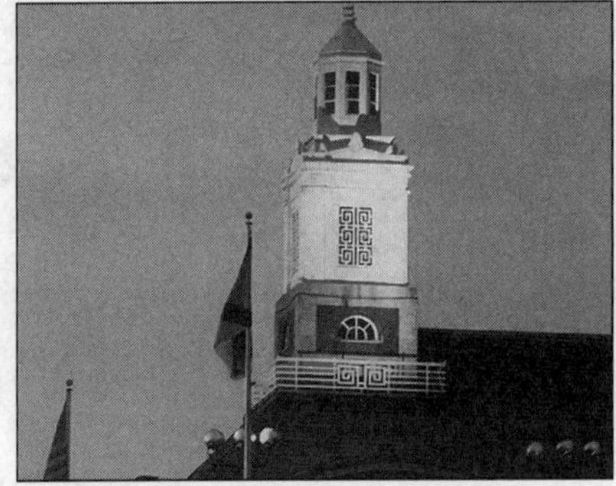

# University of Alabama School of Medicine

**Birmingham, Alabama**

Dr. Harold J. Fallon, *Dean*
Dr. George S. Hand, Jr., *Assistant Dean for Admissions*
Mark H. Martin, *Assistant Director of Medical Student Services for Financial Aid*

## ADDRESS INQUIRIES TO:

Office of Medical Student Services/Admissions
University of Alabama
School of Medicine
VH100
Birmingham, Alabama 35294-0019
(205) 934-2330; 934-8724 (FAX)

## GENERAL INFORMATION

The School of Medicine was founded in Mobile in 1859, shifted to the main campus of the University of Alabama in Tuscaloosa in 1920, and relocated in Birmingham in 1945. The University of Alabama School of Medicine, composed of the medical branches in Tuscaloosa, Birmingham, and Huntsville, was created in 1969. Birmingham is the main campus, and the Huntsville Program and the College of Community Health Sciences in Tuscaloosa are branch campuses.

## CURRICULUM

The academic program consists of a four-year sequence which provides training in basic science and clinical areas. It emphasizes the fundamentals that underlie all medical practice. Consideration is given also to the emotional, cultural, and social characteristics of patients and to the need for adapting medical care to meet their needs. Initially, basic human biology, including anatomy, physiology, biochemistry, nutrition, behavioral sciences, and neurosciences are emphasized. Second-year courses include microbiology, pharmacology, and pathology. The basic science years are completed by an integrative study of organ-system disorders and disease processes. All students are required to pass Step 1 of the USMLE at the end of the second year.

The third year and a part of the fourth year consist of required rotations through the clinical science disciplines (medicine, surgery, pediatrics, obstetrics-gynecology, family medicine/rural medicine, and psychiatry/neurology). This involves participation, under faculty supervision, in the care of patients both in the hospital and in ambulatory settings. The remainder of the fourth year is an elective or individualized experience program. All students are required to pass Step 2 of the USMLE prior to graduation.

Students complete two years of basic science course work in Birmingham; then, the clinical clerkships may be taken among the three clinical campuses during the third and fourth years. Students may choose to be assigned permanently to either Huntsville or Tuscaloosa for completion of the third and fourth years, but electives may be taken in a variety of locations.

The faculty and administration are strongly interested in attracting individuals who will train to be generalist physicians and give strong evidence of a willingness to practice in underserved areas. Curricular changes are being implemented to provide greater emphasis in the training of primary care physicians.

M.D.-Ph.D. program is available for highly qualified students who desire a career in academic medicine.

To facilitate their entry into the School of Medicine, outstanding high school seniors from Alabama who demonstrate strong motivation and maturity for the study of medicine and have earned a 3.5 GPA or better, an ACT score of 30 or higher, and/or an SAT score of 1300 or higher may apply for the Early Medical School Acceptance Program (EMSAP). Students accepted into EMSAP will enter the University of Alabama at Birmingham (UAB) and be provided with medically related experiences during their undergraduate years. In most cases, EMSAP students will be expected to complete four years of undergraduate study at UAB before beginning their medical school studies. EMSAP students will not be required to take the MCAT.

## REQUIREMENTS FOR ENTRANCE

At least 90 semester hours from an accredited institution and the MCAT are required. The MCAT should be taken during the spring before making application in early summer. A program leading to the bachelor's degree is highly recommended. Suitable major areas include the social sciences, humanities, and biological and physical sciences. It is strongly recommended that applicants also have some course work in the behavioral sciences. College work must include:

|  | *Sem. hrs.* |
| --- | --- |
| General biology or zoology | 8 |
| Inorganic chemistry (with lab) | 8 |
| Organic chemistry (with lab) | 8 |
| General physics (with lab) | 8 |
| College mathematics | 6 |
| English (composition and literature) | 6 |

## SELECTION FACTORS

Required interviews are arranged at the discretion of the Admission Committee. Alabama residents are given preference in the selection process, but nonresidents with superior academic credentials (GPA of 3.5 or higher and MCAT subtest scores which average 10 along with superior essay scores) and demonstrated evidence of nonacademic success and commitment are encouraged to apply. Nonresident students with weaker credentials should not apply. Foreign applicants must have a permanent resident visa. Alabama residents from rural areas and from minority groups are especially encouraged to apply. Race, religion, national origin, age, handicap, and sex are not factors in consideration for admission.

Acceptances were issued to 231 students (172 residents, 59 nonresidents) to obtain a class of 165 entering students (including 8 M.D.-Ph.D. students). Class characteristics include: *mean GPA 3.58, mean MCAT: VR-9.7, PS-9.6, BS-9.7; 66 females, 36 ethnic minorities. Undergraduate major,* 42 percent biology, 10 percent chemistry or biochemistry, and 24 percent from other sciences and engineering, with the remainder from a variety of fields including English, history, psychology, nursing, etc. Students came from 55 colleges and universities.

Students in good academic standing may be transferred from other U.S. allopathic medical schools for compelling reasons. Available positions are limited to attrition. Applications are not accepted from individuals attending foreign medical schools.

## FINANCIAL AID

About 76 percent of our students receive financial aid. Available loan funds are disbursed primarily on the basis of demonstrated financial need. State scholarships/loans are available in limited numbers to Alabama residents who can demonstrate economic need. Other scholarships are awarded on a merit basis. Students are advised not to seek outside employment. Summer research opportunities, supported by stipends and fellowships, are available.

## INFORMATION FOR MINORITIES

The Admission Committee attempts to identify and provide academic counseling and information to minority students early in their college careers to facilitate application processes. The School of Medicine will consider waiver of application fees for disadvantaged students, and some interviewing costs may be defrayed. A prematriculation program is provided for students who matriculate.

Public Institution

## APPLICATION AND ACCEPTANCE POLICIES FOR 1997–98 FIRST-YEAR CLASS

*School particpates in AMCAS. See Chapter 4.*

Filing of AMCAS application
    Earliest date: June 1, 1996
    Latest date: Nov. 1, 1996
School application fee after screening: $65
Oldest MCAT scores considered: 1994
Does have Early Decision Program (EDP)
    For Alabama residents only
    EDP application period: June 1–Aug. 1, 1996
    EDP applicants notified by: Oct. 1, 1996
Acceptance notice to regular applicants
    Earliest date: Oct. 15, 1996
    Latest date: Until class is filled
Applicant's response to acceptance offer
    Maximum time: 2 weeks
Requests for deferred entrance considered: Yes
Deposit to hold place in class (applied to tuition):
    $50, due with response to acceptance offer
Deposit refundable prior to: May 15, 1997
Estimated number of new entrants: 150 (12 EDP)
Starting date: Aug. 1997

## TUITION AND STUDENT FEES PER YEAR FOR 1995–96 FIRST-YEAR CLASS

Tuition                 Student fees: $2,159
    Resident: $5,708
    Nonresident: $17,124

## INFORMATION ON 1995–96 FIRST-YEAR CLASS

| Number of | In-State | Out-of-State | Total |
|---|---|---|---|
| Applicants | 578 | 1,738 | 2,316 |
| Applicants Interviewed | 405 | 149 | 554 |
| New Entrants* | 142 | 23 | 165 |

*98% took the MCAT; 97% had baccalaureate degrees.

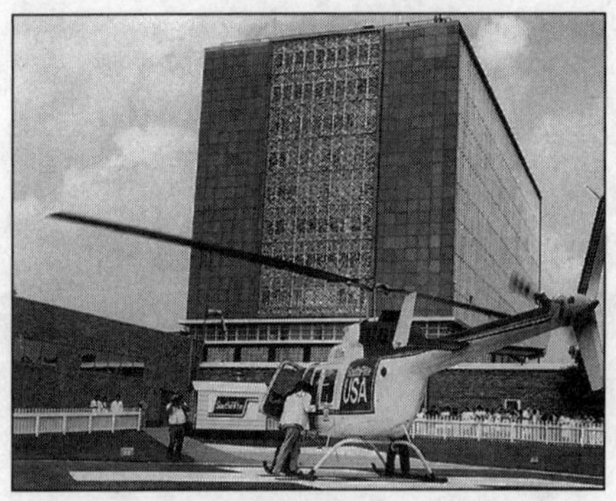

# University of South Alabama College of Medicine

## Mobile, Alabama


Dr. Albert W. Pruitt, *Dean*

Dr. Samuel J. Strada, *Senior Associate Dean*

Dr. Mark Scott, *Director for Admissions*


## ADDRESS INQUIRIES TO:


Office of Admissions, 2015 MSB
University of South Alabama
College of Medicine
Mobile, Alabama 36688-0002
(334) 460-7176; 460-6278 (FAX)


## GENERAL INFORMATION

The College of Medicine of the University of South Alabama was approved by the Board of Trustees of the university in 1967; the legislature of the state of Alabama passed a resolution authorizing the college on August 19, 1967. The college admitted a charter class of 25 students in January 1973 and a full class of 64 students in September 1973. No increase or decrease in the number of entering students is planned. The basic medical sciences are housed on the university campus in a building which was completed in March 1974. The largest site for the clinical education program is the University of South Alabama Medical Center. Operating continuously since 1831, this hospital has provided medical education for more than a century. It functions as the major physician-staffed emergency facility in South Alabama and has been named a Level I trauma center by the Alabama Committee on Trauma. Other clinical training facilities include the U.S.A. Springhill Campus, U.S.A. Cancer Center and Clinical Building, U.S.A. Health Services Building, and Searcy Hospital. Recent acquisition of two additional hospital complexes, Knollwood and Doctors Hospital, ranks the University of South Alabama as the largest medical system in our region.

## CURRICULUM

The first year is devoted to the basic sciences of anatomy, physiology, biochemistry, neuroanatomy, and embryology. However, opportunity for early introduction to clinical problems is afforded by courses such as Correlation Conferences and Medical Practice and Society. The second year includes pathology, physical diagnosis, microbiology-immunology, pharmacology, and behavioral science. Public health/epidemiology and medical genetics round out the second-year curriculum. All students are required to take and pass Step 1 of the USMLE examinations at the end of the second year. The third year is composed of clinical clerkships in medicine, surgery, pediatrics, psychiatry, obstetrics-gynecology, and family practice. The fourth year is composed of 9 rotations of four weeks each. The student is required to select one rotation each in clinical neuroscience, surgical subspecialties, ambulatory care, primary care subspecialty in medicine, pediatrics, or obstetrics-gynecology, acting internship, and an in-house elective. Three of the rotations may be used for approved extra mural experiences. Students are required to take and pass Step 2 of the USMLE examinations in September of the fourth year. An A–F (A, B, C, D, F) grading system is used with the exception of the fourth year, during which an honors/pass/fail system is used.

The philosophy of the institution is to utilize all of the existing resources, which provide opportunities for almost all of the experiences in clinical medicine. After acquiring a sound basis in scientific medicine, students then have the opportunity to select multiple tracks of study.

A combined M.D.-Ph.D. program in basic medical sciences is also offered.

## REQUIREMENTS FOR ENTRANCE

The MCAT and three years of college are required; the baccalaureate degree is highly desirable. Each applicant must have at least 90 semester hours of acceptable credit from an accredited undergraduate institution. Required courses are:

*Sem. hrs.*

| | |
|---|---:|
| General biology (with lab) | 8 |
| General chemistry (with lab) | 8 |
| Organic chemistry (with lab) | 8 |
| General physics (with lab) | 8 |
| Humanities | 8 |
| English composition and/or literature | 8 |
| College mathematics | 8 |

Calculus is highly recommended.

The University of South Alabama College of Medicine does not accept pass/fail grades for required science courses, except in the rare instance in which an applicant's college assigns only pass/fail grades.

Applicants are strongly urged to take the MCAT in the spring of the year of application and to have their basic science requirements completed at the time of application. Required course work in process or fall MCAT scores delay the processing of an application.

## SELECTION FACTORS

The Committee on Admissions will consider seriously all candidates whose undergraduate academic work and scores on the MCAT indicate that they will be able to handle the rigorous curriculum of the College of Medicine. However, consideration will be given to more than scholastic achievement alone. Applicants will be considered from the standpoint of their potential to become conscientious and capable physicians. The University of South Alabama provides equal educational opportunities and is open to all qualified students without regard to race, creed, national origin, sex, or handicap with respect to all of its programs and activities. Because the college is state-supported, preference is shown to Alabama residents; however, residents of the Mississippi Gulf Coast and Florida Panhandle qualify for in-state tuition.

Disadvantaged, rural, and minority residents of Alabama are strongly encouraged to apply. The application process consists of two stages: the preliminary AMCAS application and the final application sent when requested by the Committee on Admissions. This latter application requires recommendations, a photograph, and a $25 fee. After review of the final application, the committee will select those applicants to be invited to the campus for interviews. Fee waivers, based solely on economic need, are granted when documented.

The 64 members of the 1995 entering class came from 30 different undergraduate schools. The *average undergraduate GPA* was 3.60; *average MCAT scores,* VR-9.5, PS-9.3, BS-9.6; 90 percent *residents* of Alabama.

## FINANCIAL AID

The Office of Financial Aid coordinates the programs of assistance available to medical students demonstrating financial need. Scholarships are also available for entering freshmen and medical students who have demonstrated academic excellence and/or financial need.

A limited number of state scholarships/ loans are available to Alabama residents who can demonstrate economic need. After graduation repayment may be made by cash or by the practice of medicine in certain areas of the state for the number of years stipulated by law.

The Medical Student Summer Research Program is available to entering first-year students and rising second-year students. The participants are paid a stipend and no previous research experience is necessary. Part-time employment is available; however, students are discouraged from accepting employment during academic periods.

## INFORMATON FOR MINORITIES

The school is committed to the enrollment and education of individuals from all disadvantaged groups. For information, write Dr. Hattie M. Myles, assistant dean of special programs and student affairs.

Public Institution

## APPLICATION AND ACCEPTANCE POLICIES FOR 1997–98 FIRST-YEAR CLASS

*School participates in AMCAS. See Chapter 4.*

Filing of AMCAS application
    Earliest date: June 1, 1996
    Latest date: Nov. 15, 1996
School application fee after screening: $25
Oldest MCAT scores considered: 1993
Does have Early Decision Program
    For Alabama residents only
    EDP application period: June 1–Aug. 1, 1996
    EDP application notified by: Oct. 1, 1996
Acceptance notice to regular applicants
    Earliest date: Oct. 15, 1996
    Latest date: Until class is filled
Applicant's response to acceptance offer
    Maximum time: 2 weeks
Requests for deferred entrance considered: Yes
Deposit to hold place in class (applied to tuition):
    $50, due with response to acceptance offer
Deposit refundable prior to: May 15, 1997, if requested in writing
Estimated number of new entrants: 64 (10 EDP)
Starting date: Aug. 1997

## TUITION AND STUDENT FEES PER YEAR FOR 1995–96 FIRST-YEAR CLASS

Tuition                Student fees: $567
    Resident: $5,808
    Nonresident: $11,616

## INFORMATION ON 1995–96 FIRST-YEAR CLASS

| Number of | In-State | Out-of-State | Total |
|---|---|---|---|
| Applicants | 550 | 957 | 1,507 |
| Applicants Interviewed | 223 | 10 | 233 |
| New Entrants* | 57 | 7 | 64 |

*All took the MCAT and had baccalaureate degrees

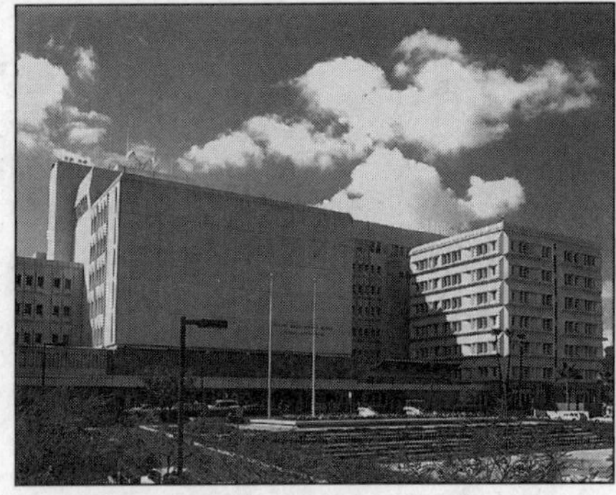

# University of Arizona
# College of Medicine

**Tucson, Arizona**

Dr. James E. Dalen, *Vice President for Health Sciences and Dean, College of Medicine*
Dr. Shirley Nickols Fahey, *Associate Dean*

## ADDRESS INQUIRIES TO:

Admissions Office, Room 2209
University of Arizona
College of Medicine
P.O. Box 245075
Tucson, Arizona 85724-5075
(520) 626-6214; 626-4884 (FAX)

## GENERAL INFORMATION

The College of Medicine enrolled its first class of students in 1967. As a professional and graduate college of the University of Arizona located adjacent to the main campus, its programs provide education and training for both the M.D. and Ph.D. degrees.

The University of Arizona Health Sciences Center complex consists of several interconnected buildings and adjoining structures on a 30-acre site north of the main campus (Basic Sciences Building, Clinical Sciences Building, Life Sciences Building, Outpatient Clinic, University Medical Center, Children's Research Center, and Arizona Cancer Center). Planned or under construction are a heart center, arthritis center, and ambulatory care clinic. The colleges of nursing and pharmacy are located south of the Basic Sciences Building. A student wing of the Basic Sciences Building houses the multi-disciplinary laboratories, anatomy laboratories, the learning resource center, lecture rooms, conference rooms, student lounge, and support facilities.

## CURRICULUM

The overall purpose of the educational program is to give students the desire for life-long learning in medicine by creating study habits that call for the continuous pursuit of knowledge and the capacity to modify previously acquired information. The program also aims to give students the skills to conduct patient care activities as well as the professional attitudes consonant with the charge to provide patients with preventive and curative advice and treatment.

Biologic, cultural, psychosocial, economic, and sociologic concepts and data are provided in the core curriculum. Increasing emphasis is placed on problem-solving ability, beginning with initial instruction and carried through to graduation. Excellence in performance is encouraged and facilitated. Awareness of the milieu in which medicine is practiced is also encouraged. The core curriculum comprises three years of required studies and one year of elective rotations. The learning environment encompasses lectures, small-group instruction, independent study, clinical clerkships, practice in physical diagnosis, computer-based instruction, and a variety of other modes for the learner. Students learn in the classroom, conference room, laboratory, clinic and physician's office, bed units of hospitals, special sites for diagnostic and therapeutic maneuvers, University Medical Center, and a variety of inpatient and outpatient settings in both Tucson and Phoenix. All medical students will participate in an educational experience with an underserved population sometime during medical school. Upon graduation the physician is equipped to continue postgraduate education in general or specialty practice, teaching, or research. A combined M.D.-Ph.D. program of study is also offered.

## REQUIREMENTS FOR ENTRANCE

All applicants must be residents of Arizona or WICHE certified and funded residents of Alaska, Montana, or Wyoming. The MCAT and a minimum of three years of college are required. Each applicant must successfully complete at least 90 semester hours (135 quarter hours) at an accredited college or university, including 30 semester hours of upper division courses. A baccalaureate degree is preferred. Applicants educated outside the United States must have completed at least two full years of study in an accredited college or university in the United States or Canada, including upper division courses, prior to application. Postbaccalaureate students should have recent courses in the required science areas. The following specific courses are required:

|  | Sem./Qtr. |
| --- | --- |
| General biology or zoology | 2/3 |
| General chemistry | 2/3 |
| Organic chemistry | 2/3 |
| Physics | 2/3 |
| English (comp. and lit.) | 2/3 |

CLEP or AP credits are not acceptable for the required courses. Applicants are strongly urged to take the MCAT in the spring of the year of application and to have their basic requirements completed at the time of application. All required courses must be completed by the spring semester prior to matriculation. Applicants are encouraged to take the required science courses that include laboratory experiences. No preference is given to any particular kind of undergraduate academic major, although applicants are encouraged to have a broad social science and/or humanities background.

## SELECTION FACTORS

Only residents of Arizona and highly qualified applicants who are WICHE certified and funded residents of western states without medical schools should apply. Applicants from states other than these will not be considered. Applicants are chosen on the basis of their ability, motivation, integrity, emotional maturity, interpersonal skills, and other personal characteristics which the Admissions Committee regards as important for prospective medical students and the successful practice of medicine. In evaluating candidates, attention is given to the entire academic record, MCAT scores, college preprofessional committee evaluations, other letters of recommendation, and personal interviews. Also considered is breadth of the undergraduate education, whether in the humanities, social sciences, or natural sciences. Applicants who are seriously considered will be interviewed at the College of Medicine. Acceptance is dependent on far more than academic achievement. Each applicant is considered from the standpoint of the applicant's potential as a physician.

Accepted students for the 1995 entering class had the following characteristics: *mean GPA,* 3.57; *sex,* 49 percent women; *residence,* 98 percent from Arizona, 2 percent WICHE; *overall acceptance rate,* 24.9 percent of those seriously considered received acceptances; and 131 acceptances were offered out of 527 applicants considered. Disadvantaged, rural, and minority residents of Arizona are strongly encouraged to apply. The College of Medicine does not discriminate on the basis of sex, age, race, creed, national origin, or handicap in its admission policies.

## FINANCIAL AID

Federal and local scholarships and loans are available to students with financial need. Eighty-seven percent of the students are receiving financial assistance. All determinations of need are made after an applicant is accepted for enrollment.

## INFORMATION FOR MINORITY AND NONTRADITIONAL STUDENTS

The College of Medicine and the Office of Minority Affairs have an active program dedicated to the recruitment, admission, education, and graduation of an increased number of individuals from underrepresented groups. The program offers the Minority Medical Education Program for pre-med students and a Summer Prematriculation Program for entering medical students. Learning specialists work closely with students during all phases of their medical education. The Commitment to Underserved People (CUP) project provides numerous opportunities to participate in neighborhood clinic settings. Tutoring, counseling, and a variety of student support services are also available. Faculty members participate in all aspects of the program.

Public Institution

## APPLICATION AND ACCEPTANCE POLICIES FOR 1997–98 FIRST-YEAR CLASS

*School participates in AMCAS. See Chapter 4.*

Filing of AMCAS application
 Earliest date: June 1, 1996
 Latest date: Nov. 1, 1996
School application fee: None
 Oldest MCAT scores considered: 1994
Does not have Early Decision Program
Acceptance notice to regular applicants
Earliest date: Jan. 30, 1997
 Latest date: Until class is filled
Applicant's response to acceptance offer
 Maximum time: 2 weeks
Requests for deferred entrance considered: Yes
Deposit to hold place in class: None
Estimated number of new entrants: 100
Starting date: July 1997

## TUITION AND STUDENT FEES PER YEAR FOR 1995–96 FIRST-YEAR CLASS

Tuition                                   Student fees: $66
 Resident: $6,960
 Nonresident: Not applicable

## INFORMATION ON 1995–96 FIRST-YEAR CLASS

| Number of | In-State | Out-of-State | Total |
|---|---|---|---|
| Applicants | 540 | 602 | 1,142 |
| Applicants Interviewed | 513 | 14* | 527 |
| New Entrants† | 98 | 2* | 100 |

*Certified WICHE applicants from Alaska, Montana, and Wyoming.
†All took the MCAT; 99% had baccalaureate degrees.

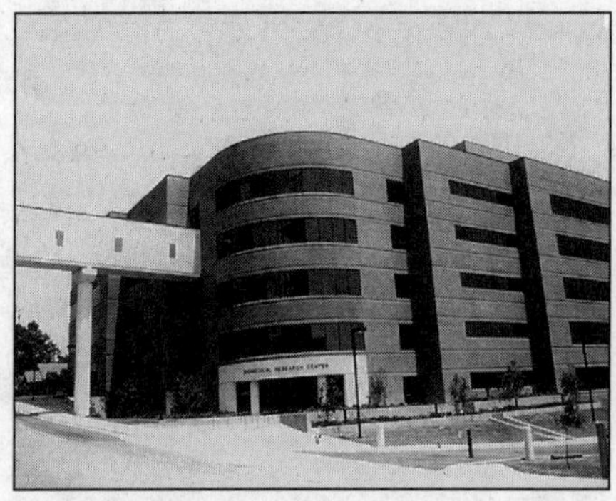

# University of Arkansas for Medical Sciences College of Medicine

**Little Rock, Arkansas**

Dr. I. Dodd Wilson, *Dean*
Linda W. Williams, *Director of Student Admissions*
Tom G. South, *Director of Financial Aid*

## ADDRESS INQUIRIES TO:

Office of Student Admissions
University of Arkansas for Medical Sciences
College of Medicine
4301 West Markham Street, Slot 551
Little Rock, Arkansas 72205-7199
(501) 686-5354; 686-5873 (FAX)
E-Mail: LWilliams@comdeanl.uams.edu
Web Site: http://www.uams.edu

## GENERAL INFORMATION

The University of Arkansas College of Medicine was established in 1879 and in 1957 occupied the present facilities along with the colleges of nursing, pharmacy, the graduate school, health-related professions, and the 400-bed University Hospital. The T. H. Barton Institute for Medical Research, a nine-story wing, was added in 1960. A building for expanded instructional and library facilities was completed in 1978, and an ambulatory care center opened in 1980. A family and community medicine clinic building was dedicated in 1986. The Arkansas Cancer Research and Treatment Center opened in 1989. Our new Biomedical Research Building and the Harvey and Bernice Jones Eye Institute opened in 1993 providing over 146,000 square feet of new laboratories, support space, and areas for patient care and education. A new facility to house our department of anatomy opened in 1995. A student union-residence building has accommodations for both single and married students. Clinical instruction is carried out in the University Hospital, two Veterans Administration hospitals (a 500-bed general hospital and a 2,000-bed neuropsychiatric hospital), the State Hospital for Nervous and Mental Diseases, and the Arkansas Children's Hospital. Certain senior electives are based at St. Vincent Infirmary, Baptist Medical Center, and community hospitals in health education centers in several Arkansas cities.

## CURRICULUM

Along with the standard courses in anatomy, biochemistry, and physiology, the first year includes a program to introduce the student to clinical contacts and concepts. This is accomplished with formal lectures in medico-socioeconomic topics, small-group discussions, and faculty-supervised interviews with patients.

The duration of the second-year program is eight months; the study consists of a standard but shortened curriculum.

The third year is a full 48 weeks with rotation through the major clinical services. This expanded clinical year provides substantial preparation for the predominantly elective fourth year, which consists of a minimum of 36 weeks to a maximum of 48 weeks of courses selected with the assistance of a faculty adviser. On- and off-campus electives are available to round out preparation for each student's career goals. The traditional grading system (A, B, C, D, F) is used throughout the first three years. Elective courses and a few selected ones in the first three years are graded as pass/fail. Opportunities are provided for students to engage in research activities and to pursue graduate courses leading to the M.S. and Ph.D. degrees.

## REQUIREMENTS FOR ENTRANCE

The MCAT and at least 90 semester hours of college work are required; a baccalaureate degree is strongly recommended. The following courses must be completed prior to matriculation:

|  | *Semesters** |
| --- | --- |
| Biology | 2 |
| General chemistry | 2 |
| Organic chemistry | 2 |
| Physics | 2 |
| Mathematics | 2 |
| English | 3 |

*Or equivalent.

Applicants who believe they have a compelling reason for being exempted from meeting any of the above requirements for admission may appeal directly to the admissions committee for a waiver.

No particular undergraduate field is given preference in the selection process; students from a variety of backgrounds are actively sought. While applicants are encouraged to follow their own interests in selecting college majors, courses such as embryology, genetics, quantitative analysis, psychology, history and logic are also recommended.

Applicants must have taken the MCAT no later than April 1993 and prior to the November 15 application deadline. Those enrolled in graduate/professional programs must have an adviser submit a letter assuring graduation prior to medical college entry in August.

## SELECTION FACTORS

Selection is based on scholastic attainment, performance on the MCAT, personal interviews with members of the faculty, and recommendations, particularly evaluations by college pre-professional advisory committees. Selection is made without regard to race, sex, creed, national origin, age or handicap. Unsuccessful applicants may reapply without prejudice.

Matriculants for the 1995 entering class had the following profile: *mean GPA,* 3.52 (97 percent above 3.0); *sex,* 40 percent women; *undergraduate major,* 80 percent in science disciplines, *average MCAT score,* 8.48.

Although applications are accepted from students who are not residents of the state of Arkansas, preference must be given to qualified resident applicants. Nonresidents who do not have a GPA of at least 3.5 (based on a 4.0 scale) and above average scores on each section of the MCAT should not apply.

## FINANCIAL AID

To date, adequate financial aid has been provided to all students in need of assistance to complete their academic programs. Such assistance comes in the form of loans and scholarship funds provided by federal, state, school, and private sources. Some form of aid is now being received by approximately 80 percent of the students. The financial status of applicants is not a factor in selection for admission.

While the University of Arkansas has no policy regarding student employment, students should not expect to be employed to the detriment of academic performance. In appropriate cases, students are assisted in obtaining employment at the university and elsewhere.

## INFORMATION FOR MINORITIES

Minority students are encouraged to apply for admission. The Office of Minority Student Affairs has developed an active recruitment and retention program. The Summer Science Program for Minority Students is available for five weeks during the summer and offers an introduction to the medical school curriculum, along with reading and study skill enrichment sessions designed to strengthen students in these areas. Beginning in 1993, a prematriculation program was implemented that has as its primary focus students who may have some problems mastering the medical college curriculum. A decelerated first or second year is offered as an option to all students who make clear and reasonable requests. Every effort is made by the faculty to assist students academically as these needs are identified. Nonrepayable financial assistance is provided, within program limits, to each student with demonstrated need.

Public Institution

## APPLICATION AND ACCEPTANCE POLICIES FOR 1997–98 FIRST-YEAR CLASS

*School participates in AMCAS. See Chapter 4.*

Filing of AMCAS application
  Earliest date: June 1, 1996
  Latest date: Nov. 15, 1996
School application fee after screening: $10
Oldest MCAT scores considered: 1993
Does not have Early Decision Program
Acceptance notice to regular applicants
  Earliest date: Dec. 15, 1997
  Latest date: Until class is filled
Applicant's response to acceptance offer
  Maximum time: 2 weeks
Requests for deferred entrance considered: Yes
Deposit to hold place in class: None
Estimated number of new entrants: 150
Starting date: Aug. 1997

## TUITION AND STUDENT FEES PER YEAR FOR 1995–96 FIRST-YEAR CLASS

| Tuition | Student fees: $783 |
| --- | --- |
| Resident: $7,334 | |
| Nonresident: $14,688 | |

## INFORMATION ON 1995–96 FIRST-YEAR CLASS

| Number of | In-State | Out-of-State | Total |
| --- | --- | --- | --- |
| Applicants | 400 | 505 | 905 |
| Applicants Interviewed | 374 | 17 | 391 |
| New Entrants* | 140 | 3 | 143 |

*All took the MCAT; 97% had baccalaureate degrees

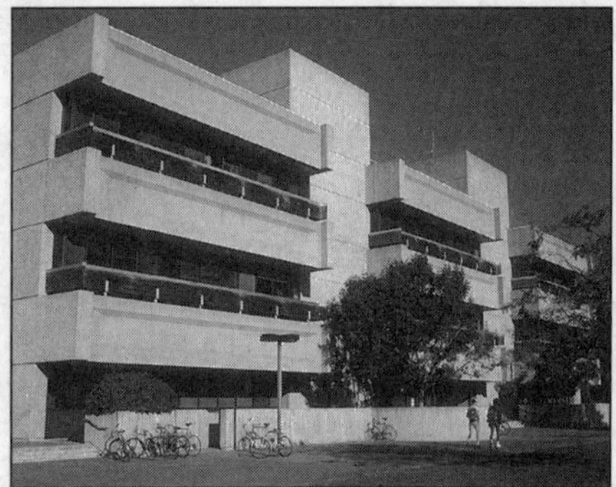

# University of California, Davis
## School of Medicine

**Davis, California**


Dr. Gerald S. Lazarus, *Dean*
Dr. Ernest L. Lewis, *Associate Dean for Student Affairs and Chair, Admissions Committee*
Edward D. Dagang, *Director of Admissions*


## ADDRESS INQUIRIES TO:

Admissions Office
University of California, Davis
School of Medicine
Davis, California 95616
(916) 752-2717

## GENERAL INFORMATION

The School of Medicine, University of California, Davis, admitted its first class in 1968. The school provides its students with a foundation of medical knowledge upon which they may proceed to careers in primary care, specialty practice, research, public health, or administration.

## CURRICULUM

The curriculum was revised in 1980 to provide a balanced blend of basic and clinical sciences. Basic science courses are emphasized during the first year and continue into the second. Early clinical exposure is provided during the first year through a continuing course entitled Introduction to Patient Evaluation. Knowledge of essential concepts and techniques is emphasized in the first year and is amplified in the second year, utilizing selected clinical problems, both functional and organic. The third and fourth years provide continued application of the principles of basic science to solving clinical problems in the setting of clinical clerkships and electives. Many courses are departmental; others are interdisciplinary, being planned and presented by course committees composed of members from a variety of academic departments and disciplines. Beginning with the first year, students are given the opportunity to take elective courses to broaden their knowledge of the health sciences.

The Davis campus affords opportunities for interaction with other schools, colleges, departments, and laboratories of the university. Research, teaching, and service are interrelated, and the biological and allied sciences are emphasized. Close relationships are enjoyed with the School of Veterinary Medicine, the California Primate Research Center, the Laboratory for Energy Related Health Research, and the Food Protection and Toxicology Center.

First- and second-year students attend basic science classes in the Medical Sciences I complex in Davis. Very early in the student's training, use is made of the clinical facilities of the 493-bed University of California, Davis, Medical Center, Sacramento. The Medical Center offers a full range of inpatient services, diagnostic services, an ambulatory care program with over 150 specialty clinics, and 24-hour major emergency medical service.

In addition to the doctor of medicine degree, UC Davis offers a variety of dual degree programs through coordination with other graduate school divisions. These advanced degrees can couple the M.D. degree to the Ph.D., M.S. and M.A. degree through the division of graduate studies of UC Davis. The M.D. degree can also be combined with an MBA through the Graduate School of Management of UC Davis, with an M.P.H. degree through the School of Public Health, University of California, Berkeley.

## REQUIREMENTS FOR ENTRANCE

The new MCAT and three years (90 semester hours or 135 quarter hours) in an accredited college or university in the United States or Canada are required. Applicants are urged to take the MCAT in the spring but no later than the summer in which the application is made. A course of study leading to a bachelor's degree is recommended.

The school believes a medical student should have a sound background in the humanities and behavioral and social sciences as well as in the physical and biological sciences. Premedical requirements must be completed by June of the year of desired entry. The following college level courses are required:

|  | *Years* |
|---|---|
| English | 1 |
| Biological sciences (with lab) | 1 |
| General chemistry (with lab) | 1 |
| Organic chemistry | 1 |

If two or more undergraduate courses are offered, the more rigorous option is recommended.

| | |
|---|---|
| Physics | 1 |

Mathematics
Course work sufficient to satisfy prerequisites for integral calculus is required.

CLEP credit is not acceptable for prerequisite courses.

## SELECTION FACTORS

The School of Medicine selects students for admission with a view to meeting the needs of society, of the medical profession, and of the school. Because the educational experience is enhanced by the interaction of students from various backgrounds, the school desires diversity in its student body. This is reflected in the school's commitment to expand opportunities in medical education for individuals from groups underrepresented in medicine as the result of social discrimination and to increase the number of physicians practicing in underserved areas. Therefore, the Admissions Committee, which is composed of individuals from a variety of cultural backgrounds and which is representative of a broad spectrum of medical sciences, evaluates applicants in terms of all relevant factors. These include academic credentials, with due regard to how they may have been affected by disadvantage experienced by the applicant; such personal traits as character and motivation; experience in the health sciences and/or the community; career objectives; and the ability of the individual to make a positive contribution to society, the profession, and the school.

Factors that will be considered are the applicant's scholastic record, MCAT performance, and reports of teachers and advisers regarding intellectual capacity, motivation, and emotional stability. Characteristics which may make such applicants particularly attractive to the Admissions Committee are outstanding nonacademic achievements, capability for independent study, maturity, and other factors which suggest good academic potential.

A personal interview will normally be required of each applicant who is accepted. Regional interviews are not normally available. Primary consideration for admission will be given to students who are legal residents of California. UC-Davis School of Medicine participates in the WICHE Professional Student Exchange Program for applicants from certain western states that do not have medical schools.

## FINANCIAL AID

A complete range of financial aid is available to medical students at the University of California, Davis: scholarships, fellowships, grants, and a variety of loans. The majority of financial aid is awarded based on demonstrated financial need. However, all accepted students are considered for university-awarded, merit-based scholarships.

Historically, students at the School of Medicine have been able to receive full financial aid funding of their calculated financial need. Due to the school's low fees and high aid availability, only a small percentage of students must borrow nondeferred interest loans. Financial aid applications are available in December or early January. Students granted an interview can request an application by mail or pick up an application when they come to UC Davis for their interview. Early application for aid is strongly recommended. Questions should be directed to the Financial Aid Office at (916) 752-6618.

## INFORMATION FOR UNDERREPRESENTED MINORITY AND FINANCIALLY DISADVANTAGED APPLICANTS

The mission of the Office of Minority Affairs is to ensure diversity in medicine for the state of California. This mission includes efforts to diversify both the student body and the faculty of the school of medicine. Thus, applications from qualified students representing groups that historically have been underrepresented in medicine are encouraged. Through an array of public and private grant funds, the office has offered a variety of supplemental assistance programs and services for these students. For more information on these resources, contact Roberto Paez, director, Office of Minority Affairs, School of Medicine, UC Davis, Davis, CA 95616; phone: (916) 752-8119.

Public Institution

### APPLICATION AND ACCEPTANCE POLICIES FOR 1997–98 FIRST-YEAR CLASS

*School participates in AMCAS. See Chapter 4.*

Filing of AMCAS application
Earliest date: June 1, 1996
Latest date: Nov. 1, 1996
School application fee after screening: $40
Oldest MCAT scores considered: 1994
Does not have Early Decision Program
Acceptance notice to regular applicants
    Earliest date: Oct. 15, 1996
    Latest date: Until class is filled
Applicant's response to acceptance offer
    Maximum time: 2 weeks
Requests for deferred entrance considered: Yes
Deposit to hold place in class: None
Estimated number of new entrants: 93
Starting date: Sept. 1997

### TUITION AND STUDENT FEES PER YEAR FOR 1995–96 FIRST-YEAR CLASS

| Tuition | Student fees: $7,837 |
| --- | --- |
| Resident: None | |
| Nonresident: $7,699 | |

### INFORMATION ON 1995–96 FIRST-YEAR CLASS

| Number of | In-State | Out-of-State | Total |
| --- | --- | --- | --- |
| Applicants | 4,612 | 879 | 5,491 |
| Applicants Interviewed | * | * | 700 |
| New Entrants† | 90 | 3 | 93 |

*Data not available.
†All took the MCAT and had baccalaureate degrees.

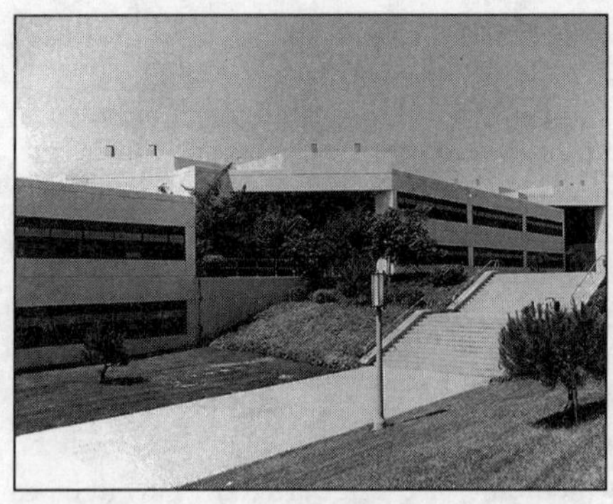

# University of California, Irvine
# College of Medicine

**Irvine, California**

Dr. Thomas C. Cesario, *Dean*
Dr. Alberto Manetta, *Senior Associate Dean, Educational Affairs*
E. Leah Parker, *Director of Admissions*

## ADDRESS INQUIRIES TO:

Office of Admissions
UCI-College of Medicine
P.O. Box 4089—Medical Education Bldg.
Irvine, California 92717-4089
(714) 824-5388; (800) 824-5388;
824-2485 (FAX)
Web Site: http://www.meded.uci.edu

## GENERAL INFORMATION

The predecessor of the University of California, Irvine (UCI) College of Medicine began as a private institution in 1896. It became part of the University of California in 1965 and was relocated to a 122-acre site on the Irvine campus in 1968, admitting the first group of medical students the same year.

Since its establishment at UCI, the college has grown extensively, attaining national recognition. Approximately 380 medical students are enrolled at the college, and over 100 students are pursuing graduate degrees in the biomedical sciences. The faculty currently includes more than 450 full-time and 1,700 voluntary members in 20 academic departments. The faculty have expertise in a wide range of biomedical subjects. Research emphasized at the college includes the following multispecialty areas: the neurosciences, oncology, cardiovascular and pulmonary diseases, medical imaging, geriatric medicine, immunology, molecular biology and human genetics, and neonatology.

The UCI Clinical Services System consists of the UCI Medical Center, off-site outpatient facilities, and numerous affiliated hospitals and clinics that participate in the educational and research programs of the college.

## CURRICULUM

The college offers a well-balanced curriculum in the clinical and basic sciences through educational and research programs in 20 academic departments. The curriculum consists of 16 instructional periods spread over four years, including a 10-week vacation period between the first and second years, and up to 12 weeks of vacation in the senior year. The core curriculum provides a body of knowledge and skills considered requisite for all those receiving the M.D. degree, regardless of their specific specialty choices.

The first two years of the curriculum are scheduled on a modified quarter system and concentrate on the sciences basic to clinical medicine and preclinical courses. The third and fourth years of the core curriculum consist of clinical clerkships and are scheduled according to 10-week quintiles. Students are also provided ample opportunity to participate in clinical and research elective courses of their choosing.

The focus of this curriculum is on active medical student participation toward the achievement of educational objectives. Demonstrations, small-group discussions, seminars, laboratory work by students, student projects oriented to problem solving, and exposure to clinical situations are integral parts of this focus.

An ongoing Academic Monitoring Program beginning with enrollment is coordinated by the Office of Student and Resident Affairs to identify students in academic difficulty early in their course work and to ensure the availability of all resources before serious academic difficulties are encountered. Faculty advisers are assigned to all students to provide academic advice through their medical school years. A Peer Tutoring Program is available to all medical students to provide tutorial assistance in the basic and clinical sciences. Study skills training and USMLE examinations review courses are also provided.

An honors/pass/fail/grading system was adopted in 1994.

A combined M.D.-Ph.D. degree is available through the Medical Scientist Program for highly qualified students who have the required academic background, research experience, and strong commitment to a career in biomedical research. Applicants to the Medical Scientist Program must notify the College of Medicine and complete a supplemental application form. In applying for the program, students must meet the admission requirements of both the College of Medicine and the Office of Research and Graduate Studies, as well as the specific admission requirements of the individual graduate program they select.

## REQUIREMENTS FOR ENTRANCE

The MCAT and a minimum of three full years of undergraduate college course work are required; however, almost all students accepted in recent years had already obtained their bachelor's degrees. The latest MCAT that can be accepted is that given in the fall of the year preceding anticipated admission.

Minimum requirements include the successful completion of the following courses with a grade of C or better:

Sem. hrs.

Biology and/or zoology . . . . . . . . . . . . . . . . . . . . . . . . . 12
  Must include one year of lower division biology
  and/or zoology plus one-half year of upper
  division courses, excluding botany.
General chemistry . . . . . . . . . . . . . . . . . . . . . . . . . . . . . 8
Organic chemistry . . . . . . . . . . . . . . . . . . . . . . . . . . . . . 8
Physics . . . . . . . . . . . . . . . . . . . . . . . . . . . . . . . . . . . . 8
Calculus . . . . . . . . . . . . . . . . . . . . . . . . . . . . (1 qtr.)
Biochemistry . . . . . . . . . . . . . . . . . . . . . . . . . . . . . . . 3

Applicants who do not meet these requirements or who do not indicate that these subjects will be completed by the date of entrance will not be considered for admission.

The Admissions Committee desires to admit students with diverse backgrounds, and no specific undergraduate major is required; however, demonstrated ability in the sciences is of great importance.

## SELECTION FACTORS

The UCI College of Medicine seeks to admit students who are highly qualified to receive training in the practice of medicine, and whose backgrounds, talents, and experiences contribute to the college's goal of achieving a broad spectrum of diversity in the student body. The Admissions Committee carefully reviews all applicants whose undergraduate record and scores on the MCAT indicate that they will be able to handle the rigorous curriculum of medical school. Careful consideration is given to applicants from disadvantaged backgrounds (that is, disadvantaged through social, cultural, and/or economic conditions). In addition to scholastic achievement, attributes deemed desirable in prospective students include indications of leadership ability and participation in extracurricular activities, such as research and medically related experience, as well as community service. Preference is given to California residents and to those applicants who are either U.S. citizens or permanent residents.

The AMCAS application is used for preliminary screening. Upon decisions of the Admissions Committee, applicants may be asked to submit additional information. Invitations for personal interviews are extended. The UCI-College of Medicine does not provide funds for interview trips; however, interview reports from other medical schools may be submitted in place of on-campus interviews.

The Admissions Committee reviews the academic records, letters of recommendation, and the results of personal interviews before making its final selections.

The 1995 entering class had the following statistics: *mean science GPA, 3.53; mean GPA, 3.56, mean MCAT 10.30.*

## FINANCIAL AID

The Office of Medical Student Financial Aid offers a variety of aid programs (scholarships, grants, and loans) to assist medical students. To qualify for assistance from most of these programs, an applicant must demonstrate financial need. Currently, 87 percent of the entering students receive aid of some type. For further information, call (714) 824-4606.

## INFORMATION FOR DISADVANTAGED APPLICANTS

Qualified applicants from disadvantaged backgrounds are encouraged to apply. The application fee may be waived to individuals granted a fee waiver by AMCAS. Programs for the recruitment and retention of disadvantaged students have been developed through the Office of Student and Resident Affairs and are supported in part by a grant from the Health Careers Opportunity Program (HCOP). For further information, call (714) 824-4603.

---

Public Institution

## APPLICATION AND ACCEPTANCE POLICIES FOR 1997–98 FIRST-YEAR CLASS

*School participates in AMCAS. See Chapter 4.*

Filing of AMCAS application
  Earliest date: June 1, 1996
  Latest date: Nov. 1, 1996
School application fee after screening: $40
  Oldest MCAT scores considered: 1994
Does not have Early Decision Program
Acceptance notice to regular applicants
  Earliest date: Nov. 15, 1996
  Latest date: Until class is filled
Applicant's response to acceptance offer
  Maximum time: 2 weeks
Requests for deferred entrance considered: Yes
Deposit to hold place in class: None
Estimated number of new entrants: 92
Starting date: Sept. 1997

## TUITION AND STUDENT FEES PER YEAR FOR 1995–96 FIRST-YEAR CLASS

Tuition                          Academic fees: $8,282
  Resident: None
  Nonresident: $7,699

## INFORMATION ON 1995–96 FIRST-YEAR CLASS

| *Number of* | *In-State* | *Out-of-State* | *Total* |
|---|---|---|---|
| Applicants | 4,656 | 533 | 5,189 |
| Applicants Interviewed | * | * | 484 |
| New Entrants† | 92 | 0 | 92 |

*Data not available.
†All took the MCAT and had baccalaureate degrees.

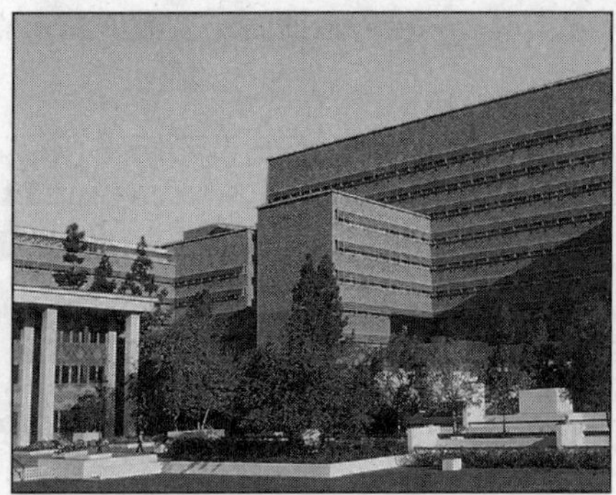

# University of California, Los Angeles
# UCLA School of Medicine

**Los Angeles, California**

Dr. Gerald Levey, *Dean*
Dr. Neil Parker, *Associate Dean for Admissions*
Lili Fobert, *Director of Admissions*

## ADDRESS INQUIRIES TO:

Office of Student Affairs
Division of Admissions
UCLA School of Medicine
Center for Health Sciences
Los Angeles, California 90095-1720
(310) 825-6081

## GENERAL INFORMATION

The UCLA School of Medicine graduated its first class in 1955. The medical school is situated on the UCLA campus. A large biomedical library and the University Medical Center are integral parts of the medical school. Close affiliation exists between the UCLA School of Medicine and the Los Angeles County Harbor/UCLA Medical Center, the Veterans Administration hospitals at West Los Angeles and Sepulveda, Cedars-Sinai Medical Center, Olive View Medical Center, and Santa Monica Hospital.

## CURRICULUM

The first two years of a four- year curriculum present a thorough knowledge of the sciences basic to medicine. An integrated approach to basic and clinical sciences is enhanced through problem-based learning in most courses of the first- and second-year curricula. Students are introduced to a holistic approach to patient care from the beginning of medical school and throughout the curriculum. The second year centers on the processes of disease, with emphasis on organ-system oriented instruction. The third and fourth years, covering 94 weeks, have a core curriculum of clinical clerkships encompassing the areas of internal medicine, surgery, obstetrics and gynecology, pediatrics, psychiatry, family practice, radiology, neurology, dermatology, and ophthalmology. Electives in the clinical continuum are designed to give students a solid foundation on which to develop and fulfill their personal interests, broaden their clinical knowledge, and give them an educational advantage in securing the clinical training calculated to best prepare them for postgraduate medical training. In 1993, UCLA initiated a pass-fail grading system with letters of distinction possible for outstanding performance.

A Medical Scientist Training Program, leading to both M.D. and Ph.D. degrees, is available for a limited number of students who desire careers in medical research. This program requires six to seven years to complete and provides rigorous research training in addition to the medical curriculum. Stipends are available for some of the students in this program.

## DREW/UCLA JOINT MEDICAL PROGRAM

Approximately 24 of the 145 students admitted each year have been admitted to the Drew/ UCLA Joint Medical Program. This program is designed to attract students who have an interest in addressing the concerns of underserved populations. Students will spend their first two years at the UCLA campus and their second two years at the Drew campus. Interested applicants should contact Charles R. Drew University of Medicine and Science, 1621 East 120th Street, Los Angeles, California 90059; or call (213) 563-4960.

## UCR/UCLA BIOMEDICAL SCIENCES PROGRAM

An additional 24 students are admitted to the UCLA School of Medicine through participation in the UCR/UCLA Biomedical Sciences Program, a cooperative venture involving the University of California, Riverside (UCR), UCLA School of Medicine, and Harbor/ UCLA Medical Center. Students follow an integrated course of study through five years on the UCR campus and the final two years of clinical studies at the UCLA School of Medicine. Qualified high school students should write to: Division of Biomedical Sciences, University of California, Riverside, Riverside, California 92521-0121; or call (909) 787-4333.

## REQUIREMENTS FOR ENTRANCE

The MCAT and three years of college are required. Ordinarily a baccalaureate degree is required, but in exceptional instances those who have completed three full academic years at an approved college or university will be considered. The required courses are:

|  | Years |
|---|---|
| English and composition | 1 |
| College physics (with lab) | 1 |
| Chemistry (with lab) | 2 |

Must include study of inorganic chemistry, quantitative analysis, and organic chemistry. (Biochemistry is highly recommended.)

| | |
|---|---|
| Biology | 2 |

One year of upper division courses should be included.

College mathematics . . . . . . . . . . . . . . . . . . . . . . . . . . . . 1
   Study of introductory calculus is highly recommended.

The study of Spanish is highly recommended.

Taking courses, such as human anatomy, that overlap in subject matter with those in medical school is not advised. However, advanced or specialized courses in biological science, such as cellular biology, are desirable.

Candidates are urged to take the MCAT in the spring rather than in the summer of the year of application.

## SELECTION FACTORS

The Admissions Committee gives preference to those applicants who present evidence of broad training and high achievement in their college education and possess in the greatest degree those traits of personality and character essential to success in medicine. Applicants whose records are judged by the Admissions Committee to qualify them for further consideration will be scheduled to have a personal interview by members of the faculty. The applications are initially reviewed on the basis of letters of recommendation, personal comments, the GPA, and MCAT scores.

In the 1995 entering class, accepted students had the following profile: *mean science GPA, 3.64; mean nonscience GPA, 3.66*. Applicants to the 1995 class had the following profile: *mean overall science GPA, 3.31; mean nonscience GPA, 3.47*.

Selections are made on the basis of individual qualifications and not on the basis of race, sex, creed, age, national origin, or handicap.

A third application is discouraged.

## FINANCIAL AID

Scholarships and loan funds from private, state, and federal sources are available to all U.S. citizens and are awarded on the basis of need and/or scholarship. Outside employment is not prohibited but is discouraged, especially in the first year.

## DISADVANTAGED APPLICANTS

The UCLA School of Medicine Admissions Committee is composed of subcommittees, one of which is devoted exclusively to the consideration of applicants who have had a disadvantaged educational or cultural background. This admissions subcommittee, which is composed of faculty and medical students, makes all recommendations for action to be taken on disadvantaged applicants, although final decisions are made by the full Admissions Committee.

---

Public Institution

### APPLICATION AND ACCEPTANCE POLICIES FOR 1997–98 FIRST-YEAR CLASS

*School participates in AMCAS. See Chapter 4.*

Filing of AMCAS application
   Earliest date: June 1, 1996
   Latest date: Nov. 1, 1996
School application fee after screening: $40
Oldest MCAT scores considered: 1995
Does not have Early Decision Program
Acceptance notice to regular applicants
   Earliest date: Jan. 15, 1997
   Latest date: Until class is filled
Applicant's response to acceptance offer
   Maximum time: 2 weeks
Requests for deferred entrance considered: Yes
Deposit to hold place in class: $100; refundable prior
   to May 15, 1997
Estimated number of new entrants: 145
Starting date: Aug. 1997

### TUITION AND STUDENT FEES PER YEAR FOR 1995–96 FIRST-YEAR CLASS

Tuition                     Academic fees: $7,864
   Resident: None
   Nonresident: $7,699

### INFORMATION ON 1995–96 FIRST-YEAR CLASS

| Number of | In-State | Out-of-State | Total |
|---|---|---|---|
| Applicants | 4,266 | 1,845 | 6,111 |
| Applicants Interviewed | 673 | 127 | 800 |
| New Entrants* | 131 | 14 | 145 |

*All took the MCAT and had baccalaureate degrees

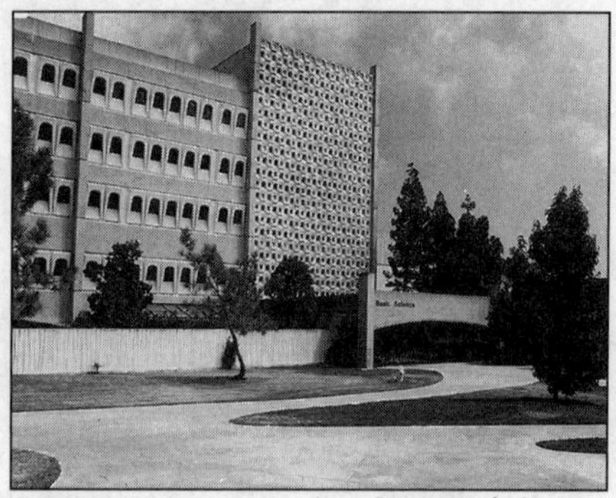

# University of California, San Diego
# School of Medicine

## La Jolla, California

Dr. John F. Alksne, *Dean*
Dr. Robert Resnik, *Associate Dean for Admissions*
Maria Lofftus, *Assistant Dean for Admissions*

## ADDRESS INQUIRIES TO:

Office of Admissions, 0621
Medical Teaching Facility
University of California, San Diego
School of Medicine
9500 Gilman Drive
La Jolla, California 92093-0621
(619) 534-3880; 534-5282 (FAX)

## GENERAL INFORMATION

The simultaneous development of the School of Medicine and the general campus at the University of California, San Diego (UCSD), has fostered implementation of innovative programs enabling the medical students to benefit from the diversity of university faculty, from a wide variety of laboratory teaching facilities, and from a broad spectrum of clinical opportunities. Located on the main campus of the university at La Jolla, the School of Medicine is surrounded by learning resources and research institutions representing all disciplines. Unusual opportunities exist for integrating instruction in medical and related sciences with the natural sciences and disciplines centering on man in his social milieu. Clinical instruction is carried on at University of California Medical Center, Veterans Administration Hospital, Naval Regional Medical Center, and eight other affiliated hospitals and clinics.

## CURRICULUM

The goal of the medical curriculum and faculty-student interactions is to develop critical, objective, conscientious physicians prepared for changing conditions of medical practice and continuing self-education.

The curriculum is divided into two major components: the core curriculum and the elective programs. These are pursued concurrently, with the core curriculum predominating in the early years. The core curriculum includes those aspects of medical education deemed essential for every medical student regardless of background or ultimate career direction. The integrated core curriculum of the first two years is designed to provide each entering student with an essential understanding of the fundamental disciplines underlying modern medicine. The core curriculum of the last two years is composed of the major clinical specialties taught in hospital settings, outpatient situations, and relevant extended-care facilities.

Each student is required to plan and complete an Independent Study Project in consultation with a member of the faculty. A written document is required in all projects. Other components are devised by the student and faculty member.

A Medical Scientist Training Program has been designed to provide the opportunity to earn both the M.D. and Ph.D. degrees over a six- to seven-year period of study for a limited number of students.

## REQUIREMENTS FOR ENTRANCE

The MCAT is required. A minimum of three years of college are required, including one full-time year at an accredited four-year university; the baccalaureate degree is preferred. The academic preparation for admission should be subject-oriented. If two or more undergraduate courses are offered, prospective applicants should select the most rigorous option. Minimal requirements are successful completion of the following courses with a grade of C or better:

*Biology:* One year of college level biology (excluding botany and biochemistry).
*Chemistry:* Two years of college level chemistry; must include one year of organic chemistry.
*Physics:* One year of college level general physics.
*Mathematics:* One year of course work; only calculus, statistics, or computer science will be considered.
*English:* Competence in speaking and writing English is required.

A broad base of knowledge is advantageous in preparing for the many roles of a physician and may include courses in: behavioral sciences, the biology of cells and development, genetics, biochemistry, English, social sciences, or conversational Spanish.

The Admissions Committee will only consider applicants who have taken the MCAT and completed the academic prerequisites.

## SELECTION FACTORS

The Admissions Committee selects applicants who have demonstrated intelligence, maturity, integrity, and dedication to the ideal of service to society and who are best suited for an educational curriculum designed to prepare students for care of the total patient either in preparation for primary care specialization or as a ground work for other fields of medicine. The school is seeking a student body with a broad diversity of backgrounds and interests reflecting our diverse population. The Admissions Committee has no preference as to undergraduate major but does prefer students with evidence of broad training and in-depth achievement in a particular area of knowledge, whether in the humanities, social sciences, or natural sciences.

Preference is necessarily afforded to California residents, and consideration is given only to applicants who are either U.S. citizens or permanent residents. Candidates are evaluated on the nature and depth of scholarly and extracurricular activities undertaken, their academic record, performance on the MCAT, letters of recommendation, and personal interviews. The Admissions Committee interview evaluates the applicants' abilities and skills necessary to satisfy the nonacademic or technical standards established by the faculty and the personal and emotional characteristics that are necessary to become an effective physician. The UCSD School of Medicine participates in the WICHE Professional Student Exchange Program for applicants from certain western states without medical schools.

Accepted students for the 1995 entering class had the following credentials: *mean GPA,* 3.65; *sex,* 45 percent women; *residence,* 93 percent from California; *undergraduate major,* 43 percent in biology or chemistry, with the remainder in the physical sciences, humanities, and social sciences; overall formal application and acceptance rates, 45 percent of those students interviewed received acceptances, and 265 acceptances were offered to obtain a class of 122 students.

## FINANCIAL AID

Financial aid in the form of scholarships, grants, loans, and work opportunities is offered to help students in need of financial assistance. Approximately three- quarters of the students receive financial assistance during their four years of study. Medical Scientist Training Program participants may receive full tuition and a stipend for up to six years. An application form for financial aid is sent to every accepted student upon request.

## DISADVANTAGED APPLICANTS

The UCSD School of Medicine is committed to expanding the educational opportunities for applicants coming from disadvantaged educational or economic backgrounds. This institutional commitment is expressed through a prematriculation summer program, tutorial support programs, and financial aid assistance.

---

Public Institution

## APPLICATION AND ACCEPTANCE POLICIES FOR 1997–98 FIRST-YEAR CLASS

*School participates in AMCAS. See Chapter 4.*

Filing of AMCAS application
    Earliest date: June 1, 1996
    Latest date: Nov. 1, 1996
School application fee after screening: $40
Oldest MCAT scores considered: 1993
Does not have Early Decision Program
Acceptance notice to regular applicants
    Earliest date: Oct 15, 1996
    Latest date: Until class is filled
Applicant's response to acceptance offer
    Maximum time: 2 weeks
Requests for deferred entrance considered: Yes
    Deposit to hold place in class: None
Estimated number of new entrants: 122
Starting date: Sept. 1997

## TUITION AND STUDENT FEES PER YEAR FOR 1995–96 FIRST-YEAR CLASS

Tuition            Academic fees: $8,239
  Resident: None
  Nonresident: $7,699

## INFORMATION ON 1995–96 FIRST-YEAR CLASS

| *Number of* | *In-State* | *Out-of-State* | *Total* |
|---|---|---|---|
| Applicants | 4,178 | 1,386 | 5,564 |
| Applicants Interviewed | * | * | 594 |
| New Entrants† | 114 | 8 | 122 |

*Data not available.
†All took the MCAT and had baccalaureate degrees

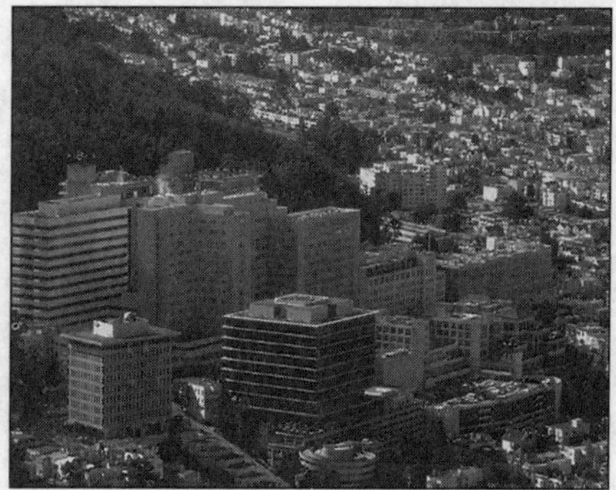

# University of California, San Francisco School of Medicine

## San Francisco, California

Dr. Haile T. Debas, *Dean*
Dr. Michael V. Drake, *Associate Dean for Admissions and Student Programs*
Kathleen Ryan, *Admissions Officer*

## ADDRESS INQUIRIES TO:

School of Medicine, Admissions
C-200, Box 0408
University of California, San Francisco
San Francisco, California 94143
(415) 476-4044

## GENERAL INFORMATION

The University of California, San Francisco (UCSF), School of Medicine, established as the Toland Medical College in 1864, became affiliated with the University of California in 1873. Clinical instruction is carried out at University of California Hospitals, San Francisco General Hospital, Veterans Administration Hospital, Mount Zion Hospital, and 33 other hospitals.

## CURRICULUM

During the first two years, core instruction in the basic sciences is offered by the preclinical departments. Early clinical correlation is introduced both in the basic science courses and in clinical courses. Emphasis is placed on small-group teaching. During the first year, students learn medical problem solving in the beginning of the year, and they begin patient experiences during the introduction to clinical medicine course. In the last two years the various clinical departments provide 52 weeks of core clerkships, which teach students the basic techniques of clinical medicine. An additional 34 weeks of clinical and basic science courses must be elected from a wide range of offerings at UCSF Medical Center and other hospitals.

The grading system is pass/not pass. Honors recognition is assigned on an individual basis in third- and fourth-year courses of three units or more.

There are numerous opportunities for students to engage in research. They include the joint degree programs, Student Research Fellowship Program, research electives, and various opportunities offered at UCSF and other institutions. Students who wish to do research should consult with the assistant dean of student research.

Special programs are available for students who wish to earn the M.D. degree jointly with the M.S., M.P.H., or Ph.D. degree. In addition, through the Medical Scientist Training Program, approximately eight students in each class may obtain the M.D. and Ph.D. degrees in six or more years of study.

The Joint Medical Program, sponsored by the University of California at Berkeley and San Francisco, is a five-year graduate and professional program leading to M.S. and M.D. degrees. The goal of the graduate segment (three years at Berkeley) is to develop students' abilities to approach problems of health and disease that require in-depth training in a variety of disciplines. Basic science and introductory clinical courses are enriched by individually structured master's degree programs in selected areas of the medical sciences or in the social sciences pertinent to health care. Upon the student's completion of the Berkeley phase of the program, including a master's thesis, an M.S. degree in health and medical sciences is awarded. Students then transfer to UCSF for the remainder of their training for the M.D. degree. The size of each class is limited to 12 students. Details are available from: Graduate Office, Health and Medical Sciences Program, 570 University Hall, #1190 University of California, Berkeley, California 94720; telephone (415) 642-5671.

## REQUIREMENTS FOR ENTRANCE

The MCAT and a minimum of three years of college are required. A baccalaureate degree is strongly recommended but not required. The MCAT must be taken within two years of application but no later than August of the year prior to matriculation. However, applicants are strongly urged to take the test the preceding spring rather than the summer.

Applicants must complete 135 quarter units (90 semester units) of acceptable transfer college credit by June of the year of desired entry. These courses must be completed at an accredited institution; moreover, only 105 acceptable quarter units may be transferred from a junior college. Courses must include:

|  | Qtr. hrs. |
| --- | --- |
| Biology or zoology (with lab) | 12 |
| Must include vertebrate zoology. | |
| General chemistry (with lab) | 12 |
| Organic chemistry | 8 |
| Physics (with lab) | 12 |

Survey courses in the sciences are not acceptable as fulfilling the requirements in science.

It is to the applicant's advantage to complete the above prerequisites before taking the MCAT and filing an application.

## SELECTION FACTORS

The School of Medicine welcomes applicants from all backgrounds and does not discriminate on the basis of race, color, national origin, sex, sexual orientation, handicap, or age.

Selection is based on an appraisal of both intellectual and personal characteristics which the Admissions Committee regards as desirable for prospective medical students and physicians. Based on these considerations, a limited number of applicants (550–600) are selected for interview. Personal interviews are required of applicants who pass the second screening. Regional interviews are not available.

Successful applicants tend to have strong academic records; firm and clear motivation for medicine which is manifested in their work experience, activities, or interests; and outstanding personal qualities. Academic performance is evaluated in relation to background, with the aim of determining the influence of external factors on this parameter. Since preference is given to California residents, only nonresidents with superior qualifications are encouraged to apply. Foreigners who are not permanent residents of the United States should not apply unless they have superior qualifications and adequate funding for their medical education and living expenses.

Some statistics of the 1995 entering class were: *mean cumulative GPA, 3.68; mean science GPA, 3.73; mean MCAT scores, VR-11, PS-11, BS-11;* 51 percent women; *nonwhite ethnic groups,* 54 percent; *underrepresented minority groups,* 30 percent.

## FINANCIAL AID

A limited number of scholarships are awarded to entering students on the basis of scholarship and/or need. General financial support is awarded through the Student Financial Services Office. Aid packages consist of a combination of loans, grants-in-aid, and scholarships.

## INFORMATION FOR MINORITIES

The School of Medicine has a long-standing commitment to increasing the number of physicians who are members of minority groups which are underrepresented in the medical profession. As a result, over the last 30 years UCSF has had one of the highest minority enrollment and graduation rates of continental U.S. medical schools. In addition, the medical school welcomes applications from socioeconomically disadvantaged persons, regardless of race.

---

Public Institution

## APPLICATION AND ACCEPTANCE POLICIES FOR 1997–98 FIRST-YEAR CLASS

*School participates in AMCAS. See Chapter 4.*

Filing of AMCAS application
   Earliest date: June 1, 1996
   Latest date: Nov. 1, 1996
School application fee after screening: $40
Oldest MCAT scores considered: 1995
Does not have Early Decision Program
Acceptance notice to regular applicants
   Earliest date: Nov. 15, 1996
   Latest date: Until class is filled
Applicant's response to acceptance offer
   Maximum time: 2 weeks
Requests for deferred entrance considered: Yes
Deposit to hold place in class: None
Estimated number of new entrants: 141
Starting date: Sept. 1997 (June 1997 for
   Joint Medical Program)

## TUITION AND STUDENT FEES PER YEAR FOR 1995–96 FIRST-YEAR CLASS

Tuition                          Academic Fees: $7,696
   Resident: None
   Nonresident: $7,699

## INFORMATION ON 1995–96 FIRST-YEAR CLASS

| *Number of* | *In-State* | *Out-of-State* | *Total* |
|---|---|---|---|
| Applicants | 3,221 | 2,665 | 5,886 |
| Applicants Interviewed | * | * | 521 |
| New Entrants† | 108 | 33 | 141 |

*Data not availabe.
†All took the MCAT and had baccalaureate degrees.

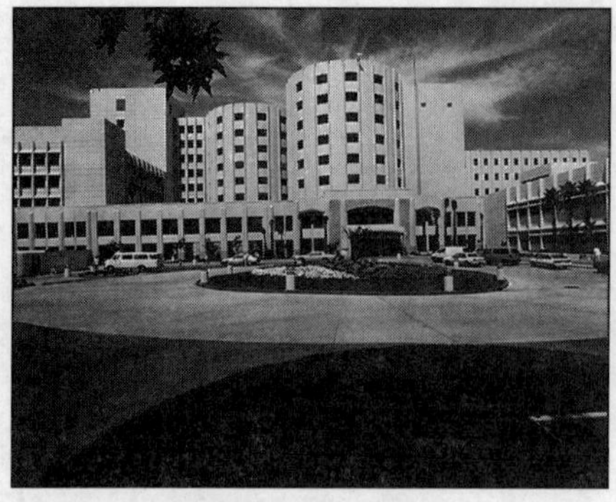

# Loma Linda University
# School of Medicine

Loma Linda, California

Dr. Brian S. Bull, *Dean*
Dr. John Thorn, *Associate Dean for Admissions*
Marilyn Dietel, *Financial Aid Officer*

## ADDRESS INQUIRIES TO:

Associate Dean for Admissions
Loma Linda University
School of Medicine
Loma Linda, California 92350
(909) 824-4467; 824-4146 (FAX)

## GENERAL INFORMATION

The School of Medicine was organized in 1909 at Loma Linda. The campus includes basic science facilities and the Loma Linda University Medical Center. Also used for clinical instruction are Loma Linda Behavioral Medicine Center, Loma Linda University Community Medical Center, Jerry L. Pettis Memorial Veterans Hospital, Riverside General Hospital, and the White Memorial Medical Center in Los Angeles. San Bernardino County General Hospital, Kaiser Foundation Hospital, and Glendale Adventist Medical Center are also affiliated with the School of Medicine and are utilized for undergraduate and postgraduate clinical training.

Objectives of the School of Medicine include providing the student with a solid foundation of medical knowledge, assisting the student in the attainment of professional skills, and motivating investigative curiosity and a desire to participate in the advancement of knowledge. The school endeavors to reinforce interest in the practical application of Christian principles through service to humanity. Our responsibility is to facilitate the formation of Christian physicians, educated to serve as generalists or specialists providing competent whole-person care to individuals, families, and communities.

## CURRICULUM

The major objective of the School of Medicine is to prepare students who will be well grounded in the science and art of medicine and who also will be prepared after further training for the practice of general medicine or any specialty.

The first two years are primarily devoted to the study of the basic medical sciences, including the relationship to pathology and clinical application, and introduction to physical diagnosis and human behavior. The last two years provide clinical rotations in the major areas of medical practice: surgery, internal medicine, pediatrics, obstetrics-gynecology, family medicine, preventive medicine, and psychiatry. Elective time is available for various types of additional educational experience in the clinical or research areas to prepare students in their selection of postgraduate medical education.

Qualified students, interested in a career in academic medicine, may earn an M.S. or Ph.D. degree along with the M.D. degree. Six to seven years are required to complete this program.

Performance of students is evaluated by means of standard or scaled scores. The grading system is on a pass/fail basis.

## REQUIREMENTS FOR ENTRANCE

The MCAT and a minimum of three years (90 semester hours or 135 quarter hours) of collegiate preparation in an accredited college or university in the United States or Canada are required. Preference is given to applicants who will have completed the baccalaureate degree prior to matriculation. No major is preferred, but a broad educational background is encouraged; however, demonstrated ability in the sciences is important. Rejected applicants may reapply and usually will receive the same consideration as first-time applicants.

Required courses are:

*Sem./Qtr. hrs.*

General biology or zoology (with lab) . . . . . . . . . . . . . . 8/12
General or inorganic chemistry (with lab). . . . . . . . . . . . 8/12
Organic chemistry (with lab). . . . . . . . . . . . . . . . . . . . . 8/12
Physics (with lab) . . . . . . . . . . . . . . . . . . . . . . . . . . . . 8/12
English
Equivalent to satisfy baccalaureate degree requirement.

CLEP and pass/fail performances are not acceptable for the required courses.

Applicants are urged to take the MCAT in the spring of the year of application and to have the basic requirements completed at the time of application.

## SELECTION FACTORS

The Admissions Committee seeks candidates who have demonstrated the greatest potential for becoming capable physicians. A strong academic background is needed in preparation for medical studies. While special attention is given to the performance in science courses, candidates should also have a solid foundation in the humanities, social sciences, and human behavior.

The Admissions Committee looks for applicants who demonstrate problem-solving skills, critical judgment, and the ability to pursue independent study and thinking. In evaluating academic achievements, the Admissions Committee considers such factors as the difficulty of the program, the need to work, social and cultural hardship, and participation in meaningful extracurricular activities. For nonacademic qualifications, the committee looks for a commitment to medicine, judgment, a positive attitude, ability to make decisions, emotional stability, and integrity.

The School of Medicine is owned and operated by the Seventh-day Adventist church; therefore, preference for admission is given to members of this church. However, it is a firm policy of the Admissions Committee to admit each year a number of nonchurch related applicants who have demonstrated a strong commitment to Christian principles. No candidate is accepted on the basis of religious affiliation alone. The school does not discriminate on the basis of race, sex, age, or handicap.

After receipt of the AMCAS application, each applicant is requested to submit the supplementary form and supply preprofessional faculty evaluations and/or personal letters of recommendation. Invitations for an interview  are extended to selected applicants on the medical school campus and on a regional basis at selected locations throughout the country.

Applicants with an outstanding academic record and with a particular interest in Loma Linda University School of Medicine are encouraged to apply through the Early Decision Program (EDP). Contact the associate dean for admissions prior to submitting AMCAS application.

Final selection is made by the Admissions Committee on the basis of overall scholastic record, personal character qualifications, and promise of success as a physician. Matriculated students for the class of 1995 had a mean overall GPA of 3.64.

## FINANCIAL AID

The School of Medicine has limited loan funds available through the Student Finance Office. All aid is awarded on the basis of a uniform needs analysis. Financial aid information is provided to all accepted students. In view of the costs of a medical education, students are urged to plan their financial program carefully.

Private Institution

## APPLICATION AND ACCEPTANCE POLICIES FOR 1997–98 FIRST-YEAR CLASS

*School participates in AMCAS. See Chapter 4.*

Filing of AMCAS application
 Earliest date: June 1, 1996
 Latest date: Nov. 1, 1996
School application fee to all applicants: $55
Oldest MCAT scores considered: 1994
Does have Early Decision Program (EDP)
 EDP application period: June 1–Aug. 1, 1996
 EDP applicants notified by: Oct. 1, 1996
Acceptance notice to regular applicants
 Earliest date: Dec. 1, 1996
 Latest date: Until class is filled
Applicant's response to acceptance offer
 Maximum time: 30 days
Requests for deferred entrance considered: Yes
Deposit to hold place in class (applied to tuition):
 $100, due with response to acceptance offer
Deposit refundable prior to: May 15, 1997
Estimated number of new entrants: 150 (10 EDP)
Starting date: Aug. 1997

## TUITION AND STUDENT FEES PER YEAR FOR 1995–96 FIRST-YEAR CLASS

Tuition $22,788         Student Fees: 0

## INFORMATION ON 1995–96 FIRST-YEAR CLASS

| Number of | In-State | Out-of-State | Total |
|---|---|---|---|
| Applicants | 2,572 | 2,480 | 5,052 |
| Applicants Interviewed | * | * | * |
| New Entrants† | 84 | 75 | 159 |

*Data not available.
†All took the MCAT and had baccalaureate degrees.

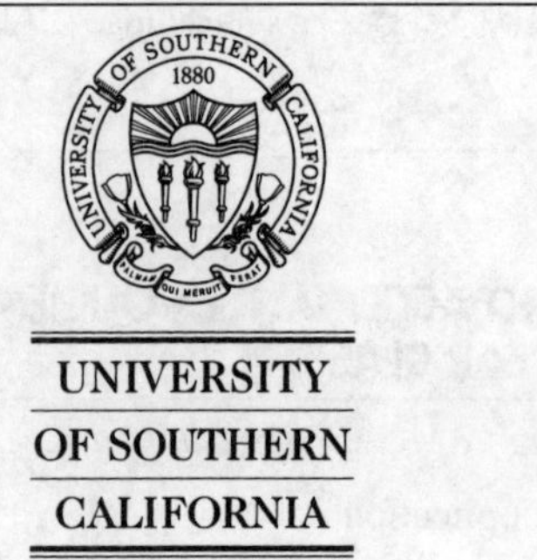



# University of Southern California School of Medicine

**Los Angeles, California**

Dr. Stephen J. Ryan, *Dean*
Arleen Marx, *Assistant Dean for Admissions*

## ADDRESS INQUIRIES TO:

Office of Admissions
University of Southern California
School of Medicine
1975 Zonal Avenue
Los Angeles, California 90033
(213) 342-2552
E-Mail: medadmit@hsc.usc.edu

## GENERAL INFORMATION

The University of Southern California (USC), a privately supported, nondenominational, coeducational university, established its School of Medicine in 1885. The 30-acre campus is located directly across the street from its chief teaching hospital, the 2,105-bed Los Angeles County+USC Medical Center. In addition to the Medical Center (largest teaching center in the United States), clinical facilities include the 275-bed USC University Hospital, USC/Norris Comprehensive Cancer Center, Doheny Eye Institute, Childrens Hospital of Los Angeles, Rancho Los Amigos Hospital, Orthopedic Hospital, Hospital of the Good Samaritan, Barlow Respiratory Hospital, California Medical Center, Huntington Memorial Hospital, Presbyterian Intercommunity Hospital, House Ear Institute, Veterans Administration Outpatient Clinic, and White Memorial Medical Center.

## CURRICULUM

Students are progressively involved in patient care beginning with patient contact during the first semester of the first year. An important feature is Introduction to Clinical Medicine, a course which begins in the freshman year and runs through the sophomore year. Doctor-patient relationships and interviewing are presented during the first year and physical diagnosis and history-taking are discussed in the second. Groups of approximately six to seven students are led by a faculty member who serves as clinical tutor to these students for their first two years.

Basic sciences are taught largely in an organ system approach. Appropriate material in the basic sciences is presented during the study of these systems; patients are observed and examined for clinical illustration of the subject under discussion. In this way the student is better able to understand and retain the basic scientific principles of medicine.

In the second year the student studies the pathologic aspects of medicine, also predominantly in an organ system approach. In addition, a student may begin an investigative project sponsored by a department. The final two years are designed as a continuum of two calendar years. Each student's program is individually designed to include 46 weeks of required clerkships (i.e., medicine, general surgery, obstetrics-gynecology, pediatrics, psychiatry, neurology, and surgical specialties), 18 weeks of selective clerkships at USC (which include a 6-week clerkship in ambulatory medicine), and 15 weeks of free electives. In addition, 6 weeks are set aside for "Spring Basic Science and Clinical Rotation" and one additional week for "Senior Week" (to include a "Physician in Society" course, which will examine issues relating to the practicing physician).

Grading is on an honors, pass, and not pass basis. Required clerkships include a near honors grading category.

## SPECIAL PROGRAMS

Students have an opportunity to engage in clinical or basic research through voluntary participation in a summer fellowship program between the freshman and sophomore years.

The school sponsors an M.D.-Ph.D. program for those interested in obtaining these degrees jointly. A special fifth-year option is available for students who wish to pursue a research project and may be considering a career in academic medicine. A baccalaureate-M.D. program is offered and described in Chapter 9.

## REQUIREMENTS FOR ENTRANCE

The MCAT and a minimum of four full years or 120 semester hours of academic work at an accredited college or university at the time of matriculation. Course work must include the following subjects:

|  | *Sem./Qtr.* |
|---|---|
| Biology (with lab) | 2/3 |
| Inorganic chemistry (with lab) | 2/3 |
| Organic chemistry (with lab) | 2/3 |
| General physics (with lab) | 2/3 |

Additionally, a course in basic molecular biology and 30 semester hours (or quarter equivalent) of course work in the social sciences, humanities, and English composition are required. Facility in the principles of higher mathematics and basic statistics and in the use of computers as a tool for independent learning is recommended.

Applicants are strongly urged to take the MCAT in the spring of the year of application and to have their basic science requirements completed at the time of application.

Foreign students must have completed at least one year of study in an accredited university or college in the United States prior to application.

Individuals who have discontinued studies in medical school for academic reasons are not eligible to apply.

## SELECTION FACTORS

The Admissions Committee seriously considers candidates whose academic achievement and MCAT performance indicate their ability to satisfactorily complete the rigorous cirriculum of the medical school. Favorable consideration also reflects additional factors including motivation and evidence of qualities deemed desirable for the study and practice of medicine, significant achievements in nonacademic pursuits, and demonstrated commitment to service and community. This assessment is not influenced by race, creed, gender, nationality, residency, age or handicap.

Receipt of the application from AMCAS is acknowledged. All candidates are requested to complete the supplemental application and arrange for submission of letters of recommendation. Interview selection is based upon careful evaluation of the application and all supporting documentation. Interviews are required of all applicants under serious consideration and are granted only by invitation of the Admissions Committee.

The 1995 entering class had a mean GPA of 3.47 and mean MCAT scores of 10 in each category. Women comprised 42 percent of the class which came from 45 colleges and universities and 17 states. The mean age was 24 (range 20–38). Fourteen students had advanced degrees.

## FINANCIAL AID

A variety of university scholarships and loans are available to supplement federal and state programs. Awards are based on need as demonstrated through a financial statement. Approximately 75 percent of students receive some type of financial assistance. Student employment during the academic year is discouraged. For additional information, contact Linda Lewis, director of financial aid, (213) 342-1016.

## INFORMATION FOR MINORITIES

The Office of Minority Affairs provides supportive services to minority medical students, including organized tutorial assistance, group and individual counseling, community support and interdepartmental communication. It also serves to create a warm environment where all students feel a sense of belonging. The office is involved in the active recruitment of qualified minority applicants for the health professions. Potential applicants are encouraged to contact Althea Alexander, assistant dean, (213) 342-1050.

---

Private Institution

### APPLICATION AND ACCEPTANCE POLICIES FOR 1997–98 FIRST-YEAR CLASS

*School participates in AMCAS. See Chapter 4.*

Filing of AMCAS application
   Earliest date: June 1, 1996
   Latest date: Nov. 1, 1996
School application fee to all applicants: $70
Oldest MCAT scores considered: 1995
Does have Early Decision Program (EDP)
   EDP application period: June 1–Aug. 1, 1996
   EDP applicants notified by: Oct. 1, 1996
Acceptance notice to regular applicants
   Earliest date: Jan. 1, 1997
   Latest date: Until class is filled
Applicant's response to acceptance offer
   Maximum time: 2 weeks
Requests for deferred entrance considered: Yes
Deposit to hold place in class (applied to tuition):
   $100, due with response to acceptance offer
Deposit refundable prior to: May 15, 1997
Estimated number of new entrants: 150
Starting date: Aug. 1997

### TUITION AND STUDENT FEES PER YEAR FOR 1995–96 FIRST-YEAR CLASS

Tuition $26,520        Student fees: $1,232

### INFORMATION ON 1995–96 FIRST-YEAR CLASS

| Number of | In-State | Out-of-State | Total |
|---|---|---|---|
| Applicants | 4,346 | 2,142 | 6,488 |
| Applicants Interviewed | * | * | 800 |
| New Entrants† | * | * | 150 |

*Data not available.
†All took the MCAT and had baccalaureate degrees.

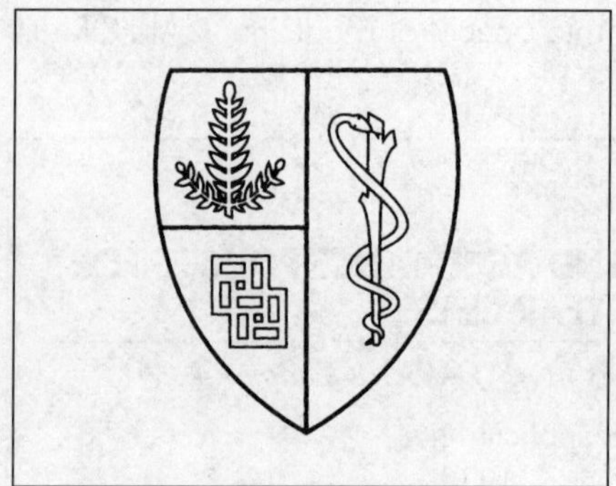

# Stanford University School of Medicine

**Palo Alto, California**

Dr. Eugene A. Bauer, *Dean*
Dr. Norman Blank, *Director of Admissions*
Judy Colwell, *Assistant Director of Admissions*

## ADDRESS INQUIRIES TO:

Office of Admissions
Stanford University
School of Medicine
851 Welch Road-Room 154
Palo Alto, California 94304-1677
(415) 723-6861; 725-4599 (FAX)
Web Site: http://www.stanford.edu/

## GENERAL INFORMATION

The Stanford University Hospital and School of Medicine, established in San Francisco in 1908, were relocated on the university campus at Palo Alto in 1959. Association with several local hospitals (totaling over 3,000 beds) provides facilities for comprehensive clinical training, and the school offers opportunities in many areas of fundamental and clinical research.

## CURRICULUM

The curriculum aims to develop students' capacities for innovative leadership in clinical practice and to maximize their opportunities to prepare for careers in research and teaching in the various branches of clinical and social medicine and biomedical sciences. The curricular plan affords wide opportunities for academic, research, and cultural activities in the medical school and university.

The required curriculum includes work in the basic medical sciences and clinical experiences in medicine, surgery, pediatrics, gynecology-obstetrics, and psychiatry. All M.D. candidates must satisfactorily complete at least 13 quarters of academic work. Fees for additional quarters are nominal. Students are encouraged to plan for a five-year course of study in order to include research activities, teaching assistantships, and a variety of elective courses both in the medical school and in other schools of the university in their educational enrichment plans. Thus, the time spent in medical school may vary with the individual student's background and study plans. Courses are graded pass/fail.

Stanford offers many opportunities for study in depth in the preclinical and clinical disciplines. Students with strong interests in careers in medical research should inquire from the Office of Admissions about the Medical Scientist Training Program (MSTP) or the training programs in cancer biology, immunology, medical information sciences, neurosciences, or pharmacology. These federally funded programs enable selected students to pursue research and course work leading to both the M.D. and Ph.D. degrees. Students request MSTP application forms on the supplementary application to the School of Medicine. Applications for other programs are also supplied on request to the specific department.

The medical school offers a summer matriculation program for new matriculants who qualify on the basis of minority or disadvantaged status.

## REQUIREMENTS FOR ENTRANCE

The MCAT is required, preferably taken in the spring but no later than late summer of the year of application. A baccalaureate degree is preferred but not required. Applicants seeking admission under unusual circumstances should contact the Office of Admissions. The minimal entry requirements are:

|  | *Years* |
|---|---|
| Biological science (with lab) | 1 |
| Chemistry, including organic chemistry (with labs) | 2 |
| Physics (with lab) | 1 |

Courses in calculus, physical chemistry, behavioral sciences, and particularly in biochemistry are strongly recommended.

An undergraduate major in any field is acceptable, provided the candidate presents a record of outstanding achievement. Breadth of education and/or experience in the humanities and social sciences and knowledge of a foreign language are desirable.

## SELECTION FACTORS

Stanford's educational milieu fosters rigorous scholarship and encourages students to develop investigative and innovative approaches to problems in medicine. The school seeks applicants who have a strong humanitarian commitment and whose originality, creativity, and independent, critical thinking best equip them for this environment.

Stanford does not discriminate against applicants on the basis of race, religion, national origin, sex, marital status, age, or disability. The applicant's state of residence is irrelevant in the selection process. No preference is given to California residents. Foreign applicants must have completed a minimum of one year of study in a U.S., Canadian, or United Kingdom accredited college or university.

Acceptances are based upon standards of merit, and no quotas of any kind play a role in the evaluation or selection process.

In recent years, applicants granted admission have had a mean GPA of about 3.6 and mean MCAT scores as follows: *VR*-10, *PS*-11, *BS*-11. Applicants whose MCAT scores are below the national mean are highly unlikely to be admitted to the medical school.

The application fee applies to students who return the supplemental application and will be waived for applicants who have obtained a fee waiver from AMCAS. Otherwise, fee waiver requests must be accompanied by a supporting statement from the dean or financial aid officer.

Application during the summer or very early fall is strongly encouraged.

## FINANCIAL AID

Acceptance is independent of the applicant's financial status, and Stanford makes every effort to ensure that students are not excluded from the school for financial reasons. Approximately 80 percent of the students receive some sort of financial assistance. Available loan and grant funds are allocated to candidates on the basis of need, as determined by needs analysis (see Part 1). All students are considered to be parental dependents. Eligibility for aid is assessed according to budgets that are standardized for various living situations. Any expenses in excess of the standard budget are reviewed separately. As many legitimate expenses as possible will be covered subject to availability of funds.

Accepted candidates who are neither American citizens nor permanent residents are not eligible for federal financial aid nor are they eligible for institutional-based financial aid programs at Stanford.

Teaching assistantships and research opportunities, for which students receive a salary and a tuition grant, can reduce the indebtedness of students who receive financial aid. However, such employment should not be viewed as a guaranteed way to meet expenses.

Applicants should submit the needs analysis form as soon as possible after February 1 so that, if requested, a preliminary estimate of the award can be provided by the Financial Aid Office. Application forms for financial aid are made available to all applicants who reach the interview stage. The telephone number for the Financial Aid Office is (415) 723-6958.

## INFORMATION FOR MINORITIES AND WOMEN

Because minorities and women are underrepresented in medicine, especially in academic medicine, Stanford seeks to recruit and educate underrepresented minority and women students. Thus, applications from these students are strongly encouraged.

Private Institution

## APPLICATION AND ACCEPTANCE POLICIES FOR 1997–98 FIRST-YEAR CLASS

*School participates in AMCAS. See Chapter 4.*

Filing of AMCAS application
    Earliest date: June 1, 1996
    Latest date: Nov. 1, 1996
School application fee after screening: $55
    Oldest MCAT scores considered: 1994
Does have Early Decision Program (EDP)
    EDP application period: June 1–Aug. 1, 1996
    EDP applicants notified by: Oct. 1, 1996
Acceptance notice to regular applicants
    Earliest date: Oct. 15, 1996
    Latest date: Until class is filled
Applicant's response to acceptance offer
    Maximum time: 2 weeks
Requests for deferred entrance considered: Yes
Deposit to hold place in class: None
Estimated number of new entrants: 86 (2 EDP)
Starting date: Sept. 1997

## TUITION AND STUDENT FEES PER YEAR FOR 1995–96 FIRST-YEAR CLASS

Tuition $24,375          Student fees: $607

## INFORMATION ON 1995–96 FIRST-YEAR CLASS

| Number of | In-State | Out-of-State | Total |
|---|---|---|---|
| Applicants | 2,858 | 4,148 | 7,006 |
| Applicants Interviewed | 292 | 338 | 630 |
| New Entrants* | 48 | 38 | 86 |

*All took the MCAT and had baccalaureate degrees.

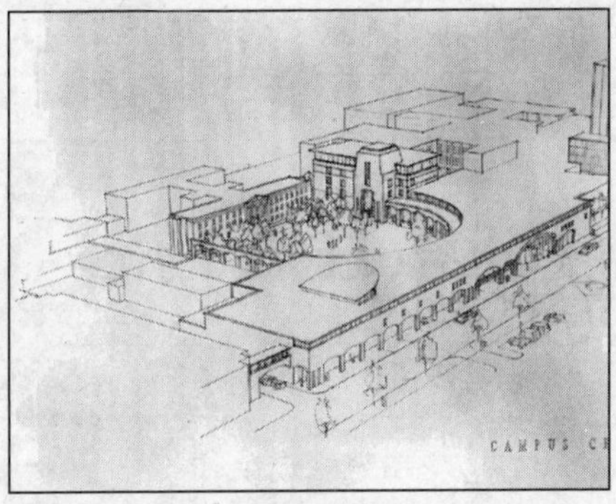

# University of Colorado School of Medicine

**Denver, Colorado**

Dr. Richard D. Krugman, *Dean*
Dr. Maureen J. Garrity, *Associate Dean for Admissions*
Jane Nakata, *Director of Financial Aid*

## ADDRESS INQUIRIES TO:

Medical School Admissions
University of Colorado
School of Medicine
4200 East 9th Avenue, C-297
Denver, Colorado 80262
(303) 270-7361; 270-8494 (FAX)
(Note: After Sept. 1996, the phone prefix will be
315 rather than 270.)

## GENERAL INFORMATION

The University of Colorado School of Medicine admitted its first students in 1883. The School of Medicine is a part of the University of Colorado Health Sciences Center, located in Denver. The Health Sciences Center also includes the schools of dentistry, nursing, pharmacy, and the graduate school. Basic science and clinical opportunities for the medical students are located throughout the Denver area in a number of hospitals and clinics and rural health experiences are found throughout the state of Colorado. Although no official student housing is provided, the school is located in a neighborhood with a wide range of housing choices.

The medical school is home for approximately 1,200 full-time and 2,000 volunteer faculty members. In addition to educating students and participating in research, the faculty assumes considerable responsibility for patient care. Opportunities for student research and a variety of extracurricular activities are available.

## CURRICULUM

The curriculum is designed to provide the scientific and clinical background to prepare graduates for the practice of medicine. Most of the basic science courses are taught during the first two years. Primary Care I, II, and III is a course taught over the first three years and is designed to introduce students to clinical problems early in their medical education. Students spend two to three days each month with a physician/preceptor who is practicing in one of the primary care areas. The third and fourth years consist of clinical clerkships with required clerkships primarily in the third year and electives primarily in the fourth year.

## REQUIREMENTS FOR ENTRANCE

The MCAT and a baccalaureate degree or at least 120 semester hours of college credit with a major leading to a degree are required. The MCAT must be taken before the November 15 application deadline. The following courses are required:

*Sem. hrs.*

General biology or zoology (with lab) . . . . . . . . . . . . . . . . . 8
General chemistry (with lab) . . . . . . . . . . . . . . . . . . . . . . . 8
Organic chemistry (with lab) . . . . . . . . . . . . . . . . . . . . . . . 8
General physics (with lab) . . . . . . . . . . . . . . . . . . . . . . . . . 8
College mathematics . . . . . . . . . . . . . . . . . . . . . . . . . . . . . 6
   Should include at least college level algebra
   and trigonometry or the equivalent by means
   of advanced placement.
English literature or equivalent . . . . . . . . . . . . . . . . . . . . . . 6
English composition or creative writing
   or equivalent . . . . . . . . . . . . . . . . . . . . . . . . . . . . . . . . . 3

Calculus and a quantitative mathematically oriented physics course are recommended as a valuable conceptual basis for understanding rates of change in physiological processes.

The literature and English composition requirements are based on the recognized need of the future physician to have skill in communication.

In order to receive credit for any advanced placement, the subject matter credited must be listed on the official college transcript.

## SELECTION FACTORS

Places are offered to the applicants who appear to the Committee on Admissions to be the most highly qualified in terms of intellectual growth and achievement, character, motivation, maturity, and emotional stability. For this assessment, college grades, MCAT scores, recommendations from college instructors and others, and personal interviews are used. Interviews are arranged for applicants who have a good chance of being accepted, and no applicant will be accepted without a personal interview.

Of the approximately 130 places in each class, more than 85 percent will be awarded to Colorado residents. Colorado residents from rural areas and from minority groups are especially encouraged to apply. Thereafter, preference will be given to applicants from certain western states participating in the WICHE program and to applicants from other states who have high GPAs and MCAT scores.

A wide variety of undergraduate majors are considered acceptable in the selection of applicants and no special preferences are given to science majors over nonscience majors. However, demonstration of good performance in the required science courses is essential. Accepted students for the 1995 entering class had the following statistics: *mean GPA* 3.6, *mean MCAT* 9.7, *mean age* 26 years, 43 percent women, 20 percent underrepresented minorities.

An Early Decision Program exists for a limited number of students with strong academic credentials who have decided that they wish to apply only to the University of Colorado School of Medicine. Applicants must have taken the spring MCAT prior to applying to be considered for the Early Decision Program.

The medical school has an active M.D.-Ph.D. combined-degree program for qualified applicants who combine medical school with intensive scientific training. Information about this program may be obtained by calling (303) 270-8986. Graduate study and research for the doctoral degree are pursued after the student has completed the basic science curriculum in the first two years. Medical students not in the combined-degree program may also be provided with research opportunities in the basic science or clinical departments.

If places open up in the second or third year classes, transfer applications are accepted. Although in most years there is at least one place, there are rarely more than two or three openings. Applicants who are currently in good standing in allopathic United States medical schools and who are Colorado residents are given preference for any open places.

The University of Colorado School of Medicine does not discriminate on the basis of race, sex, creed, national origin, age, or disability. Financial status is not a factor in the selection of applicants.

## FINANCIAL AID

The medical school participates in the federal aid programs and also has available a number of other scholarship and loan funds which are distributed on the basis of financial need. Colorado student grant funds are available for Colorado residents. Financial aid questions should be directed to (303) 270-8364.

## INFORMATION FOR MINORITIES

The University of Colorado encourages applications from qualified minority group students. Acceptance is determined by the Committee on Admissions and is based on the same type of criteria that apply to nonminority applicants. The committee carefully considers the student's social, economic, and educational background. It is possible for some disadvantaged students to have application fees and interview costs defrayed. Detailed information may be obtained by contacting the Center for Multicultural Enrichment at (303) 270-8558.

---

Public Institution

### APPLICATION AND ACCEPTANCE POLICIES FOR 1997–98 FIRST-YEAR CLASS

*School participates in AMCAS. See Chapter 4.*

Filing of AMCAS application
    Earliest date: June 1, 1996
    Latest date: Nov. 15, 1996
School application fee to all applicants: $70
Oldest MCAT scores considered: 1992
Does have Early Decision Program (EDP)
    EDP application period: June 1–Aug. 1, 1996
    EDP applicants notified by: Oct. 1, 1996
Acceptance notice to regular applicants
    Earliest date: Oct. 15, 1996
    Latest date: Varies
Applicant's response to acceptance offer
    Maximum time: 2 weeks
Requests for deferred entrance considered: Yes
Deposit to hold place in class (applied to tuition, fees, or other student obligations during last term): $200, due with response to acceptance offer.
Deposit refundable prior to: July 1, 1997
Estimated number of new entrants: 130 (5 EDP)
Starting date: Aug. 1997

### TUITION AND STUDENT FEES PER YEAR FOR 1995–96 FIRST-YEAR CLASS

Tuition            Student fees: $1,768
    Resident: $10,382
    Nonresident: $47,794

### INFORMATION ON 1995–96 FIRST-YEAR CLASS

| Number of | In-State | Out-of-State | Total |
|---|---|---|---|
| Applicants | 755 | 2,320 | 3,075 |
| Applicants Interviewed | 524 | 248 | 772 |
| New Entrants* | 106 | 23 | 129 |

*All took the MCAT; 98% had baccalaureate degrees.

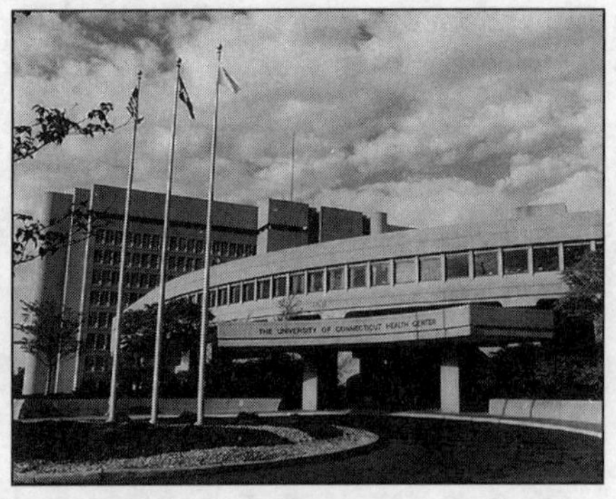

# University of Connecticut School of Medicine

**Farmington, Connecticut**

Dr. Peter Deckers, *Dean*
Keat Sanford, *Assistant Dean, Director of Admissions and Student Records*
Patricia Freedman, *Director of Financial Aid*

## ADDRESS INQUIRIES TO:

Office of Admissions and Student Affairs
University of Connecticut
School of Medicine
263 Farmington Avenue, Rm. AG-062
Farmington, Connecticut 06030-1905
(860) 679-2152; 679-1282 (FAX)
E-Mail: sanford@nso1.uchc.edu
Web Site: http://www.uchc.edu

## GENERAL INFORMATION

Established in 1968 as a unit of the University of Connecticut, the School of Medicine occupies the University of Connecticut Health Center complex in Farmington. The Health Center includes under one roof the School of Medicine and School of Dental Medicine, the 230-bed University Hospital and Ambulatory Unit, and the 130,000-volume Stowe Library. Clinical training programs exist in eight affiliated hospitals in the greater Hartford area and 11 allied community hospitals.

## CURRICULUM

The curriculum plan for medical students is based on a multidepartmental approach. Basic medical sciences are taught from an organ system approach. Normal structure/function is presented first followed by pathophysiology and therapeutic approaches. Patient contract begins in year one as part of the clinical medicine curriculum. Students learn medical history taking, physical diagnosis, and various other aspects of the physician-patient relationship. In addition, students participate in a longitudinal ambulatory clinical experience throughout all four years. In the third year, the students rotate through ambulatory and in-patient activities in each of the major clinical disciplines. In the fourth year, students complete clinical rotations in emergent and urgent care and have 5 months of electives. To aid individual development, students are assigned significant amounts of free time during the first two years and a wide choice of elective subjects in the clinical years. The NBME examinations are required of all students. The grading system is strictly pass/fail; there are no class rank scales or class standing. The third-year grading system is honors and pass/fail.

## REQUIREMENTS FOR ENTRANCE

The MCAT and three years of college are required; four years of college and the baccalaureate degree are recommended. Prerequisite courses are:

|  | Sem. hrs. |
|---|---|
| General biology or zoology (with lab) | 8 |
| General chemistry (with lab) | 8 |
| Organic chemistry (with lab) | 8 |
| General physics (with lab) | 8 |

The level of these required courses should be equal to courses for those majoring in these respective fields.

The School of Medicine supports the view that a broad liberal arts education provides the best background for those entering the medical profession. It will be difficult for students to master the programs in medicine unless they are adept in the use of the English language and in the handling of quantitative concepts. It is strongly recommended, therefore, that students include courses in their undergraduate curriculum that will provide them with a broad liberal arts background and aid them in the future development of their communicative and quantitative skills.

## SELECTION FACTORS

The aim of the University of Connecticut School of Medicine is to accept qualified Connecticut residents, with special effort to include those at a disadvantage by reason of economic background or race. This assumes that places will be offered only to those whose achievements and/or capabilities are consistent with the rigor and high standards of the school's educational programs. A few exceptionally qualified out-of-state residents will be considered. An Early Assurance Program is available. Occasionally, a couple of transfer positions are available in the third year.

The factors considered by the Admissions Committee are the applicant's career and clinical specialty interests, achievements, ability, motivation, and character. The applicant's GPA and MCAT scores are considered along with difficulty of the academic program, evidence of academic achievement beyond the regular course work, and evidence of intellectual growth and development. Additional consideration is given for nonacademic activities and involvements and for letters of recommendation.

Requests to consider MCAT scores older than three years are handled individually. Personal interviews are arranged only at the request of the Admissions Committee. The 1995 entering class had a mean GPA of 3.5 and a mean MCAT of 29.

The University of Connecticut policy prohibits discrimination in education, in employment, and in the provision of services on account of race, religion, sex, age, marital status, national origin, ancestry, sexual orientation, disabled veteran status, physical or mental disability, mental retardation, other specifically covered mental disabilities, and criminal records that are not job related, in accordance with provisions of the Civil Rights Act of 1964, Title IX Education Amendments of 1972, the Rehabilitation Act of 1973, the Americans with Disabilities Act, and other existing federal and state laws and executive orders pertaining to equal rights.

## FINANCIAL AID

Financial aid is available in three forms: scholarships; long-term, low-interest loans; and short-term, no-interest emergency loans. Eligibility for all programs is primarily based on demonstrated need. A limited number of part-time jobs are available. Approximately 80 percent of the students receive financial aid during the four-year educational period. Financial need is not considered relevant to the admissions process. A student's financial need is assessed after admission, and every effort is made to meet the student's minimum financial requirements. Further information is available from Patricia Freedman, director of financial aid.

## MINORITY AFFAIRS

The School of Medicine recruits minority group and disadvantaged applicants nationally through the Office of Minority Student Affairs. Minority applications are reviewed by the same general procedure for all applications and by the full Admissions Committee. Candidates for admission receive a full and sensitive review and are selected on a competitive basis. Minority candidates invited for an interview meet with the staff of the Office of Minority Student Affairs who answer questions in an informal setting. The School of Medicine has developed summer enrichment programs for high school and college students from groups traditionally underrepresented in American medicine in order to expand the pool of minority applicants to medical school. Information about enrichment programs may be obtained by writing to the Office of Minority Student Affairs or by calling at (860) 679-3483.

Tutorial and counseling assistance is available to all students. The financial aid package is constructed on the basis of individual need, and every effort is made to meet this need. Application fees may be waived for disadvantaged students.

Public Institution

## APPLICATION AND ACCEPTANCE POLICIES FOR 1997–98 FIRST-YEAR CLASS

*School participates in AMCAS. See Chapter 4.*

Filing of AMCAS application
   Earliest date: June 1, 1996
   Latest date: Dec. 15, 1996
School application fee to all applicants: $60
Oldest MCAT scores considered: 1993
Does have Early Decision Program (EDP)
   EDP application period: June 1–Aug. 1, 1996
   EDP applicants notified by: Oct, 1, 1996
Acceptance notice to regular applicants
   Earliest date: Oct. 15, 1996
   Latest date: Until class is filled
Applicant's response to acceptance offer
   Maximum time: 2 weeks
Requests for deferred entrance considered: Yes
Deposit to hold place in class (applied to tuition):
   $100, due with response to acceptance offer
Deposit refundable prior to: May 15, 1997
Estimated number of new entrants: 80 (8 EDP)
Starting date: Aug. 1997

## TUITION AND STUDENT FEES PER YEAR FOR 1995–96 FIRST-YEAR CLASS

Tuition               Student fees: $3,300
   Resident: $8,050
   Nonresident: $18,400

## INFORMATION ON 1995–96 FIRST-YEAR CLASS

| Number of | In-State | Out-of-State | Total |
|---|---|---|---|
| Applicants | 446 | 2,890 | 3,336 |
| Applicants Interviewed | 272 | 127 | 399 |
| New Entrants* | 71 | 10 | 81 |

*All took the MCAT and had baccalaureate degrees.

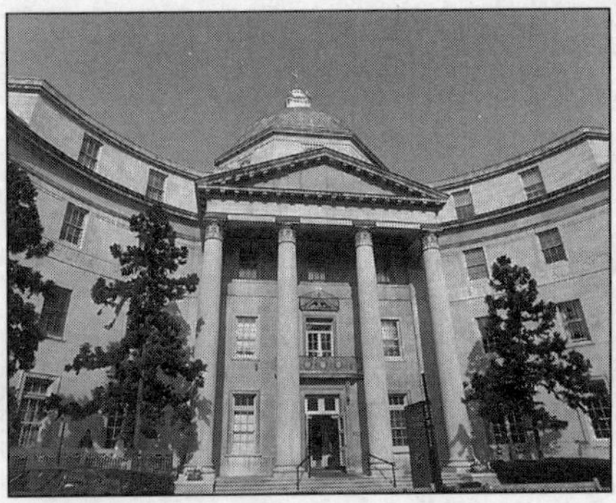

# Yale University School of Medicine

**New Haven, Connecticut**

Dr. Gerard N. Burrow, *Dean*
Dr. Thomas L. Lentz, *Assistant Dean for Admissions*
Pamela J. Nyiri, *Director of Financial Aid*

## ADDRESS INQUIRIES TO:

Office of Admissions
Yale University
School of Medicine
367 Cedar Street
New Haven, Connecticut 06510
(203) 785-2643; 785-3234 (FAX)
E-Mail: medicalschool.admissions@quickmail.yale.edu
Web Site: http://info.med.yale.edu/medadmit

## GENERAL INFORMATION

The Yale University School of Medicine was established by passage of a bill in the Connecticut General Assembly in 1810 granting a charter for the Medical Institution of Yale College. The Yale-New Haven Medical Center is composed of the School of Medicine, the School of Nursing, and the Yale-New Haven Hospital. The West Haven Veterans Hospital, Connecticut Mental Health Center, Yale Psychiatric Institute, Hospital of St. Raphael, and Waterbury Hospital are also used for instruction. The Yale Medical Library has an extensive collection of current and historical medical literature.

## CURRICULUM

The educational objective of the School of Medicine is to develop physicians who are highly competent and compassionate practitioners of the medical arts, schooled in the current state of knowledge of both medical biology and patient care. It is hoped that Yale-trained physicians will establish a lifelong process of learning the medical, behavioral, and social sciences by independent study. The aim is to produce physicians who will be among the leaders in their chosen field, whether it be in the basic medical sciences, academic clinical medicine, or medical practice in the community. Belief in the maturity and responsibility of students is emphasized by creating a flexible program, through anonymous examinations and the elimination of grades, and by encouraging independent study and research. The program allows considerable freedom for planning according to the ability and interests of the student.

The first two years of the Yale School of Medicine are spent building a foundation in the basic sciences. The first year emphasizes normal biological form and function. The second-year curriculum emphasizes the study of disease. Throughout both years, a patient-doctor course meets weekly to teach physical diagnosis and the art of talking with patients. The third year is almost entirely devoted to clinical clerkships with forty-five weeks of study in clerkships required for graduation. The fourth year is devoted to electives, a required primary care clerkship, and completion of the thesis work.

The thesis, a requirement since 1839, is an essential part of the curriculum and is designed to develop critical judgment, habits of self-education, and application of the scientific method to medicine. The thesis, based on original research in an area of the student's choosing, gives students the opportunity to work closely with faculty who are distinguished scientists, clinicians, and scholars.

A combined M.D.-Ph.D. Program is available for qualified applicants with a strong motivation towards a career in academic medicine and the biomedical sciences. Support is made available through the Medical Scientist Training Program. The M.D.-Ph.D. Program is flexible and normally takes seven to eight years to complete. Application should be made with supplemental forms included in the School of Medicine application packet.

## REQUIREMENTS FOR ENTRANCE

It is recommended that students enter medical school after four years of study in a college of arts and sciences or institute of technology. Students holding advanced degrees in science or other fields are also considered. Foreign students must have completed at least one year of study in an American college prior to application. Students who have been refused admission on three prior occasions are ineligible to apply for admission to the first-year class. The MCAT and satisfactory completion of the following courses are required.

*Sem. hrs.*

General biology or zoology (with lab) . . . . . . . . . . . . . . . 6–8
General or inorganic chemistry (with lab) . . . . . . . . . . . . 6–8
Organic chemistry (with lab) . . . . . . . . . . . . . . . . . . . . . . 6–8
General physics (with lab) . . . . . . . . . . . . . . . . . . . . . . . . 6–8

Acceptable courses in these subjects usually extend over one year and are given credit for six to eight semester hours. The medical faculty has no preference as to a major field for undergraduate study but recommends that students advance beyond the elementary level in their field of study. Students entering college with a strong background in the sciences, as demonstrated by advanced placement, are encouraged to substitute advanced science courses for the traditional requirements listed above.

Yale University School of Medicine does not participate in AMCAS. Application requests should be sent directly to the Office of Admissions.

## SELECTION FACTORS

The Committee on Admissions in general seeks to admit students who best suit the philosophies and goals of the school, which include providing an education in the scholarly and humane aspects of medicine and fostering the development of leaders who will advance medical practice and knowledge. It also seeks to ensure an adequate representation of women and minority groups and a diversity of interests and backgrounds. Yale University School of Medicine does not discriminate on the basis of race, sex, religion, national origin, age, handicap, or sexual orientation.

In considering applicants, the committee views the individual as a whole, taking into consideration each student's academic record, MCAT scores, premedical committee evaluations, letters of recommendation, outside accomplishments, personal qualities, and suitability for Yale.

Interviews are arranged only by invitation of the admissions committee. A large number of applicants have attained a high level of academic achievement as indicated by grades and test scores. Activities and accomplishments are of considerable importance in distinguishing candidates as individuals and demonstrating the ability to make significant independent contributions. The admissions committee also considers personal attributes thought to be important in a physician and suitability for the Yale program of medical education.

## FINANCIAL AID

The school discourages excessive outside work and provides scholarship awards and loans for those who have serious financial needs. Financial aid applications will be mailed on or around January 1. All applicants for financial aid will be required to participate in FAFSA. A supplemental needs analysis will be required for students applying for institutional funds. This application will require student, spouse, and family financial statements.

## INFORMATION FOR MINORITIES

Yale University School of Medicine seeks to obtain an adequate representation of all minority groups and encourages qualified minority students to apply. Applicants invited for interviews will have the opportunity to meet with minority students and faculty to learn about the school. The Committee on Admissions includes minority members.

Further information may be obtained from Dr. Forrester Lee, Assistant Dean for Multicultural Affairs.

Private Institution

## APPLICATION AND ACCEPTANCE POLICIES FOR 1997–98 FIRST-YEAR CLASS

Filing of application
    Earliest date: June 1, 1996
    Latest date: Oct. 15, 1996
School application fee to all applicants: $55
Oldest MCAT scores considered: 1993
Does have Early Decision Program (EDP)
    EDP application period: June 1–Aug. 1, 1996
    EDP applicants notified by: Oct. 1, 1996
Acceptance notice to regular applicants
    Earliest date: March 15, 1997
    Latest date: Until class is filled
Applicant's response to acceptance offer
    Maximum time: 3 weeks
Requests for deferred entrance considered: Yes
Deposit to hold place in class (applied to tuition):
    $100, due with response to acceptance offer
Deposit refundable prior to: May 15, 1997
Estimated number of new entrants: 100 (5 EDP)
Starting date: Sept. 1997

## TUITION AND STUDENT FEES PER YEAR FOR 1995–96 FIRST-YEAR CLASS

Tuition: $23,300          Student fees: $175

## INFORMATION ON 1995–96 FIRST-YEAR CLASS

| Number of | In-State | Out-of-State | Total |
|---|---|---|---|
| Applicants | 146 | 3,286 | 3,432 |
| Applicants Interviewed | 34 | 766 | 800 |
| New Entrants* | 11 | 90 | 101 |

*All took the MCAT; 99% had baccalaureate degrees.

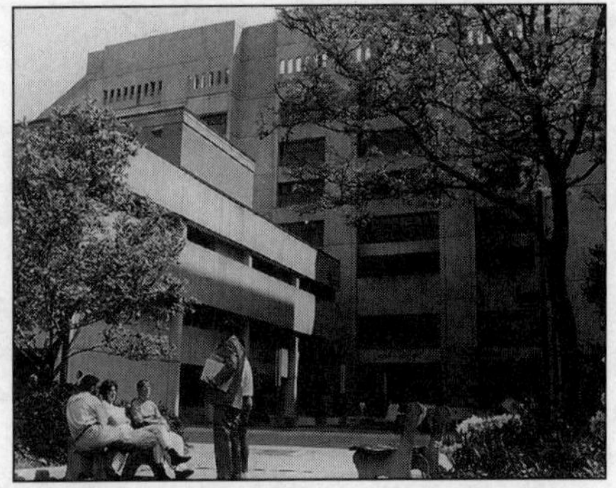

# George Washington University
# School of Medicine and Health Sciences

**Washington, D.C.**

Dr. Robert I. Keimowitz, *Dean for Academic Affairs*
Dr. John F. Williams, *Associate Dean for Admissions*
Charles Carpenter, *Director of Financial Aid*

## ADDRESS INQUIRIES TO:

Office of Admissions
George Washington University
School of Medicine and Health Sciences
2300 Eye Street, N.W., Room 615
Washington, D.C. 20037
(202) 994-3506

## GENERAL INFORMATION

Classes were first held in the School of Medicine of the George Washington University (GWU) in 1825. By 1973 modern facilities, including Ross Hall (a research and basic sciences center) and a medical library with a sophisticated audio visual department, were in operation near the University Hospital and clinics. The University Hospital provides clinical teaching and research opportunities; the clinics provide ambulatory experience in the medical and surgical specialties. The teaching services of the Children's Hospital National Medical Center, Fairfax Hospital, Holy Cross Hospital, National Naval Medical Center, St. Elizabeths Hospital, Veterans Administration Hospital, and Washington Hospital Center are available to students, under the direction of the faculty.

## CURRICULUM

The curriculum is designed to provide students a medical education comprehensive enough to prepare them for generalist careers and offer them the exposure on which to base career selection. The faculty's objectives include imparting to students a substantial body of information, while stressing the attitude of compassion, the skill of problem solving, the habit of self-education, and a high regard for the acquisition of new knowledge, both basic and applied. Emphasis is placed on education through cooperative effort, not through competition.

An innovative change was made to the M.D. curriculum and introduced in the fall of 1993. This program, the Practice of Medicine (POM), integrates the building blocks of a traditional medical education—a strong foundation of basic and clinical sciences—by interweaving them throughout the four-year curriculum. Gone is the conventional distinction between two years of basic sciences followed by two years of patient care. The first phase of this new course places every student with a practicing clinician every other week throughout Years I and II. On alternate weeks, clinical assessment skills (including learning to take a history and do the core physical examination) will be taught and evaluated.

Clinical clerkships offered under close supervision begin in the third year. Choice of courses is largely elective during the fourth year. The honors/pass/conditional/fail system is used for grading.

A joint program offered through GW's Columbian College and Graduate School of Arts and Sciences and the School of Medicine and Health Sciences is the Seven-Year Integrated B.A.-M.D. program. This program is designed for high school honor students of high ability and maturity who have already decided to become physicians and want to accomplish that goal in a shorter time and at a lower overall cost without seriously sacrificing the breadth of knowledge gained from a liberal arts education. Another joint program—an eight-year integrated engineering M.D. program—is available through the School of Engineering and the School of Medicine and Health Sciences.

An M.D.-master's of public health degree program and M.D.-Ph.D. program is also available to medical students. Course work can begin the summer preceding medical school matriculation.

## REQUIREMENTS FOR ENTRANCE

The MCAT and three years of college are required. Ninety semester hours of credit applicable toward a B.A. or B.S. in an approved college is the minimal requirement, although most selected students have completed four years of college.

Required courses are:

|  | *Sem. hrs.* |
|---|---|
| Biology and/or zoology (with lab) | 8 |
| Inorganic chemistry (with lab) | 8 |
| Organic chemistry (with lab) | 8 |
| Physics (with lab) | 8 |
| English composition and literature | 6 |

With the exception of these specific requirements, applicants are urged to follow their personal interests in developing a premedical course of study. Applicants with an undergraduate emphasis in the arts, humanities, and social sciences are welcomed.

## SELECTION FACTORS

The first step in the selection procedure is an overall evaluation based on data contained in the AMCAS and supplemental applications. This evaluation screens applicants on the basis of grades (taking into account the college of origin as well as improvement in performance in later years); MCAT scores; pertinent extracurricular, health related research, and work experiences; and evidence of non-scholastic accomplishments. Evidence of good performance in recent, relevant course work is to an applicant's advantage. Some additional consideration is given to applicants from the District of Columbia and its metropolitan area as well as to applicants from the university's undergraduate school. The next phase of the selection procedure depends on careful examination of personal comments and letters of recommendation. The most promising applicants are then invited for a personal interview either at the school or with a regional interviewer. The last phase includes the review by the Committee on Admissions of the entire dossier. The last phases are designed to select from students who are academically well prepared and those with motivational and personal characteristics that the committee considers important in future physicians. Many qualified reapplicants are accepted each year. There is no discrimination in the selection process because of race, sex, religion, age, marital status, handicap, or national or regional origin.

The 158 members of the 1995 entering class came from 66 different undergraduate schools. The mean undergraduate GPA was 3.4, although there was great variability about the average. Some other characteristics of the 1995 entering class were: *undergraduate major,* 28 percent in non-science fields; *graduate degrees,* 19 students; *gender,* 86 women; *geographic,* generally proportional to applications from across the country.

## FINANCIAL AID

Information regarding financial aid is available at the time of interview. Although responsibility for arranging the financing of a medical education must rest with the student, the financial aid officer will provide information and assistance to try to help students meet their needs. Limited merit-based admissions scholarships are available. Students are not encouraged to seek part-time employment.

Because of the restrictions placed on funds, financial aid can rarely be obtained by non-U.S. citizens. This fact will have to play a role in the Committee on Admissions' deliberations on such candidates. Ability to pay expenses is not a consideration for U.S. citizens and permanent residents.

## INFORMATION FOR MINORITIES

Qualified minority group applicants are invited and encouraged to apply. Under appropriate circumstances the school's supplemental application fee will be waived. Regional interviews can be arranged to help contain application costs for disadvantaged students. Tutorial assistance can be arranged for students in academic need.

Private Institution

### APPLICATION AND ACCEPTANCE POLICIES FOR 1997–98 FIRST-YEAR CLASS

*School participates in AMCAS. See Chapter 4.*

Filing of AMCAS application
 Earliest date: June 1, 1996
 Latest date: Nov. 1, 1996
School application fee to all applicants: $55
Oldest MCAT scores considered: 1994
Does have Early Decision Program (EDP)
 EDP application period: June 1–Aug. 1, 1996
 EDP applicants notified by: Oct. 1, 1996
Acceptance notice to regular applicants
 Earliest date: Oct. 15, 1996
 Latest date: Until class is filled
Applicant's response to acceptance offer
 Maximum time: 2 weeks
Requests for deferred entrance considered: Yes
Deposit to hold place in class: None; a tuition
 prepayment of $2,500 is required by July 1, 1997
Estimated number of new entrants: 150 (2 EDP)
Starting date: Aug. 1997

### TUITION AND STUDENT FEES PER YEAR FOR 1995–96 FIRST-YEAR CLASS

Tuition: $30,200          Student fees: $732

### INFORMATION ON 1995–96 FIRST-YEAR CLASS

| Number of | D.C. | Out-of-State | Total |
|---|---|---|---|
| Applicants | 81 | 12,290 | 12,371 |
| Applicants Interviewed | 35 | 1,023 | 1,058 |
| New Entrants* | 19 | 139 | 158 |

*82% had baccalaureate degrees; 92% took the MCAT.

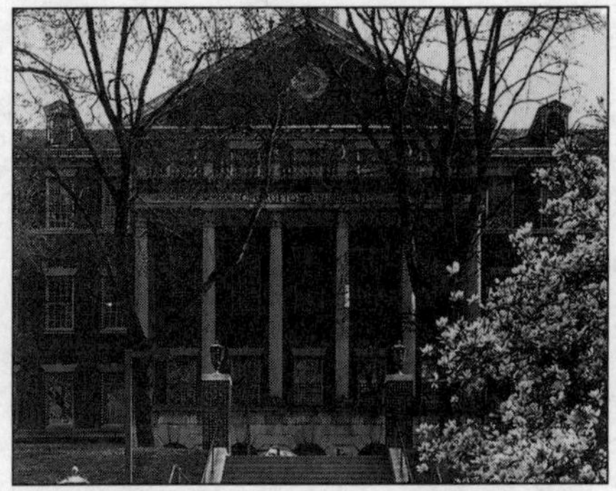

# Georgetown University School of Medicine

## Washington, D.C.

Dr. William C. Maxted, *Dean for Academic Affairs*
Karen L. Pfordresher, *Assistant Dean for Admissions and Financial Planning*

## ADDRESS INQUIRIES TO:

Office of Admissions
Georgetown University
School of Medicine
3900 Reservoir Road, N.W.
Washington, D.C. 20007
(202) 687-1154
Web Site: http://www.georgetown.edu

## GENERAL INFORMATION

The Georgetown School of Medicine, established in 1851, is a part of the oldest Catholic and Jesuit-sponsored university in the United States. Committed to training physicians in all dimensions of the delivery of humane patient care, the School of Medicine works in association with the 409-bed Georgetown University Hospital and 8 affiliated federal and community hospitals in the Washington metropolitan area. Providing an environment that promotes training and educational opportunities, the medical center includes a $23-million Concentrated Care Center with a modern 12-room surgical suite, 24 preoperative and postoperative surgical suites, and state-of-the-art emergency, x-ray, and transplant facilities. The campus also contains a modern health science library, basic and preclinical science buildings, classrooms, laboratories, and a research building.

Georgetown also offers opportunities for the overall development of its student body. The Reverend Gerard F. Yates, S.J., Memorial Field House, constructed in 1979, houses swimming facilities and jogging and multi- and single-purpose courts and offers many athletic programs. The Thomas and Dorothy Leavey Center, completed in 1988, provides a focus for faculty and student activities. It contains facilities for conferences and the performing arts and a variety of dining establishments and guest quarters.

The university is located in one of the most concentrated regions for medical research in the country. Adjacent to the hospital is the Vincent T. Lombardi Cancer Research Center. The school is near the National Institutes of Health and other nationally prominent health care and research facilities.

## CURRICULUM

Georgetown's four-year curriculum combines departmentally based basic science courses and laboratory work, prescribed clinical clerkships, multidisciplinary courses and conferences, and electives. Courses in the first two years focus on the development of fundamental knowledge concerning the body's normal and altered structure and functions. Small-group teaching and problem-based presentations have replaced a portion of the large class lectures. Exposure to patient assessment and care begins in the first year.

In the third year, clinical clerkships stress the skills required to acquire and interpret patient-based data, while the fourth year further develops skills in patient management, including rotations in ambulatory care settings. Twenty-four weeks of electives are available during this final year, four of which may be used for vacation.

A research track for medical students and a combined M.D.-Ph.D. program are also available; the Ph.D. may be taken in a basic medical science department, the neurosciences, or in philosophy-bioethics.

At Georgetown the grading system consists of honors, high pass, pass, and fail. Faculty-student review of the curriculum is an important continuing endeavor of the School of Medicine. A revised curriculum was implemented in 1991–92.

## REQUIREMENTS FOR ENTRANCE

In general, Georgetown requires the MCAT and a minimum of three years of college (90 semester hours) for consideration of admission to the School of Medicine. The baccalaureate degree is highly desirable. The minimum specific course requirements are:

|  | Sem./Qtr. |
|---|---|
| Biology (with lab) | 2/3 |
| Inorganic chemistry (with lab) | 2/3 |
| Organic chemistry (with lab) | 2/3 |
| General physics (with lab) | 2/3 |
| College mathematics | 2/3 |
| English | 2/3 |

While a solid preparation in the basic sciences is essential, a broad background in the humanities and computer science are also important. Biochemistry is strongly recommended and can be substituted for second semester organic chemistry.

Applicants should take the MCAT in the spring of the year they intend to apply to the School of Medicine and make sure that required courses will be completed. Georgetown allows six to eight hours of prerequisites to be taken during the application year. Applicants are cautioned that files are not reviewed by the Committee on Admissions until MCAT scores are received; a delay in the receipt of such credentials may delay consideration of an application.

## SELECTION FACTORS

The Committee on Admissions selects students on the basis of academic achievements, character, maturity, and motivation. There are no geographical quotas, although some preference is given to residents of the metropolitan District of Columbia area. In rendering its decisions, the Committee on Admissions evaluates the applicant's entire academic record, performance on the MCAT, college premedical advisory committee evaluations, letters of recommendation, and personal interviews.

For the 1995 entering class, 12,448 candidates applied from over 789 undergraduate colleges. The applicants who enrolled had the following characteristics: *mean GPA,* 3.58; *undergraduate major,* 46 percent in the biological sciences, 15 percent in the physical sciences, 19 percent in social sciences, 20 percent in various humanities and other majors; 42 percent women.

Georgetown requires personal interviews. These interviews are conducted on the medical center campus, and applicants are not invited to interview until all their credentials have been received and reviewed by the Committee on Admissions. Applicants are urged to submit their applications and supporting credentials as early as possible. The School of Medicine does not discriminate on the basis of race, sex, creed, age, handicap, or national or ethnic origin.

## FINANCIAL AID

Georgetown's medical school participates in federal financial aid programs and awards limited school-administered grants, scholarships, and low interest loans to students on the basis of financial need. Parents' financial information is required for all students seeking school administered aid.

Medical students at Georgetown are expected to take responsibility for their financial affairs in meeting deadlines for both tuition payment as well as in applying for financial aid. Loan indebtedness counseling is an important function of the Office of Student Financial Planning (OSFP) as a majority of students at the School of Medicine incur substantial educational debt. Candidates for admission are strongly encouraged to contact the OSFP with questions about financial aid.

## INFORMATION FOR MINORITIES

In 1995 the School of Medicine had a minority enrollment, (including African American, Mexican American, mainland Puerto Rican, and native American students) totaling 9.7 percent of the entering class. Questions about programs and opportunities for qualified minority applicants should be addressed to Dr. Arthur Hoyte, director, Office of Programs for

Minority Student Development. The Georgetown Experimental Medical Studies (GEMS) Program is a one-year postbaccalaureate program for qualified underrepresented minority students. Priority consideration is given to residents of the District of Columbia. For more information, write or telephone Joy Williams, GEMS Program coordinator, at (202) 687-1406.

---

Private Institution

### APPLICATION AND ACCEPTANCE POLICIES FOR 1997–98 FIRST-YEAR CLASS

*School participates in AMCAS. See Chapter 4.*

Filing of AMCAS application
    Earliest date: June 1, 1996
    Latest date: Nov. 1, 1996
School application fee to all applicants: $60
Oldest MCAT scores considered: 1993
Does not have Early Decision Program (EDP)
Acceptance notice to regular applicants
    Earliest date: Oct. 15, 1996
    Latest date: Until class is filled
Applicant's response to acceptance offer
    Maximum time: 3 weeks
Requests for deferred entrance considered: Yes
Deposit to hold place in class (applied to tuition):
    $100, due March 15, 1997 or within 3 weeks of
    acceptance
Deposit refundable prior to: May 1, 1997
Partial tuition repayment due June 1, 1997
Estimated number of new entrants: 165
Starting date: Aug. 1997

### TUITION AND STUDENT FEES PER YEAR FOR 1995–96 FIRST-YEAR CLASS

Tuition: $23,625

### INFORMATION ON 1995–96 FIRST-YEAR CLASS

| Number of | D.C. | Out-of-State | Total |
|---|---|---|---|
| Applicants | 62 | 12,386 | 12,448 |
| Applicants Interviewed | * | * | 1,960 |
| New Entrants† | 2 | 163 | 165 |

*Data not available.
†All had baccalaureate degrees; 96.4% took the MCAT.

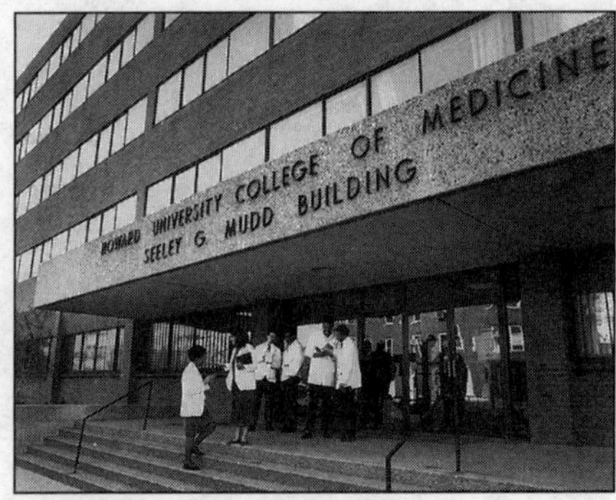

# Howard University
# College of Medicine

**Washington, D.C.**

Dr. Floyd J. Malveaux, *Dean*
Ann Finney, *Admissions Officer*
Sterling M. Lloyd, Jr., *Assistant Dean for Student Affairs*

## ADDRESS INQUIRIES TO:

Admissions Office
Howard University
College of Medicine
520 W Street, N.W.
Washington, D.C. 20059
(202) 806-6270; 806-7934 (FAX)

## GENERAL INFORMATION

The Howard University College of Medicine is the oldest and largest historically black medical school in the United States and the 36th oldest of all 125 medical schools in this country. Initially established as a medical department, the college opened in 1868 with eight students and seven faculty members. The medical department's primary goal then remains the college's today: to train students to become competent, compassionate physicians who will provide care in medically underserved communities.

In 1871, Howard University graduated its first medical class, consisting of two black men and three white men. One woman was graduated the following year. Subsequent classes throughout the College of Medicine's history have been similarly cosmopolitan in accordance with the spirit and intention of Howard University's founders. The college proudly cites its long history of training men and women of all races and ethnic origins, religions, creeds, nationalities and economic backgrounds.

The college has more than 4,000 living alumni, including approximately 25 percent of all black practicing physicians in this country. During the first half of this century, the college contributed nearly half of the black physicians in the United States.

The 300-bed Howard University Hospital was completed in 1975. It is the college's primary teaching hospital for medical students and is used for postgraduate training in the various specialties of medicine. Medical students also serve clerkships at the District of Columbia General Hospital, St. Elizabeths Hospital, Walter Reed Army Medical Center, U.S. Naval Medical Center, the Washington Veterans Administration Medical Center, Greater Southeast Community Hospital, Providence Hospital, the National Rehabilitation Hospital, the Washington Hospital Center, and Prince George's Hospital Center.

## CURRICULUM

The curriculum is designed to provide a firm basis for the science and art of medicine and to provide effective integration of basic science concepts, clinical application, and research. Students are presented the essential knowledge and skills necessary for the practice of medicine in courses which are required of all medical students. In addition, time is provided in the schedule for students to pursue areas of their interest through elective courses.

The required disciplines of the first and second years include gross and developmental anatomy, histology and cell structure, biochemistry, physiology, pathology, pharmacology, medical genetics, psychiatry, biometrics and epidemiology, and microbiology. In addition to these, three interdisciplinary courses are offered in the first year: basic neuroscience and introduction to patient care I and II. During the second year, the interdisciplinary courses are offered as pathophysiology of organ systems, and the principles of physical diagnosis in introduction to patient care III.

The third and fourth years consist of blocks of instruction in a continuum of clerkships and examinations in various clinical subjects. During the fourth year, opportunity is available for additional clinical or research experience through 20 or 24 weeks of required electives.

A five-year curriculum is offered to students who demonstrate during their first semester of enrollment or by the end of the January neuroscience course that they are having difficulty meeting the demands of the four-year curriculum and need additional time to meet the requirements for satisfactory performance. This curriculum, which does not require additional courses, includes changes in the scheduling of courses in the four-year curriculum to accommodate the one-year extension.

Satisfactory performance is required in all courses for promotion and graduation. Students are required to pass Step 1 of the USMLE examinations for promotion to the third year. Passing of Step 2 of the USMLE examinations is required for graduation. Grades in the College of Medicine are reported as H (honors), S (satisfactory), or U (unsatisfactory).

The Early Entry Medical Education Program (EEMEP), initiated in 1971, permits undergraduates who have completed their third year to be eligible for admission to the College of Medicine. This program allows for the reduction of the traditional total years of college and medical school to seven years. Participants in the EEMEP must have completed their premedical requirements and must present above average scores on the MCAT.

A combined B.S.-M.D. program was initiated in 1974 for students enrolling in the Howard University College of Arts and Sciences from high school. Both degrees may be obtained in a six-year period.

An M.D.-Ph.D. degree program is available in anatomy, human genetics, microbiology, biochemistry, pharmacology, physiology, biology, and chemistry.

## REQUIREMENTS FOR ENTRANCE

The MCAT is required. It is recommended that all applicants take the MCAT in the spring rather than in the fall of the year in which they apply. A minimum of 62 semester hours at an accredited U.S. or Canadian university or college is required. Course work should include:

|                        | Sem. hrs. |
| ---------------------- | --------- |
| Biology or zoology     | 8         |
| General chemistry      | 8         |
| Organic chemistry      | 8         |
| General physics        | 8         |
| College mathematics    | 6         |
| English                | 6         |

## SELECTION FACTORS

There are four major criteria used in the selection of applicants for admission to the College of Medicine: (1) character and discernible motivation for a career in medicine, (2) scholastic record, (3) results of the MCAT, and (4) letters of recommendation from preprofessional advisers and faculty. Candidates for admission and alternates are selected from those applicants who satisfy the criteria and who are most likely to serve in communities needing physician services. MCAT scores and GPAs are used for initial screening.

An invitation for an interview may be extended to an applicant after the Committee on Admissions has made a preliminary examination of the applicant's credentials and has decided that an interview is desirable. Although the total student is evaluated, the Committee on Admissions gives strongest consideration to those who have GPAs of 3.0 and above.

There are no residence restrictions. All applicants will be evaluated regardless of their sex, race, religion, national or ethnic origin, age, marital status, or handicap. In the 1995 entering class, 68 percent were black, 11 percent were Latino, 14 percent were Asian, 6 percent were foreign, and 52 percent were women.

A nonrefundable $150 enrollment fee (due with response to acceptance) is required of accepted students who have never previously enrolled at Howard University. This is in addition to the $100 refundable good faith deposit.

## FINANCIAL AID

Approximately 85 percent of the students enrolled in the College of Medicine receive some sort of financial assistance. Financial aid applicants must submit the FAFSA. Students with demonstrated need may receive school-based scholarships and loans, and those who qualify are recommended for federally guaranteed and private educational loans. Some merit awards are offered to outstanding entering freshmen and for exceptional academic performance in the medical curriculum. Some students receive scholarships and loans funded by the U.S. Public Health Service or by the military.

---

Private Institution

### APPLICATION AND ACCEPTANCE POLICIES FOR 1997–98 FIRST-YEAR CLASS

*School participates in AMCAS. See Chapter 4.*

Filing of AMCAS application
  Earliest date: June 1, 1996
  Latest date: Dec. 15, 1996
School application fee to all applicants: $25
Oldest MCAT scores considered: 1993
Does not have Early Decision Program
Acceptance notice to regular applicants
  Earliest date: Oct. 15, 1996
  Latest date: Until class is filled
Applicant's response to acceptance offer
  Maximum time: 30 days
Requests for deferred entrance considered: Yes
Deposit to hold place in class (applied to tuition):
  $100, due with response to acceptance offer
Deposit refundable prior to: May 15, 1997
Estimated number of new entrants: 110
Starting date: Aug. 1997

### TUITION AND STUDENT FEES PER YEAR FOR 1995–96 FIRST-YEAR CLASS

Tuition: $14,400          Student fees: $788

### INFORMATION ON 1995–96 FIRST-YEAR CLASS

| Number of            | D.C. | Out-of-State | Total |
| -------------------- | ---- | ------------ | ----- |
| Applicants           | 67   | 6,094        | 6,161 |
| Applicants Interviewed | 13 | 493          | 506   |
| New Entrants*        | 4    | 107          | 111   |

*All took the MCAT; 96% had baccalaureate degrees.

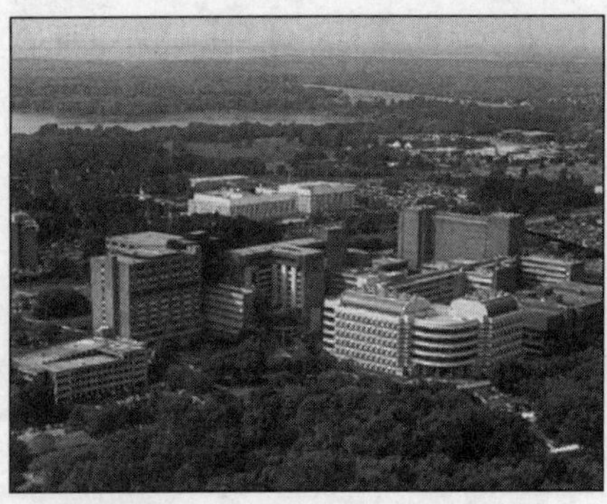

# University of Florida College of Medicine

**Gainesville, Florida**

Dr. Allen H. Neims, *Dean, College of Medicine and Associate Vice President for Clinical Affairs*
Dr. Robert Hatch, *Chair, Medical Selection Committee*
Ellen M. Parris, *Coordinator of Financial Aid*

## ADDRESS INQUIRIES TO:

Chair, Medical Selection Committee
Box 100216
J. Hillis Miller Health Center
University of Florida
College of Medicine
Gainesville, Florida 32610
(352) 392-4569; 846-0622 (FAX)
Web Site: http://www.med.ufl.edu/

## GENERAL INFORMATION

The College of Medicine, a component college of the University of Florida Health Science Center, admitted the first class in September 1956. Situated at the southeast corner of the 2,000-acre campus of the University of Florida, the College of Medicine enjoys the benefit of strong ties with other programs within the university as well as a close relationship to the other Health Science Center colleges (dentistry, health related professions, nursing, pharmacy, and veterinary medicine). The University of Florida Health Science Center complex also includes the Chandler A. Stetson Medical Science Building, the Communicore Building (library, teaching laboratories, and classrooms), the Academic Research Building, the Cancer Research Building, Shands Hospital, and the Veterans Administration Medical Center, located across the street from the Health Science Center. The University of Florida Health Science Center—Jacksonville is our urban campus. Formal educational affiliations have also been established in Ft. Lauderdale, Orlando, and Pensacola.

## CURRICULUM

The curriculum is divided into three blocks of time—preclinical basic sciences (first two years), clinical clerkships (third year), and postclerkship electives and required courses (fourth year). The required clinical clerkship rotations provide the students with experiences in eight general areas of medicine—anesthesiology, family medicine, medicine, neurology, psychiatry, obstetrics and gynecology, surgery, and pediatrics. The rotations include a 12-week interdisciplinary clerkship, which includes ambulatory clinical experience in family medicine, medicine, and pediatrics. The fourth year includes four weeks of required medicine, pediatrics, or family medicine, four weeks of required advanced pharmacology, and four weeks of required surgery. The remainder of the senior year is devoted to elective course work. Students' performance in academic course work will be evaluated by letter grades. However, some courses use a pass-fail system.

During the first summer and the elective period, students may choose involvement in biomedical or clinical research. Students may also delay a clerkship rotation to the fourth year.

Students may elect the option of taking the preclinical basic science course over a three-year period. This option might provide an opportunity for research or be advantageous to students from nonscience or disadvantaged backgrounds and who would benefit from a more moderately paced schedule.

## MEDICAL SCIENTIST TRAINING PROGRAM (M.D.-PH.D.)

This program offers an opportunity for students who are motivated toward an academic career in the medical sciences. The M.D.-Ph.D. program is designed to be flexible. Candidates for this program must satisfy admission requirements for the college of medicine and the graduate school and have significant research experience.

## JUNIOR HONORS MEDICAL PROGRAM

Students accepted into the Junior Honors Medical Program at the end of their second year of college enroll in basic medical science seminars and undergraduate courses during their third year. They become full-time medical students during their fourth year and receive a B.S. degree at the end of their fourth year from the College of Liberal Arts and Sciences. Although primarily intended for students in their second year at the University of Florida, applications from students enrolled at other colleges and universities will be considered. Further information may be obtained by writing to the director of the Junior Honors Program at the College of Medicine.

## REQUIREMENTS FOR ENTRANCE

The MCAT is required and must be taken at a time that enables scores to be received by the admissions office prior to the December application deadline to be considered for admission the following August. The student should have completed the requirements for a bachelor's degree at an accredited college or university. In exceptional instances students upon whom the degree has not been conferred may be admitted. College work must include:

|  | *Sem. hrs.* |
|---|---|
| Biochemistry | 4 |
| Biology (with lab) | 8 |
| Inorganic chemistry (with lab) | 8 |
| Organic chemistry (with lab) | 4 |
| General physics (with lab) | 8 |

## SELECTION FACTORS

Applicants will be appraised on the basis of personal attributes, academic record, evaluation of past activities, the MCAT, and personal interview. The school does not discriminate on the basis of race, sex, age, disability, creed, or national origin. Although Florida residents are given preference in admission, a limited number of nonresidents are considered each year. Nonresident applicants must demonstrate superior qualifications. The school will continue to seek minority applicants and strongly encourages members of minority groups to apply regardless of residence.

Accepted students for the 1995 entering class had the following characteristics: *mean GPA,* 3.69; *MCAT* 28; *sex,* 52 percent *female*; 14 percent *minorities;* 36 percent *nonwhite.*

## FINANCIAL AID

Every attempt is made to assist enrolled students who need financial aid. A limited number of scholarships and loan funds are available to students in need, and applications are accepted at any time. Student summer and school-year research fellowships are available. Loans and scholarships are available to qualified students with financial need.

## FLORIDA STATE UNIVERSITY PROGRAM IN MEDICAL SCIENCES

The Program in Medical Sciences is an inter-university program between Florida State University and the University of Florida College of Medicine. Thirty first-year medical students are selected by the Program Selection Committee to complete the first year of basic medical sciences curriculum at Florida State University. The program is open to all residents of Florida who complete a baccalaureate degree and fulfill the usual prerequisite course requirements. Application is through AMCAS. Early selection is open to outstanding applicants from Florida State University, University of West Florida, and Florida Agricultural and Mechanical University. The program is especially interested in selecting students who have a likelihood of practicing medicine in primary care medical specialties. Students from rural areas, underrepresented minorities, and applicants who demonstrated a dedication to service to others are encouraged to apply. During this first year experience, students gain clinical skills by serving in local health clinics, working with primary care physicians who serve as their preceptors, and completing a semester-long preceptorship at the Family Practice Residency Program at Tallahassee Memorial Regional Medical Center. Students complete the remaining three years of medical education at the University of Florida College of Medicine upon successful completion of the first-year curriculum. For further information write: Program in Medical Sciences, Florida State University, Tallahassee, FL 32306-4051; or phone: (904) 644-1855.

Public Institution

## APPLICATION AND ACCEPTANCE POLICIES FOR 1997–98 FIRST-YEAR CLASS

*School participates in AMCAS. See Chapter 4.*

Filing of AMCAS application
  Earliest date: June 1, 1996
  Latest date: Dec. 1, 1996
School application fee after screening: $20
Oldest MCAT scores considered: 1994
Does not have Early Decision Program
Acceptance notice to regular applicants
  Earliest date: Oct. 15, 1996
  Latest date: Until class is filled
Applicant's response to acceptance offer
  Maximum time: 2 weeks
Requests for deferred entrance considered: Yes
Deposit to hold place in class: None
Estimated number of new entrants: 85
Starting date: Aug. 1997

## TUITION AND STUDENT FEES PER YEAR FOR 1995–96 FIRST-YEAR CLASS

| Tuition: | Student fees: |
|---|---|
| Resident: $7,141.50 | Resident: $1,031.06 |
| Nonresident: $19,521.96 | Nonresdient: $1,650.08 |

## INFORMATION ON 1995–96 FIRST-YEAR CLASS

| *Number of* | *In-State* | *Out-of-State* | *Total* |
|---|---|---|---|
| Applicants | 1,449 | 1,105 | 2,554 |
| Applicants Interviewed | 347 | 22 | 369 |
| New Entrants* | 81 | 4 | 85 |

*All took the MCAT and had baccalaureate degrees, except the 12 entering the Junior Honors Program.

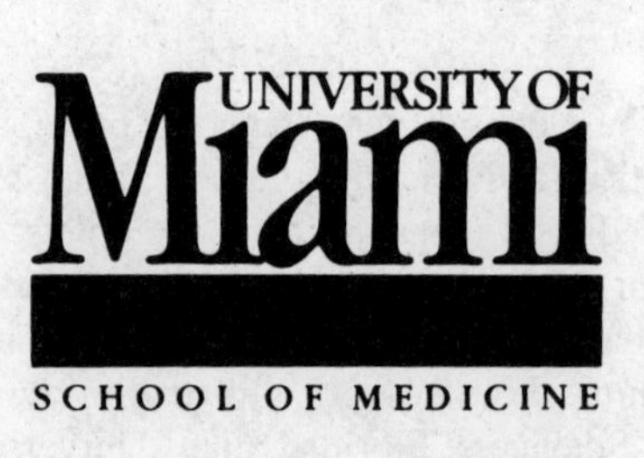

# University of Miami
# School of Medicine

**Miami, Florida**

Dr. John G. Clarkson, *Senior Vice President for Medical Affairs and Dean, School of Medicine*
Dr. R.E. Hinkley, *Associate Dean for Admissions and Enrollment Management*
Laura L. Horsley, *Assistant Dean for Student Financial Assistance*

## ADDRESS INQUIRIES TO:

Office of Admissions
University of Miami
School of Medicine
P.O. Box 016159
Miami, Florida 33101
(305) 243-6791; 243-6548 (FAX);
E-Mail: miami-md@mednet.med.miami.edu
Web Site: http://www.med.miami.edu

## GENERAL INFORMATION

The University of Miami School of Medicine is the largest and oldest medical school in the State of Florida. Since its founding in 1952, the School of Medicine has experienced a remarkable growth rate and has been the catalyst in the development of one of the largest and most comprehensive health care centers in the nation. In 1995 the school had a full-time faculty of 1,000, who held more than 450 grants and contracts to do research in a variety of fields, an annual budget of $451 million, and a total of more than 4,800 graduates.

The School of Medicine is located on the medical campus next to Jackson Memorial Hospital in the Civic Center area of Miami. Classrooms used by students during the first two years, as well as administrative offices and research laboratories, are located in the Rosenstiel Medical Sciences Building and the Glaser Medical Research Building. Jackson Memorial Hospital and the Veterans Affairs Medical Center provide the primary settings in which third- and fourth-year students acquire and hone their clinical skills. With over 50,000 admissions per year, Jackson Memorial Hospital is a unique asset, providing a complete spectrum of clinical experiences.

Also located on the medical campus and affiliated with the University of Miami School of Medicine are the Mailman Center for Child Development, the Bascom Palmer Eye Institute and Anne Bates Leach Eye Hospital, the Applebaum Magnetic Resonance Imaging Center, the Ambulatory Care Center, the UM Hospitals and Clinics, the Diabetes Research Institute, and the Ryder Trauma Center. The Sylvester Comprehensive Cancer Center is the only facility in the State of Florida to be designated as a comprehensive center by the National Cancer Institute. More than 3,000 beds are available for clinical teaching in the UM-JMH Medical Center.

## CURRICULUM

The curriculum is a well-balanced educational program, and its goal is to educate students to be knowledgeable and compassionate physicians. The first two years are devoted primarily to the basic sciences and are taught in a "block" format. The Community Clinical Experience is a course that provides students with direct patient contact and hospital experience throughout the first two years of the curriculum.

Clinical teaching in the third and fourth years is primarily at the bedside and is supported by small-group conferences. Required clerkships include medicine, primary care, obstetrics, pediatrics, psychiatry, surgery, neurology, and geriatrics. Much of the fourth year is spent in elective clerkships.

The School of Medicine has two B.S.-M.D. programs. Further information about these special programs may be obtained from the Office of Undergraduate Admissions at (305) 284-4323. The school sponsors an M.D.-Ph.D. program.

## REQUIREMENTS FOR ENTRANCE

The School of Medicine accepts U.S. citizens and permanent residents of the United States who have completed a minimum of 90 semester hours of college work exclusive of courses in military science and physical education. Credits earned at foreign institutions are not accepted. Courses specifically required are:

|  | *Sem. hrs.* |
| --- | --- |
| English | 6 |
| Chemistry (with lab) | 8 |
| Organic chemistry (with lab) | 8 |
| Physics (with lab) | 8 |
| General biology or zoology | 6 |
| Other science courses* | 6 |

*These may be distributed in the biological sciences, chemistry, physics, or mathematics. A course in biochemistry is strongly recommended and can be substituted for one semester of organic chemistry.

AP credit may be used as part of the 90 semester hour total, but the credits listed above should be graded credits. CLEP credits are not accepted.

All applicants must take the MCAT exam no later than the fall preceding the year in which they hope to enroll in the School of Medicine.

## SELECTION FACTORS

Florida residents are given preference in all admissions decisions. Nonresidents are encouraged to apply only if they have a truly superior academic record and MCAT scores or have other unique qualifications which the Committee on Admissions would find desirable. The committee gives careful consideration to many factors when evaluating candidates for admission. Some of these factors are scholastic aptitude and preparedness to study medicine, results of the MCAT, and personal factors such as maturity, dedication, motivation, interpersonal skills, and leadership ability. The 1995 entering class (138 new entrants) had the following profile: *mean GPA,* 3.62; *mean MCAT scores: VR*-9.9, *PS*-9.9, *BS*-10.0; 51 percent women, 10 percent minorities; 50 percent *biology or chemistry majors; undergraduate colleges,* 38 represented. Applicants' files are reviewed without regard to race, creed, sex, national origin, age, or handicap. A personal interview is required to complete the application process. Interviews are arranged at the initiative of the committee and are held on the medical campus.

## FINANCIAL AID

Eighty percent of all medical students receive some kind of financial aid. In 1994–95 the amount awarded totaled about $15 million. The school participates in all major federal and state programs. Several scholarships are awarded each year for academic promise and for proven financial need. Information concerning financial assistance and student budgets may be obtained by calling the Office of Student Financial Assistance at (305) 243-6211.

## INFORMATION FOR MINORITIES

The Minority Students Health Careers Motivation Program is a special seven-week summer program that provides premedical undergraduates with the opportunity to gain first-hand knowledge of the requirements of a medical education. The purpose of the program is to enlarge the pool of qualified underrepresented minorities and individuals from disadvantaged backgrounds who are interested in health careers, primarily medicine. The program gives participants a "mini" medical school experience and consists of courses in human anatomy, biochemistry, and microbiology, along with a specialized course in reading and study skills. Books, supplies, meals, and housing are provided by the program and all accepted students receive a stipend. Application forms and further information about the program may be obtained by writing to the Office of Minority Affairs or by calling at (305) 243-5998.

Private Institution

## APPLICATION AND ACCEPTANCE POLICIES FOR 1997–98 FIRST-YEAR CLASS

*School participates in AMCAS. See Chapter 4.*

Filing of AMCAS application
  Earliest date: June 1, 1996
  Latest date: Dec. 1, 1996
School application fee to all applicants: $50
Oldest MCAT scores considered: 1994
Does have Early Decision Program
  For Florida residents only
  EDP application period: June 1–Aug. 1, 1996
  EDP applicants notified by: Oct. 1, 1996
Acceptance notice to regular applicants
  Earliest date: Oct. 15, 1996
  Latest date: Until class is filled
Applicant's response to acceptance offer
  Maximum time: 3 weeks
Requests for deferred entrance considered: No
Deposit to hold place in class (applied to tuition):
  $100, due with response to acceptance offer
Deposit refundable prior to: May 15, 1997
Estimated number of new entrants: 144 (5 EDP)
Starting date: Aug. 1997

## TUITION AND STUDENT FEES PER YEAR FOR 1995–96 FIRST-YEAR CLASS

Tuition: $23,040          Student fees: $110

## INFORMATION ON 1995–96 FIRST-YEAR CLASS

| Number of | In-State | Out-of-State | Total |
|---|---|---|---|
| Applicants | 1,406 | 1,867 | 3,273 |
| Applicants Interviewed | 307 | 7 | 314 |
| New Entrants* | 136 | 2 | 138 |

*All took the MCAT; 74% had baccalaureate degrees.

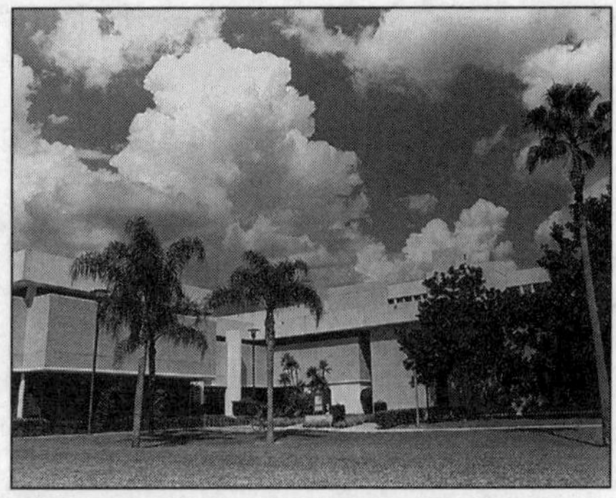

# University of South Florida College of Medicine

**Tampa, Florida**


Dr. Randolph Manning, *Associate Dean, Student Affairs*
Jay S. Layman, *Director of Admissions*
Carolyn Nicolosi, *Director of Student Affairs*


## ADDRESS INQUIRIES TO:

Office of Admissions
Box 3
University of South Florida
College of Medicine
12901 Bruce B. Downs Boulevard
Tampa, Florida 33612-4799
(813) 974-2229; 974-4990 (FAX)

## GENERAL INFORMATION

The College of Medicine, one of the three Colleges of the University of South Florida (USF) Health Sciences Center, admitted the first class of medical students in 1971. At present, the freshman class consists of 96 new students each year. In addition to the three colleges, the Health Sciences Center includes a medical science area, auditorium, cafeteria, medical library, and medical clinics. Clinical instruction for College of Medicine students is in large part based in Tampa at the USF Medical Clinics, Tampa General Hospital, James A. Haley Veterans Hospital, Tampa Unit Shriners Hospital for Crippled Children, H. Lee Moffitt Cancer Center and Research Institute, Tampa General Hospital University Psychiatry Center, and the University Diagnostic Institute. Clinical instruction is also provided at All Childrens' Hospital, Bayfront Medical Center, Bay Pines Veterans Hospital in St. Petersburg, and the Orlando Regional Medical Center.

## CURRICULUM

The four-year curriculum is designed to permit the student to learn the fundamental principles of medicine, to acquire skills of critical judgment based on evidence and experience, and to develop an ability to use principles and skills wisely in solving problems of health and disease. It includes the sciences basic to medicine, the major clinical disciplines, and other significant elements such as behavioral science, medical ethics, and human values.

The intent is to foster in students the ability to learn through self-directed, independent study throughout their professional lives. Using both ambulatory and hospital settings, students are given increasing responsibility for patient care in preparation to enter graduate medical education residencies.

Some students begin medical school with future plans such as primary care practice, clinical research, or preventive medi-cine and public health. For these students, special opportunities are available in medical school. For students seriously considering primary care, there are special opportunities to test and to reinforce this interest through a variety of existing and newly developed programs. Special programs are available for a select few students interested in an intense research career or to acquire both the M.D. and Ph.D. degrees in less time than would ordinarily be required for each separately. Likewise, it is possible for a student interested in public health, preventive medicine, epidemiology, health care systems, and related areas to achieve both an M.D. and master's in public health (M.P.H.) degree with minimal additional time. The M.P.H. degree is awarded through the College of Public Health.

## PREMEDICAL HONORS PROGRAM

This is an integrated program in which the College of Medicine will reserve certain places in the first- year medical class for superior students who satisfy the requirements for both university honors and admission to the study of medicine. All questions concerning the premedical options in university honors should be addressed to: Director of Honors, CPR 273, University of South Florida, Tampa, Florida 33620; the telephone number is (813) 974-3087.

## REQUIREMENTS FOR ENTRANCE

The MCAT is required. A minimum of three years of college or university work at a fully accredited institution is mandatory. Although the baccalaureate degree is desirable, a three-year applicant with a superior academic record and demonstrated maturity may be considered. Required courses are as follows:

*Semesters*

| | |
|---|---|
| General biology (with lab) | 2 |
| General chemistry (with lab) | 2 |
| Organic chemistry (with lab) | 2 |
| General physics (with lab) | 2 |
| Mathematics | 2 |
| English | 2 |

Applicants are strongly urged to take the MCAT in the spring of the year of application and to have their basic science requirements completed at the time of application. No applicant will be considered for admission until the application materials are complete and received in the Admissions Office.

Applications from individuals who wait to take the MCAT in the spring of the year in which they anticipate matriculating will not be considered.

## SELECTION FACTORS

The selection of students of medicine is based on character, integrity, motivation, academic achievement, emotional maturity, stability, and the applicant interview. In addition, course load and types of courses taken will be evaluated and will constitute a factor in the overall evaluation.

Although the selection process is essentially competitive, with evaluation of students by their college faculty being a significant factor, there are some general guidelines on suitability of an applicant to the college. Because the University of South Florida is a state institution, preference is given to Florida residents. In those instances where residency is in question, for tuition purposes, an applicant is requested to submit a Declaration of Domicile. *Nonresidents are discouraged from applying.*

Applicants requesting an application should clearly indicate whether or not they are Florida residents.

To be considered, Florida residents should have a minimum GPA of 3.0 or better on a 4.0 scale and a score of 8 or better on each category of the new MCAT.

The 1995 entering class profile was: *mean SGPA,* 3.7; *mean MCAT scores, OGP*-3.7; *VR*-9.5, *PS*-9.7, *BS*-9.7; *minorities,* 33 percent; *sex,* 34.4 percent female.

The Admissions Office may at its discretion invite the applicant to come for a personal interview. An invitation for an interview means only that the initial evaluation is sufficiently high to warrant further consideration by the Medical Student Selection Committee. Eligibility for admission will be determined without regard to race, creed, sex, age, religion, national origin, or handicap.

## FINANCIAL AID

The financial status of applicants does not affect their acceptance. Limited funds are available for loans and scholarships.

First-year students are not permitted to engage in outside employment. There are employment opportunities in Tampa and the surrounding area for spouses.

Questions may be addressed to Michele Williamson, director of financial aid, by telephoning (813) 974-2068.

## INFORMATION FOR MINORITIES

Events, activities, programs, and facilities of the University of South Florida are available to all without regard to race, sex, religion, national origin, Vietnam or disabled veteran status, handicap, or age, as provided by law and in accordance with its respect for personal dignity. Qualified minority applicants who are Florida residents are strongly encouraged to apply; the telephone number is (813) 974-3609.

---

Public Institution

## APPLICATION AND ACCEPTANCE POLICIES FOR 1997–98 FIRST-YEAR CLASS

*School participates in AMCAS. See Chapter 4.*

Filing of AMCAS application
  Earliest date: June 1, 1996
  Latest date: Dec. 1, 1996
School application fee to all applicants: $20
Oldest MCAT scores considered: 1993
Does have Early Decision Program (EDP)
  For Florida residents only
  EDP application period: June 1–Aug. 1, 1996
  EDP applicants notified by: Oct. 1, 1996
Acceptance notice to regular applicants
  Earliest date: Oct. 15, 1996
  Latest date: Until class is filled
Applicant's response to acceptance offer
  Maximum time: 2 weeks
Requests for deferred entrance considered: Yes
Deposit to hold place in class: None
Estimated number of new entrants: 96 (29 EDP)
Starting date: Aug. 1997

## TUITION AND STUDENT FEES PER YEAR FOR 1995–96 FIRST-YEAR CLASS

Tuition                    Student fees: $1,120
  Resident: $7,142
  Nonresident: $20,141

## INFORMATION ON 1995–96 FIRST-YEAR CLASS

| Number of | In-State | Out-of-State | Total |
|---|---|---|---|
| Applicants | 1,433 | 560 | 1,993 |
| Applicants Interviewed | 377 | 0 | 377 |
| New Entrants* | 96 | 0 | 96 |

*All took the MCAT and had baccalaureate degrees

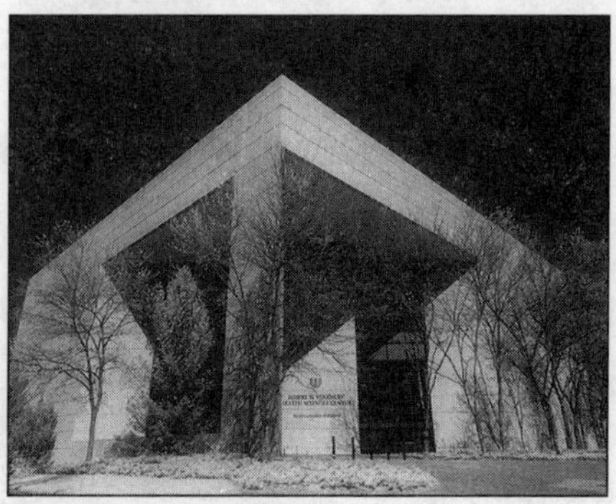

# Emory University School of Medicine

## Atlanta, Georgia


Dr. Jeffrey L. Houpt, *Dean*
Dr. John H. Stone, *Associate Dean and Director of Admissions*
Dr. Jonas A. Shulman, *Associate Dean for Medical Education/Student Affairs*


## ADDRESS INQUIRIES TO:

Medical School Admissions, Room 303
Woodruff Health Sciences Center
Administration Building
Emory University
School of Medicine
Atlanta, Georgia 30322-4510
(404) 727-5660; 727-0045 (FAX)
E-Mail: medschadmiss@medadm.emory.edu
Web Site: http://www.emory.edu/WHSC/

## GENERAL INFORMATION

The Emory University School of Medicine, a private school, was founded in 1915, resulting from several reorganizations dating from 1854 when the Atlanta Medical College was founded. Students spend the first two years primarily on the university campus. The last two years are spent in the school's teaching hospitals, in which there are more than 3,000 beds and large outpatient clinics.

Emory University is accredited by the Commission on Colleges of the Southern Association of Colleges and Schools.

## CURRICULUM

The curriculum is intended to lay a comprehensive foundation for a career in practice, teaching, research, or other medical areas. The first two years consist primarily of basic health sciences and incorporate multimedia teaching aids. Recent curricular changes include a reduction in lecture hours, a parallel increase in small-group/problem-based learning, and introduction to patients in the first year of medical school. Courses are often interdisciplinary, for example, neurobiology, molecular and human genetics, medical problem solving, patient-doctor, and human values in medicine. In the second year, students complete their basic science background and spend a major portion of their time in integrated courses in pathology, pathophysiology, and clinical methods which extend broadly into the various clinical fields. The third and fourth years are devoted exclusively to instruction in all major clinical subjects, including primary care. The 19-month period of actual coursework includes time for elective clerkships that encompass a large variety of studies at both local and distant sites.

A combined M.D.-Ph.D. degree program is available for highly qualified students interested in careers in academic medicine. This six- to seven-year program provides the in-depth clinical experience and biomedical research training necessary for future medical scientists. A five-year dual degree M.D.-M.P.H. program is also available to prepare medical students for leadership roles in public health.

## REQUIREMENTS FOR ENTRANCE

The MCAT and a minimum of three years of college are required. Ninety semester or 135 quarter hours in arts and sciences at an institution accredited by its regional association must be completed to be eligible for enrollment.

The premedical program should be aimed toward a balanced liberal education and should ensure thorough grounding in the stated requirements. Majors in the sciences or non-sciences are equally acceptable. The latter must show competence in the natural sciences and mathematics. Majors in the natural sciences or mathematics should always include subjects of broad educational value in their premedical curricula.

Specific minimum requirements are:

|  | *Sem. hrs* |
| --- | --- |
| Biology (with lab) | 8 |
| Inorganic chemistry (with lab) | 8 |
| Organic chemistry (with lab) | 8 |
| Physics (with lab) | 8 |
| English | 6 |
| Humanities, social and/or behavioral sciences | 18 |

Biochemistry is highly recommended.

Undergraduate degree credit that has been granted to the student on the basis of CLEP will be accepted provided (1) the credit appears on the official transcript and (2) CLEP credits are not the sole fulfillment of any specific course requirement listed above. CLEP credit in excess of 25 percent of a student's total undergraduate credit will not be accepted.

## SELECTION FACTORS

Approximately 50 percent of the entering class positions are filled by Georgians. Students are selected on the basis of scholastic achievement, fitness and aptitude for the study of medicine, and personal qualifications, without regard to race, sex, sexual orientation, age, disability, creed, veteran status, or national origin. All applicants must (a) present a level of scholarship above average (GPA of 3.5 or above is recommended for non-Georgians); (b) take the MCAT preferably in the spring but no later than the fall of the year of application; (c) apply through AMCAS and submit the required Emory supplemental application form and fee (this form is sent immediately upon receipt of the AMCAS application); (d) have the required evaluation(s) submitted; and (e) appear for a personal interview before the Admission Committee. Interview is by invitation and is conducted only at Emory University. Students from foreign schools must have completed at least one year of academic work in an accredited U.S. or Canadian institution. It is anticipated anyone enrolled in a graduate degree program will have completed all required work for the degree by the date of matriculation. Only students enrolled in U.S. LCME-accredited medical schools are eligible to apply for transfer to Emory's second- or third-year class. Advanced standing is not given for work completed in other professional or graduate schools.

The 1995 class had the following credentials at the time of application: *mean GPA,* 3.66; *mean MCAT scores, VR*-9.8, *PS*-9.8, *WS*-P, *BS*-9.9; *undergraduate major,* 45 percent in biology, 15 percent in chemistry, 20 percent in humanities and social/behavioral sciences, 10 percent in a nonscience combined with biology/chemistry or physics, and 10 percent in other disciplines. Other characteristics of the entering class of 114 students were: *sex,* 44.7 percent women; *non-white ethnic groups,* 33.3 percent; *underrepresented minority groups,* 13.2 percent.

## FINANCIAL AID

A limited number of scholarships and loans are available through the Financial Aid Office of Emory University. Approximately 75 percent of all the enrolled medical students receive scholarships and loans through Emory University. Most scholarships and loans are awarded on the basis of documented financial need. Application information may be requested prior to acceptance from the university Financial Aid Office. Approximately 6 percent of the students receive U.S. Armed Forces scholarships. A limited number of highly qualified students in the first-year class are awarded merit scholarships. Foreign citizens who are not permanent residents of the United States must provide and document their own funding for tuition, fees, and living expenses.

Six Robert Woodruff Fellowships, not based on need, are awarded yearly to entering students. Additional information on this competitive, merit-based program is available from the Medical School Admissions Office.

## INFORMATION FOR MINORITIES

Emory University School of Medicine is strongly committed to increasing opportunities for minority students. The Office of Minority Affairs works in conjunction with the Admission Committee and the Office of Student Affairs in the recruitment, selection, and retention of qualified minority students. Further inquiries may be addressed to Dr. Robert Lee, director of minority affairs.

Private Institution

## APPLICATION AND ACCEPTANCE POLICIES FOR 1997–98 FIRST-YEAR CLASS

*School participates in AMCAS. See Chapter 4.*

Filing of AMCAS application
   Earliest date: June 1, 1996
   Latest date: Oct. 15, 1996
School application fee to all applicants: $50
Oldest MCAT scores considered: 1991
Does not have Early Decision Program
Acceptance notice to regular applicants
   Earliest date: Oct. 15, 1996
   Latest date: Mid-March 1997
Applicant's response to acceptance offer
   Maximum time: 3 weeks
Requests for deferred entrance considered: Yes
Deposit to hold place in class (applied to tuition):
   None
Estimated number of new entrants: 110
Starting date: Late July/Aug. 1997

## TUITION AND STUDENT FEES PER YEAR FOR 1995–96 FIRST-YEAR CLASS

Tuition: $20,280        Student fees: $430

## INFORMATION ON 1995–96 FIRST-YEAR CLASS

| *Number of* | *In-State* | *Out-of-State* | *Total* |
|---|---|---|---|
| Applicants | 716 | 7,896 | 8,612 |
| Applicants Interviewed | 205 | 671 | 876 |
| New Entrants* | 60 | 54 | 114 |

*All took the MCAT and had baccalaureate degrees

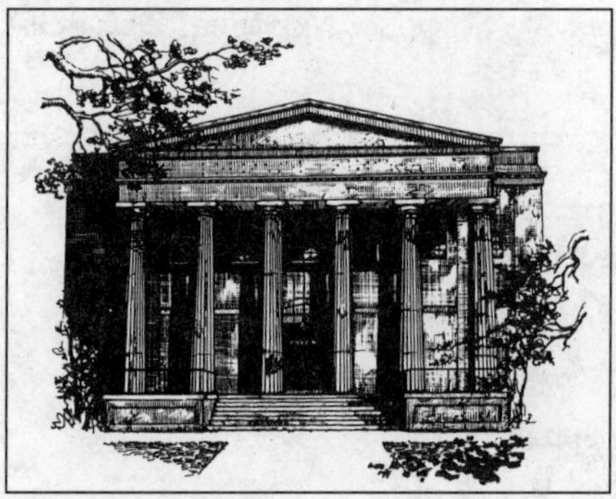

# Medical College of Georgia
# School of Medicine

**Augusta, Georgia**

Dr. Darrell G. Kirch, *Dean*
Dr. Mary Ella Logan, *Associate Dean for Admissions*
Sandra D. Fowler, *Director of Student Financial Aid*

## ADDRESS INQUIRIES TO:

Dr. Mary Ella Logan
Associate Dean for Admissions
School of Medicine
Medical College of Georgia
Augusta, Georgia 30912-4760
(706) 721-3186; 721-0959 (FAX)

## GENERAL INFORMATION

The School of Medicine of the Medical College of Georgia was founded in 1828 and is the nation's 11th oldest medical school. The institution is a separate university under the Georgia Higher Education System and consists of five schools: medicine, allied health, dentistry, graduate studies, and nursing.

The Medical College of Georgia Hospital and Clinics is the primary clinical teaching facility. Other hospitals in Augusta and in cities throughout the state have affiliate agreements with the Medical College of Georgia to provide clinical teaching facilities.

## CURRICULUM

During the first year (Phase I), students study the structure and functions of the human body through courses in anatomy, cell biology and development, biochemistry, neuroscience, and physiology. Courses in humanities, community medicine, behavioral science/psychiatry, and a patient-doctor clinical experience introduce students to ethical and interpersonal aspects of the practice of medicine. Contact with patients begins with physical diagnosis and patient-doctor courses during the first year.

During the second year (Phase II), emphasis is placed on clinical problem solving and pathophysiology through courses in pathology, pharmacology, reproduction, and clinical microbiology. Introduction to clinical medicine and physical diagnosis emphasize clinical problem solving and bedside skills in preparation for the clinical clerkships. A student led, faculty facilitated problem-based learning course emphasizes skills of case-based, self-directed learning, development of information retrieval and analysis skills, group dynamics, and evaluation.

Interdepartmental cooperation and clinical relevance are stressed throughout the first two years. During part of the first year, two afternoons a week are available for electives.

During Phase III, students are required to take 18 months of academic work, which must include 12 months of basic clerkships in the departments of medicine, surgery, obstetrics and gynecology, family medicine, pediatrics, and neuroscience. The remaining 6 months consist of an acting internship and electives.

Students are required to pass Step 1 of USMLE at the end of their second year and Step 2 of the USMLE prior to graduation.

## REQUIREMENTS FOR ENTRANCE

The MCAT and three years of undergraduate college work leading to a baccalaureate degree in an institution accredited by its regional association are required. However, preference is given to students who will have completed the baccalaureate degree prior to enrollment at the School of Medicine.

College work must include:

|  | *Years* |
| --- | --- |
| Biology (with lab) | 1 |
| Inorganic chemistry (with lab) | 1 |
| Advanced chemistry (with lab) | 1 |
|   Must include one semester or two quarters of organic chemistry. | |
| Physics (with lab) | 1 |
| English (Sufficient to satisfy baccalaureate degree requirements.) | |

Biochemistry is highly recommended.

These required courses must be taken on a letter/number grading system (not pass/fail) if at all possible.

## SELECTION FACTORS

Applicants for admission to the School of Medicine are considered on the basis of academic ability and achievement; scores on the MCAT; and assessment of individual potential for meeting society's health care needs as evaluated by the premedical adviser, two personal references, and interviews with Medical College of Georgia faculty.

Preference is given to residents of Georgia. A maximum of 5 percent of the entering class may be nonresidents of Georgia. Nonresidents who wish to apply should have a minimum GPA of 3.5.

Early Decision Program applicants must take the MCAT prior to making application. All other applicants must take the MCAT no later than the fall of the year application is made.

The Admissions Committee selects the applicants to be invited to interviews by reviewing each application. Interviews are with members of the Admissions Committee and Medical College of Georgia faculty who aid in assessing the applicant's personality, motivation, and ability to make the adjustments necessary for the successful study of medicine. Applicants who did not receive at least the last two years of their undergraduate education in an accredited U.S. or Canadian institution cannot be considered. Advanced standing is not given for work completed in professional or graduate schools other than medical schools. Anyone enrolled in a graduate degree program is expected to complete all required work for the degree prior to the date of matriculation.

The Medical College of Georgia does not discriminate on the basis of age, race, sex, creed, or national origin in its admissions process.

## FINANCIAL AID

The Office of Financial Aid coordinates the programs of assistance which are available to medical students.

An applicant's financial status does not affect acceptance for admission. Information and applications may be obtained by writing the Office of Financial Aid.

## INFORMATION FOR MINORITIES

The School of Medicine at the Medical College of Georgia seeks to enroll qualified minority students. One of the primary recruiting mechanisms is a summer program designed for undergraduate college students who show academic promise and desire to study medicine. Students may apply for this program by writing to Dr. R. Allen-Noble, associate dean for special academic programs.

## GENERALIST PHYSICIAN INITIATIVE

The Generalist Physician Initiative at the Medical College of Georgia, funded in part by the Robert Wood Johnson Foundation, is an effort to graduate more physicians who choose to practice family medicine, general internal medicine, or general pediatrics. The initiative involves all aspects of medical education, from pre-entry through undergraduate and residency education, to practice entry and support of generalist physicians. It is anticipated that ultimately 50 percent of MCG graduates will select generalist residency and generalist practice.

Public Institution

## APPLICATION AND ACCEPTANCE POLICIES FOR 1997–98 FIRST-YEAR CLASS

*School participates in AMCAS. See Chapter 4.*

Filing of AMCAS application
    Earliest date: June 1, 1996
    Latest date: Nov. 1, 1996
School application fee: None
Oldest MCAT scores considered: 1994
Does have Early Decision Program (EDP)
    For Georgia residents only
    EDP application period: June 1–Aug. 1, 1996
    EDP applicants notified by: Oct. 1, 1996
Acceptance notice to regular applicants
    Earliest date: Oct. 15, 1996
    Latest date: Until class is filled
Applicant's response to acceptance offer
    Maximum time: 14 days
Requests for deferred entrance considered: Yes
Deposit to hold place in class (applied to tuition):
    $50, due with response to acceptance offer
Deposit refundable prior to: Aug. 1997
Estimated number of new entrants: 180 (45 EDP)
Starting date: Aug. 1997

## TUITION AND STUDENT FEES PER YEAR FOR 1995–96 FIRST-YEAR CLASS

Tuition                              Student fees: $249
    Resident: $4,755
    Nonresident: $14,976

## INFORMATION ON 1995–96 FIRST-YEAR CLASS

| Number of | In-State | Out-of-State | Total |
|---|---|---|---|
| Applicants | 978 | 933 | 1,911 |
| Applicants Interviewed | 470 | 26 | 496 |
| New Entrants* | 176 | 4 | 180 |

*All took the MCAT; 99% and had baccalaureate degrees

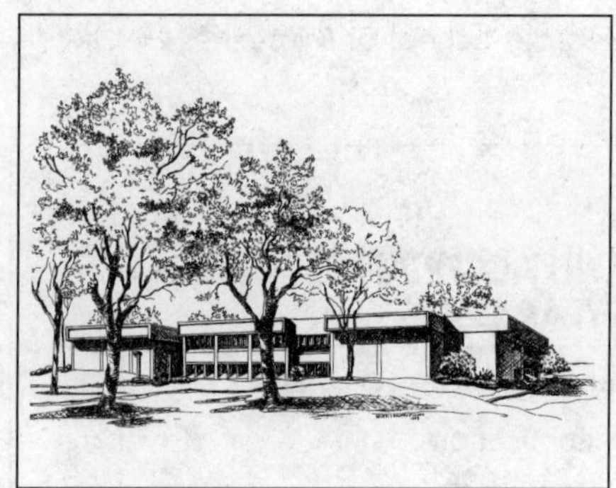

# Mercer University School of Medicine

## Macon, Georgia

Dr. W. Douglas Skelton, *Vice President for Health Affairs and Dean*
Dr. Roger W. Comeau, *Associate Dean for Admissions and Student Affairs/Registrar*
Youvette D. Hudson, *Director for Financial Aid*

## ADDRESS INQUIRIES TO:

Office of Admissions and
Student Affairs
Mercer University
School of Medicine
Macon, Georgia 31207
(912) 752-2542
E-Mail: KOTHANEK.J@GAIN.MERCER.EDU

## GENERAL INFORMATION

Mercer University School of Medicine (MUSM) admitted its charter class in August 1982. The school's mission is to educate physicians to meet the health care needs of rural and other underserved areas of Georgia. The program's educational format is that of problem-based, student-centered learning.

The medical education building is located on the campus of Mercer University and serves as the primary center for learning. In addition to multiple self-instructional facilities, it houses Mercer Health Systems, a 40-room ambulatory care facility. The Medical Center of Central Georgia, a 518-bed community hospital and family health center, serves as the primary affiliate clerkship site. Clinical teaching is also provided at the Memorial Medical Center, Inc., in Savannah, the Floyd Medical Center in Rome, Phoebe Putney Memorial Hospital in Albany, the Medical Center in Columbus, and several rural hospitals throughout Georgia.

## CURRICULUM

The first two years are divided into three phases (A, B, C) of varying lengths. While the major emphasis during these phases is placed on the acquisition and practical application of basic science knowledge, there are two other programs which are designed to prepare the students for contact with patients, private practices, and communities.

The Biomedical Problems Program is the educational vehicle for motivating students to obtain and apply the basic scientific knowledge germane to the practice of medicine. The onus of gathering this knowledge is on the individual student through a program of self-directed learning. The application occurs in small-group tutorials in which specific cases are discussed.

The Clinical Skills Program runs through Phase C and has three components. In the Community Office Practice Program (COPP), students are afforded the opportunity to observe and participate in the office of an accomplished primary care physician. During this time they practice the skills they are developing in other parts of the program. Interviewing skills provides encounters with persons who are trained to portray specific behavioral roles and give constructive feedback to the students. These sessions train the students to recognize different behaviors, establish communication, and obtain clinically useful information. The Physical Diagnosis Program trains the students in general and systems specific history-taking and physical examinations. These skills are practiced on standardized patients and in the COPP. As much as possible, this program parallels the cases in the Biomedical Problems Program.

The Community Science Program familiarizes students with a primary care practice in rural Georgia, while educating them to the health needs of individuals, families, and communities. This program extends throughout the four years culminating in a 4-week rural clerkship in Phase E (year 4).

Phase D (year 3) consists primarily of the Clerkship Program, which has six clinical rotations: internal medicine, surgery, pediatrics, obstetrics-gynecology, ambulatory family medicine, and psychiatry. In addition, there are weekly programs in radiology.

The fourth year (Phase E), while predominantly an elective year, has three required programs in addition to the rural clerkship. These are an acute or critical care clerkship, surgery subspecialties, and a substance abuse clerkship.

## REQUIREMENTS FOR ENTRANCE

The MCAT and the equivalent of three academic years or a minimum of 90 semester hours in an approved college or university are required for admission. Students are advised to balance their work in the biological sciences with courses in the social sciences and humanities. In addition, they are urged to follow their own inclinations in choosing a subject to pursue as a major. Required courses are:

|  | *Years* |
| --- | --- |
| General biology (with lab) | 1 |
| General or inorganic chemistry (with lab) | 1 |
| Organic chemistry or organic/biochemistry sequence (with lab)* | 1 |
| General physics (with lab) | 1 |

*Must include one semester or two quarters of organic chemistry. Biochemistry is highly recommended.*

## SELECTION FACTORS

The Admissions Committee accepts only applicants who are legal residents of Georgia. Each applicant must also show promise of learning effectively in Mercer's curriculum and show strong potential of practicing a medical specialty commensurate with the health care needs of rural and other underserved areas of Georgia.

In addition to the AMCAS application, a supplementary application is required. This application has a $25 fee and requests the following: two letters of recommendation or one premedical committee evaluation, a personal history (a chronological list of residences and activities since the beginning of high school), certification of Georgia residency, and a list of the required premedical courses.

Interviews are by invitation only and are held at the medical school. In making the final decisions for acceptance or rejection, the Admissions Committee considers all criteria but emphasizes strongly an applicant's potential for complying with the mission of the institution. The committee does not discriminate on the basis of race, sex, creed, national origin, age, or handicap.

The 54 students that matriculated in 1994 consisted of 30 men and 24 women; 2 students were minority, and the average age was 24.

## FINANCIAL AID

Financial aid in the form of loans and scholarships is available. Awards are made on the basis of need and merit. Although acceptance to MUSM is not based on an applicant's ability to pay, the responsibility for adequate funding rests with the student. The financial aid officer conducts financial management conferences and assists students in obtaining needed support. A MUSM Faculty-Staff Emergency Loan Fund for students is also available.

## INFORMATION FOR MINORITIES

The school is committed to the recruitment of qualified individuals from underrepresented groups and disadvantaged backgrounds.

---

Private Institution

## APPLICATION AND ACCEPTANCE POLICIES FOR 1997–98 FIRST-YEAR CLASS

*School participates in AMCAS. See Chapter 4.*

Filing of AMCAS application
   Earliest date: June 1, 1996
   Latest date: Dec. 1, 1996
School application fee after screening: $25
Oldest MCAT scores considered: 1994
Does have Early Decision Program (EDP)
   For Georgia residents only
   EDP application period: June 1–Aug. 1, 1996
   EDP applicants notified by: Oct. 1, 1996
Acceptance notice to regular applicants
   Earliest date: Oct. 15, 1996
   Latest date: Until class is filled
Applicant's response to acceptance offer
   Maximum time: 10 days
Requests for deferred entrance considered: Yes
Deposit to hold place in class (applied to tuition):
   $100, due with response to acceptance offer
Deposit refundable prior to: May 15, 1997
Estimated number of new entrants: 56 (10 EDP)
Starting date: Aug. 1997

## TUITION AND STUDENT FEES PER YEAR FOR 1995–96 FIRST-YEAR CLASS

Tuition and student fees: $18,890

## INFORMATION ON 1995–96 FIRST-YEAR CLASS

| Number of | In-State | Out-of-State | Total |
|---|---|---|---|
| Applicants | 733 | 738 | 1,471 |
| Applicants Interviewed | 188 | 0 | 188 |
| New Entrants* | 55 | 0 | 55 |

*All took the MCAT and had baccalaureate degrees

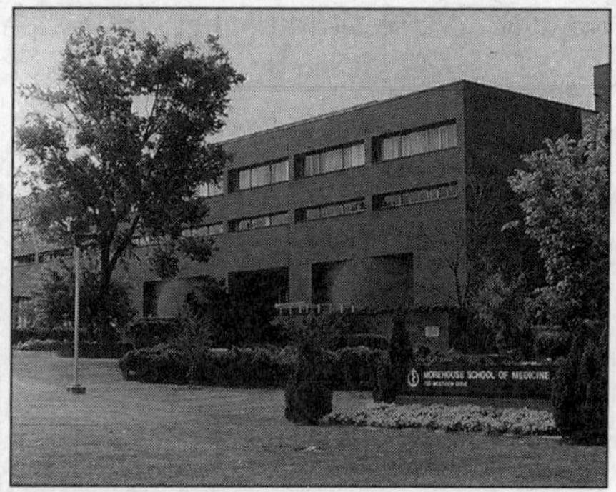

# Morehouse School of Medicine

## Atlanta, Georgia

Dr. Angela Walker Franklin, *Associate Dean for Student Affairs*
Karen A. Lewis, *Assistant Director of Admissions*
Cynthia Handy, *Director of Student Fiscal Affairs*

## ADDRESS INQUIRIES TO:

Admissions and Student Affairs
Morehouse School of Medicine
720 Westview Drive, S.W.
Atlanta, Georgia 30310-1495
(404) 752-1650; 752-1512 (FAX)

## GENERAL INFORMATION

Morehouse School of Medicine is one of three medical schools in the nation founded by historically black institutions and is the first such medical school begun in this century. The School of Medicine admitted its first students to a two-year basic medical science curriculum in September 1978. The inaugural M.D. degree class graduated in May 1985.

Basic science teaching facilities are located in the lecture halls and multidisciplinary laboratories of the Basic Medical Sciences Building, which also houses research laboratories, preclinical departments, and administrative offices. The medical education building, dedicated in May 1987, houses clinical and preclinical departments, research laboratories, study areas, and the library.

Clinical instruction takes place in affiliated hospitals and clinics, including Grady Memorial Hospital, Southwest Community Hospital, and Tuskegee Veterans Administration Medical Center (Tuskegee, Alabama). The school also administers the Area Health Education Center Program.

## CURRICULUM

An educational experience focusing both on scientific medicine and on meeting more effectively the primary health care needs of underserved inner city and rural patients is offered. The concept of the patient as a whole person is fostered through a variety of teaching experiences that relate social, environmental, emotional, and cultural factors to medical disorders.

The first two years of the curriculum emphasize an understanding of the principles, concepts, and major factual background of the basic medical sciences. Exposure to clinical medicine begins in the first year through assignment to a preceptor and increases in the second year with introduction to clinical medicine. Clinical education is continued through core clerkships during the third and fourth years with 16 weeks of electives in the senior year. The major strengths of the curriculum include small class size, a highly diversified faculty, and courses that are taught by departmental and/or interdisciplinary faculty.

All students are required to pass Step 1 and Step 2 of the USMLE examinations for promotion and graduation respectively. Student performance is evaluated primarily by letter grade. Promotion into the next year's class is recommended by the Student Academic Progress and Promotions Committee.

First-year classes begin in early July with a required summer program. Learning resources and other support services are available to all students throughout their four years. Morehouse School of Medicine also offers the Ph.D. in biomedical sciences and master's of public health degrees. Applicants interested in dual degree opprtunities must apply to each program separately.

## REQUIREMENTS FOR ENTRANCE

The MCAT and three years (at least 90 semester hours or 135 quarter hours) of accredited college work are required. It is highly recommended that the MCAT be taken in the spring of the year in which the application is made. Over the years, it has been exceptional for a student to matriculate without a baccalaureate degree.

The faculty has no preference as to the major field of undergraduate study; students should determine their fields of major study according to their personal interest. Applicants are expected to present a sound, well balanced academic background with evidence of competency in the stated requirements. Specific minimum requirements are:

|  | *Sem./Qtr. hrs.* |
| --- | --- |
| Biology (with lab) | 8/12 |
| Inorganic or general chemistry (with lab) | 8/12 |
| Organic chemistry (with lab) | 8/12 |
| Physics (with lab) | 8/12 |
| College mathematics | 6/10 |
| English (including composition) | 6/10 |

Course work in behavioral sciences is strongly recommended.

## SELECTION FACTORS

Selection of students for admission is made by the Committee on Admissions after careful consideration of many factors. These include MCAT scores, the undergraduate academic record, the extent of academic improvement, balance and depth of academic program, difficulty of courses taken, and other indicators of maturation of learning ability. Additional factors considered by the committee include the nature of extracurricular activities, hobbies, the need to work, research projects and experiences, evidence of activities which indicate concurrence with the school's mission, and evidence of pursuing interests and talents in depth. Finally, the committee looks for evidence of those traits of personality and character essential to success in medicine: compassion, integrity, motivation, and perseverance.

All information available about each applicant is considered without assigning priority to any single factor. Students are admitted on the basis of individual qualifications regardless of sex, age, race, creed, national origin, or handicap. Preferential consideration is given to qualified applicants who are residents of the state of Georgia. However, all well qualified applicants are encouraged to apply.

After receipt and preliminary screening of the AMCAS application, qualified applicants will be invited to submit a supplementary application and letters of evaluation. After review of all submitted materials, applicants who are competitive in this stage of the admissions process are invited to Atlanta for a personal interview. Interviews are arranged only by invitation of the Committee on Admissions.

Medical education requires that the accumulation of scientific knowledge be accompanied by the simultaneous acquisition of skills and professional attitudes and behavior. Technical standards have been established as a prerequisite for admission and graduation from the Morehouse School of Medicine. All courses in the curriculum are required in order to develop essential skills required to become a competent physician.

A candidate for the M.D. degree must have aptitude, abilities, and skills in five areas: observation, communication, motor, conceptual integrative and quantitative, and behavior and social.

Morehouse School of Medicine's Technical Standards for Medical School Admissions and Graduation are provided in the supplemental application packets.

## FINANCIAL AID

A broad financial aid program is available. In addition to federally insured loan programs, a number of scholarships and loans are available. Scholarships and loans are awarded on the basis of documented financial need as determined by the College Scholarship Service needs analysis system (see Part 1). Applicants with an AMCAS fee waiver can waive the $45 school application fee. Accepted applicants are eligible to apply for financial aid to the Office of Student Fiscal Affairs. Approximately 87 percent of the students receive some form of financial aid during a part or all of their four years of study. Students are discouraged from accepting outside employment because of the lack of available time during a heavy academic schedule.

Private Institution

## APPLICATION AND ACCEPTANCE POLICIES FOR 1997–98 FIRST-YEAR CLASS

*School participates in AMCAS. See Chapter 4.*

Filing of AMCAS application
    Earliest date: June 1, 1996
    Latest date: Dec. 1, 1996
School application fee to all applicants: $45
Oldest MCAT scores considered: 1994
Does have Early Decision Program (EDP)
    For residents of Georgia only
    EDP application period: June 1–Aug. 1, 1996
    EDP applicants notified by: Oct. 1, 1996
Acceptance notice to regular applicants
    Earliest date: Dec. 20, 1996
    Latest date: Until class is filled
Applicant's response to acceptance offer
    Maximum time: 2 weeks
Requests for deferred entrance considered: Yes
Deposit to hold place in class (applied to tuition):
    $100, due with response to acceptance offer
Deposit refundable prior to: May 15, 1997
Estimated number of new entrants: 35 (1 EDP)
Starting date: July 1997

## TUITION AND STUDENT FEES PER YEAR FOR 1995–96 FIRST-YEAR CLASS

Tuition: $15,750        Student fees: $1,933

## INFORMATION ON 1995–96 FIRST-YEAR CLASS

| *Number of* | *In-State* | *Out-of-State* | *Total* |
|---|---|---|---|
| Applicants | 400 | 2,530 | 2,930 |
| Applicants Interviewed | 126 | 114 | 240 |
| New Entrants* | 26 | 9 | 35 |

*All took the MCAT; 97% had baccalaureate degrees

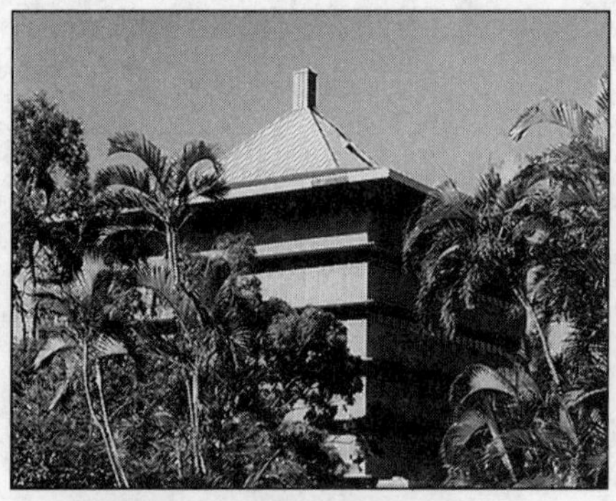

# University of Hawaii
# John A. Burns School of Medicine

**Honolulu, Hawaii**

Dr. Christian L. Gulbrandsen, *Dean*
Dr. Satoru Izutsu, *Associate Dean/Chair, Admissions Committee*
Marilyn M. Nishiki, *Admissions Officer/Registrar*

## ADDRESS INQUIRIES TO:

Office of Admissions
University of Hawaii
John A. Burns School of Medicine
1960 East-West Road
Honolulu, Hawaii 96822
(808) 956-8300; 956-9547 (FAX)
E-Mail: nishikim@jabsom.biomed.hawaii.edu

## GENERAL INFORMATION

The University of Hawaii John A. Burns School of Medicine is part of the College of Health Sciences and Social Welfare, which also includes schools of public health, nursing, and social work. The School of Medicine is based on the Manoa campus of the university in Honolulu and has some elements at nearby Leahi Hospital. It also has teaching facilities in 10 affiliated community hospitals and three primary care clinics throughout the state.

## CURRICULUM

The four-year M.D. program is taught in a problem-based curriculum. Clinical work, including principles of history-taking and physical diagnosis, behavioral science, and community medicine, begins in the first year.

Special features of the program include the following: an emphasis on primary care medicine and cross-cultural psychiatry; clinical training in community hospitals and primary care clinics (by medical school faculty); interdisciplinary training in community medicine together with students of public health, nursing, and social work; and opportunities for preceptorships in rural areas of the Hawaiian Islands and other areas of the Pacific Basin.

Beginning in September 1992, 15 students who entered the freshman class experienced about 30 percent of their academic and clinical training at community sites. This program, known as the Academic Community Partnership in Health Professions Education and funded by the Kellogg Foundation, began at the Waianae Coast Comprehensive Health Center, the Kalihi-Palama Clinic, and the Queen Emma Clinics at the Queen's Medical Center. It will eventually involve other health care facilities around the state of Hawaii.

An honors/credit/no credit grading system is used along with individual evaluations of student performance by faculty.

Requirements for Entrance. The MCAT and at least 90 college credits are required. Course work must include:

|  | Sem. hrs. |
|---|---|
| Biology (with lab) | 8 |
| Chemistry (with lab) | 4 |
| Molecular and Cell Biology (with lab) | 4 |
| Biochemistry | 4 |
| Physics (with lab) | 8 |

These courses should be vigorous and the type acceptable for students majoring in these areas. Other science courses are not required. Although many students will take upper level science courses out of interest or to fulfill the requirements of a major, breadth of education in the liberal arts is of vital importance, and work in the humanities is strongly advised. Applicants also must be fully competent in reading, speaking, and writing the English language.

## SELECTION FACTORS

All applicants are considered without discrimination as to age, sex, race, creed, national origin, or handicap. The school admits 48 students to its regular freshman class and 8 students to a special opportunity program for disadvantaged students each year. Selection depends upon the prospective medical student's character, scholarship, ideals, motivation, and aptitude. An evaluation of what the potential student might contribute to the health profession in the Pacific is an integral part of the selection process. For the limited number of applicants who reach a secondary screening level, interviews are conducted on Oahu.

The 1995 regular entering class had the following profile: *mean cumulative GPA,* 3.55; *mean MCAT scores, VR-9.0, PS-9.7, BS-9.79.*

Except as permitted in unusual situations by the Admissions Committee, applications will not be accepted from students who are currently enrolled in a graduate degree program at the University of Hawaii unless they will satisfactorily complete their degree program prior to the academic year for which they seek admission or will enroll in a joint M.D.-Ph.D. program already approved by the Ph.D. field of study.

A Liberal Studies/Doctor of Medicine program offers the option to a few University of Hawaii students early in their undergraduate studies to receive a commitment for medical school admission after completing their bachelor's degree. Such students embark on individualized programs during which they also complete the prerequisite science courses.

## FINANCIAL AID

Financial status is not a factor in considering applicants for acceptance, and, although financial aid is limited, efforts are made to assist medical students in obtaining loans and scholarships wherever possible. Because of the federal source of loan funds, they are only available to U.S. citizens. In general, students are discouraged from seeking outside employment. Approximately 60 percent of the student body currently receive financial assistance.

## INFORMATION FOR MINORITIES

The student body and faculty are cosmopolitan and include African Americans, Caucasians, Chinese, Filipinos, Hawaiians, Japanese, Koreans, Micronesians, Samoans, and others.

Public Institution

## APPLICATION AND ACCEPTANCE POLICIES FOR 1997–98 FIRST-YEAR CLASS

*School participates in AMCAS. See Chapter 4.*

Filing of AMCAS application
   Earliest date: June 1, 1996
   Latest date: Dec. 1, 1996
School application fee after screening: $50
Oldest MCAT scores considered: 1994
Does have Early Decision Program (EDP)
   For residents of Hawaii only
   EDP application period: June 1–Aug. 1, 1996
   EDP applicants notified by: Oct. 1, 1996
Acceptance notice to regular applicants
   Earliest date: Oct. 15, 1996
   Latest date: Until class is filled
Applicant's response to acceptance offer
   Maximum time: 2 weeks
Requests for deferred entrance considered: Yes
Deposit to hold place in class: None
Estimated number of new entrants: 56 (2 EDP)
Starting date: Aug. 1997

## TUITION AND STUDENT FEES PER YEAR FOR 1995–96 FIRST-YEAR CLASS

Tuition                                        Student fees: $87
   Resident: $5,996
   Nonresident: $21,030

## INFORMATION ON 1995–96 FIRST-YEAR CLASS

| Number of | In-State | Out-of-State | Total |
|---|---|---|---|
| Applicants | 259 | 1,372 | 1,631 |
| Applicants Interviewed | 180 | 53 | 233 |
| New Entrants* | 53 | 3 | 56 |

*All took the MCAT; 98% had baccalaureate degrees

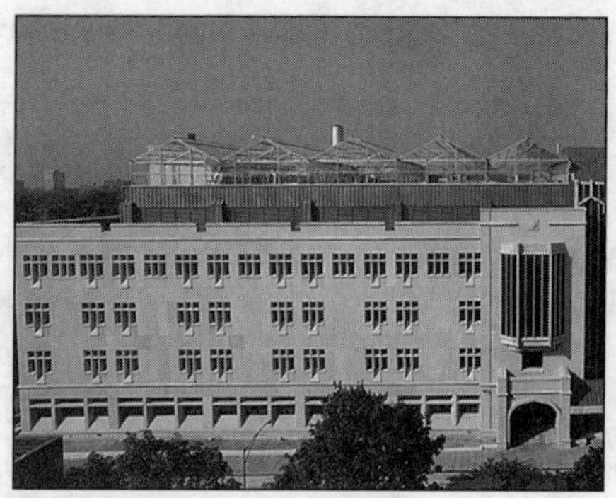

# University of Chicago
# Pritzker School of Medicine

**Chicago, Illinois**

Dr. Glenn D. Steele, *Acting Dean*
Dr. Norma Wagoner, *Dean of Students*
Sylvia Robertson, *Director of Admissions*

## ADDRESS INQUIRIES TO:

Office of the Dean of Students
University of Chicago
Pritzker School of Medicine
924 E. 57th Street, BLSC 104
Chicago, Illinois 60637-5416
(312) 702-1939; 702-2598 (FAX)

## GENERAL INFORMATION

The University of Chicago is located on the south side of Chicago in the ethnically diverse community of Hyde Park, just 12 minutes from downtown Chicago. Organized into four major divisions—biological sciences, physical sciences, humanities, and social sciences—the university is made up predominantly of graduate and professional students. In addition to the four major divisions are six professional schools including the Pritzker School of Medicine, all on one campus. Nationally, Pritzker School of Medicine is unique in that it is a part of an academic Division of the Biological Sciences. As an integral part of a world-class university, it offers medical students diverse opportunities for interdisciplinary learning and research. In this environment, the school's mission is to train academic physicians. Over 90 percent of all students engage in some form of scholarly activity prior to completing the M.D. degree, and nearly 20 percent pursue combined M.D.-Ph.D. degrees. Of graduates from 1978-87, 19.1 percent became faculty members, a figure which is consistently among the highest.

The University of Chicago Medical Center and its major affiliated institutions provide over 1,700 inpatient beds, an active outpatient service, and fully staffed state-of-the-art facilities as a basis for clinical training. In addition to rotating through the University of Chicago Hospitals, students rotate through Lutheran General Hospital, Louis A. Weiss Memorial Hospital, and MacNeal Hospital.

## CURRICULUM

The Pritzker School of Medicine is engaged in two major activities for education in the remainder of this century and the next. The first one was the completion of the Biological Sciences Learning Center and the Jules Knapp Institute for Molecular Medicine. This combined teaching and research facility serves as a visible sign of the linkages among science, teaching, and medicine in achieving the institution's mission. The Learning Center provides students and faculty a place to creatively use new methods and technologies. The Knapp Institute for Molecular Medicine houses research facilities for immunology, neurobiology, human genetics, molecular cardiology, and molecular oncology. The second one is curricular innovation. First-year students are taught clinical skills through an introduction to history taking and interviewing using standardized patients and small-group settings. In addition, students have the opportunity to explore the social, cultural, and ethical issues facing medicine with physicians from the McLean Center for Clinical Medical Ethics.

Basic science course work is horizontally integrated during the first two years, and the clinical skills course serves to bring about vertical integration with the patient as a focus. The third year is all clinical at three major sites: the University of Chicago Hospitals, Lutheran General, and MacNeal Hospital. Opportunities to increase family practice options for clinical rotations have been expanded this past year. The fourth year is all elective. Elective periods exist in all four years, and many students use them for research experiences. Pritzker is on a pass/fail grading system and does not require students to pass the USMLE for graduation.

A select number of students can pursue the M.D. and Ph.D. degrees in basic science areas with funding from the Medical Scientist Training Program or the NIH Pediatrics Growth and Development Training Grant. Other funding opportunities exist. The Program in Medicine, Arts, and the Social Sciences, funded by the Pew Foundation, is available for those desirous of Ph.D.s in nonscience areas. The M.B.A. or J.D. can be obtained if one is accepted to those schools. Every effort is made to accommodate students' requests in the development of the desired programs.

## REQUIREMENTS FOR ENTRANCE

The MCAT is required of all applicants. Applicants are required to have completed at least 90 credit hours of college level work, although a four-year baccalaureate degree is preferable. Pritzker's academic program is rigorous, and applicants are encouraged to obtain a strong course foundation in general education (English composition, mathematics, social sciences, and humanities), as well as the required science courses. The specific course requirements for admission are:

*Years*

Biology or zoology (with lab).........................1
Inorganic chemistry (with lab) ......................1
Organic chemistry (with lab) ........................1
Physics (with lab)..................................1

Pritzker has a rigorous graduate level curriculum in biochemistry, and applicants are encouraged to have a working knowledge of biochemical principles prior to matriculation. Biochemistry may be substituted for one half of the organic chemistry requirement. Officially granted Advanced Placement (AP) credit in any of the required subjects will partially fulfill Pritzker's requirements. Applicants with AP credit are expected to take advanced course work in science.

## SELECTION FACTORS

Applicants are selected solely on the basis of their ability, achievement, personality, character, and motivation. Pritzker does not discriminate on the basis of race, sex, creed, national origin, age, or handicap. The Committee on Admissions carefully selects between 600 to 700 applicants from among its large applicant pool for interviews on the Pritzker campus from early October through March. There are no residency restrictions, but about 40 percent of the entering class come from the state of Illinois. Students in the 1995 entering class had the following academic profile: average GPAs–science 3.51; cumulative 3.55; average MCAT–10.3.

## FINANCIAL AID

The Pritzker School of Medicine believes no student should be denied admission or be unable to attend for financial reasons. Scholarships and low-interest loans are made available to all students who have demonstrated need. Loans are both of the federally subsidized type and low or no interest ones from the university. Approximately 82 percent of students receive some form of financial assistance. Current levels of indebtedness for Pritzker students are below the national mean for private institutions. All accepted applicants are sent financial aid information after January 1; students seeking university loans and scholarships are required to complete the need analysis disk. Accepted applicants wishing further information may write to Jennifer Talbot, the director of financial aid, Office of the Dean of Students.

## INFORMATION FOR MINORITIES

Pritzker is particularly interested in seeking diversity among its students and is sensitive to society's needs for increasing the representation of minority men and women among physicians. Pritzker is involved in a wide ranging effort to increase minority representation at all levels. Significant strides have been made to attract students, residents, and faculty. The medical school utilizes the MED-MAR List to contact prospective students. When applicants come to Pritzker for interviews, every effort is made to provide them time with

enrolled minority students or faculty. Minority medical students who have attended Pritzker often assume strong leadership roles, both within their class and at the national level.

---

Private Institution

### APPLICATION AND ACCEPTANCE POLICIES FOR 1997–98 FIRST-YEAR CLASS

*School participates in AMCAS. See Chapter 4.*

Filing of AMCAS application
   Earliest date: June 1, 1996
   Latest date: Nov. 15, 1996
School application fee after screening: $55
Oldest MCAT scores considered: 1993
   Does have Early Decision Program (EDP)
   EDP application period: June 1–Aug. 1, 1996
   EDP applicants notified by: Oct. 1, 1996
Acceptance notice to regular applicants
   Earliest date: Oct. 15, 1996
   Latest date: Until class is filled
Applicant's response to acceptance offer
   Maximum time: 30 days
Requests for deferred entrance considered: Yes
Deposit to hold place in class (applied to tuition):
   $100, due with response to acceptance offer
Deposit refundable prior to: July 1, 1997
Estimated number of new entrants: 104 (5 EDP)
Starting date: Sept. 30, 1997

### TUITION AND STUDENT FEES PER YEAR FOR 1995–96 FIRST-YEAR CLASS

Tuition: $21,660          Student fees: $1,645

### INFORMATION ON 1995–96 FIRST-YEAR CLASS

| *Number of* | *In-State* | *Out-of-State* | *Total* |
|---|---|---|---|
| Applicants | 1,165 | 7,242 | 8,407 |
| Applicants Interviewed | 136 | 348 | 484 |
| New Entrants* | 42 | 62 | 104 |

*All took the MCAT and had baccalaureate degrees.

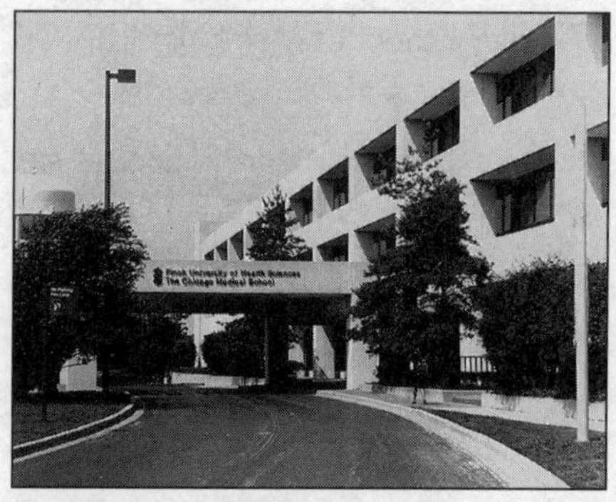

# Finch University of Health Sciences/ Chicago Medical School

## North Chicago, Illinois

Dr. Theodore Booden, *Dean, Chicago Medical School*
Kristine A. Jones, *Director of Admissions and Records*
Maryann DeCaire, *Director of Financial Aid*

## ADDRESS INQUIRIES TO:

Office of Admissions
Chicago Medical School
3333 Green Bay Road
North Chicago, Illinois 60064
(847) 578-3206/3207; 578-3284 (FAX)

## GENERAL INFORMATION

The Chicago Medical School, founded in 1912, is part of the Finch University of Health Sciences, which is located in North Chicago, Illinois. It is a private, nonsectarian, coeducational institution chartered by the state of Illinois and administered by a Board of Trustees. The Chicago Medical School is the core component of three allied units. The other units are the School of Graduate and Postdoctoral Studies, which grants degrees at the master and doctoral levels in the major basic science areas, as well as the doctorate in clinical psychology. The School of Related Health Sciences currently offers programs in physical therapy, medical technology, healthcare risk management, nutrition and clinical dietetics, and physician assistant, leading to baccalaureate and master's degrees. In addition, the university offers a BSN completion program in cooperation with Barat College, Lake Forest, Illinois, and a B.S.-M.D. accelerated honors program in engineering/medicine in conjunction with Illinois Institute of Technology. Clinical training at various levels is provided at Cook County Hospital, Edward Hines Veterans Affairs Medical Center, Mt. Sinai Hospital, North Chicago Veterans Affairs Medical Center, Illinois Masonic Medical Center, Swedish Covenant Hospital, Norwalk (Ct.) Hospital, and Lutheran General Hospital.

## CURRICULUM

To meet the changing need of the future physician, the content of the curriculum is under continual evaluation and revision. The curriculum offers students a strong foundation in both the science and practice of medicine by providing an interface between basic science and clinical science.

Currently, the four-year curriculum consists of 13 terms. Of the 6 terms of basic science, the first 3 are devoted primarily to the study of the structure and function of the human body. Many courses, including medical ethics, genetics, and biostatistics, are offered in didactic and small-group sessions. The following 3 terms are devoted to the study of disease etiology, processes, therapy, and prevention. Concomitantly, there is extensive training in physical diagnosis, medical interviewing, and history-writing. Of the last 7 terms, 48 weeks are devoted to junior clinical rotations and 36 weeks are spent in senior clinical selectives, electives, and/or basic science courses. The required junior clinical clerkships include medicine, surgery, obstetrics-gynecology, psychiatry, family medicine, pediatrics, emergency medicine, neurology, and ambulatory care medicine. The senior requirements include a medical subinternship and a primary care clerkship, plus 28 weeks of approved electives (14 of which must be done on campus). The elective period gives students an opportunity, through both intramural and extramural experiences, to explore and strengthen their personal career interests.

Along with passing all courses and clerkships, students are required to pass Step 1 and Step 2 of the USMLE examinations as a requisite for graduation.

All students are required to complete the first two years within three academic years; clinical clerkships and electives are to be completed within 2½ years. Thus, students must complete their education at the Chicago Medical School in no more than 5½ years, unless enrolled in a combined-degree program, or on an approved extended program, or on an approved leave of absence.

Combined M.D.-Ph.D. degree programs are available for students interested in biomedical or clinical research. These programs provide an opportunity for a limited number of students to pursue a program of individualized course work and research leading to the M.D. and Ph.D. degrees. Candidates who complete their Ph.D. degrees may receive full tuition scholarships for all four years of medical school and their graduate studies. Applications and additional information are available from the director, combined M.D.-Ph.D. degree program.

## REQUIREMENTS FOR ENTRANCE

The MCAT and three years of college (minimum of 135 quarter hours) are required; the baccalaureate degree is preferred. The college work must include the following:

|  | *Years* |
|---|---|
| Biology or zoology (with lab) | 1 |
| Inorganic chemistry (with lab) | 1 |

Organic chemistry (with lab) . . . . . . . . . . . . . . . . . . . . . . 1
General physics (with lab) . . . . . . . . . . . . . . . . . . . . . . . 1

Science courses beyond those required will be helpful in preparing for study in medical school; however, the applicant is expected to have a broad foundation in general education, and any major field of interest is acceptable.

## SELECTION FACTORS

Students are selected on the basis of various criteria, including scholarship, character, motivation, and educational background without regard to race, creed, religion, sex, disability, age, or national origin. One's potential for the study and practice of medicine will be evaluated on the basis of academic achievement, MCAT results, personal appraisals by a preprofessional advisory committee or individual instructors, and a personal interview, if requested by the Student Admissions Committee.

Successful applicants for the 1995 entering class had the following credentials: *mean GPA,* 3.3; *residence,* 28 percent from Illinois, with the remainder from 24 other states; *undergraduate major,* 42 percent in biology or chemistry, with the remainder from a variety of fields. Approximately 15 percent of those seriously considered matriculated.

Applicants working on advanced degrees will be considered on the same basis as all other applicants. Applicants who have not been accepted previously and who make reapplication will be treated on the same basis as first-time applicants.

## FINANCIAL AID

Limited university administered financial aid is available to students who are unable to meet school costs through family resources and major financial aid programs. Awards are made to eligible students based on the availability of funds and demonstrated financial need (expenses minus resources). The university utilizes ACT to uniformly measure student resources. Approximately 75 percent of the medical students receive financial assistance. An average award through university-administered funds is $2,500 for full need medical students.

## INFORMATION FOR MINORITIES

The school maintains an extensive recruitment and retention program for minority students. Application fees may be waived for financially disadvantaged students. Deceleration of basic science curriculum is an option available to all students with demonstrated need.

Private Institution

## APPLICATION AND ACCEPTANCE POLICIES FOR 1997–98 FIRST-YEAR CLASS

*School participates in AMCAS. See Chapter 4.*

Filing of AMCAS application
   Earliest date: June 1, 1996
   Latest date: Dec. 15, 1996
School application fee to all applicants: $65
Oldest MCAT scores considered: 1994
Does have Early Decision Program (EDP)
   EDP application period: June 1–Aug. 1, 1996
   EDP applicants notified by: Oct. 1, 1996
Acceptance notice to regular applicants
   Earliest date: Oct. 15, 1996
   Latest date: Until class is filled
Applicant's response to acceptance offer
   Maximum time: 2 weeks
Requests for deferred entrance considered: Yes
Deposit to hold place in class (applied to tuition):
   $100, due with response to acceptance offer
Deposit refundable prior to: May 15, 1997
   Estimated number of new entrants: 160 (3 EDP)
Starting date: July 1997

## TUITION AND STUDENT FEES PER YEAR FOR 1995–96 FIRST-YEAR CLASS

Tuition: $29,106        Student fees: $100

## INFORMATION ON 1995–96 FIRST-YEAR CLASS

| Number of | In-State | Out-of-State | Total |
|---|---|---|---|
| Applicants | 1,342 | 11,456 | 12,798 |
| Applicants Interviewed | 147 | 553 | 700 |
| New Entrants* | 46 | 120 | 166 |

*All took the MCAT; 99% had baccalaureate degrees.

# University of Illinois
# College of Medicine

**Chicago, Illinois**

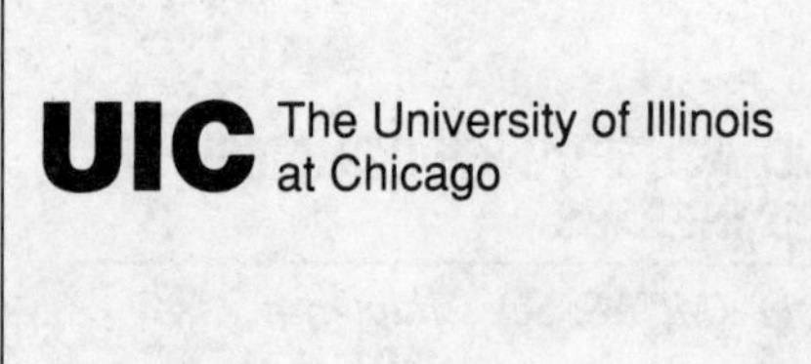


Dr. Gerald S. Moss, *Dean*
Dr. Jorge A. Girotti, *Associate Dean and Director, College of Medicine Admissions*
James Mendez, *Associate Director of Financial Aid*


## ADDRESS INQUIRIES TO:

Medical College Admissions
Room 165 CME M/C 783
University of Illinois
College of Medicine
808 South Wood Street
Chicago, Illinois 60612-7302
(312) 996-5635; 996-6693 (FAX)

## GENERAL INFORMATION

Founded in 1881 as the College of Physicians and Surgeons of Chicago, the name was changed to the University of Illinois College of Medicine in 1900. Following a reorganization of college structure approved by the Board of Trustees in 1982, the College of Medicine programs are now conducted on two educational tracks at four geographic sites. The College of Medicine at Chicago is located at the Health Sciences Center of the university. The College of Medicine at Urbana-Champaign offers a four-year medical curriculum integrated with the programs of a comprehensive campus. The College of Medicine at Peoria includes facilities in each of the hospitals in that community and a modern downtown campus. The College of Medicine at Rockford has a centrally located campus and conducts programs in each of the Rockford hospitals and in several nearby smaller communities.

## CURRICULUM

There are two separate curricular tracks within the College of Medicine. Students assigned to the Chicago campus will pursue their full four-year program of undergraduate medical education under the supervision of the faculty at that site. Students assigned for their first year of instruction to the Urbana-Champaign campus either will remain assigned to that site for the last three years or will transfer to Peoria or Rockford for the three remaining years of the program. Once students begin in either Chicago or Urbana-Champaign, transfers between curricular tracks will be limited.

Each clinical curriculum presents techniques and information necessary for examination and care for the patient, and each provides supervised experiences in a wide variety of clinical settings under direction of the faculty. Through college level faculty committees consisting of representation from all sites, the standards of quality are regularly evaluated for admissions, instruction student appraisal, and student promotion.

The college also offers a number of special programs. The Medical Scholars Program on the Urbana-Champaign campus links the medical school with over 40 other academic units, including the natural and biological sciences, social sciences, humanities, business administration, and law, so that students can earn a combined graduate and medical degree. A combined-degree program on the Chicago campus enables medical students to carry out graduate work in the basic medical sciences and public health. The Chicago, Rockford, and Peoria campuses offer independent study programs through which medical students can design their own curricula and carry out in-depth studies of health care topics in which they have a special interest.

## REQUIREMENTS FOR ENTRANCE

All candidates must take the MCAT no later than the fall test period of the academic year in which application is made. The Committee on Admissions uses in its evaluation the highest MCAT scores reported of three previous years.

Applicants must be citizens of the United States or permanent legal residents six months prior to June 1 of the AMCAS processing year.

Applicants must receive the baccalaureate degree prior to matriculation in the College of Medicine. Students may elect any major field of interest. Biology, chemistry (through organic), physics or biophysics, and behavioral science will be particularly helpful in preparing for study in the college. However, the undergraduate major may be chosen from the humanities, fine arts, or behavioral, biological, or physical sciences. Mathematics through calculus is useful for those anticipating advanced work in basic or clinical research.

Letters of recommendation are required of all applicants.

## SELECTION FACTORS

All candidates apply to the Committee on Admissions, and admitted applicants are given their choices of study sites insofar as places permit. Prospective and admitted students are provided with detailed information to help in their selection of sites.

The College of Medicine endeavors to select applicants who in the judgment of the Committee on Admissions demonstrate best the academic achievement, emotional stability, maturity, integrity, and motivation adjudged necessary for successful study and practice of medicine. The committee is interested in evidence of the applicant's capacity for mature and independent scholarship, while discouraging rigid patterns of course work. The committee will consider the quality of work of each applicant in all subject areas, the breadth of education, achievement in advanced projects, and work and extracurricular experiences that demonstrate the applicant's imagination, initiative, and creativity. The College of Medicine does not discriminate against applicants on the basis of race, creed, sex, religion, national origin, age, disability, or status as a disabled veteran or veteran of the Vietnam era.

Selection of students is based on a critical evaluation of all available data on each applicant and on the changing needs of society. The Committee on Admissions gives strong preference to candidates who are Illinois residents and who also: (1) possess a GPA of B or better, (2) have attained an MCAT score above the national mean, and (3) meet the safety and technical standards set by the college. Candidates whose formal education has been interrupted are reviewed with respect to their potential contribution to the practice of medicine and to their competitive status with other applicants. An interview of selected candidates may be required.

## FINANCIAL AID

Entering students are encouraged to provide timely application through the College of Medicine Office of Student Financial Aid for loan funds and grant-in-aid scholarship assistance based on need. Grants and scholarships to meet proven financial need are awarded each year to students from all classes. Financial aid consultation and information can be obtained by calling (312) 413-0127.

## INFORMATION FOR MINORITY AND RURAL CANDIDATES

The College of Medicine has developed programs to encourage applications from qualified individuals from medically underserved areas of Illinois. The College maintains a professional staff to provide guidance and counseling to motivated students from minority ethnic groups that are underrepresented within the physician population of Illinois (Black American, Hispanic, American Indian) and resident candidates whose backgrounds indicate potential for rural Illinois practice. The Committee on Admissions reviews all applications, and students are accepted on the basis of their potential for successfully meeting all college standards leading to the M.D. degree.

Public Institution

## APPLICATION AND ACCEPTANCE POLICIES FOR 1997–98 FIRST-YEAR CLASS

*School participates in AMCAS. See Chapter 4.*

Filing of AMCAS application
  Earliest date: June 1, 1996
  Latest date: Dec. 1, 1996
School application fee after screening: $30
Oldest MCAT scores considered: 1994
Does have Early Decision Program (EDP)
  For Illinois residents only
  EDP application period: June 1–Aug. 1, 1996
  EDP applicants notified by: Oct. 1, 1996
Acceptance notice to regular applicants
  Earliest date: Nov. 1, 1996
  Latest date: Until class is filled
Applicant's response to acceptance offer
  Maximum time: 2 weeks
Requests for deferred entrance considered: Yes
Deposit to hold place in class (applied to tuition):
  $100, due with response to acceptance offer
Deposit refundable prior to: May 15, 1997
Estimated number of new entrants: 300
Starting date: Aug. 1997

## TUITION AND STUDENT FEES PER YEAR FOR 1995–96 FIRST-YEAR CLASS

Tuition                              Student fees: $1,218
  Resident: $9,520
  Nonresident: $27,740

## INFORMATION ON 1995–96 FIRST-YEAR CLASS

| Number of | In-State | Out-of-State | Total |
|---|---|---|---|
| Applicants | 2,123 | 4,532 | 6,655 |
| Applicants Interviewed* | 0 | 0 | 0 |
| New Entrants† | 298 | 19 | 317 |

*Some special programs conduct interviews.
†All took the MCAT and had baccalaureate degrees.

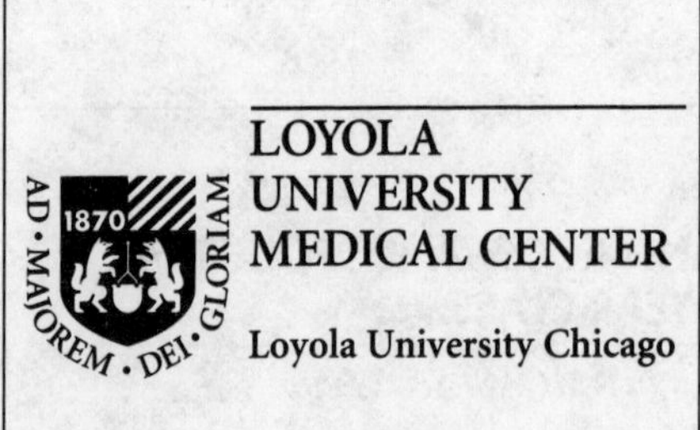


# Loyola University Chicago
# Stritch School of Medicine

## Maywood, Illinois

Dr. Daniel H. Winship, *Dean*
LaDonna E. Norstrom, *Assistant Dean, Admissions*
Donna J. Sobie, *Director, Financial Aid*

## ADDRESS INQUIRIES TO:

Office of Admissions, Room 1752
Loyola University Medical Center
Stritch School of Medicine
2160 South First Avenue
Maywood, Illinois 60153
(708) 216-3229

## GENERAL INFORMATION

Loyola University Chicago is a private university founded in 1870 by the Jesuits. It is one of the largest Catholic universities in the United States. By 1920 the university had organized several small medical colleges into a new medical school. In 1948 the school was named in honor of Samuel Cardinal Stritch, Archbishop of Chicago. In 1969 the university opened the Loyola University Medical Center, built on land given by the Veterans Administration, in Maywood, a suburban community located 12 miles west of the Chicago Loop. The medical center houses both the Stritch School of Medicine and the Foster G. McGaw Hospital. Students receive their clinical training at the 570-bed McGaw Hospital, at the 1,022-bed Hines Veterans Administration Hospital, and at a number of affiliated hospitals in the Chicago area.

## CURRICULUM

The primary purpose of the Stritch School of Medicine is to train physicians who will care for their patients with skill, respect, and compassion. The personal and intellectual development of each student is promoted through close contact with members of the faculty and administration. Students are exposed to the operation of a large medical center, where they learn in an atmosphere of cooperation and mutual assistance. The first year of the curriculum concentrates on the basic principles and processes related to the normal structure, function, and regulation of the human body. In addition, the first year includes instruction in health promotion/disease prevention, health care finance and access, medical ethics, medical/legal issues and the doctor/patient relationship. Students also have the opportunity to visit ambulatory care sites to experience the delivery of medical care in the ambulatory setting. The second year of the curriculum focuses on basic science principles related to the mechanisms of human disease, neuroscience, and the therapeutic approach to disease. Additionally, students have the opportunity to continue to develop their knowledge about human behavioral science, physical examination skills, basic clinical skills, evidence-based clinical decision making, and medical ethics and humanities. The third and fourth years are organized into clinical clerkships. The core curriculum includes medicine (20 weeks), surgery (12 weeks), pediatrics (6 weeks), psychiatry (6 weeks), family medicine (6 weeks), neurology (4 weeks), and obstetrics and gynecology (6 weeks). Students also take between 26 and 34 weeks of electives during these two years. Through these electives, they anticipate their residency training and prepare for careers in medicine suited to their particular interests and talents.

Special features of the curriculum include the Medical Humanities Program, which extends from the basic science semesters through clinical training, and the Dual Degree Program, whereby medical students can earn M.D. and Ph.D. degrees in order to prepare for careers as medical scientists and teachers.

## REQUIREMENTS FOR ENTRANCE

A bachelor's degree and the MCAT, preferably taken by the spring but no later than the fall of the year of application, are required. The following courses are required:

|                                      | *Years* |
| ------------------------------------ | ------- |
| Biology or zoology (with lab)        | 1       |
| Inorganic chemistry (with lab)       | 1       |
| Organic chemistry (with lab)         | 1       |
| Physics (with lab)                   | 1       |

A semester or quarter of biochemistry can be substituted for part of the organic chemistry requirement.

Any undergraduate major is acceptable. Applicants are expected to take challenging course work in the humanities and social sciences, and they should be able to speak and write the English language correctly.

Applicants must be U.S. citizens or hold a permanent resident visa. As a rule, applicants are limited to applying no more than twice. Applicants enrolled in advanced degree programs must expect to complete their degrees prior to matriculation.

## SELECTION FACTORS

The academic record will be evaluated for both depth and breadth of study. Circumstances, such as need to work, which affect a student's academic performance will be taken into account when the record is evaluated. The 1995 entering class had a mean GPA of 3.5. Applicants who present academic credentials which indicate they are capable of succeeding in the rigors of a medical education will be evaluated for evidence of the personal qualifications they can bring to the medical profession. Essential characteristics include an interest in learning, integrity, compassion, and the ability to assume responsibility. Of particular concern will be an applicant's exploration of the field of medicine and the nature of the motivation to enter this career. Each year approximately 600 applicants are invited to interviews with members of the Committee on Admissions. These interviews are conducted only at the medical center campus.

At least 50 percent of each entering class are residents of Illinois. Approximately 45 percent of each entering class are women, and the age range of accepted applicants is quite wide. Early submission of the AMCAS application and prompt return of all supporting material will enhance an applicant's chance of being offered a place in the class.

Loyola-Stritch recommends the Early Decision Program (EDP) for applicants with strong academic credentials and a particular interest in the school. Those considering applying through the EDP should contact the assistant dean for admissions prior to submitting their AMCAS application.

Loyola University does not discriminate on the basis of race, religion, national origin, sex, age, or handicap. The Committee on Admissions attempts to select students with diversified backgrounds for the contributions they can make to the educational process and the medical profession. Members of minority groups underrepresented in medicine are encouraged to apply.

## FINANCIAL AID

Over 90 percent of Stritch students receive some form of financial aid during the four years of medical school. Student aid is primarily in the form of loans, but limited scholarship and grant money is also available. Some students have found it possible to work during their first two years, often in jobs at the medical center. The school's financial aid office attempts to keep student debt at a manageable level through workshops on budgeting and financial planning. Applicants should contact the director of financial aid approximately one month after submitting financial aid forms.

---

Private Institution

## APPLICATION AND ACCEPTANCE POLICIES FOR 1997–98 FIRST-YEAR CLASS

*School participates in AMCAS. See Chapter 4.*

Filing of AMCAS application
    Earliest date: June 1, 1996
    Latest date: Nov. 15, 1996
School application fee after screening: $50
Oldest MCAT scores considered: 1993
Does have Early Decision Program (EDP)
    EDP application period: June 1–Aug. 1, 1996
    EDP applicatnts notified by: Oct 1, 1996
Acceptance notice to regular applicants
    Earliest date: Oct. 15, 1996
    Latest date: Until class is filled
Applicant's response to acceptance offer
    Maximum time: 2 weeks
Requests for deferred entrance considered: Yes
Deposit to hold place in class: None
Estimated number of new entrants: 130 (6 EDP)
Starting date: July 1997

## TUITION AND STUDENT FEES PER YEAR FOR 1995–96 FIRST-YEAR CLASS

Tuition: $25,600          Student fees: $409

## INFORMATION ON 1995–96 FIRST-YEAR CLASS

| Number of | In-State | Out-of-State | Total |
|---|---|---|---|
| Applicants | 1,676 | 8,670 | 10,346 |
| Applicants Interviewed | 214 | 347 | 561 |
| New Entrants* | 65 | 65 | 130 |

*All took the MCAT and had baccalaureate degrees.

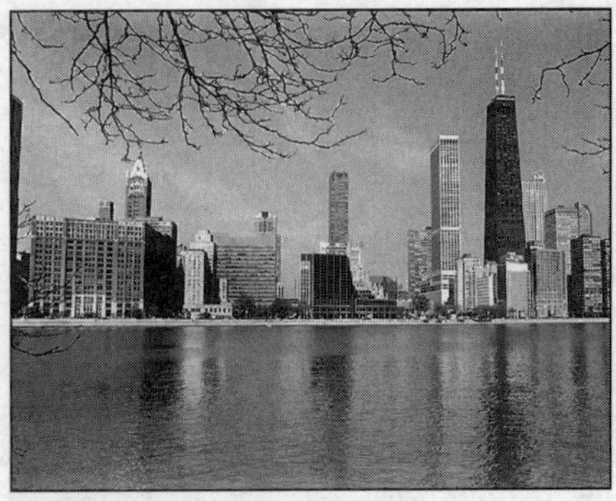

# Northwestern University Medical School

## Chicago, Illinois

Dr. Harry N. Beaty, *Dean*
Dr. Charles A. Berry, *Associate Dean for Admissions*
Delores Brown, *Assistant Dean for Admissions*

## ADDRESS INQUIRIES TO:

Associate Dean for Admissions
Northwestern University Medical School
303 East Chicago Avenue
Chicago, Illinois 60611
(312) 503-8206

## GENERAL INFORMATION

Founded in 1859, the Medical School is located on the university's lakefront Chicago campus, along with three of the McGaw Medical Center hospitals. Medical students may live on campus at Abbott Hall or Lake Shore Center. More than 2,200 full-time, part-time, and contributed services faculty members offer instruction in the basic sciences and clinical medicine. The school also offers opportunities in basic science research and clinical research. The McGaw hospitals—a group of urban, suburban, specialized, and general hospitals—are Northwestern Memorial, Children's Memorial, Evanston, and Glenbrook hospitals; Rehabilitation Institute of Chicago; and VA Lakeside Medical Center.

## CURRICULUM

Northwestern's goal is to graduate men and women who are so well grounded in both basic and clinical sciences that they can capably diagnose and treat patients in a variety of settings.

The curriculum presents the basic sciences in four integrated blocks throughout the first two years and is graded on a pass/fail system. No more than 10 hours per week are allocated to the lecture format and an additional 10 hours per week are devoted to small-group sessions; laboratory sessions and other teaching formats. The integrated block approach provides a context more in keeping with the practice of medicine. In the third year, students learn from attending physicians and residents during clinical clerkships in medicine, surgery, neurology, psychiatry, pediatrics, obstetrics and gynecology, rehabilitation medicine, and anesthesia. To help students round out their medical education and focus on career goals, the fourth year combines electives with required clerkships in medicine, ambulatory care, and two surgical subspecialties.

A combined M.D.-Ph.D. program, offered by the medical school in cooperation with the graduate school, prepares students for careers in academic medicine.

A combined M.D.-M.M. program with the Kellogg Graduate School of Management enables a student to obtain both degrees in five calendar years.

## HONORS PROGRAM

One of the oldest combined baccalaureate-M.D. programs in the country, the Honors Program in Medical Education (HPME) each year selects 60 highly motivated, talented high school graduates for a course of study leading to B.S. and M.D. degrees in seven years. A program option leading to the B.S. degree in engineering and the M.D. also is offered. Inquiries about the HPME should be directed to Dr. Stuart Spies, HPME Director, Northwestern University Medical School, 303 E. Chicago Avenue, Chicago, Illinois 60611.

## REQUIREMENTS FOR ENTRANCE

The MCAT and 135 quarter hours (90 semester hours) of undergraduate course work from an accredited college are required. U.S. citizens as well as foreign nationals should plan on taking their course work at an undergraduate institution in the United States or Canada. The medical school does not place emphasis on any major field of study. It does recommend that year-long courses in biology, general chemistry, organic chemistry, physics, and English be completed before matriculating into medical school.

Candidates are strongly urged to take the MCAT prior to submitting an application for admission. Preference will be given to applicants who will have received a bachelor's degree prior to enrollment at Northwestern University Medical School.

## SELECTION FACTORS

The medical school is committed to filling about half its positions with Illinois residents. After Illinois residents and those enrolled in the HPME are accommodated, about 50 to 60 positions remain for conventional out-of-state applicants.

All completed applications are reviewed and evaluated. Reviewers look for evidence of emotional maturity, motivation, past achievement, and character as well as academic excellence. A premium is placed on breadth of the academic program, life experiences of the individual, and clinical exposure. Applicants should be liberally educated men and women who have studied in some depth subjects beyond the conventional premedical sciences. For example, the Admissions Committee appreciates candidates who major in such subjects as history, English, or sociology and yet desire to be physicians. Panel interviews are required of all students considered seriously for acceptance; interview invitations are issued solely upon the request of the Admissions Committee and are conducted at the Medical School.

Some characteristics of the 1994 entering class were: *GPA,* 3.51; *MCAT* scores averaging about the 75th percentile nationally; *average age,* 22 (range 19-44); *sex,* 51 percent women.

The Medical School faculty has established technical performance standards. Candidates for admission should demonstrate the mental capability, moral integrity, and physical skills required to function effectively in a broad variety of laboratory and clinical situations. Northwestern University does not discriminate on the basis of race, religion, national origin, sex, age, or handicap in its educational programs or activities in accordance with civil rights legislation.

## FINANCIAL AID

Financial considerations do not influence admissions decisions. More than 60 percent of the student body have received financial aid. Support is provided primarily through national and local loan programs. Northwestern University offers an institutional loan program to international students who can find a U.S. citizen or permanent resident who is creditworthy and who is willing to be a co-signer on the loan with the student (i.e., he/she must agree to repay the loan if the student fails to do so).

Accepted applicants wishing to receive further information may write to the assistant director for financial aid, 850 N. Lake Shore Drive, Room 209, Chicago, Illinois, 60611.

## INFORMATION FOR UNDERREPRESENTED MINORITIES

The Medical School is committed to the recruitment, admission, and graduation of underrepresented minorities (African Americans, Hispanics, and American Indians). Minority faculty members and alumni participate in all aspects of the program. Applications are encouraged from underrepresented minorities. The application process and standards for acceptance are the same as those described in the preceding paragraphs; there is no separate admissions process. Students are urged to take the April MCAT and to submit their application early. Students wishing to discuss their qualifications and/or the admissions process should contact the assistant dean for admissions well in advance of applying.

Private Institution

## APPLICATION AND ACCEPTANCE POLICIES FOR 1997–98 FIRST-YEAR CLASS

*School participates in AMCAS. See Chapter 4.*

Filing of AMCAS application
    Earliest date: June 1, 1996
    Latest date: Oct. 15, 1996
School application fee after screening: $50
Oldest MCAT scores considered: 1993
Does have Early Decision Program (EDP)
    EDP application period: June 1–Aug. 1, 1996
    EDP applicants notified by: Oct 1, 1996
Acceptance notice to regular applicants
    Earliest date: Nov. 15, 1996
    Latest date: Varies
Applicant's response to acceptance offer
    Maximum time: 2 weeks
Requests for deferred entrance considered: Yes
Deposit to hold place in class: None
Deposit refundable prior to: May 15, 1997
Estimated number of new entrants: 173 (5 EDP)
Starting date: Sept. 1997

## TUITION AND STUDENT FEES PER YEAR FOR 1995–96 FIRST-YEAR CLASS

Tuition: $25,446          Student fees: None

## INFORMATION ON 1995–96 FIRST-YEAR CLASS

| Number of | In-State | Out-of-State | Total |
|---|---|---|---|
| Applicants | 1,371 | 8,151 | 9,522 |
| Applicants Interviewed | 192 | 293 | 485 |
| New Entrants* | 81 | 93 | 174 |

*All took the MCAT and had baccalaureate degrees (excluding the HPME entrants).

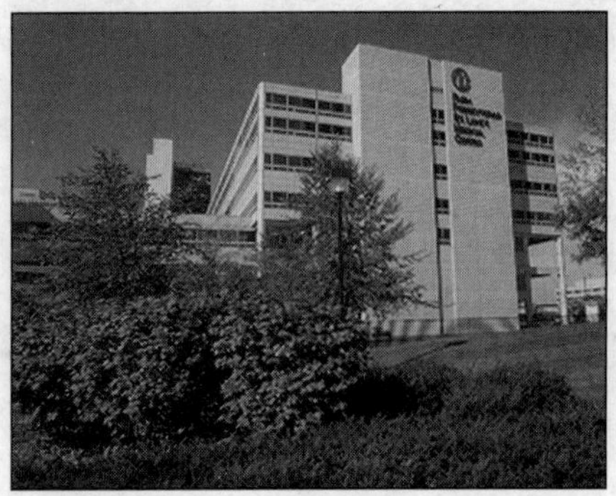

# Rush Medical College of Rush University

**Chicago, Illinois**


Dr. Erich E. Brueshke, *Dean*
Jan L. Schmidt, *Director of Admissions*
Robert Dame, *Director of Student Financial Aid*


## ADDRESS INQUIRIES TO:

Office of Admissions
524 Academic Facility
Rush Medical College of Rush University
600 South Paulina Street
Chicago, Illinois 60612
(312) 942-6913; 942-2333 (FAX)

## GENERAL INFORMATION

Rush Medical College, founded in 1837, is the oldest component of Rush University. The original medical college graduated over 10,000 physicians before closing in 1942. Rush Medical College reopened in 1971 and is part of Rush University.

Through the academic and health care network of more than a dozen affiliated hospitals and a neighborhood health center, Rush-Presbyterian-St. Luke's Medical Center serves 1.5 to 2 million people. Thus, the students of Rush University train in urban, suburban, and rural areas in a variety of socioeconomic and ethnic settings.

## CURRICULUM

Rush Medical College provides a firm background in the science of medicine and a balanced introduction to the practice of clinical medicine in a four-year curriculum designed to provide educational flexibility. A major goal of the college and its faculty is to create an environment that fosters commitments to competent and compassionate patient care and to attitudes of inquiry and lifelong learning.

In the traditional curriculum, the first year introduces students to the basic medical sciences. The second year expands the basic science background with the study of pathological processes and therapeutics. In addition, clinical skills are introduced and developed in preparation for the clinical years.

A small-group oriented problem-assisted alternative curriculum is available for 24 students in each entering class. This alternative curriculum shifts the allocation of basic science faculty effort to the preparation of effective guidebooks and to serving as expert resources for students. The guidebooks outline the basic science material, which is to be learned in an integrative fashion, and illustrate relevant problem-solving approaches, learning examinations, and appropriate reference material. Material is integrated from several disciplines for study together as a unit. Scheduled student-faculty contact hours are devoted to examining clinical problems which serve as vehicles for learning in the basic sciences and for developing clinical reasoning and interpersonal skills.

The third and fourth years consist of required core clerkships in internal medicine, surgery, obstetrics and gynecology, pediatrics, psychiatry, family practice, and neurology; a required subinternship in internal medicine, pediatrics, or family practice; and a minimum of 18 weeks of elective clerkships. Many students spend some of their elective clerkship experience in foreign countries.

Rush University offers qualified students who aspire to careers in academic medicine and research the opportunity to enroll in a combined M.D.-Ph.D. program. Ph.D. programs are offered in the Graduate College in the following areas: anatomical sciences, biochemistry, immunology, microbiology, medical physics, neurosciences, pharmacology, and physiology. Students in concurrent programs must meet the full conditions and requirements of the Graduate College, Graduate Division, and the Medical College.

Upon entering Rush Medical College, each student is assigned an academic adviser to help define goals, aid in the selection of courses of study, provide other counseling, and serve as role model and friend. This adviser will continue with the student as the student progresses through school.

## REQUIREMENTS FOR ENTRANCE

The MCAT and 90 semester hours of undergraduate work in an accredited college are required. College work must include the following science areas:

|  | *Sem. hrs.* |
|---|---|
| Biology or zoology | 8 |
| Inorganic chemistry | 8 |
| Organic chemistry | 8 |
| General physics | 8 |

Four semester hours of biochemistry may be substituted for the second semester of organic chemistry.

Sound preparation in the basic sciences is essential, but a broad background in the humanities and wide exposure to people and their problems are equally necessary.

Applicants are strongly urged to take the MCAT in the spring of the year of application; however, those who take it in the fall will also be considered.

## SELECTION FACTORS

Students who enter the Rush Medical College program are carefully selected for their intellectual and social maturity and represent a wide variety of educational and social backgrounds. Problem-solving skills, critical judgment, and the capability to pursue independent study are considered important. Majors in science and majors in other areas with demonstrated excellence in the required science courses are considered equally appropriate to a medical education at Rush Medical College. The Committee on Admissions looks for objective evidence that the applicant will be able to handle the academic demands of the medical curriculum. In evaluating academic achievement, the committee does consider factors such as the degree of difficulty of the program, the need to work, social and cultural backgrounds, and other factors that may affect the record. In the nonacademic realm, maturity, a balanced education, personal integrity, and motivational factors are considered essential determinants.

Undergraduate academic achievement, recommendations of premedical committees and/or undergraduate faculty, performance on the MCAT, and personal interviews (which are requested of those applicants who are considered competitive candidates by the Committee on Admissions) are considered in the evaluation of applicants. Only applications from U.S. citizens or permanent residents are considered. The average GPA and MCAT scores approximate those of nationally accepted applicants. All applicants are considered without regard to sex, religion, race, age, handicap, or national origin. Applicants from disadvantaged minority groups underrepresented in the medical profession are encouraged to apply. Rush will waive its application fee for any applicants receiving an AMCAS fee waiver.

## FINANCIAL AID

Determination of a financial aid award is made after acceptance into medical school. The financial aid package will consist primarily of loans. Due to limited institutional scholarship assistance, scholarship eligibility is based on parents' resources regardless of the student's age or status. Students are awarded financial aid packages to meet 100 percent of the demonstrated financial need during each year of their medical education. Approximately 80 percent of the medical students receive financial assistance from state, federal, institutional, or other sources outside the family.

Private Institution

## APPLICATION AND ACCEPTANCE POLICIES FOR 1997–98 FIRST-YEAR CLASS

*School participates in AMCAS. See Chapter 4.*

Filing of AMCAS application
    Earliest date: June 1, 1996
    Latest date: Nov. 15, 1996
School application fee to all applicants: $45
Oldest MCAT scores considered: 1993
Does have Early Decision Program (EDP)
    EDP application period: June 1–Aug. 1, 1996
    EDP applicants notified by: Oct. 1, 1996
Acceptance notice to regular applicants
    Earliest date: Oct. 15, 1996
    Latest date: Until class is filled
Applicant's response to acceptance offer
    Maximum time: 2 weeks
Requests for deferred entrance considered: Yes
Deposit to hold place in class (applied to tuition):
    $100, due with response to acceptance offer
Deposit refundable prior to: May 15, 1997
Estimated number of new entrants: 120 (10 EDP)
Starting date: Sept. 1997

## TUITION AND STUDENT FEES PER YEAR FOR 1995–96 FIRST-YEAR CLASS

Tuition: $22,944        Student fees: $1,536

## INFORMATION ON 1995–96 FIRST-YEAR CLASS

| Number of | In-State | Out-of-State | Total |
|---|---|---|---|
| Applicants | 1,736 | 3,891 | 5,627 |
| Applicants Interviewed | 400 | 100 | 500 |
| New Entrants* | 104 | 16 | 120 |

*All took the MCAT; 99% had baccalaureate degrees.

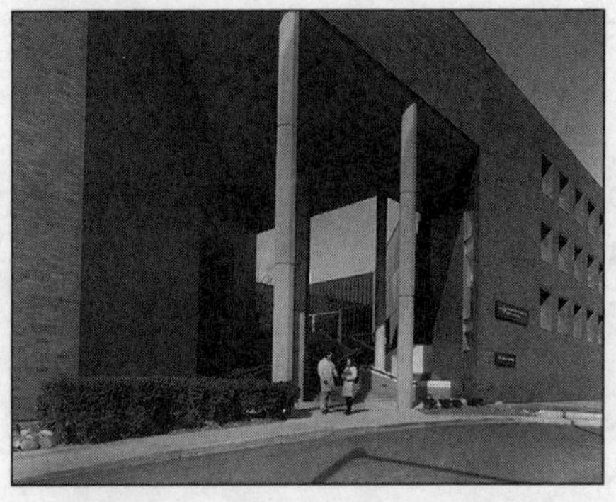

# Southern Illinois University School of Medicine

**Springfield, Illinois**

Dr. Carl J. Getto, *Dean and Provost*
Erin L. Coil, *Director of Admissions*
Nancy Calvert, *Director of Financial Aid*

## ADDRESS INQUIRIES TO:

Office of Student and Alumni Affairs
Southern Illinois University
School of Medicine
P.O. Box 19230
Springfield, Illinois 62794-1226
(217) 782-2860; 785-5538 (FAX)

## GENERAL INFORMATION

Southern Illinois University School of Medicine was established in 1969 and graduated its first class in 1975. Students spend the first 12 months of the program at the medical education facilities on the Carbondale campus and the remaining three years at the Medical Center in Springfield.

## CURRICULUM

SIU School of Medicine conducts its four-year program on two campuses. The first year occurs on SIU's Carbondale campus and takes advantage of the basic science faculty and facilities located there. The remaining three years are spent at the Medical Center in Springfield. For their basic science years, students may choose between the problem-based learning curriculum (PBLC) or the standard curriculum. Regardless of which track students choose, the curricula are organized around organ systems, and each exposes students to the sciences basic to medicine.

In the standard curriculum, the first year basic sciences concentrate on the normal functioning of the human body, while clinical medicine develops data gathering skills. The second year focuses on abnormal functioning of the human body as well as the ability to integrate history taking and physical examination skills with the underlying pathophysiology of disease. Lectures are the primary mode of delivery, although there are some laboratory and small-group sessions.

The PBLC integrates the relevant basic sciences with the necessary clinical reasoning skills through ongoing encounters with real patient problems delivered in a variety of formats, including standardized patients and paper and computer simulations. These patient problems, encountered in groups of five to seven students and a faculty tutor, serve as the primary stimuli for learning.

No matter which curriculum students choose for the first two years, they must record a passing score on the USMLE,

Step 1 before they begin 47 weeks of clinical rotations during the third year; these include the six specialties and medical humanities. Students also take a comprehensive, performance-based examination after the conclusion of the third year. Thirty-two weeks of elective study plus rotations in anesthesiology and neurology complete the program.

The grading system is honors/pass/fail.

The school also offers a six-year M.D.-J.D. program.

## REQUIREMENTS FOR ENTRANCE

Applications are accepted from all U.S. citizens and those foreign citizens possessing a permanent resident visa. A minimum of 90 semester hours of undergraduate work in an accredited degree-granting college or university are required. Foreign students are advised to have completed at least 60 semester hours of course work in the United States. Applicants are expected to have a good foundation in the natural sciences, social sciences, and humanities and to demonstrate facility in writing and speaking the English language.

To perform well on the MCAT, it is advisable to have had a minimum of two years of college chemistry (including organic), one year of physics, one year of biological or life sciences, mathematics (including statistics), and one year of English composition.

## SELECTION FACTORS

Preference is given to those with sufficient recent academic activity to demonstrate the potential for successful completion of the rigorous educational program and to those who demonstrate the necessary noncognitive characteristics of a successful medical student and physician. Although the Admissions Committee establishes no quotas, an effort is made to recruit qualified applicants from groups that have been underrepresented in the medical profession. Applicants are selected for interview according to their ability to meet the selection factors and to identify with the purpose of the School of Medicine, which is to assist the citizens of central and southern Illinois in meeting their present and future health care needs. Selected applicants are interviewed in either Springfield or Carbondale; an interview is a prerequisite to acceptance.

The School of Medicine does not discriminate on the basis of race, religion, age, sex, handicap, or national or ethnic origin in administration of its education policies, admissions policies, scholarship and loan programs, and other school administered programs.

## FINANCIAL AID

Financial assistance is made available to all students demonstrating financial need, and 88 percent of the student body receive financial aid. Only a limited number of scholarships are available. Most financial need will be met by a combination of loan funds.

Limited employment opportunities are available. Medical students are allowed to work as long as their employment commitments do not interfere with their academic progress.

## INFORMATION FOR MINORITIES

The School of Medicine sponsors the Medical Education Preparatory Program (MEDPREP) for minority and economically disadvantaged undergraduate or postbaccalaureate students. MEDPREP is a non-degree-granting program located on the Carbondale campus. Students who are admitted to the program must begin their matriculation during the term immediately preceding or following the summer semester. The MEDPREP curriculum is designed to meet students' individual preparatory needs. It consists of developmental and enrichment tutorials in small class format, preparation for the MCAT, and medical school application assistance. Additionally, students enroll in preprofessional courses offered by other departments on the campus. Personal, academic, and career counseling is also provided. Undergraduate students may participate in the program nine semesters; postbaccalaureate students may participate in the program six semesters. MEDPREP does not offer a guarantee of eventual acceptance to the School of Medicine or to any other medical school. However, careful consideration will be given to MEDPREP participant applicants by the School of Medicine and those selected medical schools working cooperatively with MEDPREP. Inquiries should be addressed to: Director, MEDPREP, Southern Illinois University School of Medicine, Carbondale, Illinois 62901.

---

Public Institution

## APPLICATION AND ACCEPTANCE POLICIES FOR 1997–98 FIRST-YEAR CLASS

*School participates in AMCAS. See Chapter 4.*

Filing of AMCAS application
 Earliest date: June 1, 1996
 Latest date: Nov. 15, 1996
School application fee after screening: $50
Oldest MCAT scores considered: 1994
Does have Early Decision Program (EDP)
 Nonresidents must apply through EDP
 or through the M.D.-J.D. program
 EDP application period: June 1–Aug. 1, 1996
 EDP applicants notified by: Oct. 1, 1996
Acceptance notice to regular applicants
 Earliest date: Oct. 15, 1996
 Latest date: Varies
Applicant's response to acceptance offer
 Maximum time: 15 days
Requests for deferred entrance considered: Yes
Deposit to hold place in class (applied to tuition):
 $100, due with response to acceptance offer
Deposit refundable prior to: May 15, 1997
Estimated number of new entrants: 72 (15 EDP)
Starting date: Aug. 1997

## TUITION AND STUDENT FEES PER YEAR FOR 1995–96 FIRST-YEAR CLASS

| Tuition | Student fees: $1,260 |
| --- | --- |
| Resident: $10,035 | |
| Nonresident: $30,105 | |

## INFORMATION ON 1995–96 FIRST-YEAR CLASS

| Number of | In-State | Out-of-State | Total |
| --- | --- | --- | --- |
| Applicants | 1,439 | 665 | 2,104 |
| Applicants Interviewed | 229 | 4 | 233 |
| New Entrants* | 72 | 0 | 72 |

*All had baccalaureate degrees; 97% took the MCAT.

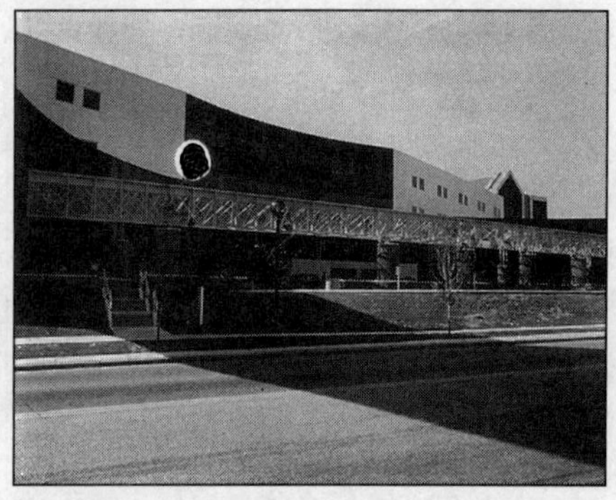

# Indiana University School of Medicine

**Indianapolis, Indiana**

Dr. Robert W. Holden, *Dean*
Dr. George T. Lukemeyer, *Chair, Admissions Committee*
Robert M. Stump, Jr., *Director of Admissions*

## ADDRESS INQUIRIES TO:

Medical School Admissions Office
Fesler Hall 213
Indiana University
School of Medicine
1120 South Drive
Indianapolis, Indiana 46202-5113
(317) 274-3772
Web Site: http://www.iupui.edu/it/medschl/home.html

## GENERAL INFORMATION

Indiana University School of Medicine, founded in 1903, is the sole institution responsible for providing medical education in the state of Indiana and operates the Indiana Statewide Medical Education System. The School has centers for medical education at Bloomington, Evansville, Fort Wayne, Gary, Lafayette, Muncie, South Bend, and Terre Haute, where students may spend their first two years of medical school. The Medical Center in Indianapolis has students enrolled in all four years of the medical curriculum.

In addition to its role and responsibilities in teaching, patient care, and service, Indiana University School of Medicine is a major academic research center.

Indiana University Medical Center includes the School of Medicine, the School of Allied Health Sciences, the School of Dentistry, the School of Nursing, research laboratories, the University Hospitals, and three other affiliated hospitals.

## CURRICULUM

The basic medical sciences are presented in the first two years. In addition, a multidisciplinary course, introduction to clinical medicine, spans the first two years. Students' skills, knowledge, and attitudes about patient care begin to take shape in this course as they encounter patients for the first time.

The Northwest Center for Medical Education's Regional Center Alternative Pathway utilizes problem-based learning methods, including small-group, case-based tutorial sessions, laboratories, and a few optional lectures to fully prepare medical students for their clinical medical education.

A 12-month clinical clerkship program at the medical center in Indianapolis occupies the third year and includes units in family medicine, internal medicine, surgery, obstetrics and gynecology, pediatrics, and psychiatry. In the fourth year, students complete clerkships in neurosensory science, radiology, and surgical specialties, and select six one-month elective units from an approved list of hundreds of choices throughout the state. With the permission of the faculty, students may arrange for elective experiences around the country and abroad.

Students are required to complete a biomedical research paper during their four-year enrollment in medical school.

Students interested in research or academic medicine may enroll in the combined-degree program and pursue a master's or Ph.D. degree in addition to the M.D. degree.

In Indianapolis, the School of Medicine's basic science departments offer combined-degree programs in anatomy, biochemistry, medical genetics, medical neurobiology, microbiology-immunology, pathology, pharmacology-toxicology, and physiology-biophysics.

The Medical Sciences Program in Bloomington offers studies in anatomy, biochemistry, pathology, pharmacology, and physiology. Also available to combined-degree students in Bloomington are studies in the humanities, law, and social and behavioral sciences as well as in the biological and physical sciences.

In cooperation with Purdue University, combined-degree programs are offered in engineering, medicinal chemistry, molecular biology, and neuroscience at the Lafayette Center for Medical Education.

## REQUIREMENTS FOR ENTRANCE

The School of Medicine recommends that students preparing for the study of medicine take a variety of courses commonly included in a traditional liberal arts and sciences curriculum.

The MCAT and a minimum of three college years (90 semester hours) are required. Physical education and ROTC courses will not be accepted as part of the 90 semester hours. The undergraduate course work must include:

|  | *Years* |
|---|---|
| Biology (with labs) | 1 |
| General chemistry (with labs) | 1 |
| Organic chemistry (with labs) | 1 |
| Physics (with labs) | 1 |

Applicants should take the MCAT in the spring prior to making application.

Although an unusually well qualified applicant is occasionally admitted after only three years of undergraduate study, the Admissions Committee shows preference to applicants who will have a baccalaureate degree prior to matriculation in medical school.

## SELECTION FACTORS

Students are offered places in the class on the basis of scholarship, character, personality, references, residence, interview, and performance on the MCAT. In addition, the medical school faculty has specified non-academic criteria (technical standards) which all applicants must meet in order to participate effectively in the medical education program and the practice of medicine.

Because the School of Medicine is state-supported, the Admissions Committee shows preference to Indiana residents in selecting the class. Nevertheless, a number of nonresidents are offered acceptances each year (39 for the 1995 entering class). The applications of nonresidents who have significant ties to the state of Indiana may be given greater consideration.

The average GPA of the 1995 entering class was 3.68/4.0. Average MCAT scores were: *VR*-9.4, *PS*-9.4, *WS*-0, *BS*-9.4.

The School of Medicine does not discriminate on the basis of race, sex, age, handicap, creed, or national origin.

## FINANCIAL AID

Scholarships and long-term, low-interest loans are available to students with financial need. There are also scholarships for students who have demonstrated academic excellence.

There is a significant scholarship for Indiana residents who commit to practicing primary care medicine in a medically underserved location.

## INFORMATION FOR MINORITIES

Applications from disadvantaged individuals and members of minority groups are encouraged.

The school recruits capable minority college students and provides counseling for high school and college students interested in the health professions. A program is available for all students who require tutorial assistance.

The School of Medicine has instituted a pre-matriculation program. Selected students are invited to participate in a two-week medical preparatory program prior to the medical school's orientation activities.

All applications are reviewed by the full Admissions Committee, which accepts students on an individual basis according to their potential and promise for medical school and for service as physicians. For additional information, please contact the Admissions Office.

---

Public Institution

## APPLICATION AND ACCEPTANCE POLICIES FOR 1997–98 FIRST-YEAR CLASS

*School participates in AMCAS. See Chapter 4.*

Filing of AMCAS application
Earliest date: June 1, 1996
Latest date: Dec. 15, 1996
School application fee after screening: $35
Oldest MCAT considered: 1993
Does have Early Decision Program (EDP)
EDP application period: June 1–Aug. 1, 1996
EDP applicants notified by: Oct. 1, 1996
Acceptance notice to regular applicants
Earliest date: Oct. 15, 1996
Latest date: Varies
Applicant's response to acceptance offer
Maximum time: 3 weeks
Requests for deferred entrance considered: Yes
Deposit to hold place in class: None
Estimated number of new entrants: 280 (50 EDP)
Starting date: Aug. 1997

## TUITION AND STUDENT FEES PER YEAR FOR 1995–96 FIRST-YEAR CLASS

Tuition            Student fees: $187
  Resident: $9,990
  Nonresident: $22,866

## INFORMATION ON 1995–96 FIRST-YEAR CLASS

| *Number of* | *In-State* | *Out-of-State* | *Total* |
|---|---|---|---|
| Applicants | 739 | 2,385 | 3,124 |
| Applicants Interviewed | 691 | 205 | 896 |
| New Entrants* | 264 | 16 | 280 |

*All took the MCAT; 98% had baccalaureate degrees.

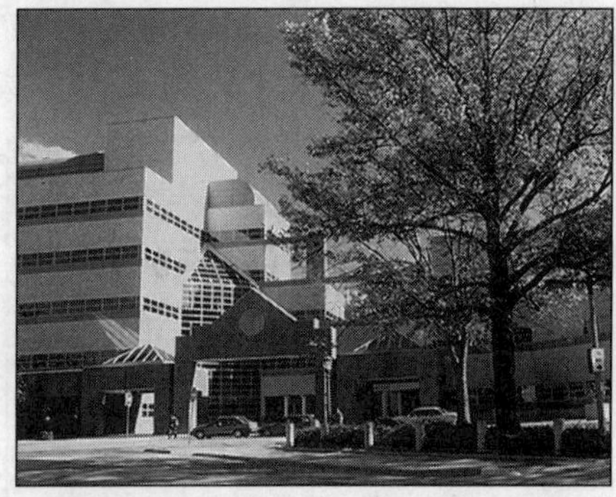

# University of Iowa College of Medicine

**Iowa City, Iowa**

Dr. Robert P. Kelch, *Dean*
Thomas C. Taylor, *Director of Admissions*
Linda G. Bissel, *Director of Financial Aid*

## ADDRESS INQUIRIES TO:

Director of Admissions
University of Iowa
College of Medicine
100 Medicine Administration Building
Iowa City, Iowa 52242-1101
(319) 335-8052; 335-8049 (FAX)
E-Mail: medical-admissions@uiowa.edu
Web Site: http://www.medadmin.uiowa.edu/osac/admiss.htm

## GENERAL INFORMATION

The College of Medicine originated in 1850 and has evolved into a major health center serving the entire state and region. The health sciences campus includes the 1,100-bed University Hospitals and Clinics, 440-bed Veterans Administration Hospital, 1,100-seat Health Sciences Library, and medical college, basic sciences, dental, nursing, and pharmacy buildings. The medical school has a full-time teaching faculty.

## CURRICULUM

A revised curriculum was introduced with the 1995 entering class. The new curriculum is intended to more efficiently incorporate advances in medical knowledge, to better prepare students to address developing health care issues, to enable students to utilize current health care delivery patterns, and to allow students and faculty to take advantage of improved instructional approaches. Problem-based and self-directed learning, clinical correlation, computer-based learning, small-group activities, and vertical integration of material are emphasized.

Year One is devoted to the investigation of the normal structure and function of the human body. Core material from the traditional basic science disciplines is presented in the first semester. The second semester is devoted to an integrated, interdisciplinary core of material arranged on an organ system basis. Year Two is devoted to the investigation of abnormal structure and function. Discipline-specific courses will again be utilized to present core material in the first half of the year. Early patient contact, an introduction to medical history taking and physical diagnosis, and coverage of emerging topic areas such as continuity of care and behavioral medicine are presented in the Foundations of Clinical Practice, a course that runs concurrently throughout the first one and one-half years of the curriculum. In the fourth semester, introduction to clinical disciplines provides students with a foundation in clinical medicine which will prepare students to perform effectively in the clinical arena.

The two clinical years of the curriculum provide a broad base of clinical experiences and training to provide the student with the essential skills and knowledge required to enter residency training. A generalist core, which includes community based primary care experiences as well as exposure to the generalist specialties and required selective segments in a variety of other specialty areas, are features of the clinical years. Ample time for electives is provided.

In order to prepare academicians in medicine, a Medical Scientist Training Program is offered which leads to both the M.D. and Ph.D. degrees over a six- to seven- year period.

## REQUIREMENTS FOR ENTRANCE

The MCAT and a minimum of 94 semester hours in an approved college are required. Completion of four years of college, including the requirements for the baccalaureate degree, is recommended. The college curriculum must include the following course work with appropriate laboratory experiences:

*Biological sciences:* A complete introductory course in the principles of animal biology or zoology and botany (but not botany alone) and one advanced course in biology.

*Chemistry:* A complete introductory course in organic chemistry, which would ordinarily follow a complete introductory course in modern general chemical principles.

*Physics:* A complete introductory course.

*Mathematics:* College algebra and trigonometry or advanced college mathematics when college algebra and trigonometry were completed in high school.

The remaining hours are chosen by the student. It is assumed that rhetoric, literature, social and behavioral science, and historical culture are generally among the courses taken as requirements for a baccalaureate degree.

Applicants for admission to the College of Medicine must demonstrate the capability to complete the entire medical curriculum, which requires proficiency in a variety of cognitive, problem-solving, manipulative, communicative, and interpersonal skills.

## SELECTION FACTORS

To be eligible for admission, the applicant must have attained at least a 2.5 GPA (based on a 4.0 scale) for all college work undertaken. Fulfillment of the basic requirements does not guarantee admission. The Admissions Committee selects those eligible applicants best qualified for the study and practice of medicine. The major factors considered are:

1. Overall undergraduate academic record as reflected in the GPA. The class has averaged 3.6.

2. Science GPA. The average has been 3.6.

3. MCAT scores. Scores have averaged 9–10 on each subtest.

4. Residence. Preference will be given to applicants with high scholastic standing who are residents of Iowa, and consideration will also be given to outstanding nonresidents.

5. Personal characteristics are evaluated by means of specially designed evaluation forms sent to each applicant to be completed by evaluators chosen by the applicant.

6. Personal interviews will be an integral part of the admissions process for the 1997 entering class. Applicants selected for interview will be contacted by the Admissions Committee.

Applications for transfer or admission with advanced standing are generally not considered.

A major in the natural sciences is not required, because the college recognizes the value of a broadly educated student body.

## FINANCIAL AID

Applicants are selected without consideration of their ability to meet the expenses of attending medical school. Students receive financial aid solely on the basis of need as calculated using the FAFSA. (See Part 1 for details.)

While students are responsible for their own financial support, the college provides information and advice on locating sources of funds. Students are urged to seek federal insured bank loans from their hometown banks. Loan and grant funds from private, state, and federal sources are available through the college.

## INFORMATION FOR DISADVANTAGED APPLICANTS

The Educational Opportunities Program (EOP) provides financial and academic assistance to educationally disadvantaged students. The program gives emphasis to groups underrepresented in American medicine. The EOP financial aid package is designed individually on the basis of need. Eligibility for the program is determined by a special committee which includes students. A prefreshman summer program includes orientation, a problem-based learning experience, a study skills program, and introductory material to other courses in the curriculum. Departmental tutors are available. Application fees and admission deposit may be defrayed for financially disadvantaged students.

---

Public Institution

## APPLICATION AND ACCEPTANCE POLICIES FOR 1997–98 FIRST-YEAR CLASS

*School participates in AMCAS. See Chapter 4.*

Filing of AMCAS application
    Earliest date: June 1, 1996
    Latest date: Nov. 1, 1996
School application fee after screening: $20
Oldest MCAT scores considered: 1991
Does have Early Decision Program (EDP)
    EDP application period: June 1–Aug. 1, 1996
    EDP applicants notified by: Oct. 1, 1996
Acceptance notice to regular applicants
    Earliest date: Oct. 15, 1996
    Latest date: Aug. 1997
Applicant's response to acceptance offer
    Maximum time: 2 weeks
Requests for deferred entrance considered: Yes
Deposit to hold place in class (applied to tuition): $50, due March 1, 1997, or within 2 weeks of acceptance offer if accepted after March 1, 1997
Deposit refundable prior to: June 15, 1997
Estimated number of new entrants: 175
Starting date: Aug. 1997

## TUITION AND STUDENT FEES PER YEAR FOR 1995–96 FIRST-YEAR CLASS

Tuition                Student fees: $172
    Resident: $8,428
    Nonresident: $22,248

## INFORMATION ON 1995–96 FIRST-YEAR CLASS

| *Number of* | *In-State* | *Out-of-State* | *Total* |
|---|---|---|---|
| Applicants | 368 | 3,145 | 3,513 |
| New Entrants* | 152 | 23 | 175 |

*All took the MCAT and had baccalaureate degrees.

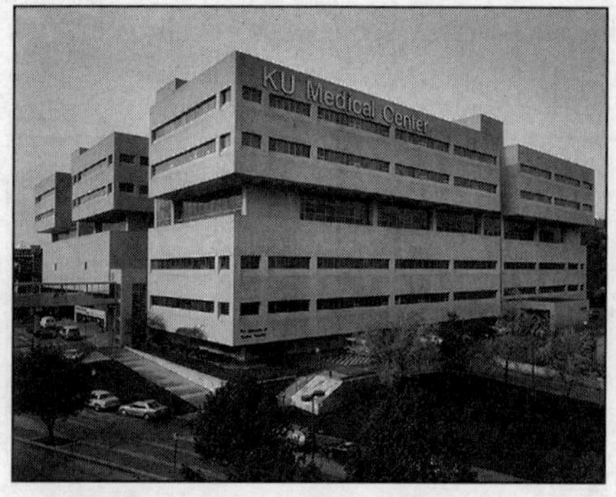

# University of Kansas School of Medicine

**Kansas City, Kansas**

Dr. Herbert Swick, *Interim Executive Dean*
Sandra J. McCurdy, *Assistant Dean for Admissions*
Sara Honeck, *Director of Student Financial Aid*

## ADDRESS INQUIRIES TO:

Assistant Dean for Admissions
University of Kansas
School of Medicine
3901 Rainbow Boulevard
Kansas City, Kansas 66160-7301
(913) 588-5245; 588-5259 (FAX)
Web Site: http://www.kumc.edu/instruction/
medicine/som.html

## GENERAL INFORMATION

The University of Kansas School of Medicine was established in 1899 with a two-year program which expanded to four years in 1906. It is located on the Medical Center campus in Kansas City, Kansas, which also houses the schools of nursing, allied health professions, and graduate studies. There are 1,500 faculty members in the School of Medicine, including 450 full-time faculty members in general and specialty medicine and the basic sciences. Full-time members actively participate in the teaching, service, and research mission of the school. Facilities at the Medical Center include the Archie R. Dykes Library of the Health Sciences, completed in 1983; the Orr-Major basic sciences facility, containing classrooms, laboratories, an auditorium, and a learning resources center, completed in 1976; the Ernst F. Lied Biomedical Research Building, completed in 1995; and the University Hospital, completed in 1979. This 485–bed hospital offers complete primary and tertiary care for patients of all ages and care for a wide range of problems from traumatic injuries to specialized care for those with chronic conditions.

The School of Medicine-Wichita was accredited in 1974, and a portion of every class completes clinical training at the four Wichita hospitals.

## CURRICULUM

The medical curriculum is designed to assist students in their acquisition of the knowledge, skills, and attitudes needed to become highly competent and caring physicians. Years 1 and 2 are traditionally formatted, with individual courses representing the basic medical science disciplines. In addition to the new ACE (Ambulatory Care Experience) program, which provides first- and second-year students with a longitudinal clinical experience in an outpatient setting, the faculty has initiated development of an interdisciplinary basic science curriculum that will incorporate increased use of small-group learning.

The curriculum of Years 3 and 4 consists of required clerkships in the core clinical areas (family medicine, medicine, surgery, pediatrics, obstetrics-gynecology, psychiatry, and geriatrics) as well as a one-month preceptorship during which each student works with a practicing Kansas physician. Clinical students choose from a large selection of basic science and clinical electives to complete a well-rounded undergraduate medical education. A comprehensive advising system assists medical students with academic counseling, professional development, and career planning.

A five-level grading system of superior, high satisfactory, satisfactory, low satisfactory, or unsatisfactory is utilized. Students must pass the USMLE Step 1 to continue their clinical training and Step 2 to graduate from the School of Medicine.

A combined M.D.-Ph.D. program in basic medical sciences is also offered. Further information and application forms may be obtained from the dean of graduate studies at the above address.

## REQUIREMENTS FOR ENTRANCE

The MCAT is required. Applicants must complete a course of study leading to a baccalaureate degree which will be conferred prior to the planned date of enrollment in medical school. The degree requirement may be modified under exceptional circumstances. Specific minimum course work requirements are:

|  | *Semesters* |
|---|---|
| General biology (with lab) | 2 |
| Inorganic chemistry (with lab) | 2 |
| Organic chemistry or organic chemistry/ biochemistry sequence (with lab) | 2 |
| Physics (with lab) | 2 |
| Calculus, statistics, or computer science | 1 |
| English | 2 |
| Sufficient credit to meet the prerequisites for a liberal arts degree. | |

Undergraduate courses should be rigorous and, in general, should be equivalent to courses taken by students majoring in those subject areas. The Admissions Committee does not give preference to a major field of study, and students are strongly advised to balance their work in the natural sciences with courses in the social sciences and humanities. No other specific courses are required.

## SELECTION FACTORS

The selection of students is made after careful consideration of the entire application, letters of evaluation from premedical faculty, and a personal interview. Each applicant's scholarship is evaluated, but it is recognized that individual capabilities and professional promise cannot always be completely measured by traditional systems of grading. Trends in academic performance, the AMCAS personal statement, impressions gained from the interview, and the record of extracurricular activities and involvement in community affairs will be assessed in considering the applicant's commitment to medicine as well as promise for the future. The University of Kansas does not discriminate on the basis of race, gender, religion, national origin, age, or handicap.

Interviews are arranged by invitation and are held in Kansas City. Secondary application materials should be returned within two weeks to receive full consideration for interview.

Qualified residents of Kansas are given first preference. The 1995 entering class was made up of 91 percent Kansans, 39 percent women, 13 percent minorities and 21 percent of the class were 25 years of age or older. The mean GPA was 3.6 with MCAT scores above the 60th percentile.

## FINANCIAL AID

Numerous loans and scholarships are available for students attending the University of Kansas School of Medicine. The majority are based on financial need, determined by filing an Application for Federal Student Aid. Over 90 percent of students receive some type of financial assistance.

A major source of assistance is the Kansas Medical Student Loan Program, which provides payment of tuition and a stipend of up to $1,500 per month. Recipients may receive loan-forgiveness by practicing primary care medicine in a small town or rural area in Kansas. Application forms and additional information can be obtained by contacting the Office of Student Financial Aid at (913) 588-5170.

## INFORMATION FOR MINORITIES

The School of Medicine has an active program dedicated to the recruitment, admission, retention, education, and graduation of increased numbers of individuals from ethnic minority groups underrepresented in the field of medicine. Several scholarships are available for qualified minority students. For additional information contact the associate dean for minority affairs at (913) 588-7285.

Public Institution

## APPLICATION AND ACCEPTANCE POLICIES FOR 1997–98 FIRST-YEAR CLASS

*School participates in AMCAS. See Chapter 4.*

Filing of AMCAS application
    Earliest date: June 1, 1996
    Latest date: Oct. 15, 1996
School application fee: $40 for nonresidents
Oldest MCAT scores considered: 1994
Does have Early Decision Program (EDP)
    EDP application period: June 1–Aug. 1, 1996
    EDP applicants notified by: Oct. 1, 1996
Acceptance notice to regular applicants
    Earliest date: Feb. 1, 1997
    Latest date: Varies
Applicant's response to acceptance offer
    Maximum time: 2 weeks
Requests for deferred entrance considered: Yes
Deposit to hold place in class (applied to tuition):
    $50, due with response to acceptance offer
Deposit refundable prior to: May 15, 1997
Estimated number of new entrants: 175 (40 EDP)
Starting date: Aug. 1997

## TUITION AND STUDENT FEES PER YEAR FOR 1995–96 FIRST-YEAR CLASS

Tuition                              Student fees: $230
    Resident: $8,572
    Nonresident: $20,756

## INFORMATION ON 1995–96 FIRST-YEAR CLASS

| Number of | In-State | Out-of-State | Total |
| --- | --- | --- | --- |
| Applicants | 445 | 2,029 | 2,474 |
| Applicants Interviewed | 360 | 76 | 436 |
| New Entrants* | 160 | 15 | 175 |

*All took the MCAT and had baccalaureate degrees.

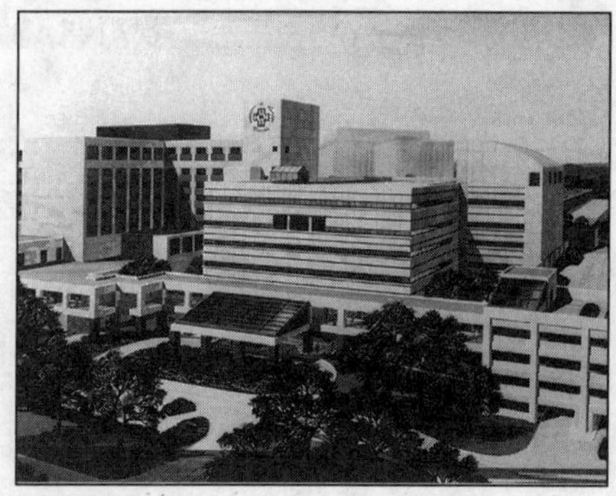

# University of Kentucky College of Medicine

**Lexington, Kentucky**

Dr. Emery A. Wilson, *Dean*
Dr. Carol L. Elam, *Assistant Dean for Admissions*
Linda A. Gilbert, *Financial Aid Coordinator*

## ADDRESS INQUIRIES TO:

Admissions, Room MN-102
Office of Education
University of Kentucky College of Medicine
Chandler Medical Center
800 Rose Street
Lexington, Kentucky 40536-0084
(606) 323-6161; 323-2076 (FAX)
Web Site: http://www.uky.edu/medicine

## GENERAL INFORMATION

Established in 1956 by the Commonwealth of Kentucky and the University of Kentucky Board of Trustees, the University of Kentucky College of Medicine admitted its first class in 1960. The College of Medicine is part of the University of Kentucky Chandler Medical Center located on the university campus in Lexington.

The medical center is comprised of five colleges: medicine, nursing, pharmacy, dentistry, and allied health professions. The majority of onsite clinical teaching occurs at the 473-bed University of Kentucky Hospital, the 662-bed Veterans Affairs Medical Center, and the Kentucky Clinic. Hospitals throughout Lexington and across the Commonwealth hold affiliation agreements with the college for clinical teaching and patient service.

Basic science teaching areas for lecture, laboratory, and small-group instruction, as well as the Medical Center Library, are located in the Medical Sciences Building. Adjacent are the Health Science Learning Center, Critical Care Center, Sanders-Brown Center on Aging, Lucille Parker Markey Cancer Center, the Mills-Davis Magnetic Resonance Imaging and Spectroscopy Center, and University of Kentucky Student Health Service.

## CURRICULUM

In a new curriculum designed to integrate basic and clinical sciences, medical students are taught the fundamental problems of human biology, how to recognize the causes of these problems, and how to prevent disease and treat patients. Year 1 of the Kentucky medical curriculum focuses on normal function of the human body (human structure, cellular structure and function, neurosciences, and human function). First-year students receive early exposure and experience in patient care through the study of interviewing, history taking, physical examination skills, and clinical decision making. In the first two years, medical students also explore principles of prevention and assess the impact of social, ethical, legal, economic, and psychological factors using case studies and small group discussions. Year 2 exposes students to abnormal functions of the human body as related to disease processes. Course work is designed to integrate studies of infectious disease, immunology, pathology, and pharmacology. Computer-based instruction reinforces basic science studies and provides linkages to clinical applications.

Clinical students work with patients in both inpatient hospital and outpatient clinic settings and are required to take medical histories, perform physical examinations on patients, and monitor laboratory tests. Year 3 of the Kentucky medical curriculum includes an integrated women's maternal and child health clerkship, along with clinical neurosciences, primary care, internal medicine, and surgery. Year 4 is highlighted by required rotations in emergency medicine, clinical pharmacology, geriatrics, rural medicine, two acting internships, and a two-month elective period.

Third-year medical students may apply for the accelerated residency programs in family medicine and general internal medicine. These programs combine the fourth-year of medical school with the first year of residency.

Selected students may opt to pursue a combined M.D.-Ph.D. in anatomy and neurobiology, biochemistry, microbiology and immunology, pharmacology, or physiology and biophysics. Combined-degree programs are also available in preventive medicine, nutritional sciences, toxicology, and biomedical engineering.

## REQUIREMENTS FOR ENTRANCE

Applicants are expected to have a broad foundation in the natural sciences, social sciences, and humanities and should demonstrate facility in writing and speaking the English language.

Applicants are strongly urged to complete their baccalaureate degrees. The MCAT is required for admission. Specific course requirements are:

|  | *Semesters* |
|---|---|
| Biology (with labs) | 2 |
| General chemistry (with labs) | 2 |
| Organic chemistry (with labs) | 2 |

Physics (with labs)............................2

English .......................................2

Emphasis is placed on written and spoken communication.

## SELECTION FACTORS

The University of Kentucky College of Medicine gives preference to qualified applicants who are residents of Kentucky. Determination of state residence is made by the registrar's office. Applicants' files are reviewed without regard to race, sex, creed, national origin, age, or handicap. Selected candidates are invited for interviews conducted at the University of Kentucky College of Medicine.

Necessary personal attributes of applicants include time management abilities, interpersonal skills, leadership, and demonstrated service to others. Admission decisions are made based upon review of academic and nonacademic factors including scholastic excellence, MCAT performance, personal attributes, breadth of experience, exposure to the profession, premedical recommendations, and admission interviews.

The students accepted for the 1995 entering class had the following profile: *mean GPA,* 3.61; *women,* 38 percent; *residence,* 95 percent; *undergraduate major,* 57 percent in the natural sciences with the remainder from the social and behavioral sciences, engineering, and liberal arts.

## FINANCIAL AID

A limited number of scholarship grants are awarded to selected students with exceptional achievement. Approximately 85 percent of the student body receives financial assistance through loans and scholarships. Institutional loan/scholarship assistance is available for eligible resident and nonresident students. Kentucky residents who plan to practice in rural Kentucky may receive aid from the Rural Kentucky Medical Scholarship Fund.

The Office of Education provides financial aid counseling and assists students in applying for aid. Only in rare circumstances are students given permission to seek employment.

## INFORMATION FOR MINORITIES

The University of Kentucky College of Medicine is committed to the recruitment and retention of underrepresented and disadvantaged students. Interested applicants are encouraged to contact the admissions office.

---

Public Institution

### APPLICATION AND ACCEPTANCE POLICIES FOR 1997–98 FIRST-YEAR CLASS

*School participates in AMCAS. See Chapter 4.*

Filing of AMCAS application
    Earliest date: June 1, 1996
    Latest date: Nov. 1, 1996
School application fee after screening: $30
Oldest MCAT scores considered: Aug. 1994
Does have Early Decision Program (EDP)
    EDP application period: June 1–Aug. 1, 1996
    EDP applicants notified by: Oct. 1, 1996
Acceptance notice to regular applicants
    Earliest date: After interview
    Latest date: Until class is filled
Applicant's response to acceptance offer
    Maximum time: 2 weeks
Requests for deferred entrance considered: Yes
Deposit to hold place in class (applied to tuition):
    $100, due with response to acceptance offer
Deposit refundable prior to: March 1, 1997
Estimated number of new entrants: 95 (30 EDP)
Starting date: Aug. 1997

### TUITION AND STUDENT FEES PER YEAR FOR 1995–96 FIRST-YEAR CLASS

Tuition                        Student fees: $389
    Resident: $8,479
    Nonresident: $18,699

### INFORMATION ON 1995–96 FIRST-YEAR CLASS

| *Number of* | *In-State* | *Out-of-State* | *Total* |
| --- | --- | --- | --- |
| Applicants | 555 | 1,743 | 2,298 |
| Applicants Interviewed | 293 | 62 | 355 |
| New Entrants* | 90 | 5 | 95 |

*All took the MCAT; 98% had baccalaureate degrees.

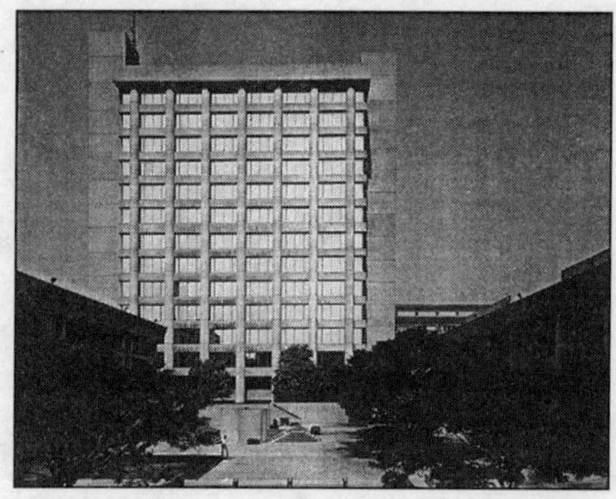

# University of Louisville School of Medicine

**Louisville, Kentucky**

Dr. Donald R. Kmetz, *Vice President for Hospital Affairs and Dean*
Libby Sklare, *Director of Admissions*
Leslie Schmidt, *Director of Financial Aid*

## ADDRESS INQUIRIES TO:

Office of Admissions
School of Medicine
Health Sciences Center
University of Louisville
Louisville, Kentucky 40292
(502) 852-5193

## GENERAL INFORMATION

The School of Medicine was established at the Louisville Medical Institute in 1833 and became affiliated with the University of Louisville in 1846. In 1970 the university became a member of the state system of higher education. In the fall of 1970 the School of Medicine moved into the Health Sciences Center, which also includes the School of Dentistry, the Health Sciences Instructional Building, and the Health Sciences Library and Commons Building. The major clinical teaching activities take place in the University Hospital and four formally affiliated hospitals, which together supply more than 1,000 teaching beds in addition to extensive outpatient services.

## CURRICULUM

The educational program includes two major components: the Core, and the Clinical Program. Revisions are instituted on an annual basis as a consequence of continuing evaluation, planning, and study by faculty and student curriculum committees.

The core consists of basic science courses and a longitudinal block course, becoming a physician, that includes topics of ethics, clinical correlation, physician-patient relationship, behavioral medicine, and the interpersonal dimension of medicine. The clinical program consists of an integrated primary care block and rotations that include family medicine, internal medicine, pediatrics, ambulatory care, community activity, surgery, OB-GYN, neurology, and psychiatry. The fourth year includes ambulatory and inpatient rotations, work in the community, and an elective experience with physician preceptorship.

Students are prepared to begin post-graduate work in primary care or medical specialties following their completion of undergraduate medical education.

Through special arrangement students may fulfill the Clinical Elective Program requirement at another approved institution. This experience permits either special work in a clinical discipline, or one of its subspecialties, or research in a clinical or preclinical science.

To assist students in their selection and to assist with guidance and counseling, there is a well organized adviser program in which each student entering the school is assigned a member of the full-time faculty.

A grade of pass or fail, a percentage score, a mean, and a median are required in all preclinical courses; a grade of pass or fail and a subjective evaluation of the student's performance are required in all clinical core courses and all clinical elective courses.

## REQUIREMENTS FOR ENTRANCE

The MCAT and three years of college are required. Applicants must have a minimum of three years (90 semester hours) of college education, exclusive of military service, physical education, and technical courses. Preference is given to applicants who will have a bachelor's degree before matriculating in the medical school. Minimal credit requirements are:

|  | *Semesters* |
|---|---|
| General biology (with lab) | 2 |
| General or inorganic chemistry (with lab) | 2 |
| Organic chemistry (with lab) | 2 |
| General physics (with lab) | 2 |
| College mathematics | 2 |
|   Or one semester of calculus | |
| English | 2 |

Regardless of major concentration, applicants should demonstrate proficiency in the required science courses.

## SELECTION FACTORS

Because the University of Louisville is a state institution, the School of Medicine gives preference to qualified residents of Kentucky. Applicants are selected on the basis of their individual merits without bias concerning sex, race, creed, national origin, age, or handicap. Admissibility is determined by the undergraduate college record, MCAT scores, recommendations of a preprofessional advisory committee, community and extracurricular activities, and personality and motivation of each applicant. A personal interview is arranged for each applicant whose credentials warrant complete exploration.

Some characteristics of students in the 1995 entering class were: *mean GPA,* 3.6; *sex,* 47 percent women; *minority,* 10 percent.

## FINANCIAL AID

Financial needs of the applicant are not a consideration in the selection process. After acceptance every effort is made to assist students in meeting their financial requirements. Approximately 90 percent of the student body receive some degree of financial aid during the academic year. Scholarships are available on a limited basis and are granted according to demonstrated financial need and scholastic and professional promise. Student Research Scholarships are available to qualified students during the summer months.

## INFORMATION FOR MINORITIES

Particular consideration is given to the evaluation of the credentials of minority applicants. The Admissions Committee is especially interested in qualified minority applicants. Scholarships are available.

Public Institution

## APPLICATION AND ACCEPTANCE POLICIES FOR 1997–98 FIRST-YEAR CLASS

*School participates in AMCAS. See Chapter 4.*

Filing of AMCAS application
  Earliest date: June 1, 1996
  Latest date: Nov. 1, 1996
School application fee after screening: $15
Oldest MCAT scores considered: 1994
Does have Early Decision Program (EDP)
  EDP application period: June 1–Aug. 1, 1996
  EDP applicants notified by: Oct. 1, 1996
Acceptance notice to regular applicants
  Earliest date: Oct. 1, 1996
  Latest date: Until class is filled
Applicant's response to acceptance offer
  Maximum time: 2 weeks
Requests for deferred entrance considered: Yes
Deposit to hold place in class (applied to tuition):
  $100, due with response to acceptance offer
Deposit refundable prior to: March 1, 1997
Estimated number of new entrants: 137 (15 EDP)
Starting date: Aug. 1997

## TUITION AND STUDENT FEES PER YEAR FOR 1995–96 FIRST-YEAR CLASS

Tuition                    Student fees: None
  Resident: $8,300
  Nonresident: $18,520

## INFORMATION ON 1995–96 FIRST-YEAR CLASS

| Number of | In-State | Out-of-State | Total |
|---|---|---|---|
| Applicants | 548 | 1,419 | 1,967 |
| Applicants Interviewed | 250 | 40 | 290 |
| New Entrants* | 124 | 13 | 137 |

*99% took the MCAT and had baccalaureate degrees.

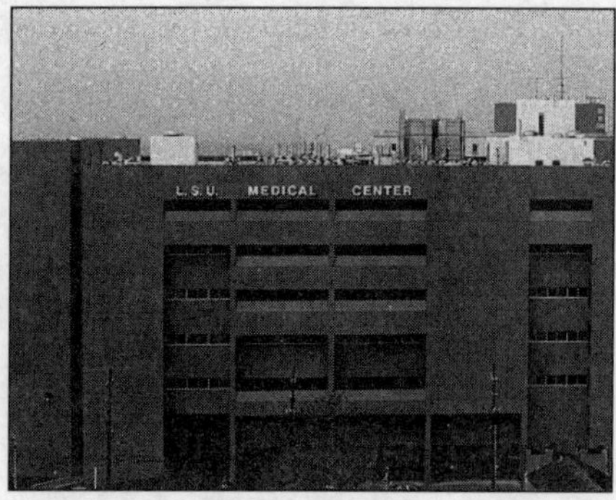

# Louisiana State University
# School of Medicine in New Orleans

**New Orleans, Louisiana**

Dr. Robert L. Marier, *Acting Dean*
Dr. John R. Ruby, *Associate Dean for Admissions*
Patrick Gorman, *Director of Student Financial Aid*

## ADDRESS INQUIRIES TO:

Louisiana State University
School of Medicine in New Orleans
1901 Perdido Street, Box P3-4
New Orleans, Louisiana 70112-1393
(504) 568-6262; 568-7701 (FAX)

## GENERAL INFORMATION

Louisiana State University School of Medicine was established in 1931 by authorization provided in the charter of Louisiana State University (LSU) and Agricultural and Mechanical College adopted in 1877. The School of Medicine is a major unit in the LSU Medical Center, which includes schools of dentistry, nursing, graduate studies, and allied health sciences. The school occupies three buildings within the medical center complex. The major teaching hospitals are the Medical Center of Louisiana in New Orleans and University Hospital. Other hospitals in the city are also used for clinical instruction and residency training. Also some residency programs and clerkships are available at the University Medical Center in Lafayette, and the Earl K. Long Hospital in Baton Rouge.

A student housing facility is available. Furnished and unfurnished apartments are available for married and single students. Regular dormitory-type space is also available.

## CURRICULUM

The first two years of the curriculum are a combination of basic sciences and clinical medicine. Introduction to patient care and contact is provided at the beginning of the second year in the introduction to clinical medicine course. Third- and fourth-year teaching is on a pure block system and is basically small-group instruction (on a conference and seminar basis) in hospitals, clinics, and private practice facilities. All third-year students are required to take a four-week clerkship in family medicine, which is given in a community physician's office. During the final year, blocks in ambulatory care, general medicine, neurosciences, special topics, and an acting internship are required. The special topics block includes nutrition, geriatrics, drug and alcohol abuse, office management, and financial planning. The remaining five months may be scheduled as electives.

Students are required to pass Step 1 of the USMLE before progressing to the third year. They must pass Step 2 prior to graduation.

An honors program is available to students who have maintained a high academic record during the first semester of school. The program entails an independent research study which should continue until graduation. In addition, a combined M.D.-Ph.D. program is available.

The curriculum is under constant evaluation and review by both faculty and students.

## REQUIREMENTS FOR ENTRANCE

The MCAT is required and must be taken at a time that enables scores to be received by the Admissions Office prior to the November application deadline to be considered for admission the following August. Applicants are strongly urged to complete the regular four-year undergraduate curriculum and take the appropriate recommended courses before entering the study of medicine. The school encourages a better balance between the natural sciences, social sciences, and the humanities.

Specific course requirements are:

|  | Sem. hrs. |
| --- | --- |
| Biology or zoology (with lab) | 8 |
| General or inorganic chemistry (with lab) | 8 |
| Organic chemistry (with lab) | 8 |
| Physics (with lab) | 8 |

Demonstrated proficiency in spoken and written English is required.

Current policy precludes acceptance of advanced placement courses for credit toward fulfilling specific requirements in the sciences (biology, chemistry, and physics). The School of Medicine does not accept pass/fail grades for required science courses.

## SELECTION FACTORS

Students are selected on the basis of character, intellectual ability, maturity, motivation, attitude, and past achievement as indicated both by excellent scholastic performance and active participation in extracurricular activities prior to entering medical school. There is no discrimination because of race, religion, sex, age, handicap, national origin, or financial status.

Students in the 1995 entering class had the following credentials: *mean science GPA,* 3.4; *sex,* 38 percent women.

The number of applications from qualified residents of Louisiana precludes the school from offering places to nonresidents. Transfer students who are nonresidents may be considered for upper level classes. Determination of state residence is provided by LSU system regulations.

Interviews are arranged by invitation from the Committee on Admissions and are conducted at the LSU Medical Center facilities.

## FINANCIAL AID

Financial assistance is available for students through several different methods. There are direct scholarship programs, state and federal loan programs, work-study programs, and employment opportunities in the New Orleans area for students in their third and fourth years. Financial assistance information is available from the Student Financial Aid Office.

## INFORMATION FOR MINORITIES

Members of minority groups are encouraged to apply. The School of Medicine's Office of Minority Affairs actively recruits minority students and provides counseling for high school and college students.

Further information may be obtained by contacting Dr. Edward Helm, assistant dean for minority affairs at (504) 568-8501 or at the above-listed address.

---

Public Institution

## APPLICATION AND ACCEPTANCE POLICIES FOR 1997–98 FIRST-YEAR CLASS

*School participates in AMCAS. See Chapter 4.*

Filing of AMCAS application
  Earliest date: June 1, 1996
  Latest date: Nov. 15, 1996
School application fee after screening: $50
Oldest MCAT scores considered: 1993
Does have Early Decision Program
  For Louisiana residents only
  EDP application period: June 1–Aug. 1, 1996
  EDP applicants notified by: Oct. 1, 1996
Acceptance notice to regular applicants
  Earliest date: Oct. 15, 1996
  Latest date: Varies
Applicant's response to acceptance offer
  Maximum time: 2 weeks
Requests for deferred entrance considered: Yes
Deposit to hold place in class (applied to tuition):
  $100, due with response to acceptance offer
Deposit refundable prior to: May 15, 1997
Estimated number of new entrants: 175 (9 EDP)
Starting date: Aug. 1997

## TUITION AND STUDENT FEES PER YEAR FOR 1995–96 FIRST-YEAR CLASS

Tuition                                Student fees: $150
  Resident: $6,776
  Nonresident: $14,676

## INFORMATION ON 1995–96 FIRST-YEAR CLASS

| *Number of* | *In-State* | *Out-of-State* | *Total* |
|---|---|---|---|
| Applicants | 891 | 521 | 1,412 |
| Applicants Interviewed | 397 | 1* | 398 |
| New Entrants† | 174 | 1* | 175 |

*Special Program with the University of New Orleans.

†All took the MCAT; 95% had baccalaureate degrees.

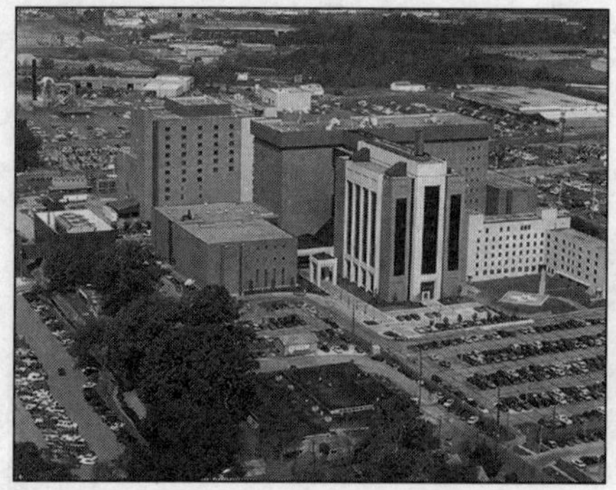

# Louisiana State University School of Medicine in Shreveport

## Shreveport, Louisiana

Dr. Ike Muslow, *Vice Chancellor and Interim Dean*
Dr. F. Scott Kennedy, *Assistant Dean for Student Admissions*
Nancy Rodwell, *Associate Director of Student Financial Aid*

## ADDRESS INQUIRIES TO:

Office of Student Admissions
Louisiana State University Medical Center
School of Medicine in Shreveport
P.O. Box 33932
Shreveport, Louisiana 71130-3932
(318) 675-5190; 675-5244 (FAX)
E-Mail: shuadm@lsumc.edu

## GENERAL INFORMATION

The Louisiana State University (LSU) School of Medicine in Shreveport, a four-year school, admitted its first class in 1969; the first M.D. degrees were awarded in 1973. Teaching takes place at the school's principal teaching hospital, Louisiana State University Hospital (675 beds), and at the affiliated Shreveport Veterans Administration Hospital (450 beds). Permanent medical school facilities, consisting of a basic and clinical science building, library, and Comprehensive Care Teaching Facility, were occupied in the winter of 1975.

## CURRICULUM

The curriculum is traditional in general features but not entirely classical in detail. It is flexible to permit experimentation without disruption. Contact with patients begins early, paralleling a thorough grounding in the basic medical sciences. In addition to short courses in radiology, psychiatry, biometry, and physical examination, live clinics throughout the first and second years serve to indicate application of the basic sciences in clinical medicine. A wide variety of elective instruction is available to first- and second-year students, and one-third of the senior year is elective time on campus or at other institutions. A program of comprehensive care is woven through all four years. The third and fourth years are essentially rotating clerkships in the clinical disciplines. A letter grading system is employed: A, B, C, D (barely pass), and F (fail).

## REQUIREMENTS FOR ENTRANCE

The MCAT and a minimum of three years of college (at least 90 semester hours) are required. A baccalaureate degree is desirable. Required courses are:

|  | *Sem. hrs.* |
|---|---|
| Biology or zoology (with lab) | 8 |
| Inorganic chemistry (with lab) | 8 |
| Organic chemistry (with lab) | 8 |
| General physics (with lab) | 8 |
| English | 6 |

Prospective applicants are strongly urged to take the MCAT by the spring prior to the year of application and to complete most of the required course work by the time of application. They should pursue their own particular interests in selecting college courses not required for admission; a broad educational background is desirable.

## SELECTION FACTORS

Admission is based upon character, motivation, intellectual ability, and achievement as judged by recommendations of premedical advisers, personal interviews with members of the faculty at the School of Medicine, college grades, and MCAT scores. In recent years, the number of applications filed by well qualified residents of Louisiana has been in excess of the number of places available. For this reason, places have not been offered to nonresidents. Determination of state residence is provided by LSU system regulations.

Accepted students for the 1995 entering class had the following credentials: *mean science GPA,* 3.4; *mean overall GPA,* 3.5; *sex,* 33 percent women (acceptance rate the same for men and women per number of applicants); *residence,* 100 percent from Louisiana; *undergraduate major,* 63 percent in biology or chemistry; undergraduate college, 23 schools represented.

The School of Medicine in Shreveport does not discriminate in applicant selection on the basis of race, sex, creed, national origin, age, or handicap.

## FINANCIAL AID

Scholarship and long-term, low-interest loan funds are available to students with financial need. In the past, no accepted students have been unable to meet their financial needs. Scholarships and loans are available to students all four years and are based on applicants showing verified need. Certain awards are given in recognition primarily of academic accomplishment and promise. The school offers summer employment to many students but does not advise employment during school sessions which would interfere with academic performance. Financial need has no bearing on an applicant's acceptance. Applications for financial assistance are furnished by the dean's office after students have been accepted and the class is firmly filled. Approximately 81 percent of the student body obtain financial aid in the form of loans.

## INFORMATION FOR MINORITIES

Applications from minority students are encouraged and will be given every consideration.

---

Public Institution

## APPLICATION AND ACCEPTANCE POLICIES FOR 1997–98 FIRST-YEAR CLASS

*School participates in AMCAS. See Chapter 4.*

Filing of AMCAS application
    Earliest date: June 1, 1996
    Latest date: Nov. 15, 1996
School application fee to all applicants: $50
Oldest MCAT scores considered: 1994
Does not have Early Decision Program
Acceptance notice to regular applicants
    Earliest date: Oct. 15, 1996
    Latest date: Until class is filled
Applicant's response to acceptance offer
    Maximum time: 2 weeks
Requests for deferred entrance considered: Yes
Deposit to hold place in class (applied to tuition):
    $100, due with response to acceptance offer
Deposit refundable prior to: May 15, 1997
Estimated number of new entrants: 100
Starting date: Aug. 1997

## TUITION AND STUDENT FEES PER YEAR FOR 1995–96 FIRST-YEAR CLASS

Tuition                  Student fees: $151
    Resident: $6,776
    Nonresident: $14,676

## INFORMATION ON 1995–96 FIRST-YEAR CLASS

| Number of | In-State | Out-of-State | Total |
|---|---|---|---|
| Applicants | 783 | 294 | 1,077 |
| Applicants Interviewed | 208 | 0 | 208 |
| New Entrants* | 101 | 0 | 101 |

*All took the MCAT; 95% had baccalaureate degrees.

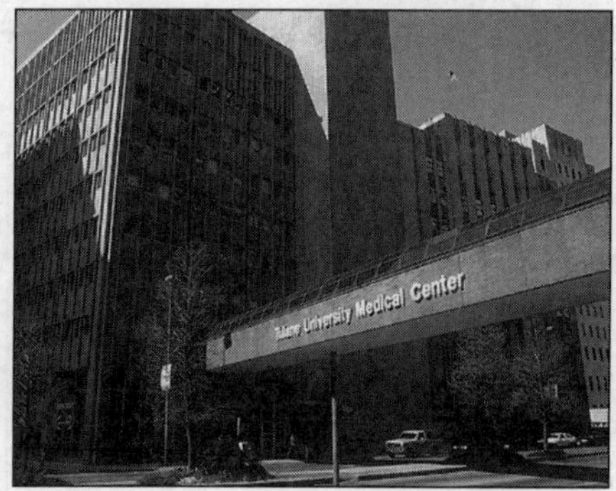

# Tulane University School of Medicine

## New Orleans, Louisiana


Dr. James J. Corrigan, Jr., *Dean*
Dr. Joseph C. Pisano, *Associate Dean*
Michael T. Goodman, *Director of Financial Aid*


## ADDRESS INQUIRIES TO:


Office of Admissions
Tulane University School of Medicine
1430 Tulane Avenue, SL67
New Orelans, Louisiana 70112-2699
(504) 588-5187; 585-6462 (FAX)
E-Mail: medsch@tmcpop.tmc.tulane.edu
Web Site: http://www.mcl.tulane.edu


## GENERAL INFORMATION

Tulane University School of Medicine, founded in 1834, is a private, nonsectarian institution located in New Orleans. Adjacent to the School of Medicine is its principal teaching hospital, Charity Hospital of New Orleans. The Tulane Medical Center Hospital and Clinic is also incorporated into the medical school teaching programs. Other affiliated teaching hospitals include eight hospitals in New Orleans and seven hospitals in other communities in Louisiana.

## CURRICULUM

The School of Medicine offers a four-year program leading to the M.D. degree. While the emphasis in the first two years is on the principles of the basic medical sciences, the goal of the first two years is helping students develop clinical problem-solving skills instead of emphasizing the transmission of facts devoid of clinical context. The program in Foundations in Medicine, which spans the first two years, is responsible for instructing students in the complex art and science of patient interaction. This objective is accomplished through lectures, small-group discussions, clinical demonstrations, visits to community health facilities, and interactions with both real patients and individuals trained as patient-instructors. The third and fourth years provide experience in clinical settings where the emphasis is on patient care and community health. Flexibility is attained throughout the four years by allowing approximately one-third of scheduled curriculum time for elective courses and selected advanced studies. Throughout all four years a number of interdisciplinary courses are offered by the combined faculties of the basic and clinical science departments. The course of study and grading methods are under review at all times by faculty and students.

Several combined-degree programs are available to medical students. Work towards a Ph.D. degree in combination with the doctorate in medicine requires concurrent enrollment in the Graduate School and the School of Medicine. Medical students may choose to concurrently enroll in the School of public Health and Tropical Medicine to complement their doctorate in medicine with an M.P.H. degree. Students wishing to obtain the M.P.H. are encouraged to begin their studies in the School of Public Health and Tropical Medicine during the summer before their matriculation into medical school.

In the summer prior to matriculation into medical school, accepted students may choose to participate in a program designed to facilitate the transition into the medical school environment. In addition to this prematriculation program called PRIME, Tulane offers a wide variety of support systems for medical students. Such support systems include an academic year tutorial program, a summer directed study program, study and test-taking skills workshops, and review programs for the USMLE.

## REQUIREMENTS FOR ENTRANCE

The MCAT and a minimum of three years of college or 90 semester hours are required. Four years of college and the baccalaureate degree are strongly recommended.

Applicants are strongly urged to take the MCAT in the spring of the year of application and to have their basic science requirements completed at the time of application. The required courses are:

|  | *Sem./Qtr. hrs.* |
|---|---|
| Biology or zoology (with lab) | 8/12 |
| Inorganic chemistry (with lab) | 8/12 |
| Organic chemistry (with lab) | 8/12 |
| General physics (with lab) | 8/12 |
| English | 6/9 |

In premedical preparation, the major program need not be in one of the science fields. Students are urged to follow their own inclinations in choosing a course of study, recognizing that a physician should have a broad educational background.

## SELECTION FACTORS

In evaluating applicants, the Committee on Admissions relies on such criteria as grade point averages, MCAT scores, faculty appraisals from the applicant's college, special accomplishments and talents, and the substance and level of courses taken in a particular college. Most successful applicants have attained a GPA of 3.5 and a composite MCAT score of 30. Because of national priorities, most students accepted must be U.S. citizens. Personal character of the highest order is required along with strong motivation, great potential, and evidence of high-level performance. Tulane University does not discriminate on the basis of race, sex, creed, age, national origin, or handicap.

All completed applications are read in full by members of the Committee on Admissions. Personal interviews are held in New Orleans, and selected applicants are invited for an interview. Following interview sessions, the committee reviews again an applicant's record during one of its regular weekly meetings. The committee holds the authority to decide whether a candidate should be accepted, rejected, or held for further evaluation at a later date.

## FINANCIAL AID

Scholarships, long-term loans, and a tuition deferment plan are available to students based on an analysis of the individual's financial needs. More than 80 percent of the students receive some form of financial assistance during their four years of study.

First-year students ordinarily are not encouraged to undertake employment during the session; this is also true for students in the other years if their scholastic standing would be jeopardized. A number of paid externships are available in the local hospitals.

## INFORMATION FOR MINORITIES

Tulane encourages qualified minority and disadvantaged students to apply. Special activities available for, but not limited to, minority students include summer enrichment programs prior to entering medical school and tutorial and counseling services for students in medical school. These services are available through MEDREP, the Student Academic Services Committee, and other groups and programs. The Committee on Admissions includes minority members, but there is no separate review for minority applicants or for any other special group.

Private Institution

## APPLICATION AND ACCEPTANCE POLICIES FOR 1997–98 FIRST-YEAR CLASS

*School participates in AMCAS. See Chapter 4.*

Filing of AMCAS application
    Earliest date: June 1, 1996
    Latest date: Dec. 15, 1996
School application fee to all applicants: $95
Oldest MCAT scores considered: 1994
Does have Early Decision Program
    EDP application period: June 1–Aug. 1, 1996
    EDP applicants notified by: Oct. 1, 1996
Acceptance notice to regular applicants
    Earliest date: Oct. 15, 1996
    Latest date: Until class is filled
Applicant's response to acceptance offer
    Maximum time: Prior to May 15, 1997
Requests for deferred entrance considered: Yes
Deposit to hold place in class (applied to tuition):
    $500, due with response to acceptance offer;
    nonrefundable
Estimated number of new entrants: 148 (10)
Starting date: Aug. 1997

## TUITION AND STUDENT FEES PER YEAR FOR 1995–96 FIRST-YEAR CLASS

Tuition: $25,791          Student fees: $1,341

## INFORMATION ON 1995–96 FIRST-YEAR CLASS

| Number of | In-State | Out-of-State | Total |
|---|---|---|---|
| Applicants | 618 | 10,528 | 11,146 |
| Applicants Interviewed | 136 | 709 | 845 |
| New Entrants* | 33 | 111 | 144 |

*All took the MCAT; 98% had baccalaureate degrees.

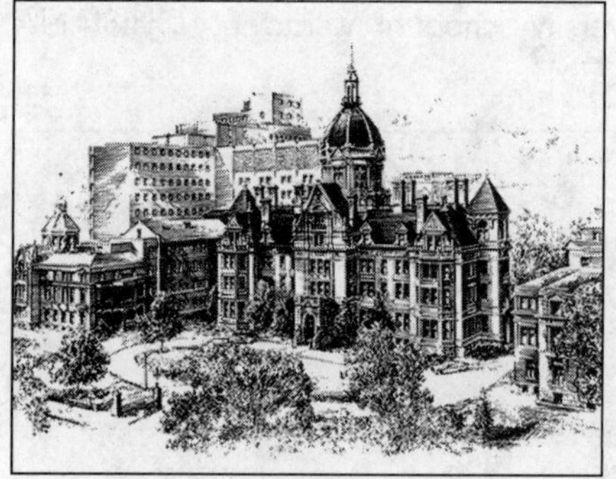

# Johns Hopkins University School of Medicine

**Baltimore, Maryland**

Dr. Michael M.E. Johns, *Dean of the Medical Faculty*
David M. Trabilsy, *Assistant Dean for Admissions*
Julie Disa, *Director of Financial Aid Services*

## ADDRESS INQUIRIES TO:

Committee on Admission
Johns Hopkins University
School of Medicine
720 Rutland Avenue
Baltimore, Maryland 21205-2196
(410) 955-3182
Web Site: http://infonet.welch.jhu.edu/education/
prospectives.html

## GENERAL INFORMATION

Johns Hopkins University School of Medicine is a private, nondenominational institution which fosters the training of medical practitioners, teachers, and biomedical scientists. The medical center provides: library facilities, the Reed Residence Hall, off-campus housing assistance, cafeterias, recreational sports in the Cooley Center, and performing arts programs.

Preclinical courses are given in the adjacent basic science complex. Medical care facilities such as the Johns Hopkins Hospital and the new Outpatient Center provide an extensive and diverse patient base for the teaching of all clinical subjects. Students also attend educational programs conducted at community hospitals in Baltimore and pursue elective experiences at other medical schools in the United States and foreign countries.

## CURRICULUM

The Johns Hopkins curriculum provides sound foundations in basic sciences and clinical medicine while retaining the flexibility required for students to identify and to develop diverse career interests.

The M.D. program includes the integration of basic sciences and clinical experiences and the expanded use of case-based small-group learning sessions. Students have contact with clinical medicine throughout the first year by working with community physicians. The physician and society course spans the four-year program and covers topics such as ethics, finances, legal and political issues, fine arts as they relate to medicine (literature, music, art), and history of medicine.

First Year: Includes integrated coverage of introductory basic sciences, neuroscience, and epidemiology.

Second Year: Study of advanced basic sciences, behavioral sciences, clinical skills, and beginning clerkships.

Third and Fourth Years: With the assistance of faculty advisors, students develop individualized programs incorporating required clerkships in major clinical areas and electives. Students may use electives for specialized clerkships, research, and public health experience.

Students interested in academic medicine can obtain combined M.D.-Ph.D. degrees by pursuing coordinated graduate studies in biochemistry and molecular biology, biological chemistry, biomedical engineering, biophysics, cell biology and anatomy, cellular and molecular medicine, epidemiology, history of medicine, human genetics, microbiology and immunology, neurosciences, pharmacology, and physiology. Candidates accepted for M.D.-Ph.D. studies can apply for financial support through the Medical Scientist Training Program which provides full tuition and stipend. Students may also enroll for special studies or seek advanced degrees in any component of the Johns Hopkins University, including the School of Hygiene and Public Health.

The Flexible Medical Admissions Program (FlexMed) provides opportunities for assured admission to college juniors, and delayed matriculation into the School of Medicine to college seniors for up to three years. FlexMed enables students to plan and pursue alternative education, research, work experience, international fellowships, or humanitarian service, which will enhance their future careers in medicine. Because FlexMed is a collaborative educational venture, students' plans for utilizing the various options must be supported by their colleges and approved by the School of Medicine. For more information on the FlexMed Program, please contact the Admissions Office.

## REQUIREMENTS FOR ENTRANCE

The MCAT is not required for admission. All applicants must provide one official score from a single Scholastic Aptitude Test (SAT), American College Test (ACT), or Graduate Record Examination (GRE) taken previously. MCAT scores must be substituted by applicants who have never taken the above tests or by applicants who feel that the MCAT best represents their standardized testing skills. The B.A. degree or equivalent is required of all students entering the School of Medicine. Students are encouraged to complete coherent studies of sciences and liberal arts consistent with their undergraduate major. Required courses are:

*Sem. hrs.*

General biology (with lab). . . . . . . . . . . . . . . . . . . . . . . . . 8
General chemistry (with lab) . . . . . . . . . . . . . . . . . . . . . . 8
Organic chemistry (with lab) . . . . . . . . . . . . . . . . . . . . . 8
General physics (with lab) . . . . . . . . . . . . . . . . . . . . . . . 8
Humanities and social and behavioral sciences . . . . . . . . 24
Calculus. . . . . . . . . . . . . . . . . . . . . . . . . . . . . . . . . . . . . 4

Advanced placement credit is acceptable for meeting the calculus requirement and maybe used to satisfy general chemistry and physics requirements when supported by one semester of advanced studies in the same discipline. Required courses must be evaluated by a traditional grading system other than pass/fail grades. CLEP credit may not be used to satisfy required courses.

Johns Hopkins does not participate in AMCAS. Application requests should be sent directly to the Committee on Admission.

Catalog and application information may be accessed on the internet at the following URL http://infonet.welch.jhu.edu under Education.

## SELECTION FACTORS

In addition to proven academic competence, previous achievements and activities help the Committee on Admission to evaluate applicants' suitability for medicine. Students who have unusual talents, strong personal qualities, demonstrated leadership, and creative abilities are sought. There are no residence requirements for U.S. citizens, and applications are invited from candidates in all sections of the country. The Johns Hopkins University complies with federal and state law prohibiting discrimination.

## FINANCIAL AID

Financial aid in the form of grants and loans is awarded solely on the basis of need. Financial considerations do not influence admissions decisions. Approximately 80 percent of matriculating students receive financial assistance. Students are awarded financial aid packages to fully meet their demonstrated financial need. Student fellowship stipends are frequently available for projects carried out in summers.

Non-U.S. citizens without permanent resident or immigrant visa status are not eligible to receive financial aid because of government restrictions on funds which support the aid program. Qualified foreign students receive final acceptance only after establishing an escrow account acceptable to the School of Medicine that is sufficient to meet all tuition, fees, and living expenses for the anticipated period of enrollment.

## INFORMATION FOR MINORITIES

The school is committed to the enrollment and education of individuals from all disadvantaged groups. For information write Dr. Roland Smoot, assistant dean for student affairs.

---

Private Institution

## APPLICATION AND ACCEPTANCE POLICIES FOR 1997–98 FIRST-YEAR CLASS

*Dates in italics are for FlexMed Junior Year Option*

Filing of application
    Earliest date: July 1, 1996; *Nov, 1, 1996*
    Latest date: Nov. 1, 1996; *Feb 1, 1997*
School application fee to all applicants: $60
Oldest MCAT scores considered: 1977
Does have Early Decision Program (EDP)
    EDP application period: July 1–Aug. 15, 1996
    EDP applicants notified by: Oct. 1, 1996
Acceptance notice to regular applicants
    Earliest date: Nov. 1, 1996; *June 1, 1997*
    Latest date: March 31, 1997; *June 1, 1997*
Applicant's response to acceptance offer
    Maximum time: 3 weeks
Requests for deferred entrance considered: Yes
    (FlexMed Senior Year Option)
Deposit to hold place in class: None
Estimated number of new entrants: 120 (5 EDP)
Starting date: Sept. 1997

## TUITION AND STUDENT FEES PER YEAR FOR 1995–96 FIRST-YEAR CLASS

Tuition: $21,800          Student fees: $1,828

## INFORMATION ON 1995–96 FIRST-YEAR CLASS

| *Number of* | *In-State* | *Out-of-State* | *Total* |
|---|---|---|---|
| Applicants | 339 | 3,371 | 3,710 |
| Applicants Interviewed | 76 | 637 | 713 |
| New Entrants* | 17 | 102 | 119 |

*All students matriculating into four-year program had baccalaureate degrees; 78% reported the MCAT.

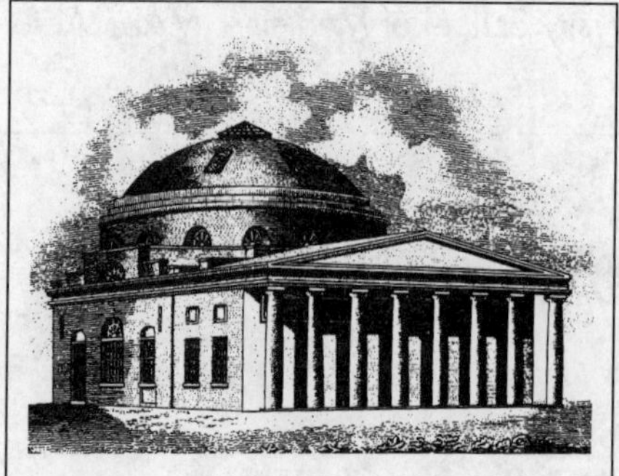

# University of Maryland School of Medicine

**Baltimore, Maryland**

Dr. Donald E. Wilson, *Dean*
Dr. Milford M. Foxwell, Jr., *Associate Dean for Admissions*
Mary S. Vansickle, *Director of Financial Aid*

## ADDRESS INQUIRIES TO:

Committee on Admissions
Room 1-005
University of Maryland
School of Medicine
655 West Baltimore Street
Baltimore, Maryland 21201
(410) 706-7478

## GENERAL INFORMATION

The University of Maryland School of Medicine is the fifth oldest medical college in the United States. It was organized in 1807 and chartered in 1808 under the name of the College of Medicine of Maryland; the first class was graduated in 1810. Among the first to erect its own hospital for clinical instruction in 1823, the University of Maryland established the first intramural residency for senior students.

Along with the other professional schools of the University of Maryland (dentistry, law, nursing, pharmacy, social work, and the graduate schools of basic sciences), the School of Medicine is located on the Baltimore City Campus, which is adjacent to the downtown Charles Center, Inner Harbor, and Oriole Park at Camden Yards.

The University of Maryland Medical System and affiliated hospitals in and around Baltimore have more than 2,300 general hospital beds for teaching purposes.

## CURRICULUM

The basic sciences during the first two years of medical school will be integrated and taught as systems, using interdisciplinary teaching with both basic and clinical science teachers. Problem-based learning was implemented throughout the freshman year in 1995–96. Contact hours have been reduced, with an emphasis on independent study with the availability of mentors and learning resources. A half-day course in Introduction to Clinical Practice will begin at the inception of the freshman year and will continue throughout the first two years, dedicated to the instruction of interviewing, physical examination, intimate human behavior, ethical issues, and the dynamics of ambulatory care. Much of this experience will be off-site in clinical settings. The clinical clerkships during the last two years of medical school will include a mandatory ambulatory month in family medicine, an emphasis on ambulatory teaching in all other disciplines, and a longitudinal half-day experience in a clinical setting in which the student will have continuity of care for patients and families.

A program offering a combined M.D.-Ph.D. is available for selected applicants. Application forms are included in the Stage II packet. After the preclinical years, M.D.-Ph.D. students perform as full-time graduate students for approximately two years, taking the required graduate courses and seminars and focusing on dissertation research. Following this period, students begin the two years of clinical clerkships, using elective time if necessary to complete Ph.D. research.

## REQUIREMENTS FOR ENTRANCE

The MCAT and at least 90 semester hours of accredited arts and science college credit are required. Preference is given to applicants who will have earned a bachelor's degree. The following courses must be completed prior to matriculation:

|  | Sem. hrs. |
| --- | --- |
| Biological sciences | 8 |
| Inorganic chemistry | 8 |
| Organic chemistry | 6 |
| General physics | 8 |
| English | 6 |

Applicants should major in the academic area of their interest. If a nonscience major is selected, sufficient science courses should be taken to acquaint the applicant with the demands of a science oriented curriculum.

The MCAT must be taken no later than the fall test period of the year in which application is made. It is required that the MCAT be taken within three years preceding the anticipated date of matriculation.

## SELECTION FACTORS

Applications are accepted from citizens and permanent residents of the United States and Canada only. All applicants from Maryland are permitted to submit a direct application (Stage II) after the AMCAS application is received. Nonresident applicants are sent a Stage II application only upon recommendation of the Committee on Admissions. The deadline for the Stage II application is December 1. Applications from nonresidents may be rejected on the basis of GPA and MCAT scores that appear on the AMCAS application.

Interviews are arranged for those applicants who appear to have the academic and personal qualities required for successful completion of the requirements for the practice of medicine. All interviews are conducted on campus. Applications may be rejected from both residents and nonresidents without an interview.

Selections are based on a careful appraisal of academic achievement, performance on the MCAT, letters of recommendation, extracurricular activities, community service, and interviews by faculty members.

Accepted students for the 1995 entering class had the following characteristics: *average GPA,* 3.5 (range 2.7–4.0); *MCAT average,* 9 (range 6–14); *undergraduate major,* about 60 percent science majors; *sex,* 50 percent women.

The University of Maryland School of Medicine does not discriminate on the basis of race, sex, creed, national origin, age, or handicap.

## FINANCIAL AID

The school makes available financial aid in the form of scholarships and loans to those students with demonstrable financial need. The amount of the award varies according to the student's needs and the level of funding available. About 70 percent of the students are receiving some degree of financial aid.

## INFORMATION FOR MINORITIES

The University of Maryland School of Medicine is committed to the recruitment and retention of underrepresented and disadvantaged students. A major focus of our recruitment effort is to provide information on admissions requirements, the admissions process, undergraduate preparation for medicine, and education opportunities including the M.D.-Ph.D. program.

All students in the above categories are encouraged to apply. The admissions procedures for minority students are the same as those for all applicants. Among the selection factors emphasized by the Admissions Committee are undergraduate or graduate GPA, MCAT scores, application essay, and personal characteristics of the applicant including work or research experience. The interview, letters of recommendation, and the applicant's life experiences help us to evaluate the subjective qualifications.

The minority recruitment coordinator, in conjunction with other support personnel, makes a special effort to provide information relevant to minority applicants. There is no fixed quota for any special group within the applicant pool. Information may be obtained from Hermione M. Hicks, director of recruitment, Room 1-005 in the Committee on Admissions Office.

---

Public Institution

## APPLICATION AND ACCEPTANCE POLICIES FOR 1997–98 FIRST-YEAR CLASS

*School participates in AMCAS. See Chapter 4.*

Filing of AMCAS application
    Earliest date: June 1, 1996
    Latest date: Nov. 1, 1996
School application fee after screening: $40
Oldest MCAT scores considered: 1994
Does have Early Decision Program (EDP)
    EDP application period: June 1–Aug. 1, 1996
    EDP applicants notified by: Oct. 1, 1996
Acceptance notice to regular applicants
    Earliest date: Oct. 15, 1996
    Latest date: Until class is filled
Applicant's response to acceptance offer
    Maximum time: 3 weeks
Requests for deferred entrance considered: Yes
Deposit to hold place in class: None
Estimated number of new entrants: 145 (10 EDP)
Starting date: Aug. 1997

## TUITION AND STUDENT FEES PER YEAR FOR 1995–96 FIRST-YEAR CLASS

Tuition                 Student fees: $1,833
    Resident: $10,751
    Nonresident: $20,851

## INFORMATION ON 1995–96 FIRST-YEAR CLASS

| Number of | In-State | Out-of-State | Total |
|---|---|---|---|
| Applicants | 1,078 | 3,567 | 4,645 |
| Applicants Interviewed | 369 | 173 | 542 |
| New Entrants* | 121 | 25 | 146 |

*All took the MCAT and had baccalaureate degrees.

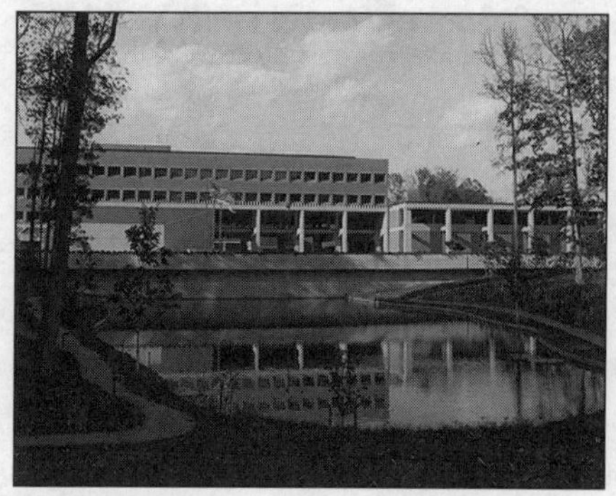

# Uniformed Services University of the Health Sciences
# F. Edward Hébert School of Medicine

## Bethesda, Maryland

Dr. Val G. Hemming, *Interim Dean*
Peter J. Stavish, LTC, MS, USA (Ret), *Assistant Dean for Admissions and
   Academic Records*
Joan C. Stearman, *Director, Office of Admissions*

## ADDRESS INQUIRIES TO:

Admissions Office, Room A-1041
Uniformed Services University
of the Health Sciences
F. Edward Hébert School of Medicine
4301 Jones Bridge Road
Bethesda, Maryland 20814-4799
(301) 295-3101; 295-3545 (FAX);
1 (800) 772-1743
Web Site: http://www.usuhs.mil

## GENERAL INFORMATION

Created by public law in 1972, the Uniformed Services
University of the Health Sciences (USUHS) was founded to
prepare young men and women for careers as health care professionals in the uniformed services. The USUHS School of
Medicine admitted its charter class in 1976. The school is
located on the grounds of the Naval Hospital in Bethesda,
Maryland. The school operates in close association with many
federal health resources located in the greater Washington,
D.C., area to provide students with a broad range of educational experiences in both the basic sciences and clinical medicine. The school's charter is to provide a comprehensive
education in medicine to select individuals who demonstrate
potential for, and commitment to, careers as medical officers
in the uniformed services.

## CURRICULUM

The school has a four-year program culminating in the doctor of medicine degree. Each of the first three academic years
is 48 weeks, and the final year runs 40 weeks. Basic science
instruction predominates in the initial two academic years,
with the final two years being devoted to clinical education.
Basic science instruction is correlated, as appropriate, both
interdisciplinarily and clinically. The integration between the
clinical and basic sciences is progressive and proceeds with
involvement in patient care activities early in the curriculum,
starting with the first semester of the freshman year. While the
overall program is designed to educate students to serve as
providers of primary health care, there is sufficient flexibility
in the curriculum to accommodate differences in interests
among students and also sufficient substances to enable graduates to pursue postgraduate activities such as research.

Elective courses are offered in clinical and research facilities
in this country and in areas of the world where diseases rarely
seen in the United States are responsible for 80 percent of the
morbidity and mortality. The curriculum also includes basic
military orientation and concentration on unique aspects of
military medicine. A conventional letter grading system is
employed to record student progress.

## REQUIREMENTS FOR ENTRANCE

Applicants must be U.S. citizens between the ages of 18
and 30 and must meet the physical and personal qualifications
for a commission in the uniformed services. Applicants cannot
be more than 30 years of age as of June 30 in the year of
matriculation. Military applicants who have the appropriate
creditable commissioned service  may be considered for a
waiver through age 35. The MCAT and a baccalaureate degree
are required.

The following courses are required:

|  | *Sem. hrs.* |
|---|---|
| General biology (with lab) | 8 |
| General or inorganic chemistry (with lab) | 8 |
| Organic chemistry (with lab) | 8 |
| Physics (with lab) | 8 |
| Calculus | 3 |
| English | 6 |

CLEP and advanced placement credits are acceptable for
required courses. However, individuals exempted from prerequisites through these programs are required to take formal
course work in the same areas at a more advanced level.

Both qualified civilians and military personnel are eligible
to apply. However, individuals who are in military service or a
program of study sponsored by the Armed Forces (including
ROTC and the service academies) must obtain a "Letter of
Approval to Apply" from their respective services before making application.

## SELECTION FACTORS

The school employs a three-stage, progressive screening
process for selecting entrants. The first stage consists of the
submission of the standard AMCAS application form; the second, the submission of supplementary materials (a premedical
committee recommendation and a personal statement describing the applicant's knowledge of and interest in a career in the

service are required); and the third, personal interviews, which are conducted at the medical school campus. Advancement in the process is competitive, based on candidates' personal and intellectual characteristics. Applicants should not send transcripts, letters of recommendation, or other such materials unless specifically requested to do so by the Committee on Admissions. The Committee on Admissions does not discriminate on the basis of sex, race, religion, marital status, or national origin. The USUHS School of Medicine is a federal institution and does not give any preference based on state of residence.

There were 3,238 applicants for the 1995 first-year class; of this total 542 were interviewed. All new entrants took the MCAT and had baccalaureate degrees. The 166 entrants had the following credentials: *mean GPA,* 3.47; *mean MCAT,* 10.1; *mean age at time of application,* 24 years; *sex,* 30 percent women; *undergraduate major,* 27 percent in biology, with engineering, biochemistry, chemistry, psychology, and physiology among others represented; residence, 20 percent from northern states, 29 percent from southern states, 44 percent from western states, 7 percent from central states. USUHS is a federal institution; preference is not given to in-state residents. These statistics are not kept.

## SERVICE BENEFITS AND MILITARY OBLIGATION

Upon entering the first-year class of the School of Medicine, the student will be commissioned and will serve on active duty in the grade of second lieutenant in either the Army or Air Force or ensign in the Navy or in the Public Health Service, receiving the appropriate pay and benefits of that grade. All incoming students will be affected by the new military retirement system if not in the military prior to August 1, 1986. The time spent in medical school is not creditable toward retirement until retirement eligibility has been established.

If current promotion policies continue, the student can expect a promotion in rank to captain in the Air Force or Army or lieutenant in the Navy or Public Health Service upon receipt of the M.D. degree. Graduates are obligated to serve on active duty as medical officers for not less than seven years as well as six years inactive ready reserve. The period of time spent in internship or residency training shall not be acceptable toward satisfying this seven-year obligation. A student who is dropped from the program for either academic deficiencies or other reasons may be required to perform active duty in an appropriate military capacity for a period equal to the time spent in the program. A disenrolled student may also be required to reimburse the government for tuition and fees. However, one year will be the minimum required active duty for persons separated from the school regardless of the time spent in the program.

## INFORMATION FOR MINORITIES

The School of Medicine has an Office of Minority Affairs. This program was designed to give competitive minority applicants whatever assistance may be necessary during the admissions process. There is no separate application or process for minority applicants.

---

Public Institution

### APPLICATION AND ACCEPTANCE POLICIES FOR 1997–98 FIRST-YEAR CLASS

*School participates in AMCAS. See Chapter 4.*

Filing of AMCAS application
    Earliest date: June 1, 1996
    Latest date: Nov. 1, 1996
School application fee: None
Oldest MCAT scores considered: 1994
Does not have Early Decision Program
Acceptance notice to regular applicants
    Earliest date: Nov. 1, 1996
    Latest date: Varies
Applicant's response to acceptance offer
    Maximum time: 2 weeks
Requests for deferred entrance considered: Yes
Deposit to hold place in class: None
Estimated number of new entrants: 165
Starting date: July 1997

### TUITION AND STUDENT FEES PER YEAR FOR 1995–96 FIRST-YEAR CLASS

There are no tuition charges for attending the USUHS. Required books, equipment, and instruments are furnished without charge. Students are required to pay for housing, food, and other expenses from their annual salary.

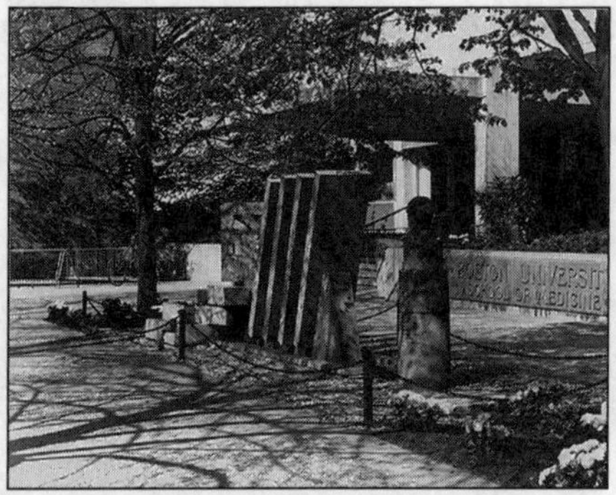

# Boston University
# School of Medicine

**Boston, Massachusetts**

Dr. Aram V. Chobanian, *Dean*
Dr. John F. O'Connor, *Associate Dean for Admissions*
Charles Terrell, *Associate Dean for Financial Management*

## ADDRESS INQUIRIES TO:

Admissions Office
Building L, Room 124
Boston University
School of Medicine
80 East Concord Street
Boston, Massachusetts 02118
(617) 638-4630

## GENERAL INFORMATION

In 1848 the New England Female Medical College was founded as the first medical college for women in the world. In 1873 the original buildings and endowment were acquired by Boston University, and the name was changed to Boston University School of Medicine. At present the School of Medicine, School of Dental Medicine, School of Public Health, Centers for Advancement in Health and Medicine, and University Hospital comprise the Boston Medical Center. All professional medical activities at Boston City Hospital are vested in the School of Medicine, and that hospital together with 21 other health care facilities affiliated with the Medical Center affords students varied and rich clinical experiences.

## CURRICULUM

The curriculum provides the opportunity to study medicine in a flexible environment that stimulates a spirit of critical inquiry and provides sound knowledge in the biological, social, and behavioral sciences. In 1992, Integrated Problems, a course using problem-based learning was added and the courses in introduction to clinical medicine reinforced. These courses link the discipline-specific work in basic sciences with applications in clinical medicine. They integrate longitudinally through the first two years.

During the first year, the basic medical sciences are emphasized in both departmental and interdisciplinary courses along with human development and community medicine.

The second-year program emphasizes the changes in normal structure and function that lead to disease. Major systems pathophysiology is presented in an integrated multidisciplinary format.

The third year represents the major clerkship year. In addition to the conventional clerkships in medicine, surgery, pedi-atrics, obstetrics, and psychiatry, a clerkship in out-patient primary care is required in either the third or fourth year.

The new curriculum includes four mandatory clerkships for the fourth year: neurology, radiology, ambulatory primary care, and home medicine. The fourth year is otherwise devoted to developing an elective program under the supervision of a faculty member. Research opportunities are available in basic science and clinical settings in an independent study program.

A dynamic generalist curriculum in the primary care disciplines of internal medicine, family practice, and pediatrics is presented throughout the four years. Faculty in nearby urban and suburban practices serve as mentors and teachers. Primary care medicine is taught in these physician's office practices, in community health centers, patients' homes, day care centers, and shelters. Experience in rural practice (in the United States and abroad) are available as electives in the fourth year.

With the approval of the promotions committee, students may complete the first-year requirements over two academic years by taking half the normal course load each year without paying any additional tuition.

In addition to the traditional M.D. degree, students may also pursue a pathway of study leading to the M.D.-Ph.D. or M.D.-M.P.H.

## REQUIREMENTS FOR ENTRANCE

Applicants are required to have a baccalaureate degree from an approved college of arts and sciences. The following courses are required:

|  | *Years* |
|---|---|
| Biology (with lab) | 1 |
| Inorganic chemistry (with lab) | 1 |
| Organic chemistry (with lab) | 1 |
| Physics | 1 |
| Humanities | 1 |
| English composition or literature | 1 |

A knowledge of a quantitation in chemistry and calculus are recommended.

Applicants are urged to acquire a broad background in the humanities and behavioral and social sciences in their college years.

All required courses must be completed before medical school work begins. If an applicant has been excused from a required college level course, another course at the same or higher level must be substituted.

The MCAT is required. Applicants are strongly urged to take the MCAT in the spring of the year of application and to have most of their basic science requirements completed at the time of application. Applicants who have not taken the MCAT by the fall of the application year will not be considered.

## SELECTION FACTORS

The Committee on Admissions chooses applicants who seem best qualified not only by scholastic record, college recommendations, and involvement in college and community activities but also by qualities of personality, character, and maturity. A personal interview is an integral part of the admissions process. Applicants who have not heard from the School of Medicine by March 1 and still wish to be considered for an interview should contact the Admissions Office. All interviews are granted at the discretion of the Committee on Admissions. The School of Medicine does not discriminate on the basis of race, sex, age, creed, or national origin.

No deferments are permitted.

If places are available, applications for transfer may be requested in January.

## FINANCIAL AID

The school is committed to equal financial access for all students demonstrating need. It, therefore, initiated a series of low-interest student revolving loan funds in 1975. Since that time it has tried to mitigate the cycle of mounting market-rate debt.

Student assistance is available to students in all years of the medical school curriculum; 52 percent of the student body receive institutional assistance; 90 percent receive institutional and/or outside support assistance. The school's Office of Student Financial Management administers its portfolio of 50 revolving loans, assists students in securing aid from outside sources, conducts debt management seminars and activities, conducts all required entrance and exit interviews, and provides daily student financial management information. Grant aid is minimal, equaling 5 percent of student aid in full-need cases. All assistance is based upon need. Upon acceptance students are automatically sent a student assistance response card which generates all necessary forms and information. Financial need is not considered in the admissions process.

## INFORMATION FOR MINORITIES

Programs for the recruitment and support of minority students have been developed through the Office of Minority Affairs. One of these programs allows students to take special summer courses in anatomy, biochemistry, and knowledge acquisition skills prior to matriculation in the fall. Minority applications are processed through the regular Committee on Admissions in consultation with the Office of Minority Affairs. It is possible to have application fees defrayed.

Private Institution

## APPLICATION AND ACCEPTANCE POLICIES FOR 1997–98 FIRST-YEAR CLASS

*School participates in AMCAS. See Chapter 4.*

Filing of AMCAS application
   Earliest date: June 1, 1996
   Latest date: Nov. 15, 1996
School application fee to all applicants: $95
Oldest MCAT scores considered: 1994
Does have Early Decision Program (EDP)
   EDP application period: June 1–Aug. 1, 1996
   EDP applicants notified by: Oct. 1, 1996
Acceptance notice to regular applicants
   Earliest date: Feb. 1997
   Latest date: Until class is filled
Applicant's response to acceptance offer
   Maximum time: 2 weeks
Requests for deferred entrance considered: No
Deposit to hold place in class (applied to tuition):
   $500, due June 15, 1997; nonrefundable
Estimated number of new entrants: 135 (3 EDP)
Starting date: Aug. 1997

## TUITION AND STUDENT FEES PER YEAR FOR 1995–96 FIRST-YEAR CLASS

Tuition: $30,300        Student fees: $375

## INFORMATION ON 1995–96 FIRST-YEAR CLASS

| Number of | In-State | Out-of-State | Total |
|---|---|---|---|
| Applicants | 774 | 10,989 | 11,763 |
| Applicants Interviewed | 248 | 966 | 1,214 |
| New Entrants* | 43 | 92 | 135 |

*All took the MCAT; 71.8% had baccalaureate degrees (excluding students from seven-year program).

# Harvard Medical School

**Boston, Massachusetts**

Dr. Daniel C. Tosteson, *Dean*
Dr. Gerald S. Foster, *Associate Dean for Admissions; Chair, Committee on Admissions*
Theresa J. Orr, *Assistant Dean and Director of Admissions and Financial Aid*

## ADDRESS INQUIRIES TO:

Admissions Office
Harvard Medical School
25 Shattuck Street
Boston, Massachusetts 02115-6092
(617) 432-1550; 432-3307 (FAX)
E-Mail: HMSADM@warren.med.harvard.edu

## GENERAL INFORMATION

Harvard Medical School was established in 1782. It has occupied its present site in the Longwood Avenue Quadrangle since 1906. Adjacent are the Harvard School of Public Health, the Harvard School of Dental Medicine, and the Francis A. Countway Library. Clinical teaching is carried out in several general and specialized hospitals. These include Massachusetts General, Brigham and Women's, Children's, Beth Israel, New England Deaconess, Massachusetts Eye and Ear, Mount Auburn, and Cambridge hospitals. The Massachusetts Mental Health Center and the McLean Hospital are psychiatric facilities. The Harvard Community Health Plan and other community-based health centers provide additional opportunities for patient care, teaching, and research. Other affiliated institutions are the West Roxbury and Brockton VA Medical Centers, the Shriners Burns Institute, and the Spaulding Rehabilitation Hospital. Vanderbilt Hall provides living facilities and a dining hall for single students. Apartments for married students may be found nearby.

## PROGRAMS

The New Pathway Program is designed to accommodate the variety of interests, educational backgrounds, and career goals that characterize the student body. The curriculum of this program reflects the changes implemented in 1987. Basic science and clinical content are interwoven throughout the four years. In the first and second years, a problem-based approach that emphasizes small-group tutorials and self-directed learning is complemented by laboratories, conferences, and lectures. Students are expected to analyze problems, locate relevant material in library and computer based resources, and develop habits of lifelong learning and independent study.

Clinical clerkships and a wide variety of elective courses and research opportunities are available at Harvard Medical School, its affiliated hospitals, Harvard University, and the Massachusetts Institute of Technology (M.I.T.). One hundred thirty-five students are admitted to this program each year.

A second M.D. Pathway is the Harvard– M.I.T. Division of Health Sciences and Technology Program (HST). This program was established jointly by the faculties of these two institutions. The curriculum of this program is designed for the student with a strong interest and background in quantitative science. Courses in the first two years are taught both at Harvard Medical School and M.I.T. with faculty drawn from both institutions. The curriculum is in a semester format. HST students join students of the New Pathway Program for their clinical rotations. Thirty students are admitted to this program each year.

The M.D.-Ph.D. program exists for qualified applicants who wish to integrate medical school and intensive scientific training. Graduate study and research for the Ph.D. are pursued through one of the basic science departments or committees of the Division of Medical Sciences, other departments of the Harvard Graduate School of Arts and Sciences, or the Graduate School of Science and Engineering at M.I.T.

Other joint programs are offered in collaboration with the Harvard School of Public Health and the John Fitzgerald Kennedy School of Government.

## ACADEMIC SOCIETIES

All students are assigned to one of five academic societies. The societies offer the perspective of smaller groupings of students and faculty who will work together during their time at Harvard Medical School. Each society has a home base in the Medical Education Center—a new teaching facility.

## REQUIREMENTS FOR ENTRANCE

The MCAT and at least three years of college are required. Students are rarely accepted without a baccalaureate degree.
*Biology*—One year with laboratory experience. Courses taken should deal with the cellular and molecular aspects as well as the structure and function of living organisms.
*Chemistry*—Two years with laboratory experience. Full-year courses in general (or inorganic) and organic chemistry meet this requirement. Other options that adequately prepare students for the study of biochemistry and molecular biology in medical school will be acceptable.
*Physics*—One year.
*Mathematics*—One year of calculus.

*Expository writing*—One year. May be met with writing, English, or nonscience courses that involve expository writing.

*HST Program*—Requirements are the same as above except that calculus through differential equations and calculus based physics is required. A course in biochemistry is encouraged.

A variety of course formats and combinations that provide equivalent preparation will be accepted. Advanced placement credits may be used to satisfy the calculus requirement and one semester of the chemistry and physics requirements for the New Pathway program. In addition to the writing requirement, at least 16 credit hours should be completed in non-science courses. No preference is shown toward students majoring in the sciences over students majoring in nonscience areas.

Foreign students must have completed at least one year of study in an approved college or university in the United States or Canada before applying. Foreign students who do not have a baccalaureate or advanced degree from an institution in the United States are rarely accepted for admission.

Students who have been enrolled in medical school or who have been refused admission by us on two prior occasions are ineligible to apply.

## SELECTION FACTORS

Academic excellence is expected. For the 1995 entering class, the average GPA was 3.8, and the average MCAT scores were VR-10.8, PS-11.8, and BS-11.7. Other factors considered include the essay, out-of-classroom activities, and life experiences. Research and community work and comments contained in letters of recommendation are considered. We look for evidence of integrity, maturity, humanitarian concerns, leadership potential, and an aptitude for working with people. Interviews are scheduled selectively and include regional interviews for those applicants who are unable to come to Boston.

The Committee on Admissions welcomes applications from qualified students representing groups that historically have been underrepresented in medicine. Harvard Medical School is committed to the enrollment of a diverse body of talented students who will reflect the character of the American people whose health needs the medical profession must serve.

The 1995 entering class came from 55 different colleges. Fifty-one percent were women, and 16 percent were underrepresented minorities.

## FINANCIAL AID

The financial needs of a candidate are not considered during the selection process. All financial aid is awarded on the basis of need. A vigorous effort is made to assist accepted applicants in meeting their medical education costs through loans, medically related employment, and scholarships.

---

Private Institution

## APPLICATION AND ACCEPTANCE POLICIES FOR 1997–98 FIRST-YEAR CLASS

Filing of application
   Earliest date: June 1, 1996
   Latest date: Oct. 15, 1996
School application fee to all applicants: $70
Oldest MCAT scores considered: 1991
Does not have Early Decision Program
Acceptance notice to regular applicants
   Latest date: Feb. 28, 1997
Applicant's response to acceptance offer
   Maximum time: 3 weeks
Requests for deferred entrance considered: Yes
Deposit to hold place in class: None
Estimated number of new entrants: 165
Starting date: Sept. 1997

## TUITION AND STUDENT FEES PER YEAR FOR 1995–96 FIRST-YEAR CLASS

Tuition: $23,200          Student fees: $1,519

## INFORMATION ON 1995–96 FIRST-YEAR CLASS

| *Number of* | *In-State* | *Out-of-State* | *Total* |
|---|---|---|---|
| Applicants | 698 | 3,216 | 3,914 |
| Applicants Interviewed | 219 | 837 | 1,056 |
| New Entrants* | 13 | 152 | 165 |

*All took the MCAT and had baccalaureate degrees.

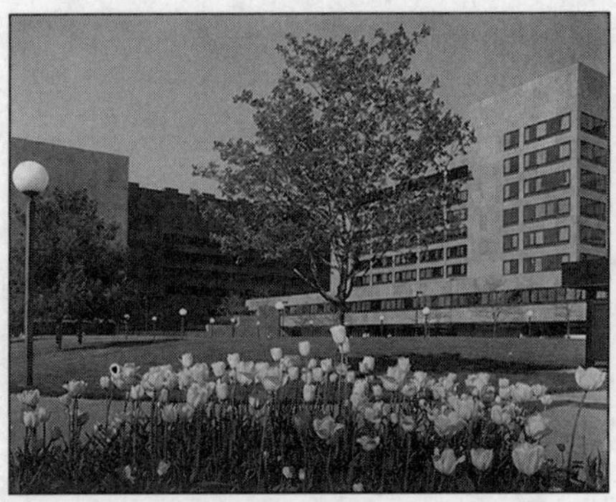

# University of Massachusetts Medical School

## Worcester, Massachusetts


Dr. Aaron Lazare, *Chancellor/Dean*
Dr. Michele P. Pugnaire, *Associate Dean for Admissions*
Judith L. Case, *Director of Financial Aid*


## ADDRESS INQUIRIES TO:

Associate Dean for Admissions
University of Massachusetts Medical School
55 Lake Avenue, North
Worcester, Massachusetts 01655
(508) 856-2323
E-Mail: Admissions@banyan.ummed.edu
Web Site: http://www.ummed.edu:8000/

## GENERAL INFORMATION

The University of Massachusetts Medical School is located on the Worcester campus in a facility which combines basic and clinical sciences with a 370-bed hospital. Clinical teaching is conducted in the University of Massachusetts Medical Center and in affiliated community hospitals in Worcester, Springfield, and Pittsfield. The Massachusetts Biotechnology Research Park, which also houses the medical school's Program in Molecular Medicine, is adjacent to the campus.

## CURRICULUM

The University of Massachusetts Medical School (UMMS) is committed to training physicians in a wide range of medical disciplines and also emphasizes training for practice in general medicine and the primary care specialties, in the public sector, and in underserved areas of Massachusetts.

Major curriculum reform is underway, and the new educational program stresses interdisciplinary learning and integration of basic and clinical science, with special attention to clinical correlation of the subject matter. Emphasis in the first year is on normal structure and function. There is a three-week field clerkship in family, community, and preventative medicine and a course in human genetics. Emphasis in the second year is on the etiology of disease, pathophysiology, pharmacology, and clinical diagnosis. Epidemiology, biostatistics, and psychiatry are also introduced.

In 1995, a new two-year multidisciplinary course on the Physician, Patient, and Society will incorporate the disciplines of medical interviewing. biomedical ethics, informatics, epidemiology, and preventive medicine. Led by senior faculty in the first year, students interview patients and participate in small groups designed to consider medical problem solving, as well as the societal and cultural aspects of health and illness.

The third and fourth years are a continuum of required clinical clerkships and both clinical and research electives. The new curriculum will weave elements of the Physician, Patient, and Society course into the clinical curriculum by offering one-week "selective" courses between month-long clerkship or electives.

The faculty of the Medical School also encourages medical students to participate in research programs in basic and clinical science departments. A combined M.D.-Ph.D. program in basic medical sciences is also offered.

## REQUIREMENTS FOR ENTRANCE

The MCAT is required. A baccalaureate degree is required. Required courses are:

|  | *Years* |
|---|---|
| Biology (with lab) | 1 |
| Inorganic chemistry (with lab) | 1 |
| Organic chemistry (with lab) | 1 |
| Physics (with lab) | 1 |
| English | 1 |

Credit for any secondary school course may be given only if such credit appears on the college transcript. Applicants may major in the areas of either sciences or humanities, and in either case independent study is encouraged. Students able to do so are encouraged to take such courses as biochemistry, calculus, statistics, sociology, or psychology. Applicants are encouraged to complete the basic science requirements by the time of application since consideration will be delayed if required courses are in progress.

## SELECTION FACTORS

Current policy limits admission to students who are Massachusetts residents. The Committee on Admissions bases its evaluation of applicants on academic ability and achievement, scores on the MCAT, and such factors as extracurricular achievement, maturity, motivation, and character as these are reflected in letters of recommendation from preprofessional advisory committees and other persons. Interviews are arranged by invitation only. Applicants are selected on the basis of their individual merits without regard to race, sex, creed, national origin, age, or disability. UMMS has a set of technical standards for admission and promotion, which are available upon request. All supplementary materials must be received by December 15.

Accepted students for the class entering August 1995 had the following credentials: *science GPA,* approximately 3.5; *sex,* 53 percent women; *undergraduate major,* 60 percent in science and 40 percent in nonscience.

## FINANCIAL AID

Students whose financial need cannot be met by personal and family resources or available outside funds should apply for school-administered financial aid. The deadline for receipt of all application materials in the Financial Aid Office is mid to late March. Incoming students are mailed financial aid applications as they are accepted. Students accepted after December 31 are given approximately six weeks to complete the entire financial aid application.

The financial aid application comprises the University of Massachusetts Worcester Financial Aid Application Form, the FAFSA, the Profile Form of the College Scholarship Service, parental and student federal income tax returns and W-2 forms, student state income tax return, and financial aid transcripts from all educational institutions previously attended.

Financial aid funds are disbursed in accordance with institutional packaging policy established by the Student Affairs Committee. Approximately 75 percent of the student body receive some form of financial assistance. The institution offers scholarship, loan, and/or employment opportunities to its students.

The University of Massachusetts Medical School offers all students, regardless of financial need, the option of entering into a learning contract. The learning contract gives students the option of paying the full tuition at the time of enrollment, deferring payment of a portion (currently two-thirds) of tuition until after residency training, or canceling the deferred payment of tuition by fulfilling a two-year period of service obligation to the Commonwealth of Massachusetts. Graduates must begin repayment no later than the earlier of the following: the sixth month after completing residency training or seven years after graduation. Service to the Commonwealth may be provided by the practice of primary care medicine anywhere in the Commonwealth, the practice of medical specialties in underserved areas in the Commonwealth, or another activity of particular benefit to the Commonwealth. For students who choose not to provide service, payment will be financed at eight percent interest; interest begins accruing after completion of the medical internship. Payment may not exceed eight years.

## INFORMATION FOR MINORITIES

We encourage applications from members of minority groups who are legal residents of Massachusetts. Contact the Office of Minority and Community Academic Programs for additional information on special programs for minority students.

---

Private Institution

## APPLICATION AND ACCEPTANCE POLICIES FOR 1997–98 FIRST-YEAR CLASS

*School participates in AMCAS. See Chapter 4.*

Filing of AMCAS application
   Earliest date: June 1, 1996
   Latest date: Nov. 1, 1996
School application fee to all applicants: $50
Oldest MCAT scores considered: 1993
Does have Early Decision Program (EDP)
   For Massachusetts residents only
   EDP application period: June 1–Aug. 1, 1996
   EDP applicants notified by: Oct. 1, 1996
Acceptance notice to regular applicants
   Earliest date: Oct. 15, 1996
   Latest date: Varies
Applicant's response to acceptance offer
   Maximum time: 2 weeks
Requests for deferred entrance considered: Yes
Deposit to hold place in class (applied to tuition):
   $100, due with response to acceptance offer
Deposit refundable prior to: May 15, 1997
Estimated number of new entrants: 100 (10 EDP)
Starting date: Aug. 1997

## TUITION AND STUDENT FEES PER YEAR FOR 1995–96 FIRST-YEAR CLASS

Tuition                Student fees: $1,720
   Resident: $8,792
   Nonresident: N/A

## INFORMATION ON 1995–96 FIRST-YEAR CLASS

| Number of | In-State | Out-of-State | Total |
|---|---|---|---|
| Applicants | 930 | 596 | 1,526 |
| Applicants Interviewed | 417 | 0 | 417 |
| New Entrants* | 100 | 0 | 100 |

*All took the MCAT and had baccalaureate degrees.

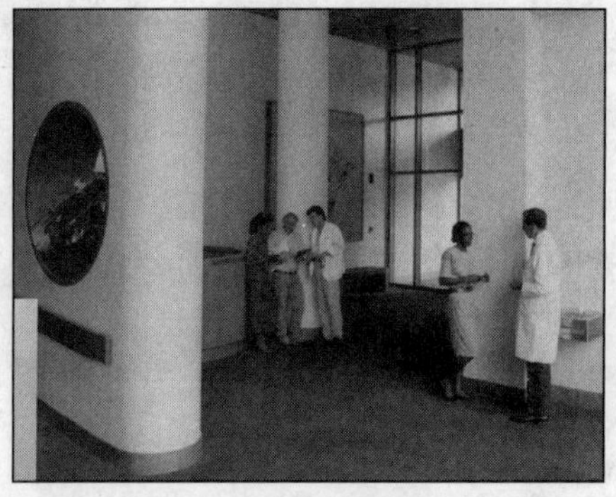

# Tufts University School of Medicine

**Boston, Massachusetts**

Dr. John Harrington, *Acting Dean*
Thomas M. Slavin, *Director of Admissions*
Gail E. Mance, *Director of Financial Aid*

## ADDRESS INQUIRIES TO:

Office of Admissions
Tufts University
School of Medicine
136 Harrison Avenue
Boston, Massachusetts 02111
(617) 636-6571

## GENERAL INFORMATION

Tufts University was founded in 1852 as a liberal arts college in Medford, Massachusetts, and has since grown into a modern university whose School of Medicine was established in Boston in 1893. The medical school is located within a health sciences complex which includes the dental school, veterinary school, Sackler School of Graduate Biomedical Sciences, Sackler Center for Health Communications, Nutrition Center, and the New England Medical Center. The medical school buildings, located in the center of Boston, house the preclinical departments, research laboratories, administrative offices, seminar rooms, lecture rooms, and the library. Close association of the School of Medicine with 30 plus hospitals affords ample facilities for clinical experience.

## CURRICULUM

The initial phase of the curriculum focuses on the biology of cells and their constituent molecules followed by a segment dealing with the structure and development of tissues and organs. This is followed by the functions of the organs and the organism and its environment. The biology of normal cells, tissues, and organs is presented before the students are exposed to the pathological manifestations of these components. The curriculum also includes those aspects of the non-biological sciences that are relevant to health care delivery and patient care, such as nutrition, health care economics, family medicine, ethics, and history of medicine. The program also emphasizes problem solving and critical, analytical discussion in small groups instead of rote learning based on a large number of lectures. A strong emphasis on the use of problem-based learning, a teaching based on case studies, is an aspect of the curriculum. The cases chosen have been closely coordinated with the material from the ongoing segments of the curriculum but provide opportunities for student learning in a wide range of areas, including ethics, socioeconomics, history, culture,

and the physician-patient relationship. The Preclinical Elective Program is designed to encourage students to pursue outside interests and talents as well as to foster meaningful faculty-student relationships. Students can explore opportunities in basic science, clinical medicine, or community aspects of medicine. In addition, faculty are able to work more closely with students and to serve as role models, mentors, and informal advisers.

The third year consists of rotations through the major clinical specialties and an elective period.

The fourth year consists of a minimum of eight four-week rotations. Five of these eight must be taken at Tufts-affiliated hospitals; of these, two must be ward service rotations and one must be the clinical specialties rotation. Beyond these requirements, students are free to schedule approved learning experiences as part of their elective rotations at the Tufts-associated hospitals or elsewhere in the United States or abroad.

Tufts offers a combined M.D.-M.P.H. program, leading to the awarding of both degrees in four years. The program is fully accredited by the Council on Education for Public Health and provides basic grounding in epidemiology and biostatistics, health planning and management, environmental health, and the behavioral sciences. A public health field experience and advanced coursework are essential parts of the program, which is fully integrated into the medical curriculum.

Tufts, in collaboration with Northeastern and Brandeis Universities, now offers a combined M.D.-M.B.A. degree in health management. The changing nature of the nation's health care system has created a demand for physicians who are trained to plan and manage these changes in the best interests of patients, health care organizations, and the community. The curriculum is designed to provide students with a foundation in business problem-solving skills and knowledge in health care management. M.D.-M.B.A. candidates will begin their studies the summer before the start of medical school and devote the summer between the first and second years of medical school to M.B.A. courses.

Tufts also offers an M.D.-Ph.D. program.

## REQUIREMENTS FOR ENTRANCE

The MCAT and a minimum of three years of college are required. Preference is given to applicants who will receive a bachelor's degree before matriculation. College credits must include:

|  | *Years* |
|---|---|
| Biology (with lab) | 1 |
| Inorganic chemistry (with lab) | 1 |
| Organic chemistry (with lab) | 1 |
| Physics (with lab) | 1 |

## SELECTION FACTORS

The selection of candidates for admission to the first year is based not only on performance in the required premedical courses, but also on the applicant's entire academic record and extracurricular experiences. Letters of recommendation and additional information supplied by the applicant are reviewed for indications of promise and fitness for a medical career. Personal interviews are a prerequisite for admission and are only granted by invitation of the Admissions Committee.

Tufts has a strong commitment to affirmative action and seeks to provide an atmosphere of nondiscrimination for members of minority groups as well as an accessible campus and support services for persons with disabilities.

Tufts accepts transfers from other American, LCME-accredited medical schools into the second- and third-year classes in years when vacancies have been created by attrition. The number of seats available has traditionally been extremely limited. In some years, no transfer openings are available.

## FINANCIAL AID

Up to 75 percent of students participate in the federal government's student loan programs at some time during their four years of study. Additionally, limited scholarship and loan assistance are available directly from Tufts for students who qualify on the basis of need. Approximately 33 percent of the students receive financial aid directly from Tufts at some time during their four years of study.

There are no rules prohibiting outside employment; however, first- and second-year students are urged not to seek outside work. Some opportunities for part-time employment are available in the various hospitals and in the medical school.

In situations of extreme financial need, the $75 application fee may be waived if AMCAS has first granted a similar waiver.

Private Institution

## APPLICATION AND ACCEPTANCE POLICIES FOR 1997–98 FIRST-YEAR CLASS

*School participates in AMCAS. See Chapter 4.*

Filing of AMCAS application
    Earliest date: June 1, 1996
    Latest date: Nov. 1, 1996
School application fee to all applicants: $75
Oldest MCAT scores considered: 1993
Does have Early Decision Program (EDP)
    EDP application period: June 1–Aug. 1, 1996
    EDP applicants notified by: Oct. 1, 1996
Acceptance notice to regular applicants
    Earliest date: Dec. 1, 1996
    Latest date: Until class is filled
Applicant's response to acceptance offer
    Maximum time: 2 weeks
Requests for deferred entrance considered: Yes
Deposit to hold place in class (applied to tuition):
    $100, due with response to acceptance offer
Deposit refundable prior to: May 15, 1997
Estimated number of new entrants: 165 (3 EDP)
Starting date: Aug. 1997

## TUITION AND STUDENT FEES PER YEAR FOR 1995–96 FIRST-YEAR CLASS

Tuition: $28,800      Student fees: $330

## INFORMATION ON 1995–96 FIRST-YEAR CLASS

| *Number of* | *In-State* | *Out-of-State* | *Total* |
|---|---|---|---|
| Applicants | 788 | 10,746 | 11,534 |
| Applicants Interviewed | 179 | 659 | 838 |
| New Entrants* | 52 | 124 | 176 |

*All took the MCAT and had baccalaureate degrees.

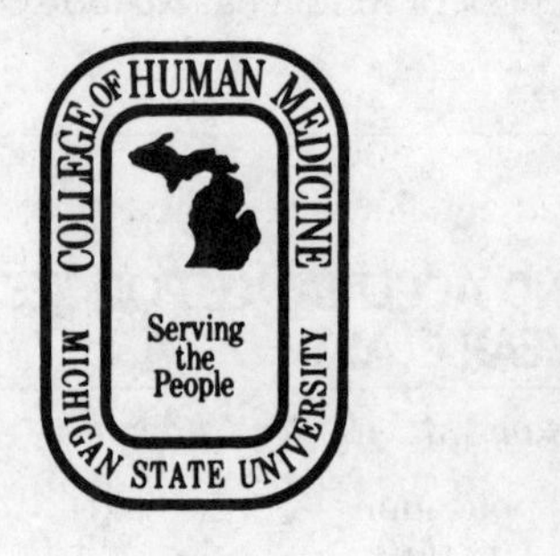

# Michigan State University
# College of Human Medicine

**East Lansing, Michigan**

Dr. William S. Abbett, *Dean*
Jane M. Smith, *Director of Admissions*
Dr. Wanda D. Lipscomb, *Director of Prematricular Programs*

## ADDRESS INQUIRIES TO:

College of Human Medicine
Office of Admissions
A-239 Life Sciences
Michigan State University
East Lansing, Michigan 48824-1317
(517) 353-9620; 432-0021 (FAX)
E-Mail: MDAdmissions@msu.edu
Web Site: http://35.8.145.179/

## GENERAL INFORMATION

The College of Human Medicine is a four-year medical school with all the advantages of a large university setting and a small college atmosphere (entering class size is 106). The mission of the College of Human Medicine is to educate excellent physicians who are caring, compassionate, and humane; primary care physicians who practice family medicine, internal medicine, and pediatrics; and physicians who work to make quality health care a reality for everyone, including underserved rural and inner city populations in Michigan. M.D.-Ph.D. programs are available.

## CURRICULUM

The curriculum is divided into three blocks organized around a commitment to the integration of the basic biological, behavioral, and social sciences; a developmental approach to learning; early teaching of clinical skills; and clinical training utilizing a community-based approach.

Block I is a three-semester experience comprising the first year in which fundamental basic science concepts and principles are presented in a structured, discipline-based format. Basic clinical skills teaching begins, along with a mentor group experience and opportunity to participate in independent as well as supplementary learning experiences (many utilizing computer formats). A clinical correlations course integrates basic science information, connects these sciences to medicine, and models a team approach to the practice of medicine.

Block II is a 2½-semester experience comprising the second year in which advanced basic science concepts are organized in an integrated, problem-based format. Emphasis is on small-group instruction and problem solving. A clinical context for learning basic science concepts is also provided. Clinical skills

training continues along with special topics seminars which deal with contemporary issues in society and medicine.

Block III is a six-semester experience comprising the third and fourth years and is spent in one of six Michigan communities associated with the college. Students live in the community during their required clinical clerkships and their experiences are in a variety of hospital and ambulatory care settings. Students have options of completing elective clerkships in other locations including third world countries. Community physicians work closely with community-based members of the college to provide a unique learning environment. The required clinical clerkships include a family practice/primary care clerkship with exposure to the comprehensive and continuous care of patients and families.

## REQUIREMENTS FOR ENTRANCE

The MCAT and a minimum of three years of accredited college education are required. In the 1995 entering class, all had B.A. or B.S. degrees and 13 percent held graduate or professional degrees.

A specific academic major is not a critical factor for admission; a solid background in the arts, humanities, or social sciences will be of as much value to the future doctor as strong preparation in the biosciences.

Specific course requirements are:

*Sem./Qtr. hrs.*

| | |
|---|---|
| Biological sciences (with lab) | 6/9 |
| Lab must be 2 semester or 3 term credits. | |
| Inorganic and organic chemistry (with lab) | 8/12 |
| Lab must be 3 semester or 5 term credits. | |
| Physics (with lab) | 6/9 |
| English composition and literature | 6/9 |
| Psychology and/or sociology | 6/9 |
| Nonscience areas | 18/27 |

May include English and psychology/sociology requirements.

## SELECTION FACTORS

All application materials are reviewed prior to an initial decision. Applicants are required to submit an autobiographical statement specifying their reasons for wishing to be a physician as well as their reasons for selecting Michigan State University (MSU). Because MSU is a state-assisted institution, enrollment of nonresidents is limited. No more than 20 percent of the entering class is from outside the state of Michigan.

The college seeks to admit a class that is not only academically competent but also one that reflects both the rural and urban character of Michigan, while representing a wide spectrum of personalities, backgrounds, talents, and motivations. Students who have the desire and aptitude to become physicians but who have experienced unequal educational opportunities because of social, cultural, or racial reasons are especially encouraged to apply.

From the over 3,600 applicants reviewed by the Committee on Admissions, approximately 400 applicants will be invited to Interview Day at the East Lansing campus for interviews with faculty and medical students. Selection is based on many factors, including the GPA, both year to year and cumulative; MCAT scores; fit with the school's primary care mission; autobiographical statement; relevant work experience in health-related and other occupations or positions; interviewers' assessments of motivation, ability to communicate, problem-solving ability, maturity, and suitability for the MSU program; state of residence; and potential to contribute to the overall quality of the entering class.

In addition to selecting students for the main campus program, the Committee on Admisions admits six students to the Upper Peninsula (UP) Medical Education Program. The UP Program is an innovative project of the College of Human Medicine established to meet the special health care needs of patients in remote, medically underserved rural areas of Michigan through training physicians committed to primary care. Students interested in the UP Program are encouraged to take the April MCAT and apply early. In addition, MSU is a recipient of one of the seven Kellogg initiatives in health professions education, which provides expanded opportunities for training in both a university setting and a community health structure. Further information is available from the Office of Admissions.

## FINANCIAL AID

Information about specific scholarships and about financial aid can be obtained from the Office of Financial Aids, 150 Administration Building. Acceptance to the class is not based on the individual's ability to pay. However, financial aid is limited, and the responsibility for adequate funding must rest with the student.

MSU provides limited financial aid for students who show strong desire and aptitude for becoming physicians but have previously been denied equal education opportunities for social, cultural, or racial reasons.

## INFORMATION FOR MINORITIES

Although the College of Human Medicine does not have a separate review for minority applicants, minority and other non-traditional students have been very competitive, and the college has a substantial enrollment of such students. The 1995 entering class had an underrepresented minority enrollment of approximately 32 percent, which included African American, Mexican American, mainland Puerto Rican, and Native American Indian students. The college also offers a postbaccalaureate program, Advanced Baccalaureate Learning Experience (ABLE), for a few selected students. Questions about the prematricular programs should be addressed to the director of prematricular programs. Questions about services afforded to minority students should be addressed to the director of admissions.

---

Public Institution

### APPLICATION AND ACCEPTANCE POLICIES FOR 1997–98 FIRST-YEAR CLASS

*School participates in AMCAS. See Chapter 4.*

Filing of AMCAS application
   Earliest date: June 1, 1996
   Latest date: Nov. 15, 1996
School application fee to all applicants: $50
Oldest MCAT scores considered: 1994
Does have Early Decision Program (EDP)
   EDP application period: June 1–Aug. 1, 1996
   EDP applicants notified by: Oct. 1, 1996
Acceptance notice to regular applicants
   Earliest date: Oct. 15, 1996
   Latest date: Varies
Applicant's response to acceptance offer
   Maximum time: 2 weeks
Requests for deferred entrance considered: Yes
Deposit to hold place in class: $50, due with response to acceptance offer
Deposit refundable prior to: May 15, 1997
Estimated number of new entrants: 106 (12 EDP)
Starting date: Aug. 1997

### TUITION AND STUDENT FEES PER YEAR FOR 1995–96 FIRST-YEAR CLASS

Tuition (3 semesters)      Student fees: $856
   Resident: $14,556
   Nonresident: $31,038

### INFORMATION ON 1995–96 FIRST-YEAR CLASS

| *Number of* | *In-State* | *Out-of-State* | *Total* |
|---|---|---|---|
| Applicants | 1,266 | 2,453 | 3,719 |
| Applicants Interviewed | 286 | 144 | 430 |
| New Entrants* | 79 | 25 | 104 |

*99% took the MCAT; all had baccalaureate degrees.

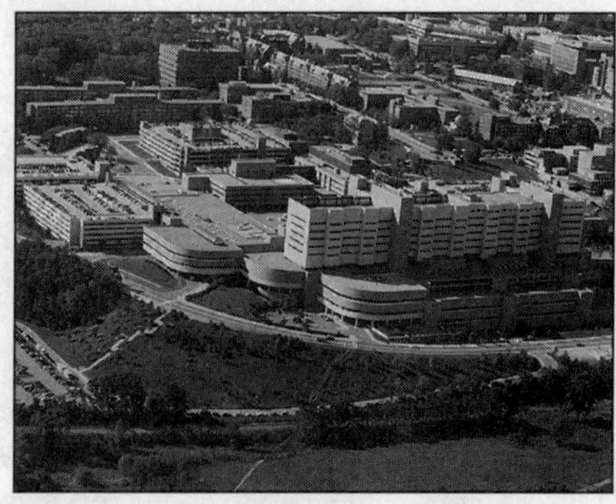

# University of Michigan Medical School

## Ann Arbor, Michigan


Dr. Giles G. Bole, *Dean*
Dr. Paul W. Gikas, *Assistant Dean and Chairman, Admissions Committee*
Wilma Porter, *Director of Financial Aid*


## ADDRESS INQUIRIES TO:

Admissions Office
M4130 Medical Science I Building
University of Michigan Medical School
Ann Arbor, Michigan 48109-0611
(313) 764-6317; 764-4542 (FAX)

## GENERAL INFORMATION

The University of Michigan was founded in 1817, and the first class of medical students matriculated in 1850. The history of the school includes the distinction of the nation's first university-owned hospital. Today, the medical center occupies 30 buildings and 84 acres of land, the world's largest one-site complex devoted to health education, research, and patient care. The university hospitals, with 888 beds and numerous ambulatory care settings, treat more than one-half million patients each year. Instructional sites also include nearby St. Joseph Mercy Hospital, Veteran's Administration Hospital, Oakwood Hospital and Clinics, and William Beaumont Hospital.

## CURRICULUM

The curriculum is designed to provide the medical science and clinical background necessary for all physicians. The individuality of each student's education and learning styles is recognized. A new curriculum was implemented in 1992. There is a strong emphasis on basic science and clinical learning throughout the program. In the first two years, the faculty have incorporated more clinically relevant content and have expanded clinical instruction with basic science integration. A course called "Introduction to the Patient" is taught in the first two years, along with the fundamentals of each of the basic sciences. In the clerkship (third and fourth) years, students participate in weekly conferences that demonstrate clinical cases and provide relevant basic science material in a clinical context. All third-year medical students will complete a four-week family practice clerkship in addition to a three-month longitudinal (1/2-day per week) primary care experience during the quarter they are assigned to internal medicine. All courses offered in the first year are graded on a pass/fail basis. In subsequent years, faculty assign students a grade of honors, high pass, pass, or fail. Students are required to pass the USMLE, Step 1, before promotion to the clinical phase in the third year, and are required to pass USMLE, Step 2, before graduation.

Opportunities exist for individual research summer programs or for special research fellowships. Students also have the option to pursue a combined M.D.-Ph.D. curriculum either as a fellow in the Medical Scientist Training Program (MSTP) or as a graduate student in one of the basic science departments. Another option is a combined M.D.-M.P.H. in one of the graduate programs of the School of Public Health.

Personal and academic counseling, academic enrichment programs, tutorial services, and career counseling are offered through various units of the medical school. A 6-week summer prematriculation program is also available, designed to enhance students' academic preparedness for medical school and provide a review of content areas such as biochemistry and anatomy.

## REQUIREMENTS FOR ENTRANCE

The MCAT and a minimum of 90 semester hours of university work are required. Grades below C in required courses are not acceptable. The specific course requirements are:

|  | Sem. hrs. |
| --- | --- |
| Biology (with lab) | 6 |
| General/inorganic and organic chemistry (with lab) | 8 |
| Biochemistry | 3 |
| Physics (with lab) | 6 |
| English composition and literature | 6 |
| Nonscience/humanities | 18 |

## SELECTION FACTORS

The Admissions Committee has the responsibility to select from each year's applicants those whose talents, skills, interests, and personal fitness indicate they will succeed in the study and practice of medicine. As part of a state university, the Medical School gives some preference to applicants who are residents of Michigan.

The Admissions Committee considers that all information pertaining to the ability, personality, and character of the applicant is relevant. Scores on the MCAT are given serious attention. Most accepted applicants have at least a B-plus undergraduate average. The mean undergraduate GPA for students admitted in 1995 was 3.6. Reports from college instructors, especially those who have had considerable experience in evaluating premedical students, are important. While only three years of undergraduate work are required, the Admissions Committee gives preference to applicants who will have completed four years by the time of matriculation.

Interviews are offered to selected students based on review of submitted information in their application and supporting documents. The interview is usually held in Ann Arbor. All students are considered on the basis of individual qualifications.

The committee does not accept applications from students who have not had at least one year, and preferably two years, of their premedical training at an accredited U.S. or Canadian college. Foreign nationals must have a permanent resident visa in the United States.

Any applicant who has been enrolled previously in a medical school in a program leading to the M.D. degree must be in good standing and eligible for reentry to that school in order to be considered for admission to the University of Michigan Medical School. The Medical School cannot accept transfer students from other medical schools or health care programs.

The Medical School participates in the Early Decision Program. To be eligible for consideration an applicant must be highly qualified.

## FINANCIAL AID

Application for financial aid may be initiated following acceptance to the Medical School. Loan funds and some scholarships are available to assist registered students with tuition expense and a share of their living expenses. It is the goal of the Financial Aid Committee that no students should be required to interrupt their education solely for financial reasons.

## INFORMATION FOR MINORITIES

Applications from members of the ethnic minority groups which are underrepresented in medicine are encouraged. An Opportunity Award Program authorized by the regents of the university provides a degree of financial support for economically disadvantaged students. Premedical students may participate in a Summer Biomedical Research Program for Minority Students (313/763-1296).

Public Institution

## APPLICATION AND ACCEPTANCE POLICIES FOR 1997–98 FIRST-YEAR CLASS

*School participates in AMCAS. See Chapter 4.*

Filing of AMCAS application
    Earliest date: June 1, 1996
    Latest date: Nov. 15, 1996
School application fee to all applicants: $50
Oldest MCAT scores considered: 1993
Does have Early Decision Program (EDP)
    EDP application period: June 1–Aug. 1, 1996
    EDP applicants notified by: Oct. 1, 1996
Acceptance notice to regular applicants
    Earliest date: Dec. 1, 1996
    Latest date: Until class is filled
Applicant's response to acceptance offer
    Maximum time: Varies
Requests for deferred entrance considered: Yes
Deposit to hold place in class (applied to tuition):
    $100, due with response to acceptance offer
Deposit refundable prior to: May 1, 1997
Estimated number of new entrants: 165 (5 EDP)
Starting date: Aug. 1997

## TUITION AND STUDENT FEES PER YEAR FOR 1995–96 FIRST-YEAR CLASS

Tuition        Student fees: $176
    Resident: $16,040
    Nonresident: $25,140

## INFORMATION ON 1995–96 FIRST-YEAR CLASS

| *Number of* | *In-State* | *Out-of-State* | *Total* |
|---|---|---|---|
| Applicants | 1,123 | 4,750 | 5,873 |
| Applicants Interviewed | 311 | 332 | 643 |
| New Entrants* | 100 | 65 | 165 |

*All took the MCAT and had baccalaureate degrees.

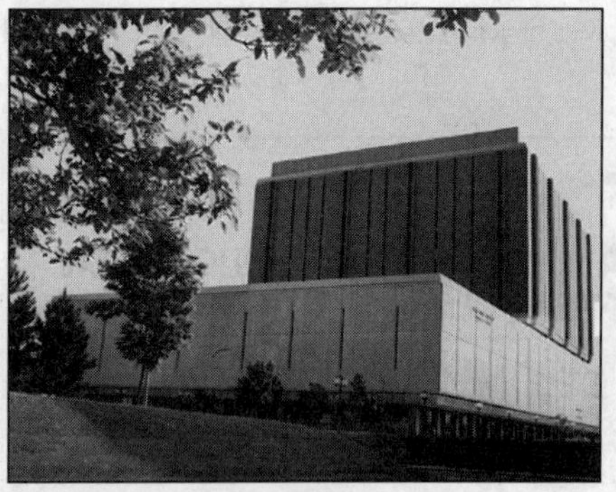

# Wayne State University
# School of Medicine

**Detroit, Michigan**

Dr. Robert J. Sokol, *Dean*
Dr. James Collins, *Assistant Dean for Admissions*
Laurinda Osterbur, *Assistant Director, Financial Aid*

## ADDRESS INQUIRIES TO:

Director of Admissions
Wayne State University
School of Medicine
540 East Canfield
Detroit, Michigan 48201
(313) 577-1466; 577-1330 (FAX)
Web Site: http://med.wayne.edu:82/admiss/admiss.htm

## GENERAL INFORMATION

The School of Medicine, which originated in 1868, is the oldest component of Wayne State University. It is located in the 236-acre Detroit Medical Center. This center is composed of a basic science building (Scott Hall), containing modern teaching facilities for the first two years of medical school; the Shiffman Medical Library; the Lande Medical Research Building; the Elliman Clinical Research Building; C. S. Mott Building; Harper-Grace, Hutzel, and Children's hospitals; Detroit Receiving Hospital and University Health Center (an ambulatory care facility); the Rehabilitation Institute; and the Veterans Administration Hospital. The Detroit Medical Center hospitals are the major clinical teaching and treatment units of the school. In addition, the medical school is affiliated with Sinai, Saint John, William Beaumont, Oakwood, Providence, and Saint Joseph Mercy hospitals.

## CURRICULUM

The curriculum is divided into four academic periods which are in sequence 9, 10, 12, and 8 months in duration. The major subjects for these respective periods are normal human biology, pathology, pharmacology, and introduction to clinical medicine, clerkships, and medical electives. Year I is primarily disciplinary, and Year II is initially disciplinary progressing to an organ systems approach. Year III focuses on clinical clerkships. The elective period, senior year, allows students an opportunity to define a major portion of their own academic program within a general structure under the guidance of faculty advisors.

A wide range of opportunities are offered for students to engage in research, basic and clinical, as well as graduate degree programs (M.S. and Ph.D.) in combination with an M.D. program. Students must pass the USMLE Step 1 to be promoted into Year III.

## REQUIREMENTS FOR ENTRANCE

The MCAT is required in addition to a baccalaureate degree or its equivalent; however, the Committee on Admissions is prepared to review the records of third-year students with unusual academic attainment. The MCAT should be taken during the year of application, preferably in the spring. Recommended courses for medical school and MCAT preparation are:

|  | *Sem. hrs.* |
|---|---|
| General biology or zoology (with lab) | 12 |
| Inorganic chemistry (with lab) | 8 |
| Organic chemistry (with lab) | 8 |
| General physics (with lab) | 8 |
| English | 8 |

Besides a strong preparation in the basic sciences, a broad educational background in a liberal arts-oriented program is desirable. Applicants are encouraged to select subjects that will contribute substantially to a broad cultural background.

## SELECTION FACTORS

The Committee on Admissions will select those applicants who, in its judgment, will make the best students and physicians. Consideration is given to the entire record, MCAT scores, college recommendations, and interview results as these reflect the applicant's personality, maturity, character, and suitability for medicine. The mean GPA for students admitted in 1995 was approximately 3.50. Special consideration is given to candidates from areas where there is a shortage of physicians.

As a state-supported school, the institution must give preference to Michigan residents; however, out-of-state applicants are encouraged to apply. An applicant's residency is determined by university regulations. Students whose educational backgrounds include work outside the United States must have completed two years of course work at a U.S. or Canadian college. Interviews are required but only scheduled with those applicants who are given serious consideration.

It is the intent of the Committee on Admissions to make final selections by March 1; therefore, students are urged to apply by November 1.

There is no discrimination on the basis of race, color, sex, national origin, religion, age, sexual orientation, marital status, or physical challenges.

## FINANCIAL AID

Scholarships, loans, and grants are awarded on the basis of academic performance, financial need, and available funding. Students may borrow through various loan programs up to the amount of total school-related costs and living expenses. Loans not based on demonstrated financial need are also available. Although the primary responsibility for financing a medical education rests with the student and the student's family, the School of Medicine will assist students with unmet need as funds are available. Short-term loans may be made for emergency purposes after registration.

Financial aid awards administered by the School of Medicine are made by the financial aid officer based on federal guidelines and those established by the Committee on Financial Aid and Scholarships, which includes student representation.

The College Work-Study Program and other medically oriented jobs are generally available to eligible students for the summer break.

Accepted students are mailed applications and updated financial aid information in February preceding matriculation. Additional information is available from the financial aid officer. Financial aid seminars are held for incoming students and their families. Financial aid appointments and information are available by calling (313) 577-1039.

## INFORMATION FOR MINORITIES

Wayne State University School of Medicine is committed to the recruitment and retention of underrepresented minority and disadvantaged applicants. The school supports a one-year post-baccalaureate program for disadvantaged medical school applicants from Michigan who have been denied admission but who appear to have the potential for academic success. The program consists of premedical science courses, study skills training, personal adjustment counseling, academic tutoring, and an introduction to the first-year medical school curriculum. Successful students are admitted to the School of Medicine. Through the minority recruitment office, the school also administers the Incoming Freshman Summer Program for minority students who are admitted to the freshman class. Additionally, college and high school premedical preparatory programs are offered. For information write Julia Simmons, director, minority recruitment and prematriculation programs.

---

Public Institution

## APPLICATION AND ACCEPTANCE POLICIES FOR 1997–98 FIRST-YEAR CLASS

*School participates in AMCAS. See Chapter 4.*

Filing of AMCAS application
  Earliest date: June 1, 1996
  Latest date: Dec. 15, 1996
School application fee to all applicants: $30
Oldest MCAT scores considered: 1992
Does have Early Decision Program (EDP)
  EDP application period: June 1–Aug. 1, 1996
  EDP applicants notified by: Oct. 1, 1996
Acceptance notice to regular applicants
  Earliest date: Oct. 15, 1996
  Latest date: Until class is filled
Applicant's response to acceptance offer
  Maximum time: 3 weeks
Requests for deferred entrance considered: Yes
Deposit to hold place in class (applied to tuition):
  $50, due with response to acceptance offer,
  nonrefundable
Estimated number of new entrants: 256 (35 EDP)
Starting date: Aug. 1997

## TUITION AND STUDENT FEES PER YEAR FOR 1995–96 FIRST-YEAR CLASS

Tuition                          Student fees: $350
  Resident: $9,566
  Nonresident: $19,061

## INFORMATION ON 1995–96 FIRST-YEAR CLASS

| Number of | In-State | Out-of-State | Total |
|---|---|---|---|
| Applicants | 1,417 | 2,992 | 4,409 |
| Applicants Interviewed | 665 | 184 | 849 |
| New Entrants* | 230 | 17 | 247 |

*All took the MCAT and had baccalaureate degrees.

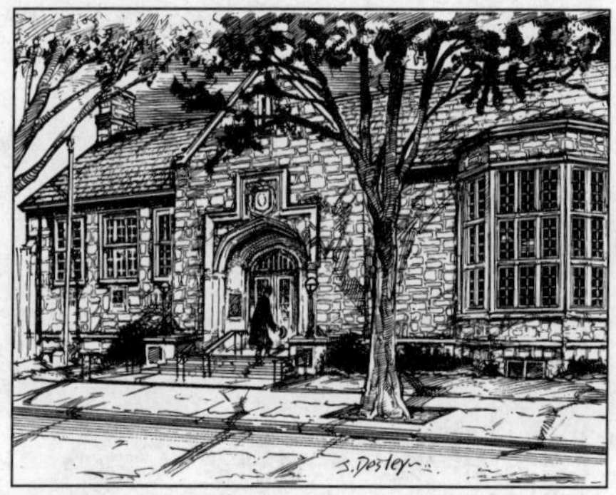

# Mayo Medical School

**Rochester, Minnesota**

Dr. Burton A. Sandok, *Dean*
Dr. Roger W. Harms, *Associate Dean for Student Affairs*
Marion K. Kelly, *Assistant Dean for Student Affairs*

## ADDRESS INQUIRIES TO:

Mayo Medical School
200 First Street, S.W.
Rochester, Minnesota 55905
(507) 284-3671; 284-2634 (FAX)
Web Site:
http://www.mayo.edu/education/mms/MMS_home_page.html

## GENERAL INFORMATION

Mayo Medical School is an integral part of Mayo Foundation and Mayo Clinic, the world's largest group practice of medicine. Minnesota residents receive grants from the state of Minnesota to diminish tuition expenses. In recognition of our three-site campus, Mayo foundation extends the same benefits to residents of the state of Florida and Arizona.

Resources of MMS include a diverse patient population of more than 390,000 registrants each year, four affiliated hospitals with facilities for clinical and basic research, primary care facilities including several rural health centers, and affiliations with physicians who practice in surrounding communities. The faculty is drawn from the clinical and scientific staff of Mayo Clinic with locations in Rochester, MN; Jacksonville, FL; and Scottsdale, AZ.

## CURRICULUM

The curriculum is designed to emphasize the integration of basic and clinical sciences throughout all four years. Governance of the curriculum is centralized and structured around learning objectives such as the Scientific Foundations of Medical Practice; the Clinical Experiences; and the Patient, Physician, and Society. Through this mechanism, longitudinal oversight of teaching of the basic and clinical sciences can be assured and integration facilitated.

In the first year, basic sciences are taught with clinical correlation emphasizing the normal function of the cell and organ systems. Simultaneous with this learning is the introduction to clinical skills culminating in the ability to perform a history and examination on a Mayo patient by the end of the first year. Preceptor experiences throughout the first year in Continuity of Care keep the focus on the patient.

The second year is devoted to an introduction to the core clinical sciences while completing the introduction of the basic scientific underlayment of clinical practice. Emphasis here is more on pathophysiology of the organ systems as students explore the use of basic clinical skills.

The third year is devoted to honing skills in all of the basic clinical clerkships, moving beyond the level of acquiring accurate information to the level of synthesis and diagnosis. Clinical experiences at Mayo have always been both ambulatory and in the hospital. Because of the small class size and more than one thousand physician faculty, in most cases these experiences occur as one-on-one assignments for staff of the Mayo Clinic. One third of the third year is an opportunity to explore the realm of scientific investigation, as every Mayo student completes a research endeavor of his or her own choice under the mentorship of an experienced Mayo investigator. Aproximately 175 Mayo scientists in 37 disciplines offer research experiences in which the students participate.

The fourth year has been carefully designed to produce students who have a well-structured completion of their undergraduate education leading to a physician who is prepared to enter any realm of medicine. Included are a sub internship in internal medicine or pediatrics; electives, within guidelines, to assure exposure to surgical disciplines; child patients. A social medicine elective to understand the role of community in the mission of medicine is also required. Integrated into the fourth-year curriculum is a three week return to the classroom to explore issues in preventive medicine, biomedical ethics, palliative medicine, and clinical pharmacology. The remainder of the fourth year is fully elective to allow students to customize their learning to meet individual goals.

Formal evaluations are recorded as honors, pass, marginal pass or fail, but are supplemented by narrative comments from the faculty. Merit scholarship renewal is dependent upon achieving a grade of pass or better in every course, but remediation is always available. Individual support and tutoring is available to all students.

A combined-degree program leading to the M.D.-Ph.D. is available for six members of the entering class. This joint effort with the Mayo Graduate School allows a student to be fully prepared for clinical practice as well as have all the tools for a career in scientific research. Another program in cooperation with the Mayo Graduate School of Medicine is available for two candidates with the D.D.S. degree who are seeking an M.D. degree and certification in oral and maxillofacial surgery. Stipend support and tuition waiver are included for these programs.

All students attending Mayo Medical School are supported by scholarship funds which significantly reduce the tuition burden to attend. In addition to participation in federal student assistance programs, Mayo has its own loan program and need-based grant program which are available to help offset educational expenses.

## REQUIREMENTS FOR ENTRANCE

A baccalaureate degree is required, but no major field is preferred. The MCAT must have been taken within three years of application. College work must include:

|  | *Years* |
|---|---|
| Biology and/or Zoology | 1 |
| Inorganic Chemistry | 1 |
| Organic Chemistry | 1 |
| A course in Biochemistry | |
| Physics (with lab) | 1 |

Mayo Medical School looks for students with excellent academic records in a breadth of educational experiences. We value diversity of talents within the class, but expect candidates to have a lifelong commitment to service. Experiences which demonstrate unique gifts along with deep commitment are evaluated in the application process.

## SELECTION FACTORS

In evaluating candidates, the entire academic record, results of the MCAT, careful reading of the candidates personal statement, and letters of recommendation are utilized in the initial steps. A standardized telephone interview is utilized in lieu of a secondary application for those candidates who have the academic credentials. A great deal of weight is placed on the personal interview in Rochester. Evidence of integrity, adaptability, maturity, leadership, and humanitarian concern are essential. Appointment notification occurs roughly every six weeks throughout the admissions process, though appointments may be given any time up to the time classes begin in August.

Foreign applicants without a permanent resident visa cannot be considered for appointment.

Some characteristics of the students accepted for the 1995 entering class were: *mean GPA,* 3.73; *mean MCAT scores,* above 10 in all categories; *gender,* 46 percent women, *underrepresented minorities,* 14 percent.

Mayo does not discriminate on the basis of race, sex, creed, national origin, age, or handicap in its educational programs or activities in accordance with civil rights legislation.

## FINANCIAL AID

An aggressive grant and scholarship program allows us to offer every student significant financial support. Forty-five percent of entering students receive a full-tuition scholarship, and a merit scholarship program reduces the cost to all students. Mayo Medical School has an aggressive affirmative action grant program. All matriculants who are underrepresented minorities in medicine are eligible to receive Outstanding Achievement Awards, resulting in full-tuition scholarships. All scholarships are forfeited by students holding appointments at other schools after May 15, 1997. Evidence of withdrawal from other institutions must be provided by that date. Mayo provides an attractive institutional loan program. Comprehensive health care coverage is included in tuition. There are no student fees. Further information may be obtained by telephoning the financial aid office at (507) 284-4839.

---

Private Institution

### APPLICATION AND ACCEPTANCE POLICIES FOR 1997–98 FIRST-YEAR CLASS

*School participates in AMCAS. See Chapter 4.*

Filing of AMCAS application
    Earliest date: June 1, 1996
    Latest date: Nov. 1, 1996
School application fee to all applicants: $60
Oldest MCAT scores considered: 1993
Does have Early Decision Program (EDP)
    EDP application period: June 1–Aug. 1, 1996
    EDP applicants notified by: Oct. 1, 1996
Acceptance notice to regular applicants
    Earliest date: Oct. 15, 1996
    Latest date: Until class is filled
Applicant's response to acceptance offer
    Maximum time: 2 weeks
Requests for deferred entrance considered: Yes
Deposit to hold place in class (applied to tuition):
    $100, due with response to acceptance offer
Deposit refundable prior to: May 15, 1997
Estimated number of new entrants: 42 (2 EDP)
Starting date: Aug. 1997

### TUITION AND STUDENT FEES PER YEAR FOR 1995–96 FIRST-YEAR CLASS

Tuition               Student fees: None
    Residents of Arizona, Florida, and
      Minnesota: $9,925*
    Nonresident: $19,800*

### INFORMATION ON 1995–96 FIRST-YEAR CLASS

| *Number of* | *In-State* | *Out-of-State* | *Total* |
|---|---|---|---|
| Applicants | 423 | 3,482 | 3,905 |
| Applicants Interviewed | 57 | 375 | 432 |
| New Entrants† | 11 | 31 | 42 |

*Merit scholarships reduce effective tuition to $4,800 for residents of MN, AZ, and FL and $9,900 for nonresidents.

†All took the MCAT and had baccalaureate degrees.

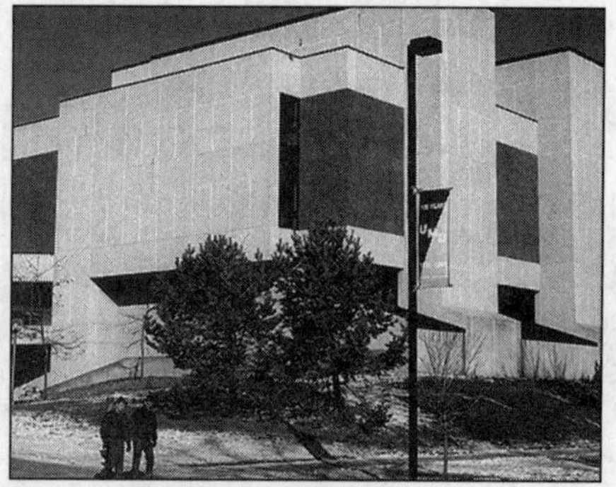

# University of Minnesota—Duluth School of Medicine

## Duluth, Minnesota

Dr. Ronald D. Franks, *Dean*
Dr. Lillian Repesh, *Assistant Dean for Admissions and Student Affairs*
Dina Flaherty, *Financial Aid Liaison*

## ADDRESS INQUIRIES TO:

Office of Admissions, Room 107
University of Minnesota—Duluth
School of Medicine
10 University Drive
Duluth, Minnesota 55812
(218) 726-8511; 726-6235 (FAX)
E-Mail: JCARLSIO@ub.d.umn.edu
Web Site: http://www.d.umn.edu/medweb

## GENERAL INFORMATION

The University of Minnesota—Duluth (UMD) School of Medicine admitted its first class of 24 students in September 1972 to a two-year basic medical and clinical sciences program. After these first two years, students are automatically transferred to the University of Minnesota Medical School at Minneapolis under an established, noncompetitive mechanism for completion of their training.

The UMD School of Medicine has established affiliation agreements with the St. Mary's and Miller-Dwan medical centers and St. Luke's Hospital of Duluth. These institutions afford medical students access to health care systems that provide patients from the northern regions of Minnesota, Wisconsin, and Michigan with care for various medical problems.

The full-time teaching faculty consists of 45 basic and clinical science members. The part-time and voluntary clinical sciences faculty includes over 250 area physicians who represent all of the major medical specialties. Their close interactions with the full-time faculty in presenting the curriculum ensures a practical as well as an academic approach toward training physicians.

## CURRICULUM

The two-year curriculum is designed to prepare students for future medical practice through careful and integrated instruction in basic, clinical, and behavioral sciences. Under the guidance of the volunteer clinical faculty, students have early exposure to patients, learning accurate medical history-taking and physical examination skills. Ample time is also devoted to basic science-clinical correlations allowing a student to utilize the basic sciences as they apply to clinical medicine. In addition, each student is paired with a family physician in a

required preceptorship arrangement. During the first year, this entails meeting with the preceptor for at least 10 hours per quarter. In the second year, students spend three consecutive days each quarter with their preceptors in small towns throughout Minnesota.

## REQUIREMENTS FOR ENTRANCE

The MCAT and completion of all requirements for a bachelor's degree must be completed by the time of matriculation. Applicants are strongly urged to take the MCAT in the spring of the year of application and to have their premedical course requirements completed at the time of application. The processing of an application may be delayed if MCAT scores or grades from required courses in process are not included in the original application.

Required courses are:

|  | Sem./Qtr. hrs. |
|---|---|
| General biology or zoology (with lab) | 8/12 |
| General physics (with lab) | 8/12 |
| General/inorganic chemistry (with lab) | 8/12 |
| Organic chemistry (with lab) | 8/12 |
| English composition | 6/9 |
| Humanities | 8/12 |

At least one course must be upper division level.

| Behavioral sciences | 8/12 |
|---|---|

At least one course must be upper division level.
Calculus or upper level statistics

A course in biochemistry is strongly recommended.

Beyond these requirements, applicants are strongly encouraged to broaden their education by taking courses in non-science areas that will provide intellectual stimulation. Applicants are also encouraged to become exposed to people and their problems and to learn about the medical profession.

## SELECTION FACTORS

The University of Minnesota is committed to the policy that all persons shall have equal access to its programs, facilities, and employment without regard to age, race, creed, sex, national origin, veteran's status, sexual preference, or handicap. As a state-supported school, strongest preference for selection is given to legal residents of Minnesota. Consideration will also be given to applicants from Douglas, Ashland, Bayfield, Burnett, Iron, Price, Sawyer, and Washburn

Counties of Wisconsin, and the Canadian Province of Manitoba and underrepresented minority applicants, regardless of residency, who wish to become family practice physicians in a small-town setting. Applicants from other states will not be considered for admission. Transfer requests are not considered.

For each applicant, the Committee on Admissions consider the entire academic record, including trends in performance, scores from the MCAT, and responses to a questionnaire prepared by the committee. If an applicant is selected from this initial screening, the individual is then invited to the Duluth campus for interviews by two full-time committee members. During this visit, the candidate is invited to have lunch with a current medical student. Letters of evaluation are requested of all interviewed applicants.

In keeping with the mandated goals set by the Minnesota legislature at the school's inception, the committee is seeking persons with personal and background traits which indicate a high potential for becoming a family physician in a small town or rural setting. There is no prejudice for or against the reapplicant. If possible, reapplicants are encouraged to identify any liabilities and rectify them before reapplying through AMCAS. Individuals who are not accepted have the opportunity to review the application with the admissions officer to try to pinpoint the reasons(s) for the action. Admissions requests for advanced standing cannot be considered because of the nature of the curriculum.

The following information pertains to the 1995 entering class: *overall acceptance rate,* 74 acceptances offered to obtain a class of 50 students; mean GPA, 3.56; *mean MCAT scores, VR*-9.2, *PS*-9.0, *BS*-9.5; *sex,* 24 women; *residence,* 90 percent from Minnesota; *undergraduate major,* 70 percent in biology or chemistry, with the remainder from a variety of fields.

## FINANCIAL AID

Financial aid is based on the demonstrated need of the student. A number of loans are available through the University Financial Aid Program, and there is limited scholarship aid. To date, no one who has been accepted has discontinued medical studies because of financial need. About 93 percent of the students are eligible for and receive financial assistance.

## INFORMATION FOR MINORITIES

The school accepts the principles of affirmative action and recognizes the need to provide minority group members with the opportunity to study medicine. Academic and cultural support, particularly for American Indians, is provided through the Center for American Indian and Minority Health and through a program called Native Americans into Medicine.

Public Institution

## APPLICATION AND ACCEPTANCE POLICIES FOR 1997–98 FIRST-YEAR CLASS

*School participates in AMCAS. See Chapter 4.*

Filing of AMCAS application
 Earliest date: June 1, 1996
 Latest date: Nov. 15, 1996
School application fee after screening: $50
Oldest MCAT scores considered: 1994
Does have Early Decision Program (EDP)
 EDP application period: June 1–Aug. 1, 1996
 EDP applicants notified by: Oct. 1, 1996
Acceptance notice to regular applicants
 Earliest date: Oct. 15, 1996
 Latest date: Varies
Applicant's response to acceptance offer
 Maximum time: 2 weeks
Requests for deferred entrance considered: Yes
Deposit to hold place in class (applied to tuition):
 None
Estimated number of new entrants: 50
Starting date: Aug. 1997

## TUITION AND STUDENT FEES PER YEAR FOR 1995–96 FIRST-YEAR CLASS

Tuition*          Student fees: $586
 Resident: $14,616
 Nonresident: $29,112

## INFORMATION ON 1995–96 FIRST-YEAR CLASS

| Number of | In-State | Out-of-State | Total |
|---|---|---|---|
| Applicants | 609 | 996 | 1,605 |
| Applicants Interviewed | 191 | 29 | 220 |
| New Entrants† | 44 | 6‡ | 50 |

*Resident tuition will be granted to higher-ability minority nonresidents.

†All took the MCAT and had baccalaureate degrees.

‡Underrepresented minorities.

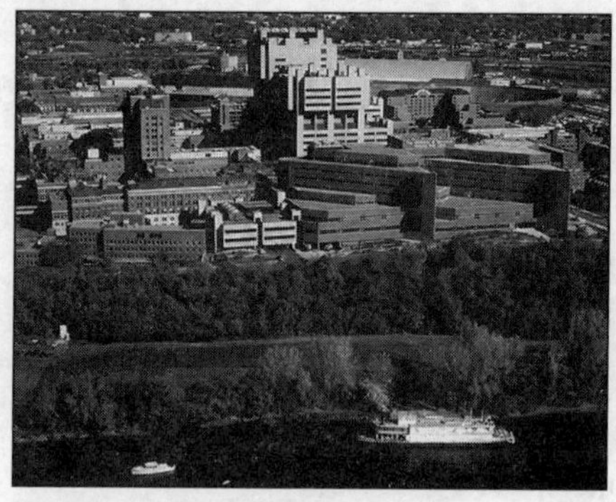

# University of Minnesota
# Medical School—Minneapolis

**Minneapolis, Minnesota**

Dr. Frank B. Cerra, *Dean*
Dr. Donald W. Robertson, *Associate Dean/Admissions*
B. J. Gibson, *Financial Aid Officer*

## ADDRESS INQUIRIES TO:

Office of Admissions and Student Affairs
Box 293-UMHC
University of Minnesota Medical School
420 Delaware Street, S.E.
Minnespolis, Minnesota 55455-0310
(612) 624-1122; 626-6800 (FAX)
Web Site: http://www.med.umn.edu/

## GENERAL INFORMATION

Founded in 1888, the University of Minnesota Medical School is located on the Minneapolis campus of the University of Minnesota. This proximity to disciplines basic or related to medicine provides unique opportunities for interchange of information, techniques, and personnel. The Medical School is a unit of the University of Minnesota Health Sciences Center and has a close working relationship with other units, including dentistry, nursing, and pharmacy. Most of the major hospitals in the Minneapolis-St. Paul area are affiliated with the Medical School. These, together with the University Hospital, a part of the Health Sciences Center, provide teaching facilities for medical students.

## CURRICULUM

A major feature of the curriculum is a well organized required course sequence in the first and second years and flexibility of the schedule in the third and fourth years. The first-year program is comprised of courses which form a basis for the continued study of medicine: anatomy, biochemistry, physiology, microbiology, and pathology. Relevance of these areas is reinforced through a series of clinical correlations. In the summer, students are introduced to topics in clinical medicine, including genetics and human behavior, and begin to acquire skills in clinical diagnosis. In the second year, pathology and pharmacology provide the framework for continued study of basic sciences, and pathophysiology is emphasized in organ system courses. Clinical skills are broadened through work in clinical medicine, in the primary care fields of medicine, pediatrics, and family practice, and in neurology. The program in the third and fourth years includes four quarters of required externships and experiences, two quarters of electives, and two quarters of free time. Students are encouraged to undertake research and are urged to develop goals and pur-

sue personal and special interests in medical education. A faculty adviser is selected during the second year. The adviser assumes an important role in assisting students in achieving their own special educational goals. Flexibility of scheduling in the third and fourth years provides the opportunity to pursue other clinical/academic interests.

A seven-year M.D.-Ph.D. program is offered to combine the breadth of medical education with the depth of a rigorous graduate research program for superior students seeking a career in academic medicine.

## REQUIREMENTS FOR ENTRANCE

The MCAT and a bachelor's degree from an approved college or university are required. Applicants are urged to take the MCAT in the spring of the year of application and to complete all of the required science courses before taking the MCAT or making application.

Required courses are:

|  | *Quarters* |
|---|---|
| General biology or zoology (with lab) | 2 |
| General or inorganic chemistry (with lab) | 2 |
| Organic chemistry (with lab) | 2 |
| General physics (with lab) | 3 |
| English | 3 |
| Behavioral sciences, social sciences, or other liberal arts courses | (27 qtr. hrs.) |
| Calculus or upper level statistics | |

Course work in biochemistry, genetics, psychology, and liberal arts subjects is strongly recommended.

## SELECTION FACTORS

Although scholastic aptitude is necessary in order to complete studies in medical school, neither high grades nor high MCAT scores alone or in combination are adequate to obtain admission. The Admissions Committee is looking for candidates who demonstrate the greatest promise of becoming competent physicians. Evidence of personal integrity, maturity, creativity, motivation for medicine, the ability to work cooperatively with others, and a sense of dedication in service to others are factors which will be evaluated by the committee. These qualities and attitudes will be evaluated by several means, including letters of evaluation, the scope and nature of extracurricular activities, the breadth of undergraduate education, and personal interview. The committee will look at all aspects of the applicant's entire academic record, including trends in the scholastic performance.

Although preference is given to legal residents of the state of Minnesota, applicants from other states are encouraged to apply if they have a high level of scholastic aptitude and have shown industriousness, creativity, and an interest in research. The school does not discriminate on the basis of race, sex, creed, disability, or national origin.

Applicants not accepted in two successive years are rarely accepted on future applications unless there have been major improvements in both their academic and nonacademic credentials.

Accepted students for the 1995 entering class had the following statistics: *mean GPA,* 3.56; *sex,* 48 percent women; *residence,* 92 percent from Minnesota; *overall acceptance rate,* 10 percent, 284 acceptances out of 2,917 applicants to obtain a class of 185 freshmen.

Interviews are required before any applicant is accepted, and the Admissions Committee will notify applicants if an appointment is to be made for an interview.

All applications must be submitted through AMCAS, and students are urged to submit their application to AMCAS as soon as possible after completing their last quarter or semester of work following their third year of college. Early Decision Program applications from academically qualified students are encouraged.

Transfer students are accepted into the third year only and usually only from the two-year medical school at the University of Minnesota—Duluth.

An advanced admission program accepts a limited number of highly academically qualified students after their second year of college to enter the Medical School after completion of the bachelor's degree. Information is available from the Medical School.

## FINANCIAL AID

Long-term loans are available to students with demonstrable financial need. All applicants for financial aid must submit an ACT-FFS needs analysis. Long-term loans and some scholarship money are available through the Medical School Financial Aid Office.

## INFORMATION FOR MINORITIES

Nonresident minority students may qualify for resident tuition. The school is committed to the recruitment, enrollment, and education of minority groups underrepresented in medicine.

---

Public Institution

### APPLICATION AND ACCEPTANCE POLICIES FOR 1997–98 FIRST-YEAR CLASS

*School participates in AMCAS. See Chapter 4.*

Filing of AMCAS application
  Earliest date: June 1, 1996
  Latest date: Nov. 15, 1996
School application fee after screening: $50
Oldest MCAT scores considered: 1994
Does have Early Decision Program (EDP)
  EDP application period: June 1–Aug. 1, 1996
  EDP applicants notified by: Oct. 1, 1996
Acceptance notice to regular applicants
  Earliest date: Nov. 15, 1996
  Latest date: May 15, 1997
Applicant's response to acceptance offer
  Maximum time: 2 weeks
Requests for deferred entrance considered: Yes
Deposit to hold place in class: None
Estimated number of new entrants: 175 (20 EDP)
Starting date: Sept. 1997

### TUITION AND STUDENT FEES PER YEAR FOR 1995–96 FIRST-YEAR CLASS

Tuition                    Student fees: $586
  Resident: $14,616
  Nonresident*: $29,112

### INFORMATION ON 1995–96 FIRST-YEAR CLASS

| Number of | In-State | Out-of-State | Total |
| --- | --- | --- | --- |
| Applicants | 816 | 2,101 | 2,917 |
| Applicants Interviewed | 571 | 125 | 696 |
| New Entrants† | 171 | 14 | 185 |

*Resident tuition may be granted to higher-ability minority and disadvantaged nonresidents.

†All had baccalaureate degrees; 91% took the MCAT.

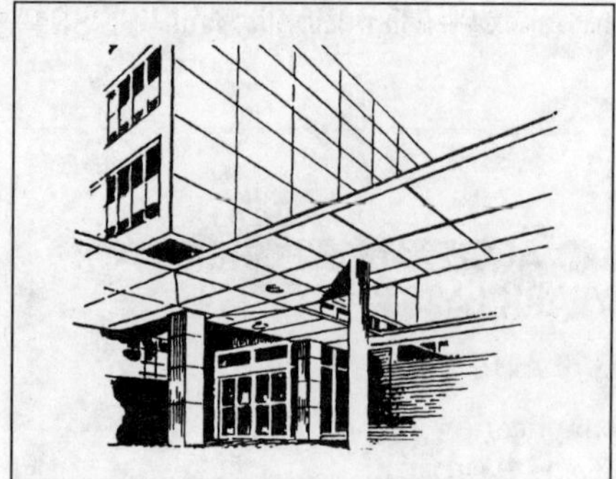

# University of Mississippi School of Medicine

**Jackson, Mississippi**


Dr. A. Wallace Conerly, *Dean*
Dr. Virginia H. Read, *Chairman, Admissions Committee*
Dr. Billy M. Bishop, *Director, Student Services and Records*


## ADDRESS INQUIRIES TO:

Chairman, Admissions Committee
University of Mississippi
School of Medicine
2500 North State Street
Jackson, Mississippi 39216-4505
(601) 984-5010; 984-5008 (FAX)

## GENERAL INFORMATION

The School of Medicine, created by a special act of the Board of Trustees in June 1903, operated as a two-year school in Oxford until 1955, when it expanded to four years and moved to the University of Mississippi Medical Center in Jackson. The medical center complex includes the School of Medicine, School of Nursing, School of Health Related Professions, School of Dentistry, Graduate Programs in the Medical Sciences, and the 593-bed University Hospital. Newest campus facilities are the Verner S. Holmes Learning Resource Center, which houses the Rowland Medical Library and the Division of Learning Resources, and an $18-million acute services addition to the teaching hospital. Clinical instruction is also carried out in the Veterans Administration Hospital, Mississippi State Hospital, and McBryde Rehabilitation Center for the Blind.

## CURRICULUM

In the first year, the courses in anatomy, biochemistry, physiology, and psychiatry/behavioral science are reinforced with a program of clinical correlation which introduces the student to presentation of patients and clinical concepts. The second-year student has courses in biostatistics, epidemiology, genetics, microbiology, pathology, pharmacology, psychiatry/behavioral science, and the conjoint course, introduction to clinical medicine. The third-year students rotate through family medicine, obstetrics-gynecology, pediatrics, psychiatry, medicine, and surgery for clinical instruction in these areas. The fourth year consists of a minimum of eight clinical clerkships (blocks), each one calendar month in length. Required blocks include core blocks in internal medicine, obstetrics-gynecology, pediatrics, and surgery. Of the required senior courses, internal medicine is largely an inpatient experience with an ambulatory component provided in medicine clinics at the Veterans Administration Medical Center or University Hospital. The required course in obstetrics-gynecology is largely ambulatory, but includes some inpatient experience in the labor and delivery suite. Of the core months required in pediatrics and surgery, one must be an inpatient clerkship. An additional ambulatory block is required. A fourth-year course in a senior seminar, which covers topics in medical ethics, medical economics and related issues, is required. The remaining months are available for elective experiences which the students select with the counsel adviser and the dean's office.

## REQUIREMENTS FOR ENTRANCE

The MCAT and three years of college are required. Each applicant must have a minimum of 90 semester hours from an accredited college, excluding physical education, military training, and certain professional courses. However, preference is given to applicants who will have completed all requirements for a baccalaureate degree prior to matriculation.

The required courses are:

|  | Sem./Qtr. hrs. |
|---|---|
| General biology or zoology (with lab) | 8/12 |
| Inorganic or general chemistry (with lab) | 8/12 |
| Organic chemistry (with lab) | 8/12 |
| General physics (with lab) | 8/12 |
| Advanced science | 8/12 |
| Mathematics | 6/9 |
| English | 6/9 |

Science courses for nonscience majors or survey courses are not acceptable for fulfilling the science requirements. Eight semester hours of advanced science must be taken in a senior college.

Students who qualify by placement tests for a more advanced course in mathematics must take a semester course of calculus I rather than algebra and trigonometry.

The student is advised to develop proficiency in a specific area and acquire a background in the humanities and behavioral sciences in undergraduate school.

## SELECTION FACTORS

Selection of applicants is made on a competitive basis without regard to age, sex, race, creed, national origin, marital status, handicap, or veteran status. The Admissions Committee selects students who are best qualified on the basis of a demonstration of scholastic aptitude and personal achievement with due consideration of other factors. Major considerations are academic performance, MCAT results, motivation for medicine, and such personal characteristics as maturity, integrity, and stability. Additional factors are the recommendation of the premedical advisers or committee and impression on personal interview. Strong preference is given to residents of Mississippi. Interviews are arranged at the discretion of the Admissions Committee.

The mean GPA for the 1995 entering class was 3.6.

## FINANCIAL AID

Accepted students may apply for financial aid. The school participates in federal scholarship programs and federal loan programs, such as Health Professions Student Loan Program, Perkins Loan Program, and Stafford Student Loan Program. Eligible students may also apply for limited scholarship funds provided by private donors. Additional financial aid is available through the American Medical Association Education and Research Foundation loan program and the Mississippi State Medical Education Scholarship Loan Program, which was established by the state legislature. In the latter program, Mississippi resident medical students who contract to practice in Mississippi may borrow up to $6,000 per school year or $24,000 in four years. Minority students are assisted by the National Medical Fellowship, Inc., program. A limited number of prizes and scholarships are awarded to outstanding students. Four dean's awards, renewable annually, are awarded each year to the freshmen with the highest academic achievement at the end of the first year. Although the study of medicine is considered a full-time occupation, students who maintain satisfactory academic standing may apply for part-time jobs in the medical center.

## INFORMATION FOR MINORITIES

The Admissions Committee recognizes the serious need for minority physicians and encourages minority students to apply for admission. Further information on the various aspects of the minority program may be obtained by writing to the director, minority student affairs.

Public Institution

## APPLICATION AND ACCEPTANCE POLICIES FOR 1997–98 FIRST-YEAR CLASS

*School participates in AMCAS. See Chapter 4.*

Filing of AMCAS application
    Earliest date: June 1, 1996
    Latest date: Nov. 1, 1996
School application fee: None
Oldest MCAT scores considered: 1993
Does have Early Decision Program (EDP)
    For Mississippi residents only
    EDP application period: June 1–Aug. 1, 1996
    EDP applicants notified by: Oct. 1, 1996
Acceptance notice to regular applicants
    Earliest date: Oct. 15, 1996
    Latest date: Until class is filled
Applicant's response to acceptance offer
    Maximum time: 15 days
Requests for deferred entrance considered: Yes
Deposit to hold place in class (applied to tuition):
    $50 for residents, due with response to
    acceptance offer
Deposit refundable prior to: May 15, 1997
Estimated number of new entrants: 100 (10 EDP)
Starting date: Aug. 1997

## TUITION AND STUDENT FEES PER YEAR FOR 1995–96 FIRST-YEAR CLASS

Tuition                 Student fees: $115
    Resident: $6,600
    Nonresident: $12,600

## INFORMATION ON 1995–96 FIRST-YEAR CLASS

| Number of | In-State | Out-of-State | Total |
|---|---|---|---|
| Applicants | 308 | 322 | 630 |
| Applicants Interviewed | 210 | 0 | 210 |
| New Entrants* | 100 | 0 | 100 |

*All took the MCAT and had baccalaureate degrees.

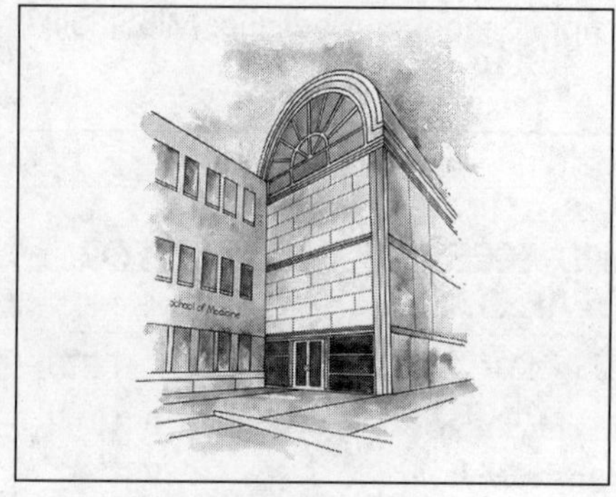

# University of Missouri—Columbia School of Medicine

## Columbia, Missouri

Dr. Lester R. Bryant, *Dean*
Dr. Robert N. McCallum, *Assistant Dean for Student Programs*
Conway A. Jones, *Financial Aid Coordinator*

## ADDRESS INQUIRIES TO:

Shari L. Swindell, *Admissions and Recruitment Coordinator*
Office of Admissions
MA202 Medical Sciences Building
University of Missouri—Columbia
School of Medicine
One Hospital Drive
Columbia, Missouri 65212
(573) 882-2923; 884-4808 (FAX)
E-Mail: SHARI_L._SWINDELL@
MUCCMAIL.MISSOURI.EDU
Web Site: http://www.miaims.missouri.edu/som

## GENERAL INFORMATION

The University of Missouri—Columbia School of Medicine was established in 1872 as a two-year medical school. In 1956 the curriculum was expanded to its present four-year program. Located on the Columbia campus of the University of Missouri, the Health Sciences Center includes the University Hospital, Mid-Missouri Mental Health Center, Harry S. Truman Veterans Administration Hospital, Medical Sciences Building, J. Otto Lottes Health Sciences Library, Howard A. Rusk Rehabilitation Center, Mason Institute of Ophthalmology, Cosmopolitan International Diabetes Center, and Ellis-Fischel Cancer Center. Students have a total of 1,000 hospital beds available for patient care. Outpatient clinics include the University Clinics, the Green Meadows Clinics, and the Crossroads West Clinics and rural primary care clinics within 35 miles of Columbia. The School of Medicine also maintains affiliations with various other health institutions across the state.

## CURRICULUM

The educational program of the School of Medicine was completely revised in 1993, to emphasize a strong foundation in the basic sciences, problem solving, clinical skills and early experiences with patients and role-model physicians, self-directed learning/life-long learning, and the attitudes essential to competent and compassionate patient care.

Each of the first two years has four 10-week blocks with two components—Basic Science/Problem Based Learning (BSci/PBL) and Introduction to Patient Care (IPC). BSci/PBL focuses on eight patient cases per block integrating basic sci-

ences, clinical concepts, and psychosocial aspects of medicine. Lectures and labs correlate with the cases. Students engage in problem solving and collaborative learning as they work in groups of eight with a faculty tutor. In IPC, students develop the clinical skills and critical thinking needed for the clinical experiences in the third and fourth years.

The third year features six 8-week required clerkships in internal medicine, surgery, child health, psychiatry/neurology, obstetrics and gynecology, and family medicine. The fourth year has three 8-week required advanced clinical selectives from a surgical area, a medical area and one other selective. Also required in the fourth year are 8 weeks of advanced biomedical science and 12 weeks of general electives. Students with an interest in rural practice some of their third-year clerkships, fourth-year clinical selectives and general electives at a rural clinical center. Students with a special interest in biomedical research follow the physician-scholar track by engaging in guided research in the basic sciences including summer research experiences, a post-sophomore fellowship and using fourth-year electives and selectives for research leading to a graduate degree.

The School of Medicine uses a multilevel grading system with satisfactory/unsatisfactory in the first year, honors/satisfactory, unsatisfactory in the second year and honors/letter of commendation/satisfactory/unsatisfactory in the third and fourth years.

Students must pass the USMLE Step 1 prior to their fourth year and Step 2 to graduate.

## REQUIREMENTS FOR ENTRANCE

Applicants are required to take the new MCAT (1993 or later preferred) and to have earned a minimum of 90 semester hours (exclusive of physical education and military science) from a recognized college or university. Nearly all successful applicants will have completed a bachelor's degree. Specific courses required for admission are:

|  | *Sem.* |
| --- | --- |
| English composition | 2 |
| May include writing-intensive courses. | |
| College-level math or calculus | 1 |

|  | *Hrs.* |
| --- | --- |
| General biology (with lab) | 8 |
| Inorganic chemistry (with lab) | 8 |

Organic chemistry (with lab) . . . . . . . . . . . . . . . . . . . . . . 8
General physics (with lab) . . . . . . . . . . . . . . . . . . . . . . . 8

Because medical training requires a rigorous background in the sciences, only those courses required for science majors may be used to meet the admissions requirements; introductory survey courses are not acceptable. A course in biochemistry is strongly recommended. Applicants are also strongly encouraged to pursue a broad-based education, including courses in the humanities, social sciences, and oral and written communication. The entering class typically shows a wide range of undergraduate fields of concentration.

## SELECTION FACTORS

The Committee on Admisssions is composed of faculty members, community physicians, and medical students. Strong selection preference is given to Missouri residents.

Personal interviews are required for admission. Selection for interview is based upon academic performance, MCAT scores, the AMCAS application, and letters of recommendation. Both academic qualifications and nonacademic attributes are important in the admission process. The committee assesses such personal characteristics as maturity, motivation, social concern, leadership ability, and commitment. Demographic factors may be considered.

Successful applicants for the 1995 entering class had the following credentials: *mean science GPA,* 3.6; *mean GPA,* 3.6; *undergraduate major,* 68 percent in sciences; *sex,* 49 percent women; *minorities,* 2 percent; *Early Decision Program acceptance,* 11 percent; *overall acceptance rate,* 122 acceptances were offered to obtain a class of 96.

The School of Medicine participates in the Early Decision Program (EDP) with eligibility requirements reviewed annually by the Admissions Committee. Potential EDP applicants are encouraged to call for updated requirements before application.

The School of Medicine does not discriminate on the basis of race, sex, creed, national origin, age, handicap, religion, or status as a Vietnam-era veteran in the admission or access to or treatment or employment in its programs and activities.

## FINANCIAL AID

Students are admitted to the School of Medicine without regard to financial circumstances. After acceptance, prospective students are mailed the necessary forms to complete the financial aid process. The school participates in the federal scholarship and loan programs. The institutional scholarship program is primarily need-based. Institutional long-term loans are available to third- and fourth-year students. The school also operates an emergency short-term loan program for all grade levels. For more information, contact the School of Medicine Financial Aid Office at (314) 882-2923.

## INFORMATION FOR MINORITIES

The University of Missouri is committed to the recruitment and education of minority, disadvantaged, and nontraditional applicants. The School of Medicine annually sponsors summer programs for minority high school students and for minority undergraduate students interested in health care professions.

---

Public Institution

### APPLICATION AND ACCEPTANCE POLICIES FOR 1997–98 FIRST-YEAR CLASS

*School participates in AMCAS. See Chapter 4.*

Filing of AMCAS application
　　Earliest date: June 1, 1996
　　Latest date: Nov. 1, 1996
School application fee: None
Oldest MCAT scores considered: 1993
Does have Early Decision Program (EDP)
　　For Missouri residents only (some exceptions)
　　EDP application period: June 1–Aug. 1, 1996
　　EDP applicants notified by: Oct. 1, 1996
Acceptance notice to regular applicants
　　Earliest date: Dec. 15, 1996
　　Latest date: Varies
Applicant's response to acceptance offer
　　Maximum time: 2 weeks
Requests for deferred entrance considered: Yes
Deposit to hold place in class (applied to tuition):
　　$100, due with response to acceptance offer
Deposit refundable prior to: May 15, 1997
Estimated number of new entrants: 96 (10 EDP)
Starting date: Aug. 1997

### TUITION AND STUDENT FEES PER YEAR FOR 1995–96 FIRST-YEAR CLASS

Tuition　　　　　　　　　　Student fees: $528
　　Resident: $13,216
　　Nonresident: $26,579

### INFORMATION ON 1995–96 FIRST-YEAR CLASS

| Number of | In-State | Out-of-State | Total |
|---|---|---|---|
| Applicants | 572 | 761 | 1,333 |
| Applicants Interviewed | 258 | 3 | 260 |
| New Entrants* | 91 | 1 | 92 |

*91% had baccalaureate degrees; 88% took the MCAT.

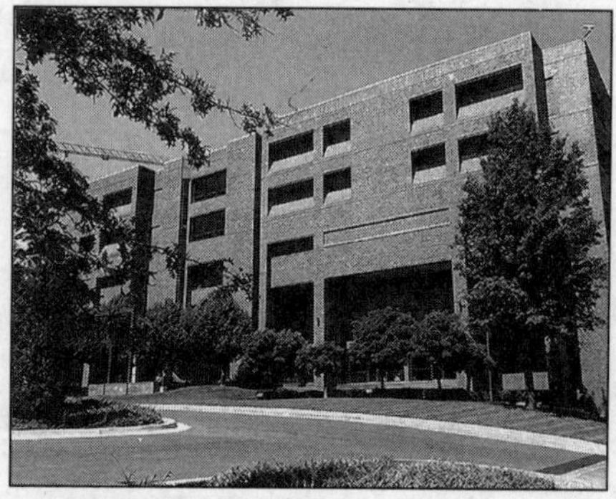

# University of Missouri—Kansas City School of Medicine

**Kansas City, Missouri**

Dr. James J. Mongan, *Dean*
Melvin Tyler, *Director of Admissions*
Patrick McTee, *Director of Student Financial Aid*

## ADDRESS INQUIRIES TO:

Council on Selection
University of Missouri—Kansas City
School of Medicine
2411 Holmes
Kansas City, Missouri 64108
(816) 235-1870; 235-5277 (FAX)
Web Site: http://research.med.umkc.edu

## GENERAL INFORMATION

The Board of Curators of the University of Missouri authorized the establishment of a medical school at the University of Missouri—Kansas City in 1969. Located on a 135-acre Hospital Hill campus, the medical school is near both the schools and colleges of the university and affiliated community hospitals.

## CURRICULUM

The School of Medicine, in combination with the College of Arts and Sciences and the School of Biological Sciences, offers a year-round program leading to baccalaureate and M.D. degrees in six calendar years. The student is required to complete both degrees and has the freedom to major in any department of the School of Biological Sciences or the College of Arts and Sciences.

*The program is designed primarily for high school seniors who are entering college.* They are permitted to obtain 30 semester hours of credit through the advanced placement program or the CLEP subject area examinations. To receive the baccalaureate degree, the student must complete 120 semester hours of credit.

The fundamental objective of the program is to provide students with a broad liberal arts education and to prepare physicians who are committed to providing comprehensive health care.

Under the guidance of a clinician-scholar, called a docent, small groups of first- and second-year students are introduced to medicine in several community hospitals where they can observe patients and their problems.

During the first two years of the program, the student is occupied predominantly with arts and sciences course work, with about one-fourth of the time being devoted to introduction to medicine courses. After these two years the student

advances, with the approval of the Council on Evaluation, to Year 3 of the six-year program.

During the last four years of the curriculum the student, with guidance from a docent and education assistant, plans a program for meeting the curriculum requirements. Two months of each year are spent with the docent unit on an inpatient internal medicine rotation. The remaining eight or nine months are spent in a number of other required and elective course offerings in the basic and clinical sciences and the humanities and social sciences. Students spend two academic terms in arts and sciences course work during the last four years of the program.

Basic, clinical, and behavioral science information is presented and emphasized throughout the six-year program. Thus, each student is expected to acquire a firm and broad base of information in each of these major content areas.

The academic program provides the medical student with a realistic working knowledge of community health problems and resources. The school provides an environment for learning medicine which is enhanced by the strong student support system.

An alternative path is available for extended study, and a combined eight-year baccalaureate-M.D.-Ph.D. degree program is open to a small number of highly qualified individuals.

## REQUIREMENTS FOR ENTRANCE

Applicants for admission to Year 1 of the six-year baccalaureate-medical program must meet the admission requirements of both the University of Missouri—Kansas City and the School of Medicine. Applicants must graduate from an accredited U.S. high school and demonstrate the ability to perform successfully at the college level, based on a combination of high school rank and scores on the American College Test (ACT).

A student admitted to the combined program at UMKC is expected to meet the following high school course requirements (one unit equals one year in class): four units of English; four units of mathematics; three units of science, including one unit of biology and one unit of chemistry; three units of social studies; one unit of fine arts; two units of a single foreign language; and one-half unit of computer science. Applicants are strongly encouraged to pursue an extensive and challenging course of study.

Only a limited number of positions become available at levels above the first year of the program. *Applications to the Year-3 level will be considered only from applicants who have a baccalaureate or advanced degree and are residents of Missouri or adjacent counties of Kansas.*

## SELECTION FACTORS

The criteria for selection are:

1. Applicant's academic potential is judged by quality of high school courses, rank in high school class and scores on the ACT. In the 1995–96 entering class, the average ACT score fell at the 93rd percentile, and the average rank in class was at the 93rd percentile.

2. Personal qualities evaluated include maturity, leadership, stamina, reliability, motivation for medicine, range of interests, interpersonal skills, compassion, and job experience.

The Council on Selection carefully reviews all applicants to this program. Applicants who appear to be well qualified are invited for interviews at the medical school campus. If invited, the applicant is notified in writing and will be required to be present at the scheduled date and time of the interview.

Students are considered on the basis of their individual qualifications without regard to race, creed, sex, or national origin. Since we are a combined B.A.-M.D. program we do not accept transfer students.

## FINANCIAL AID

There is a variety of financial assistance available to all medical students. Further information and applications for financial aid may be obtained from: Student Financial Aid Office, University of Missouri—Kansas City, 4825 Troost Avenue, Kansas City, Missouri 64110. Application should be made prior to March 15 of the year for which the student is applying.

## INFORMATION FOR MINORITIES

The University of Missouri—Kansas City offers assistance to disadvantaged students. Further information is available from Dr. Reaner Shannon, director, Office of Minority Affairs, or Kim Huggett, coordinator, Council on Selection, University of Missouri—Kansas City School of Medicine.

---

Public Institution

## APPLICATION AND ACCEPTANCE POLICIES FOR 1997–98 FIRST-YEAR CLASS

*Year 1 of six-year program.*

Filing of application
    Earliest date: Aug. 1, 1996
    Latest date: Nov. 15, 1996
School application fee to all applicants: $25 (in-state)
    $50 (out-of-state)
Does not have Early Decision Program
Acceptance notice to regular applicants
    Earliest date: Apr. 1, 1997
    Latest date: Varies
Applicant's response to acceptance offer
    Maximum time: by May 1, 1997
Requests for deferred entrance considered: No
Deposit to hold place in class (applied to tuition):
    $100, due with response to acceptance offer
    Deposit refundable prior to: May 15, 1997
Estimated number of new entrants: 100
Starting date: Aug. 1997

## TUITION AND STUDENT FEES PER YEAR FOR 1995–96 FIRST-YEAR CLASS

Tuition*                     Student fees: $480
    Resident: $12,460
    Nonresident: $25,654

## INFORMATION ON 1995–96 FIRST-YEAR CLASS

| Number of | In-State | Out-of-State | Total |
|---|---|---|---|
| Applicants | 419 | 348 | 767 |
| Applicants Interviewed | 276 | 89 | 365 |
| New Entrants | 87 | 17 | 104 |

*These figures apply to Year 1 of the six-year program.

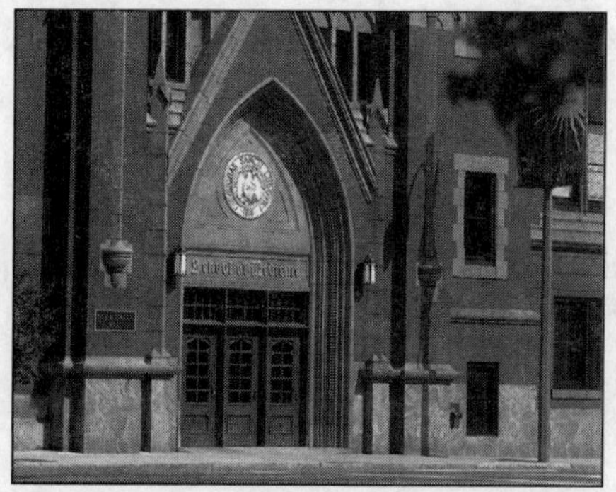

# Saint Louis University School of Medicine

## St. Louis, Missouri


Dr. Patricia Monteleone, *Dean*
Dr. William C. Mootz, *Acting Dean of Admissions*
Mary B.W. Fenton, *Assistant Dean, Student Financial Planning*


## ADDRESS INQUIRIES TO:

Nancy McPeters
Admissions Committee
Saint Louis University
School of Medicine
1402 South Grand Boulevard
St. Louis, Missouri 63104
(314) 577-8205; 577-8214 (FAX)

## GENERAL INFORMATION

Saint Louis University is a privately endowed, coeducational institution founded by the Jesuits in 1818. The first faculty of medicine was appointed in 1836, and the school assumed its general present form in 1903. Today the Saint Louis University School of Medicine includes the University Hospital, the School of Medicine (Schwitalla Hall, Doisy Medical Research Facility, and Margaret McCormick Doisy Learning Resources Center), Firmin Desloge Towers, Bordley Pavilion, David P. Wohl Memorial Mental Health Institute, Cardinal Glennon Hospital for Children, SLU-Anheuser Busch Eye Institute, Doctors' Office Building, Institute of Molecular Virology, School of Nursing, and School of Allied Health. Major teaching affiliations include Deaconess Medical Center, DePaul Medical Center, St. John's Mercy Medical Center, St. Mary's Health Center, and the St. Louis Veterans Administration hospitals.

## CURRICULUM

The school builds its clinical training offerings upon a rigorous grounding in the fundamental basic sciences of medicine. Thus, the M.D. degree curriculum follows the classical structure of two years devoted largely to a complete exposure to the basic and behavioral sciences, with problem-solving and clinical correlation, followed by two years of both structured and elective experiences in the clinical disciplines of medicine. The objective is to graduate a humanistic physician who is well qualified to embark upon postgraduate training in a selected discipline, but with a base of fundamental knowledge from which to conduct a lifetime of learning. Distinctive aspects of the program include:

1. Multidepartmentally oriented courses in medical communication skills, human sexuality, nutrition, emergency medicine, and working with dying patients and their families.

2. Novel use of a clinical simulation complex, which affords medical students a systematic and controlled introduction to virtually all of the skills required of them in the clinical phase of their education. The Crimmins Complex is used in the physical diagnosis course for sophomore medical students, in the medical communication skills courses, and by individual undergraduate medical students and residents for independent study.

3. Multiple clinical training sites offering a variety of patients from different social backgrounds.

4. A flexible senior year enabling students to design a significant portion of their program in collaboration with faculty advisers. National and international elective experiences are available to the senior medical student.

5. Opportunity to participate in a combined M.D.-Ph.D. program, in which qualified medical students undertake graduate studies leading to the Ph.D. in one of the basic science disciplines. Students interested in research may opt to receive the M.D. with distinction in research degree.

## REQUIREMENTS FOR ENTRANCE

Saint Louis University School of Medicine encourages applications from students who have demonstrated a high level of academic achievement and who manifest in their personal lives those human qualities which are required for a career of service to society. Specific academic requirements include the MCAT and a minimum of 90 semester hours (135 quarter hours) in undergraduate arts and science courses. Most accepted applicants complete a baccalaureate degree of at least 120 semester hours (180 quarter hours) from an accredited college or university. Specific course requirements are:

|  | Sem. hrs. |
| --- | --- |
| General biology or zoology (with lab) | 8 |
| Inorganic chemistry (with lab) | 8 |
| Organic chemistry (with lab) | 8 |
| Physics (with lab) | 8 |
| English | 6 |
| Other humanities and behavioral sciences | 12 |

Biochemistry is strongly recommended.

Applicants are expected to have pursued one area of knowledge or discipline in depth. The Admissions Committee does not favor any specific major in its decisions.

Suitable areas of concentration include the behavioral sciences, humanities, and natural sciences.

## SELECTION FACTORS

The selection of candidates is based upon demonstrated intellectual ability and personal qualifications, including motivation, character, emotional maturity, stability, and personality. There is no discrimination on the basis of race, color, sex, age, national origin, religion, sexual orientation, disability, or veteran status. All university policies, practices, and procedures are administered in a manner consistent with our Catholic Jesuit identity. There are no geographical restrictions or quotas for American citizens. All applicants receive serious consideration, and some additional attention is given to applicants from Saint Louis University.

Students for the 1995 entering class had the following average academic credentials: *SMGPA,* 3.64; *overall GPA,* 3.66; *mean MCAT Scores,* VR-9.8, PS-10.0, BS-10.2, WS-Q; *sex,* 36 percent women; *residence,* 28 percent from Missouri, 27 states represented; *undergraduate major,* 60 percent in life sciences, 18 percent in chemistry.

## FINANCIAL AID

Loan and scholarship aid is available and is awarded on the basis of financial need. Information on the financial status of parents is required of all students seeking "university aid." Primary responsibility for arranging the financing of medical education rests with the students or their families.

A financial aid information packet is sent to all accepted applicants. This packet contains the need analysis form, suggestions on aid, explanation of federal programs, and the application form for financial assistance from Saint Louis University.

## INFORMATION FOR MINORITIES

The School of Medicine seeks to obtain a better representation of all minority groups that are significantly underrepresented in the medical profession and of the African-American group, in particular. All minority students are encouraged to apply.

Private Institution

## APPLICATION AND ACCEPTANCE POLICIES FOR 1997–98 FIRST-YEAR CLASS

*School participates in AMCAS. See Chapter 4.*

Filing of AMCAS application
   Earliest date: June 1, 1996
   Latest date: Dec. 15, 1996
School application fee to all applicants: $100
Oldest MCAT scores considered: 1992
Does have Early Decision Program (EDP)
   EDP application period: June 1–Aug. 1, 1996
   EDP applicants notified by: Oct. 1, 1996
Acceptance notice to regular applicants
   Earliest date: Oct. 15, 1996
   Latest date: Until class is filled
Applicant's response to acceptance offer
   Maximum time: 2 weeks
Requests for deferred entrance considered: Yes
Deposit to hold place in class (applied to tuition):
   $100, due with response to acceptance offer
Deposit refundable prior to: May 15, 1997
Estimated number of new entrants: 151 (8 EDP)
Starting date: Aug. 1997

## TUITION AND STUDENT FEES PER YEAR FOR 1995–96 FIRST-YEAR CLASS

Tuition: $24,200        Student fees: $1,024

## INFORMATION ON 1995–96 FIRST-YEAR CLASS

| *Number of* | *In-State* | *Out-of-State* | *Total* |
|---|---|---|---|
| Applicants | 398 | 4,909 | 5,307 |
| Applicants Interviewed | 184 | 1,146 | 1,330 |
| New Entrants* | 42 | 110 | 152 |

*All took the MCAT and had baccalaureate degrees.

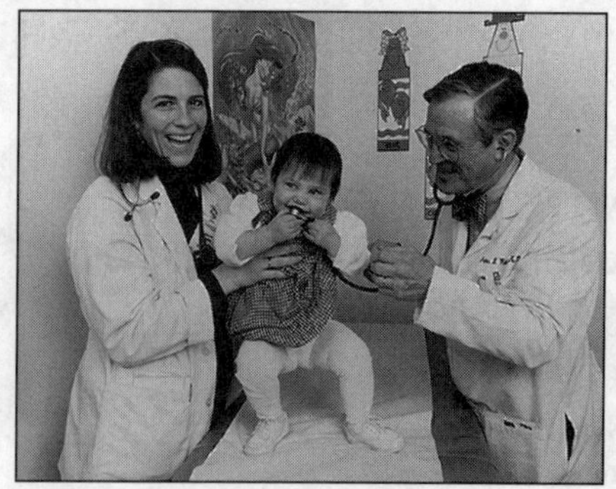

# Washington University School of Medicine

**St. Louis, Missouri**

Dr. William A. Peck, *Dean and Vice-Chancellor for Medical Affairs*
Dr. W. Edwin Dodson, *Associate Dean for Admissions*
John F. Walters, *Assistant Dean and Director of Financial Aid*

## ADDRESS INQUIRIES TO:

Office of Admissions
Washington University
School of Medicine
660 South Euclid Avenue, #8107
St. Louis, Missouri 63110
(314) 362-6857; 362-4658 (FAX)
E-Mail: wumscoa@molly.wustl.edu
Web Site: http://medschool.wustl.edu/admissions/

## GENERAL INFORMATION

In 1891, the Saint Louis Medical College, which had been founded in 1842, became the Medical Department of Washington University. In 1899, the Missouri Medical College, which had been in operation since 1840, joined Washington University, thus uniting the two oldest medical schools west of the Mississippi River as the Medical Department of Washington University.

Clinical teaching facilities are provided by Barnes-Jewish Hospital and St. Louis Children's Hospital, both located in the Washington University Medical Center, with a total capacity of 2,071 patient beds. Other teaching facilities include St. Louis Regional Medical Center, John Cochran Veterans Administration Medical Center, Malcolm Bliss Mental Health Center, Ellis Fischel Cancer Center, and Shriners Hospital for Crippled Children. Since 1993, the medical school has been affiliated with BJC Health System, the largest academically-linked health care system in the country.

Basic science teaching facilities are located in the lecture halls and multidisciplinary laboratories of the McDonnell Medical Sciences Building. The Clinical Sciences Research Building houses research laboratories for the school's clinical departments, the Howard Hughes Institute, and elaborate animal care facilities.

## CURRICULUM

The curriculum provides students with a stimulating education, both in the science and the art of clinical medicine. Instruction is by lecture, small-group interactive sessions with faculty, including problem-based exercises and self-directed learning using computers and other resources led by faculty facilitators. Medical humanities and ethics are integrated into the four years of medical training. Throughout the curriculum, serious consideration is given to the sociological and cultural concerns of the patient and to the necessity of adapting medical care to their needs.

Patient contact begins in the first semester of the first year. Courses address the broad issues of normal structure and function of humans with emphasis on neuroscience, cell biology, and genetics. The effect of disease on bodily structure and function characterize the second-year curriculum. Expanded clinical experience is integrated with course work in pathology, pathophysiology, and pharmacology. Core clinical clerkships occupy the entire third year with increasing emphasis on ambulatory medicine. The fourth year is a full year of electives planned and selected by the student with faculty guidance.

For students who care to participate, there are abundant opportunities to engage in basic and clinical research through summer research fellowships and research electives. A five-year M.A. and M.D. degrees program is available for students desiring a full year of research training. A six-year Medical Scientist Training Program permits students seeking a career in academic medicine to obtain both M.D. and Ph.D. degrees. Much of the basic research in the school is conducted under the aegis of the division of biology and biomedical sciences. Formed over two decades ago, this multi- departmental collaboration recognizes that the intellectual substance of scientific pursuit transcends the traditional departmental structure found in many other medical schools.

A tutorial program is available to any student in the school who needs academic assistance. A pass/fail grading system is used in the first year; an honors/high pass/pass/fail grading system is used thereafter.

## REQUIREMENTS FOR ENTRANCE

Accepted applicants must present evidence of superior intellectual ability and achievement, completion of at least 90 semester hours of course work in an approved college or university, satisfactory performance on the MCAT, and attributes necessary for a productive career in medicine.

Mathematics, physics, and chemistry provide the tools for modern biology, medicine, and the biological basis of patient care. Accordingly, premedical education should include a minimum of the following courses:

|  | *Years* |
|---|---|
| Biological science | 1 |
| General or inorganic chemistry | 1 |

Organic chemistry . . . . . . . . . . . . . . . . . . . . . . . . . . . . . . 1
Physics . . . . . . . . . . . . . . . . . . . . . . . . . . . . . . . . . . . . . . 1
Mathematics . . . . . . . . . . . . . . . . . . . . . . . . . . . . . . . . . . 1
Through differential and integral calculus.

Prerequisites are subject to waiver by the Committee on Admissions. The development of the intellectual talents of an individual often involves the in-depth pursuit of some areas of knowledge in humanities, social sciences, or natural sciences. A diversified background of cultural development is encouraged.

## SELECTION FACTORS

Students are selected on the basis of character, attitude, interest, intellectual ability, motivation, maturity, and past achievement as indicated both by superior scholastic work and active participation in extracurricular activities prior to entering medical school. Washington University policies and programs are nondiscriminatory, and full consideration is given to all applicants without regard to sex, age, race, handicap, sexual preference, creed, or national or ethnic origin. Minority group students are strongly encouraged to apply.

Students in the 1995 entering class had the following credentials: *mean science GPA,* 3.77; *mean nonscience GPA,* 3.80; *mean total GPA,* 3.78; *mean MCAT scores—VR-*10.7, *PS-*11.8, *BS-*11.7; *sex,* 51 percent women; *undergraduate major,* 38 percent in biological sciences or preprofessional studies, 23 percent in chemistry or biochemistry, 12 percent in physics or engineering, 27 percent in a variety of other fields of study.

Early submission of the AMCAS application permits its prompt evaluation by the Committee on Admissions. All applicants are invited to complete their application with letters of evaluation and additional personal information. Selected applicants are invited for interview. All accepted applicants are interviewed.

## FINANCIAL AID

The financial resources of an applicant do not enter into the admission selection process. Immediately upon notification of acceptance, the applicant may file for consideration for financial aid. An award decision is usually made within two weeks following receipt of the completed forms. Awards are based on documented financial need and consist of both scholarships and loans.

## INFORMATION FOR MINORITIES

The school is committed to the recruitment, enrollment, education, and graduation of an increased number of individuals from underrepresented groups. For information write to the director of minority medical student admissions.

Private Institution

## APPLICATION AND ACCEPTANCE POLICIES FOR 1997–98 FIRST-YEAR CLASS

*School participates in AMCAS. See Chapter 4.*

Filing of AMCAS application
    Earliest date: June 1, 1996
    Latest date: Nov. 15, 1996
School application fee to all applicants: $50
Oldest MCAT scores considered: 1994
Does not have Early Decision Program
Acceptance notice to regular applicants
    Earliest date: Oct. 15, 1996
    Latest date: Until class is filled
Applicant's response to acceptance offer
    Maximum time: 2 weeks
Requests for deferred entrance considered: Yes
Deposit to hold place in class (applied to tuition):
    $100, due with response to acceptance offer
Deposit refundable prior to: May 15, 1997
Estimated number of new entrants: 120
Starting date: Aug. 1997

## TUITION AND STUDENT FEES PER YEAR FOR 1995–96 FIRST-YEAR CLASS

Tuition: $25,170          Student fees: None

## INFORMATION ON 1995–96 FIRST-YEAR CLASS

| Number of | In-State | Out-of-State | Total |
|---|---|---|---|
| Applicants | 301 | 6,713 | 7,014 |
| Applicants Interviewed | 59 | 914 | 973 |
| New Entrants* | 12 | 110 | 122 |

*All took the MCAT and had baccalaureate degrees.

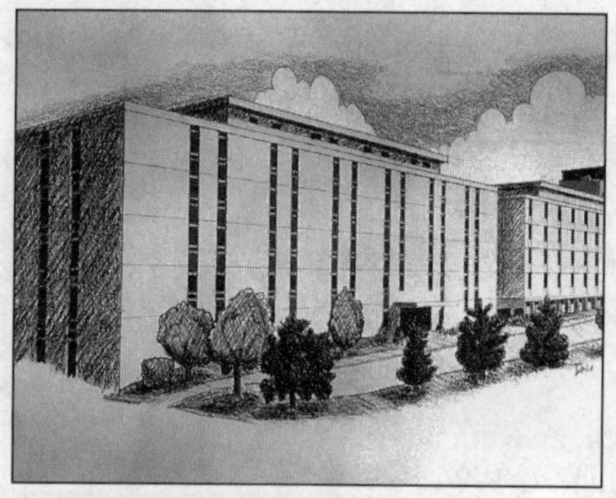

# Creighton University School of Medicine

## Omaha, Nebraska

Dr. Thomas J. Cinque, *Dean*
James L. Glass, *Director, Medical School Admissions*
Tanya T. Avant, *Financial Aid Coordinator*

## ADDRESS INQUIRIES TO:

Office of Admissions
Creighton University School of Medicine
2500 California Plaza
Omaha, Nebraska 68178
(402) 280-2798; 280-1241 (FAX)

## GENERAL INFORMATION

The Creighton University School of Medicine, a Jesuit institution, was opened 100 years ago in October 1892, 14 years after the opening of the parent university. Its plant includes four units that provide all facilities for research, basic science, and preclinical teaching. St. Joseph's Hospital, accommodating 403 patients, is the principal teaching hospital of the medical school. Clinical instruction is also carried out in the Children's Memorial, Veterans Administration, and Bergan Mercy hospitals. Clinical services are also conducted at several other area hospitals and the Boys Town Institute for Communication Disorders in Children. The Bio-Information Center, located on the west campus north of the hospital, contains a multimedia self-instructional component, a biomedical communication center, an educational services unit, and the traditional library facilities.

## CURRICULUM

A new curriculum, designed for the twenty-first century is being introduced in the summer of 1996. The educational program will be divided into four components. Component One, Biomedical Fundamentals, will serve as the foundation of the educational program followed by more complex basic science information presented in a clinically relevant context in Component Two. This component will consist of a series of organ-based and disease-based courses. Component Three consists of redesigned required core clerkships emphasizing basic medical principles, primary care, and preventive medicine. Component Four will provide additional responsibilities for patient care and a 12-week block of critical care medicine; the 24 weeks of electives will provide subinternship experience and at least four weeks of an implied in-depth basic science experience. Clinical experience will be a prominent part of the curriculum in all components, beginning with the physical diagnosis instruction in the first year and with students assigned to longitudinal clinic throughout the curriculum. The curriculum will also integrate ethical and societal issues into all four components. Instructional methodology will utilize case-based small-group sessions, and computer assisted instruction in all components. A close faculty/student relationship provides for mentoring and advising of students in choosing courses that will broaden their background for a career in medicine, as well as satisfying their special interest. Competency-base evaluation is used in all components, and the students are graded on a pass/fail/honors system.

## REQUIREMENTS FOR ENTRANCE

The MCAT and three years (at least 90 semester hours) of accredited college work are mandatory. Preference is given, however, to holders of the baccalaureate degree. Applicants may take the MCAT in the fall of the year preceding their entry into medical school. All requirements for admission must be completed by June prior to entry. Course work must include:

*Sem. hrs.*

General biology (with lab). . . . . . . . . . . . . . . . . . . . . . . . . . . 8
Inorganic chemistry (with lab). . . . . . . . . . . . . . . . . . . . . . . . 8
Organic chemistry (with lab) . . . . . . . . . . . . . . . . . . . . . 8-10
General physics (with lab). . . . . . . . . . . . . . . . . . . . . . . . . . 8
English . . . . . . . . . . . . . . . . . . . . . . . . . . . . . . . . . . . . . . . . 6

Although no additional science courses are required, applicants may pursue a baccalaureate program with a science major or with a major in any field of liberal arts (except for military science) appropriate to their interest, such as English, foreign language, history, political science, or sociology. Up to 27 hours of credit are accepted under CLEP and/or advanced placement programs.

## SELECTION FACTORS

Consideration will be given to all of the qualities considered to be necessary in a physician. Intellectual ability and curiosity, emotional maturity, honesty, and proper motivation, in addition to proven scholastic ability, are of the utmost importance. The preprofessional committee evaluations and letters of recommendation are equally important.

The school reserves the right to require a formal interview of every applicant selected before it finalizes the acceptance. The interview usually will be held on the university campus.

There are no restrictions placed on applicants because of race, religion, sex, national or ethnic origin, age, handicap, or status as a disabled veteran or veteran of the Vietnam era. Candidates are not restricted by state of residence, but preference is given to students from states that do not have medical schools. Preference is also given to applicants who have undertaken their preprofessional education at Creighton University.

Because the cumulative and science GPAs of the 112 candidates selected for the 1995 entering class were 3.67 and 3.49, respectively, it is suggested that no candidate apply whose GPA in either situation is below 3.5. Other characteristics of the 1995 entering class were: *sex*, 32 percent women; *undergraduate major*, 85 percent in science.

The AMCAS application is the principal source of information on the candidates. Additional information is requested upon receipt of the AMCAS form.

## FINANCIAL AID

In addition to federally insured student loan programs and funds available from major foundation grants, a limited number of scholarships and fellowships are available for upperclassmen and for a few well qualified entering students. Scholarship aid is awarded primarily on the basis of personal financial need.

Approximately 87 percent of the students receive some form of financial aid during a part or all of their four years of study. Students are discouraged from accepting outside employment because of the lack of available time during a heavy academic schedule, but spouses of students usually have no difficulty in finding employment in the Omaha metropolitan area.

## INFORMATION FOR MINORITIES

Consideration is given to applications from American black, American Indian, Mexican American, and mainland Puerto Rican candidates. Special summer courses and tutorial services are available to the candidates should the need arise. The school application fee will be waived if AMCAS has first waived its charges. Financial aid in the form of grants and long-term loans is available on the basis of proven need.

---

Private Institution

## APPLICATION AND ACCEPTANCE POLICIES FOR 1997–98 FIRST-YEAR CLASS

*School participates in AMCAS. See Chapter 4.*

Filing of AMCAS application
    Earliest date: June 1, 1996
    Latest date: Dec. 1, 1996
School application fee to all applicants: $50
Oldest MCAT scores considered: 1993
Does have Early Decision Program (EDP)
    EDP application period: June 1–Aug. 1, 1996
    EDP applicants notified by: Oct. 1, 1996
Acceptance notice to regular applicants
    Earliest date: Oct. 1, 1996
    Latest date: Until class is filled
Applicant's response to acceptance offer
    Maximum time: 2 weeks
Requests for deferred entrance considered: Yes
Deposit to hold place in class (applied to tuition):
    $100, due with response to acceptance offer
Deposit refundable prior to: March 1, 1997
Estimated number of new entrants: 110 (20 EDP)
Starting date: Aug. 1997

## TUITION AND STUDENT FEES PER YEAR FOR 1995–96 FIRST-YEAR CLASS

Tuition: $23,434          Student fees: $402

## INFORMATION ON 1995–96 FIRST-YEAR CLASS

| Number of | In-State | Out-of-State | Total |
|---|---|---|---|
| Applicants | 273 | 8,799 | 9,072 |
| Applicants Interviewed | * | * | 455 |
| New Entrants† | 18 | 94 | 112 |

*Data not available.

†All took the MCAT and had baccalaureate degrees.

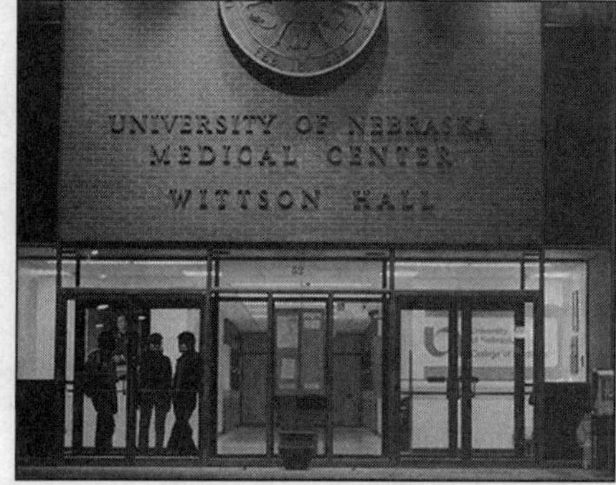

# University of Nebraska College of Medicine

**Omaha, Nebraska**

Dr. Harold M. Maurer, *Dean*
Dr. Jeffrey W. Hill, *Assistant Dean of Admissions*
Judith D. Walker, *Director of Financial Aid*

## ADDRESS INQUIRIES TO:

Office of Admissions
University of Nebraska College of Medicine
Room 5021 Wittson Hall
600 South 42nd Street
Omaha, Nebraska 68198-6585
(402) 559-6140; 559-6840 (FAX)
Web Site: http://www.unmc.edu/

## GENERAL INFORMATION

The University of Nebraska College of Medicine celebrated its centennial in the academic year 1980–81. Medical education has been continuous in Omaha since students first entered the Omaha Medical College in the fall of 1880.

The University of Nebraska Medical Center includes colleges of dentistry, medicine, nursing, and pharmacy, a school of allied health, University Hospital, University Outpatient Services, University Geriatric Center, Eppley Cancer Research Institute, and C. Louis Meyer Children's Rehabilitation Institute. These facilities are supplemented by direct teaching affiliations with the Veterans Hospital and eight private hospitals, two of which are on the medical center campus. Students, thus, have access to facilities with a total of approximately 2,800 teaching beds. Preceptorships in family practice are conducted in 69 locations in all parts of the state.

## CURRICULUM

The goal of the College of Medicine is to develop the knowledge and skills that foster attitudes appropriate for doctors of medicine. The college provides a sound basis for support of career choices in medical practice, teaching, research, or administration by stimulating students to obtain a background of basic information, a command of the language of biomedical science, a mastery of the skills necessary for clinical problem-solving, a habit of self-education, and a sympathetic understanding of the behavior of healthy and sick people. The college is particularly oriented toward training physicians to meet all the health care needs of the citizens of Nebraska.

A new integrated curriculum was introduced for students starting in the fall 1992 (graduating class of 1996). The goals are as follows: (1) Increase the number of primary care physicians for the state of Nebraska; (2) Continue to develop competency in biomedical science; (3) Encourage a balance between the acquisition of knowledge and the development of professional attitudes and skills; (4) Cultivate a learning atmosphere that encourages enthusiasm, altruism, idealism, and professional behavior; (5) Develop an appropriate balance between didactic and self-directed learning; (6) Encourage a teaching approach that fosters lifelong learning skills and promotes intellectual curiosity; (7) Integrate more fully the subject materials and improve basic science/clinical correlations; and (8) Provide early exposure to patient care.

During the first two years students will be exposed to a mix of basic science and clinical subject material presented in integrated cores of material, rather than in the traditional presentation of courses by department (e.g., anatomy, biochemistry). A significant emphasis on problem-solving situations will complement the traditional didactic lecture format. From the first week of medical school, students will have an opportunity to work with patients in a supervised clinical setting. Ample free time has been set aside during the day so that students can do in-depth studies in particular areas or pursue other interests.

During the final two years, students have clinical exposures to various medical disciplines such as family medicine, internal medicine, pediatrics, surgery, psychiatry, and obstetrics-gynecology. This is supplemented by basic science correlations and selectives in basic science areas reinforcing the interrelationships of basic and clinical sciences.

A five point letter grading system (A, B, C, D, F) is used. For promotion, students must maintain a 2.0 average for the freshman and sophomore years and a 2.5 average for the junior and senior years.

## REQUIREMENTS FOR ENTRANCE

The MCAT and a minimum of 90 semester hours (three years of college work) in an accredited college are required. However, to provide an opportunity for in-depth study, the completion of a college major or baccalaureate degree is strongly recommended. The undergraduate program must include:

|  | *Sem. hrs.* |
| --- | --- |
| Biology (with lab) | 8–10 |
| General chemistry (with lab) | 8–10 |
| Organic chemistry (with lab) | 8–10 |
| Physics (with lab) | 8–10 |
| Humanities and/or social sciences | 12–16 |

Minimum of three or four courses.

Calculus or statistics
English composition or writing course

In addition to meeting specific requirements, applicants are encouraged to adopt an educational goal that includes exploring areas of personal interest. In view of the rapidly broadening scope of medicine, a well-rounded education is considered optimum preparation. The requirements are consistent with that belief.

## SELECTION FACTORS

Selection is based on a total assessment of each candidate's motivation, interests, character, demonstrated intellectual ability, previous academic record and its trends, personal interview, scores on the MCAT, and general fitness and promise for a career in medicine. Admission is based on individual qualifications without regard to age, sex, sexual preference, race, national origin, handicap, or religious or political beliefs. Academic credentials are evaluated on the basis of course level and load, involvement in cocurricular activities or employment, and other influential factors. Cutoff levels for GPAs or for scores on the MCAT are not utilized; however, applicants are reminded of the competition for entrance and are advised to be realistic. Personal attributes are assessed through letters of reference and in the interview.

Strong preference is given to residents of Nebraska, but a limited number of students from other states may be accepted. The University of Nebraska encourages, in particular, students from rural areas, small towns, or disadvantaged backgrounds to apply. The potential for service to underserved communities is taken into consideration during the preadmission evaluation.

Accepted students for the 1995 entering class had the following credentials: *mean* GPA, 3.63; *sex,* 38 percent women; *undergraduate major,* approximately 70 percent science majors.

## FINANCIAL AID

Some scholarships are available each year. A few may be granted to entering freshmen. Several fellowships and assistantships are available to students who desire to take one or two years of graduate study or research in the basic sciences. Loan funds have been increased through efforts of physicians in Nebraska, fraternal organizations, and friends of the college. Approximately 60 percent of the students receive some financial aid.

## INFORMATION FOR MINORITIES

The University of Nebraska College of Medicine is committed to increasing the number of physicians from ethnic groups presently underrepresented in the medical profession. Applications are encouraged from resident and nonresident black Americans, American Indians, mainland Puerto Ricans, and Mexican Americans. The accomplishments of applicants will be evaluated with due consideration given to their background. The college makes every effort to retain minority students. Specific information is available from the director of multicultural affairs.

Public Institution

## APPLICATION AND ACCEPTANCE POLICIES FOR 1997–98 FIRST-YEAR CLASS

*School participates in AMCAS. See Chapter 4.*

Filing of AMCAS application
 Earliest date: June 1, 1996
 Latest date: Nov. 15, 1996
School application fee to all applicants: $25
Oldest MCAT scores considered: 1991
Does not have Early Decision Program
Acceptance notice to regular applicants
 Earliest date: Jan. 3, 1997
 Latest date: Varies
Applicant's response to acceptance offer
 Maximum time: 2 weeks
Requests for deferred entrance considered: No
Deposit to hold place in class (applied to tuition):
 $100, due within 30 days of acceptance offer
Deposit refundable prior to: May 15, 1997
Estimated number of new entrants: 120
Starting date: Aug. 1997

## TUITION AND STUDENT FEES PER YEAR FOR 1995–96 FIRST-YEAR CLASS

Tuition                              Student fees: $1,141
 Resident: $10,500
 Nonresident: $20,300

## INFORMATION ON 1995–96 FIRST-YEAR CLASS

| Number of | In-State | Out-of-State | Total |
| --- | --- | --- | --- |
| Applicants | 399 | 1,255 | 1,654 |
| Applicants Interviewed | 399 | 45 | 444 |
| New Entrants* | 119 | 0 | 119 |

*All took the MCAT; 98% had baccalaureate degrees.

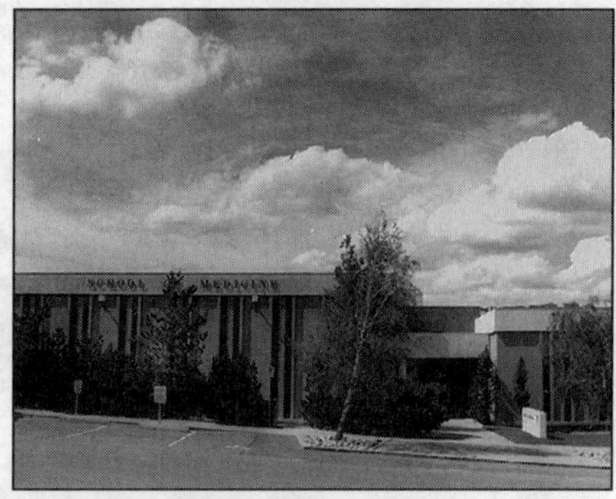

# University of Nevada School of Medicine

**Reno, Nevada**


Dr. Robert M. Daugherty, Jr., *Dean*
Dr. Jerry R. May, *Associate Dean for Admissions and Student Affairs*
Peggy Dupey, *Financial Aid Officer*


## ADDRESS INQUIRIES TO:


Office of Admissions and Student Affairs
University of Nevada
School of Medicine
Mail Stop 357
Reno, Nevada 89557
(702) 784-6063; 784-6096 (FAX)
E-Mail: ekirk@scs.unr.edu


## GENERAL INFORMATION

The University of Nevada School of Medicine is a state-supported, community-based, university-integrated school which relies heavily on community physicians as teachers and community health facilities as sites for the majority of its clinical education. The school is dedicated to selecting individuals with diverse backgrounds who will learn to be compassionate and competent physicians. Students study comprehensive health care delivery considering the needs of the individual, the family, and the community.

## CURRICULUM

The first two years of the program are concentrated in classrooms and laboratories on the Reno campus. The curriculum emphasizes biomedical and behavioral sciences basic to medicine. Basic science disciplines are often integrated with each other and with clinical problems to promote the learning of problem-solving skills. Also, a clinical correlation course which explores the basics of biomedical ethics is taught.

In addition to courses in community health, anatomy, behavioral sciences, microbiology, biochemistry, pharmacology, physiology, cell biology, and pathology, students learn the basic physician skills of interviewing, obtaining a medical history, and performing a physical examination on patients. Throughout the first and second years, students spend time with a physician to observe medical practice in the office setting and clinic settings.

There are also opportunities to participate in basic and clinical science research. The third and fourth years of the curriculum include experiences in community hospitals and physicians' offices in family medicine, internal medicine, obstetrics and gynecology, pediatrics, psychiatry, and surgery. These two years concentrate on the major clinical specialties of medicine and are a combination of required rotations and elective time. Rotations and electives are offered in Reno, Las Vegas, and rural Nevada; ample opportunity for elective experience out of state also exists.

Individualized M.D.-Ph.D. programs are offered to students, depending upon the specific interest area.

One mission of the school is to train primary care physicians for the state of Nevada. Curricular changes that give students early exposure to physicians in family medicine, general internal medicine, and general pediatrics are being initiated. In addition, clinical problem solving will be correlated with the basic science course work and ambulatory based primary care experiences. Ambulatory care will continue to be a focus throughout the clinical curriculum.

## REQUIREMENTS FOR ENTRANCE

The MCAT and a minimum of three years of college work (90 semester hours) are required. The MCAT must be taken prior to the November 1 application deadline. The Admissions Selection Committee strongly recommends completion of a baccalaureate degree prior to matriculation in medical school.

Applicants are encouraged to have a broad educational background and to enroll in an in-depth course curriculum that will lead to a discipline-oriented major, e.g., biology, English, psychology. However, no specific major is favored over any other. In addition to academic course work, people-oriented activities and health care exposure are important.

Course work must include:

|  | *Sem. hrs.* |
| --- | --- |
| Biology | 12 |
| Must include 3 sem. hrs. of upper division credit. | |
| Inorganic chemistry | 8 |
| Organic chemistry | 8 |
| Physics | 8 |
| Behavioral Sciences | 6 |
| Must include 3 sem. hrs. of upper division credit. | |

In fulfillment of the behavioral sciences requirement students should take courses that deal with the psychological stages of the life cycle (e.g., human growth and development, adolescence, aging, human sexuality, abnormal psychology, family dynamics, or medically oriented sociology). Correspondence, CLEP, AP, and/or pass/fail or audit in lieu of a letter grade is not acceptable for the above required courses.

A demonstrated competency in English composition and expression is required. Generally, students are expected to satisfy the English composition requirements of their undergraduate institution.

Supplementary courses strongly recommended but not required for admission include history, literature, philosophy, ethics, and computer sciences.

Accepted students are responsible for completing all prerequisite course work prior to matriculation.

## SELECTION FACTORS

Candidates are evaluated on the basis of academic performance; results of the MCAT; the nature and depth of scholarly, extracurricular, and health care related activities during college years (excellence and balance of the natural sciences, social sciences, and humanities); academic letters of evaluation; and the personal interview, if requested by the Admissions Selection Committee. Interviews are held in Reno or Las Vegas.

A high priority is given to residents of Nevada. A small number of nonresident applicants are considered each year who have strong residential ties to Nevada (that is, parents' residence, medical catchment area) or residents of Alaska, Idaho, Montana, or Wyoming (western rural states without medical schools). Individuals who do not meet the residential requirements should not apply.

Matriculants for the 1995 entering class had the following profile: *undergraduate major,* 90 percent in science (includes premedical majors), with the remainder from a variety of majors; *mean age,* 24; *sex,* 40 percent female; *mean GPA,* 3.6; *mean MCAT,* 9.4.

The Admissions Selection Committee encourages applicants of both genders and from all socioeconomic, racial, religious, and educational backgrounds. Applications from members of minority groups are encouraged.

Transfer positions to the second and third years are based on availability. Applications will only be accepted from individuals in good standing from accredited U.S. medical schools and applicants who have a strong residential tie to Nevada. Applications will not be accepted from students attending foreign medical schools.

Resident and nonresident applications for the EDP are encouraged.

## FINANCIAL AID

A limited number of loans and scholarships are available to medical students. Awards are made on the basis of need and merit. More than 80 percent of Nevada's medical students receive some type of financial assistance.

## INFORMATION FOR MINORITIES

The School of Medicine is committed to the recruitment, selection, and retention of underrepresented minorities. Residents of the state of Nevada and individuals who meet the nonresident criteria who are from minority and disadvantaged backgrounds are encouraged to apply. A small number of scholarships are available for underrepresented minority students.

---

Public Institution

### APPLICATION AND ACCEPTANCE POLICIES FOR 1997–98 FIRST-YEAR CLASS

*School participates in AMCAS. See Chapter 4.*

Filing of AMCAS application
   Earliest date: June 1, 1996
   Latest date: Nov. 1, 1996
School application fee after screening: $45
Oldest MCAT scores considered: 1993
   Does have Early Decision Program (EDP)
   EDP application period: June 1–Aug. 1, 1996
   EDP applicants notified by: Oct. 1, 1996
Acceptance notice to regular applicants
   Earliest date: Jan. 15, 1997
   Latest date: Varies
Applicant's response to acceptance offer
   Maximum time: 2 weeks
Requests for deferred entrance considered: Yes
Deposit to hold place in class: None
Estimated number of new entrants: 52
Starting date: Aug. 1997

### TUITION AND STUDENT FEES PER YEAR FOR 1995–96 FIRST-YEAR CLASS

Tuition          Student fees: $1,894
   Resident: $6,821
   Nonresident: $17,976

### INFORMATION ON 1995–96 FIRST-YEAR CLASS

| Number of | In-State | Out-of-State | Total |
|---|---|---|---|
| Applicants | 241 | 981 | 1,222 |
| Applicants Interviewed | 172 | 28 | 200 |
| New Entrants* | 47 | 5 | 52 |

*All took the MCAT and had baccalaureate degrees.

# Dartmouth Medical School

**Hanover, New Hampshire**

Dr. Andrew G. Wallace, *Dean*
Susan Hart Malin, *Director of Admissions*
Nanci G. Cirone, *Director of Financial Aid*

## ADDRESS INQUIRIES TO:

Admissions
Dartmouth Medical School
7020 Remsen, Room 306
Hanover, New Hampshire 03755-3833
(603) 650-1505; 650-1614 (FAX)

## GENERAL INFORMATION

Dartmouth Medical School, the fourth oldest medical school in the United States, is a component of the Dartmouth-Hitchcock Medical Center (DHMC), which includes the Mary Hitchcock Memorial Hospital, the Norris Cotton Cancer Center, and the White River Junction (VT) Veterans Administration Hospital. The Lahey-Hitchcock Clinic, whose northern division is headquartered at DNMC, is the nation's third largest multi-specilty group practice. DHMC, a state-of-the-art facility located on a 225-acre campus, serves a patient population of 1.5 million people. It includes 429 beds in two five-story in-patient towers, a diagnostic and treatment center, an ambulatory care building, the cancer center, and the Borwell Research Building. Additional clinical teaching sites include the Brattleboro Retreat (VT), the Family Medical Institute of Augusta (ME), Martin Luther King Memorial Hospital in Los Angeles, Hartford Hospital (CT), the Tuba City Indian Health Service Hospital (AZ), and numerous primary care sites in Maine, New Hampshire, and Vermont. The C. Everett Koop Institute at Dartmouth was founded in 1992. Dr. Koop serves as the institute's senior scholar. A faculty of over 900 offers all students the opportunity for individually based instruction.

## CURRICULUM

Dartmouth's curriculum is currently undergoing revision, with changes to continue over the next several years. The "New Directions" curriculum is designed to integrate the study of basic and clinical sciences throughout medical school. The curriculum's hallmarks are longitudinal experiences in both the basic and clinical sciences, introduction to the ambulatory care setting in the earliest weeks of study, extended participation in small-group learning, close working relationships with faculty members, and increased opportunities for independent learning. The first year includes the Longitudinal Clinical Experience (LCE), a course that pairs students with faculty practitioners in local communities. Clinical training in the LCE alternates with biweekly, small-group tutorials on the DMS campus. A major course in the second year is the Scientific Basis of Medicine, an interdisciplinary pathophysiology course which integrates, through lectures, seminars, and problem-based learning, the basic sciences with a broad introduction to the mechanisms of disease and the principles of clinical medicine. In the third year, students begin a series of clinical clerkships in Inpatient and Outpatient Medicine, Inpatient and Outpatient Pediatrics, Inpatient and Outpatient OB/GYN, Inpatient Surgery and Surgical Selectives, Inpatient Psychiatry, and Outpatient Family Medicine. The fourth year includes a clerkship in Neurology plus four short courses (Clinical Pharmacology; Advanced Medical Sciences; Health, Society and the Physician; and Advance Cardiac Life Support), but is largely tailored to students' individual needs and interests through substantial elective opportunities.

Entering class size at Dartmouth is 86. Sixty-six students follow the four-year curriculum at DMS and receive the M.D. degree from Dartmouth. Up to twenty students, admitted jointly by Dartmouth and the Brown University School of Medicine, spend the first two years at Dartmouth and the last two years studying at Brown. The Brown-Dartmouth students are awarded the M.D. from Brown.

DMS offers an M.D.-Ph.D. program which provides a comprehensive academic, intellectual, and financially supportive environment enabling highly-qualified students to pursue an M.D. and a Ph.D. in any of the degree-granting departments of the medical school and the college. A joint M.D.-M.B.A. program is offered through DMS and Dartmouth's Amos Tuck School of Business Administration. In addition, graduate degrees are available through Dartmouth's Center for the Evaluative Clinical Sciences.

## REQUIREMENTS FOR ENTRANCE

Except in unusual circumstances, all candidates are expected to present MCAT scores. Where possible, the spring MCAT is recommended and helps the Admissions Committee to proceed expeditiously with the review of an application.

Specific courses required at college level are:

|  | *Sem. hrs.* |
| General biology | 8 |
| Inorganic chemistry | 8 |
| Organic chemistry | 8 |
| Physics | 8 |
| Calculus | 3 |

Proficiency in written and oral English is required. At least three years of study at a Canadian or American college or university is required.

In general, the demonstration of competence in an area of study is a more important criterion than the particular discipline. Hence, students are encouraged to major in the field of their special interest and, if possible, to pursue independent investigation in that field. Students majoring in nonsciences who have demonstrated ability in science are encouraged to apply.

## SELECTION FACTORS

The decision of the Admissions Committee depends on appraisal of the entire application, including a thorough evaluation of personal and intellectual qualifications. Rigid cutoff points and inflexible criteria are avoided. Individuals holding or working toward advanced degrees are selected by the same criteria as are other applicants. Dartmouth Medical School is a national institution enrolling students from across the country.

All applicants in the final group from which the class is chosen are interviewed in Hanover. A limited number of applicants are selected for interview and invited throughout the academic year.

It is the long-standing policy of Dartmouth Medical School to support equality of opportunity for all persons regardless of race or ethnic background, and no student shall be denied admission or financial aid or be otherwise discriminated against because of age, disability, race, creed, religion, sex, sexual orientation, or national origin.

Application for the Brown-Dartmouth program is initiated at Dartmouth. All applicants invited for interviews receive a form on which to indicate their program choices. In selecting applicants for the joint program, the admission policies and standards of both institutions are observed. Successful applicants are offered acceptance to only one program at a time. Letters of acceptance state the program to which the student has been admitted and are binding.

## FINANCIAL AID

Admission decisions are made without regard to financial need. All accepted applicants with documented need are offered financial aid packages which fully meet their need. Approximately three quarters of the students receive financial aid, usually as a combination of scholarship and loan or through federally supported service programs. Scholarships and loans are awarded on the basis of need as documented on the FAFSA, the Need Access form, and the DMS financial aid application (see Part 1).

Application fee waiver is granted to individuals who have received an AMCAS fee waiver. Applicants who are neither U.S. citizens nor permanent residents should be aware that financial support for foreign students is extremely limited.

## INFORMATION FOR MINORITIES

Applications from members of ethnic minority groups underrepresented in American medicine are encouraged. The number of minority students at DMS is growing: 18 percent of one of the current classes are members of underrepresented minority groups, although 10 or 12 percent has been more typical. Martha Regan-Smith, M.D., Ed.D. is assistant dean for minority affairs.

---

Private Institution

### APPLICATION AND ACCEPTANCE POLICIES FOR 1997–98 FIRST-YEAR CLASS

*School participates in AMCAS. See Chapter 4.*

Filing of AMCAS application
    Earliest date: June 1, 1996
    Latest date: Nov. 1, 1996
School application fee to all applicants: $55
Oldest MCAT scores considered: 1994
Acceptance notice to regular applicants
    Earliest date: Dec. 15, 1996
    Latest date: Until class is filled
Applicant's response to acceptance offer
    Maximum time: 2 weeks
Requests for deferred entrance considered: Yes
Deposit to hold place in class: None
Estimated number of new entrants: 86
Starting date: Aug. 1997

### TUITION AND STUDENT FEES PER YEAR FOR 1995–96 FIRST-YEAR CLASS

Tuition: $22,810          Student fees: $3,900

### INFORMATION ON 1995–96 FIRST-YEAR CLASS

| *Number of* | *In-State* | *Out-of-State* | *Total* |
| --- | --- | --- | --- |
| Applicants | 80 | 7,966 | 8,046 |
| Applicants Interviewed | 26 | 514 | 540 |
| New Entrants* | 12 | 79 | 91 |

*All had baccalaureate degrees; 92% took the MCAT.

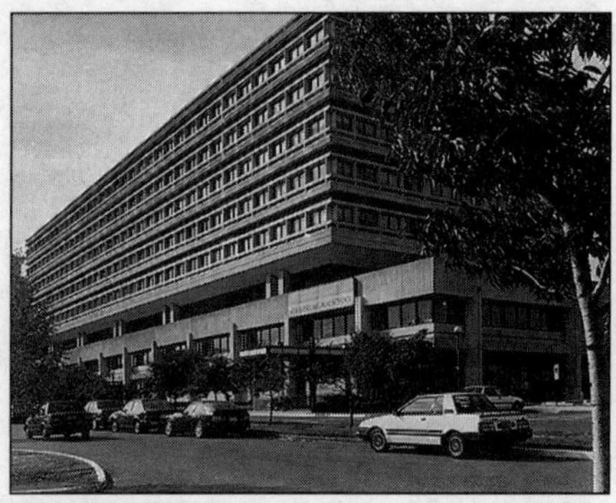

# University of Medicine and Dentistry of New Jersey New Jersey Medical School

## Newark, New Jersey

Dr. Ruy V. Lourenço, *Dean*
Dr. George F. Heinrich, *Assistant Dean for Admissions*
Michael Katz, *Director of Financial Aid*

## ADDRESS INQUIRIES TO:

Director of Admissions
UMDNJ-New Jersey Medical School
185 South Orange Avenue
Newark, New Jersey 07103
(201) 982-4631; 982-7986 (FAX)

## GENERAL INFORMATION

The New Jersey Medical School of the University of Medicine and Dentistry of New Jersey (UMDNJ-NJMS) moved into facilities situated in Newark in 1977. A $350-million complex contains the teaching-research Biomedical Science Building, a hospital, an ambulatory care center, a library, a dental school, and a community mental health center.

Major clinical instruction is carried out at the University Hospital, East Orange Veterans Administration Hospital, Beth Israel Hospital, United Hospitals of Newark, and Hackensack University Medical Center.

## CURRICULUM

During the first two years a thorough coverage of the basic medical sciences is implemented through a modified curriculum with departmental and integrated interdepartmental studies. New courses in problem-based learning and the art of medicine have been introduced with the de-emphasis of lectures and the increase in small-group sessions. A broad program of clinical correlations occurs throughout all the basic sciences. Introductory courses in clinical sciences, physical diagnosis, psychiatry, public health, and preventive and community medicine are presented during the first two years of the curriculum. The third year is spent in rotations through all of the clinical departments. This is a closely supervised comprehensive endeavor in which the student acquires the basic knowledge and techniques of clinical medicine. Instruction is carried out mainly in small groups and individual instruction. The fourth year is devoted to advanced required work and elective programs. The required courses are emergency medicine, neurology, an acting internship, and the practice of medicine course, which brings together the ethical, legal, and social factors that are part of total patient care. A curriculum task force is now in the process of making significant changes in our curriculum to make these years a continuum of education. This revision provides more flexibility for students to select the order of their clinical rotations and will include a clerkship in family medicine. This is consistent with NJMS's commitment to emphasize primary care specialties.

UMDNJ-NJMS has established accelerated baccalaureate-M.D. degree programs in conjunction with Boston University, Drew University, Montclair State University, New Jersey Institute of Technology, Stevens Institute of Technology, the Richard Stockton College of New Jersey, and Trenton State College. Inquiries may be directed to UMDNJ-NJMS or the admissions offices at the undergraduate schools.

## REQUIREMENTS FOR ENTRANCE

The MCAT and a minimum of three years of college (90 credit hours) are required. Three-year applicants with good credentials are encouraged to apply.

The minimum requirements are:

| | *Sem. hrs.* |
|---|---|
| Biology or zoology (with lab) | 8 |
| Course work must be exclusive of botany and invertebrate zoology. | |
| Organic chemistry (with lab) | 8 |
| Other chemistry (with lab) | 8 |
| Inorganic, physical, analytical chemistry or biochemistry will satisfy the requirement. | |
| General physics (with lab) | 8 |
| English | 6 |

A course in mathematics is recommended but not required.

Specific requirements may be waived or imposed at the discretion of the Admissions Committee in any individual case.

The Admissions Committee urges all candidates to prepare themselves further by completing courses in social or cultural fields and generally broadening their academic backgrounds. Candidates who are not premedical or science majors are given equal consideration if they have demonstrated academic excellence in the course requirements listed above.

Advanced standing programs may be available. An M.D.-Ph.D. option is open to all students who are accepted into the medical school. New Jersey Medical School offers a limited number of Academic Excellence Scholarships for entering first-year students.

## SELECTION FACTORS

Students are selected on the basis of scholastic achievement, fitness and aptitude for the study of medicine, and other personal qualifications. Since success in medicine depends on a number of related factors in a student's development, of which scholastic accomplishments are only a part, the Admissions Committee also gives consideration to the use of language, special aptitudes, mechanical skill, stamina, perseverance, and motivation.

New Jersey Medical School applies no GPA or MCAT cutoff levels in its selection process. It must be remembered, however, that competition is very keen, and applicants who are high in all determinable categories often receive the highest priority for acceptance. There are no restrictions as to race, creed, sex, national origin, age, or handicap.

Accepted students in the 1995 entering class had the following profile: *average* GPA, 3.40; *gender,* 30 percent women; *residence,* 16 nonresidents; *disadvantaged minorities,* 22 students.

Applications from nonresidents are accepted. However, with the large number of qualified New Jersey residents, only the most outstanding nonresident applicants have been successful.

## FINANCIAL AID

No questions of financial need are involved in the selection of students. All students who are accepted and wish to matriculate are advised to contact the financial aid officer immediately to discuss aid and fill out all necessary forms. All aid is given on the basis of financial need as assessed by an outside source. The needs analysis is usually adjusted upward to reflect costs in the northeastern United States. Approximately 70 percent of the students receive some form of financial aid. The Financial Aid Office extends itself to help all students in financial need.

The $100 deposit may be waived in cases of financial hardship.

## INFORMATION FOR MINORITIES

NJMS has a longstanding strong commitment to the recruitment of minority applicants. A special summer program is open to economically and educationally disadvantaged students who have been accepted, as well as to others in various stages of their undergraduate careers. Information is available from James Foster, assistant dean for student affairs.

NJMS is proud to have received the 1994 Outstanding Community Service Award by the AAMC.

Public Institution

## APPLICATION AND ACCEPTANCE POLICIES FOR 1997–98 FIRST-YEAR CLASS

*School participates in AMCAS. See Chapter 4.*

Filing of AMCAS application
    Earliest date: June 1, 1996
    Latest date: Dec. 1, 1996
School application fee to all applicants: $50
Will accept MCAT scores from any year
Does have Early Decision Program (EDP)
    For exceptional New Jersey residents only
    EDP application period: June 1–Aug. 1, 1996
    EDP applicants notified by: Oct. 1, 1996
Acceptance notice to regular applicants
    Earliest date: Oct. 15, 1996
    Latest date: Until class is filled
Applicant's response to acceptance offer
    Maximum time: 2 weeks
Requests for deferred entrance considered: Yes
Deposit to hold place in class (applied to tuition):
    $100, due with response to acceptance offer
Deposit refundable prior to: May 15, 1997
Estimated number of new entrants: 170 (3 EDP)
Starting date: Aug. 1997

## TUITION AND STUDENT FEES PER YEAR FOR 1995–96 FIRST-YEAR CLASS

Tuition                              Student fees: $1,100
    Resident: $13,295
    Nonresident: $17,445

## INFORMATION ON 1995–96 FIRST-YEAR CLASS

| Number of | In-State | Out-of-State | Total |
|---|---|---|---|
| Applicants | 1,410 | 2,911 | 4,321 |
| Applicants Interviewed | 539 | 256 | 795 |
| New Entrants* | 154 | 16 | 170 |

*All took the MCAT; 98% had baccalaureate degrees.

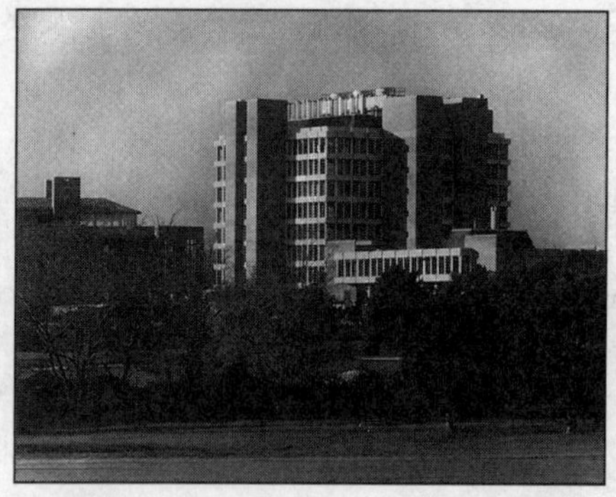

# University of Medicine and Dentistry of New Jersey
# Robert Wood Johnson Medical School

**Piscataway, New Jersey**


Dr. Harold L. Paz, *Dean*
Dr. David Seiden, *Associate Dean for Admissions and Student Affairs*
Helen S. Vlachakis, *Associate Director of Financial Aid*


## ADDRESS INQUIRIES TO:

Office of Admissions
UMDNJ-Robert Wood Johnson Medical School
675 Hoes Lane
Piscataway, New Jersey 08854-5635
(908) 235-4576; 235-5078 (FAX)
Web Site: http://www2.umdnj.edu/rwjms.html

## GENERAL INFORMATION

Robert Wood Johnson Medical School, formerly known as Rutgers Medical School, was named after the former president and chairman of the board of Johnson & Johnson Company and the benefactor of the Robert Wood Johnson Foundation.

The Basic Science Building is located adjacent to the science campus of Rutgers University. The Institute of Mental Health Sciences, which houses the Department of Psychiatry, adjoins the building. Facilities shared with Rutgers University include the Library of Science and Medicine, the Center for Advanced Biotechnology and Medicine, and the Environmental and Occupational Health Science Institute.

Robert Wood Johnson University Hospital in New Brunswick is the major teaching facility. A major teaching affiliation with the Cooper Hospital/University Medical Center in Camden also exists. These two centers, supplemented by affiliations with community hospitals in central New Jersey, provide the Medical School with a full complement of diverse clinical training facilities.

The Medical School has a division at Camden. Separate applications are not required. All students receive their basic education at the Piscataway campus. Students who matriculate in the Camden program receive their clinical education at the Camden campus.

## CURRICULUM

The curriculum is newly revised. It provides for an early introduction to patient care, an integration of clinical skills into the preclinical curriculum, and the opportunity for self-directed learning within the context of a rigorous basic science education during the first two years. Multiple learning modalities are used including lectures, laboratory exercises, small-group discussions, and computer-assisted instruction. During the first two years, in addition to the traditional basic sciences, there are courses in ethics, case-based learning, clinical pre-

vention, clinical pathophysiology, human genetics, and community and environmental medicine, among others. The third-year curriculum consists of an introduction to the clinical experience followed by six 8-week clerkships in medicine, surgery, family medicine, psychiatry, obstetrics-gynecology, and pediatrics. There is also a formative clinical skills assessment at the beginning of the third year and a summative clinical skills assessment at the end of the year. The fourth-year curriculum includes an advanced clerkship in ambulatory medicine, an advanced clerkship in surgery, neurology, a subinternship, and a minimum of 12 weeks of electives. Grades are reported as honors, high pass, pass, low pass, and fail. Students must pass USMLE Step 1 prior to entering the third year and must pass USMLE Step 2 prior to graduation.

In conjunction with the graduate program in public health, a combined M.D.-M.P.H. program is available. Combined M.D.-Ph.D. programs are available in the medical school and in conjuction with Rutgers University. Financial support that includes both tuition remission and stipends is available throughout the seven-year program.

## REQUIREMENTS FOR ENTRANCE

The MCAT and a minimum of three years of college consisting of 90 semester hours of college work (exclusive of military and physical education) are required. The MCAT must be taken within the four years preceding application and no later than the fall of the year of application. The following undergraduate courses are required:

|  | *Semesters* |
|---|---|
| Biology or zoology (with lab) | 2 |
| Inorganic chemistry (with lab) | 2 |
| Organic chemistry (with lab) | 2 |
| Physics (with lab) | 2 |
| College mathematics | 1 |
| English | 2 |

Must include one semester of a college writing course. College-approved "writing intensive courses" may substitute for English.

Robert Wood Johnson Medical School places high value on a balanced undergraduate education. While this balance will vary with the background and interests of the individual, it is expected that applicants will have exposed themselves to course work in the humanities, the behavioral sciences, and liberal arts as well as the premedical sciences. In addition, applicants may be asked to demonstrate competence in written English.

Students capable of superior performance in any academic field, whether in the sciences or humanities, should feel free to pursue their intellectual interests in depth, provided only that they can do well in the required courses mentioned above. The Admissions Committee may waive or impose specific requirements at its discretion. Ordinarily, applicants must be U.S. citizens or permanent residents to be eligible for admission.

## SELECTION FACTORS

Applicants are considered without regard to race, religion, or sex. Preference for admission, however, is given to bona fide residents of New Jersey. While no set number exists, the school accepts a small percentage of the class from outside New Jersey. Consequently, competition in this category is keen, and nonresident applicants must present superior credentials.

Admission is determined on the basis of academic achievement in a balanced undergraduate education, results of the MCAT, preprofessional committee evaluations, other recommendations, character, motivation, and personal interview. Applications from qualified members of racial minority groups are encouraged. Interviews are arranged by invitation.

Accepted students for the 1995 entering class had a mean GPA of 3.45 (ten percentile-2.91, ninety percentile-3.89). Women comprised 44 percent of the class.

## FINANCIAL AID

Accepted students who believe they will need financial aid are encouraged to request information and application forms from the Financial Aid Office. About 77 percent of the student body received some sort of financial assistance during the 1995–96 academic year. Financial aid is awarded on the basis of evaluated need computed by an approved needs analysis method. All awards consist of a package of loans and grants when funds are available. Funds have been allocated for freshman scholarships, which are renewable annually.

## INFORMATION FOR MINORITIES

UMDNJ-Robert Wood Johnson Medical School is committed to the education and training of minority physicians. Applications from both in-state and out-of-state candidates are welcome, and ample financial aid assistance is offered. Numerous support services are available, including a pre-enrollment summer program for accepted students. A summer Biomedical Careers Program for undergraduates interested in health care careers is also offered. Further information is available from Betty Treadwell-Oglesby.

---

Public Institution

## APPLICATION AND ACCEPTANCE POLICIES FOR 1997–98 FIRST-YEAR CLASS

*School participates in AMCAS. See Chapter 4.*

Filing of AMCAS application
    Earliest date: June 1, 1996
    Latest date: Dec. 1, 1996
School application fee to all applicants: $50
Oldest MCAT scores considered: 1992
Does have Early Decision Program (EDP)
    EDP application period: June 1–Aug. 1, 1996
    EDP applicants notified by: Oct. 1, 1996
Acceptance notice to regular applicants
    Earliest date: Oct. 15, 1996
    Latest date: Until class is filled
Applicant's response to acceptance offer
    Maximum time: 2 weeks
Requests for deferred entrance considered: Yes
Deposit to hold place in class (applied to tuition):
    $50, due with response to acceptance offer
Deposit refundable prior to: May 15, 1997
Estimated number of new entrants: 138 (6 EDP)
Starting date: Aug. 1997

## TUITION AND STUDENT FEES PER YEAR FOR 1995–96 FIRST-YEAR CLASS

Tuition                             Student fees: $1,187
    Resident: $13,295
    Nonresident: $17,445

## INFORMATION ON 1995–96 FIRST-YEAR CLASS

| Number of | In-State | Out-of-State | Total |
|---|---|---|---|
| Applicants | 1,452 | 3,184 | 4,636 |
| Applicants Interviewed | 593 | 157 | 750 |
| New Entrants* | 120 | 18 | 138 |

*All took the MCAT and had baccalaureate degrees.

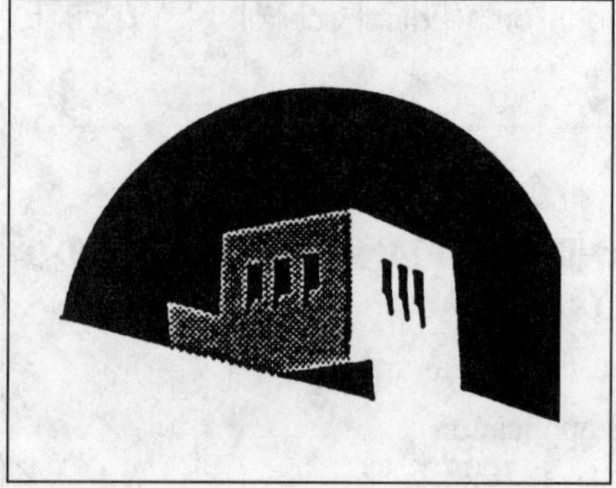

# University of New Mexico
# School of Medicine

## Albuquerque, New Mexico

Dr. Paul B. Roth, *Dean*
Dr. Diane J. Klepper, *Associate Dean for Admissions and Student Affairs*
Mitzi Vigil, *Financial Aid Coordinator*

## ADDRESS INQUIRIES TO:

Office of Admissions and Student Affairs
University of New Mexico
School of Medicine
Basic Medical Sciences Building, Room 107
Albuquerque, New Mexico 87131-5166
(505) 277-4766; 277-2755 (FAX)

## GENERAL INFORMATION

The establishment of a school of the basic medical sciences was authorized by the regents and the faculty of the University of New Mexico (UNM) in 1961. The first entering class of 24 students was enrolled in September 1964, and progress to the full four-year program was approved by the New Mexico State Legislature in 1966.

The medical school facilities are located on the north campus of the university and include a basic medical sciences building, biomedical research facility, medical center library, UNM Mental Health Center, UNM Children's Psychiatric Hospital, family practice center, Center for Non-Invasive Diagnosis, and an international cancer center. The 368-bed University of New Mexico Hospital serves as the major teaching hospital of the medical school, with additional teaching at the 462-bed Regional Federal Medical Center in Albuquerque. The faculty numbers 535, with 408 full-time appointments.

The School of Medicine is a professional and graduate school of the university. In addition to providing education in the basic and clinical sciences for the doctor of medicine degree, opportunities are available for work leading to a doctor of philosophy degree. Medical education at the resident and postgraduate levels is offered through the university's teaching hospitals.

## CURRICULUM

The University of New Mexico School of Medicine implemented a new curriculum in the fall of 1993, which incorporated aspects of its prior educational innovations from the Conventional Curriculum Track, Primary Care Curriculum, and Health of the Public Program. It will be fully implemented for all four years in 1997.

The goals of the new curriculum are to graduate physicians who: are excited and enthusiastic about learning; have assumed a major responsibility for their continued learning; have the ability to define problems, formulate questions, and carry out scholarly inquiry; are skilled in self and peer assessment; have a broad perspective on the importance of human biology, behavior, environment, culture and social setting, in the health of individuals and of populations.

Educational innovations include the following: the integration of the basic and clinical sciences throughout undergraduate medical education; early clinical skills training and community-based learning; the incorporation of a population and behavioral perspective into the clinical years; and peer teaching and computer-assisted instruction.

Student assessment will value mastery of knowledge, writing skills, critical appraisal, interpersonal and clinical skills, teaching ability, and peer and self-assessment. Assessment will be competency-based and cumulative.

## REQUIREMENTS FOR ENTRANCE

The MCAT and three years of college are required. A college program leading to the bachelor's degree from an accredited college of arts and sciences is ordinarily recommended.

Minimum course requirements are:

*Sem. hrs.*

General biology (with lab). . . . . . . . . . . . . . . . . . . . . . . . . . 8
General or inorganic chemistry (with lab) . . . . . . . . . . . . . 8
Organic chemistry (with lab) . . . . . . . . . . . . . . . . . . . . . . . 8
General physics . . . . . . . . . . . . . . . . . . . . . . . . . . . . . . . . . 6

The following courses are strongly recommended: biochemistry, calculus, and Spanish.

## SELECTION FACTORS

All applicants for first-year positions must apply through AMCAS. All New Mexico applicants will be sent additional application materials upon receipt of their application from AMCAS. Nonregional applicants, including WICHE and former New Mexico residents, must apply through the Early Decision Program to receive any consideration for admission. Those who pass an initial screening process will be sent full application materials and invited for interviews.

Selection is based upon scholastic achievement, performance on the MCAT, personal interviews with members of the Admissions Committee, and recommendations of a college professional advisory committee. The University of New Mexico is committed to providing equal educational and employment opportunities regardless of sex, marital or parental status, race, religion, age, or physical handicap. Preference is given to residents of New Mexico and next to applicants who are residents of western states which participate in the WICHE program.

To guide applicants in considering application to the School of Medicine, the following information is provided on the 1995 applicant pool: 1,283 total applicants, 100 accepted, 73 matriculated; 352 New Mexico applicants, 93 accepted, 66 matriculated; 34 WICHE applicants, 1 accepted, 1 matriculated; 897 non-regional applicants, 6 accepted, 6 matriculated. Some characteristics of the 1995 entering class were: *average GPA,* 3.54 (95 percent above 3.0); *average MCAT* 9.00; *sex,* 63 percent women; *ethnic minorities,* 30 percent. All students offered acceptance were interviewed at this school.

## FINANCIAL AID

The school makes available financial aid in the form of loans and scholarships to those students with demonstrated financial need. The amount of award varies according to the student's need and the level of funding available. A short-term, no-interest loan fund is available to all students in need of immediate financial help. The Student Affairs Office assists all students in locating necessary funds to support their medical education.

## INFORMATION FOR MINORITIES

The School of Medicine is committed to the recruitment, selection, and retention of qualified Black and Hispanic residents of New Mexico and American Indian residents of New Mexico and the Navajo Nation. The Office of Cultural and Ethnic Programs, directed by Dr. Roberto Gomez, offers several programs to support the above commitment. Additional information may be obtained by contacting the Office of Cultural and Ethnic Programs at (505) 277-2728.

Private Institution

## APPLICATION AND ACCEPTANCE POLICIES FOR 1997–98 FIRST-YEAR CLASS

*School participates in AMCAS. See Chapter 4.*

Filing of AMCAS application
  Earliest date: June 1, 1996
  Latest date: Nov. 15, 1996
School application fee after screening: $25
Oldest MCAT scores considered: 1991
Does have Early Decision Program (EDP)
Nonresidents must apply through EDP
  EDP application period: June 1–Aug. 1, 1996
  EDP applicants notified by: Oct. 1, 1996
Acceptance notice to regular applicants (EDP)
  Earliest date: Mar. 15, 1997
  Latest date: Varies
Applicant's response to acceptance offer
  Maximum time: 4 weeks
Requests for deferred entrance considered: Yes
Deposit to hold place in class: None
Estimated number of new entrants: 73 (23 EDP)
Starting date: Aug. 1997

## TUITION AND STUDENT FEES PER YEAR FOR 1995–96 FIRST-YEAR CLASS

Tuition                              Student fees: $32
  Resident: $4,867
  Nonresident: $13,954

## INFORMATION ON 1995–96 FIRST-YEAR CLASS

| Number of | In-State | Out-of-State | Total |
|---|---|---|---|
| Applicants | 252 | 931 | 1,283 |
| Applicants Interviewed | 345 | 21 | 366 |
| New Entrants* | 66 | 7 | 73 |

*All took the MCAT; 97% had baccalaureate degrees.

# Albany Medical College

## Albany, New York

Dr. Richard H. Edmonds, *Interim Dean*
Sara J. Kremer, *Director of Admissions and Registrar*
Tor Shekerjian, *Director of Financial Aid*

## ADDRESS INQUIRIES TO:

Office of Admissions, A-3
Albany Medical College
47 New Scotland Avenue
Albany, New York 12208
(518) 262-5521; 262-5887 (FAX)

## GENERAL INFORMATION

Founded in 1839, the Albany Medical College is one of the oldest medical schools in the country. The college is coeducational, nondenominational, and privately supported.

The college buildings and those of the 674-bed Albany Medical Center Hospital are physically joined in one large complex that comprises Albany Medical Center. The hospital is both a community hospital for people of the immediate area and a tertiary diagnostic and treatment center for over two million residents of eastern New York and western New England. Additional clinical facilities are provided by the Albany Veterans Administration Medical Center, the Capital District Psychiatric Center, and other affiliated hospitals located nearby.

## CURRICULUM

The Albany Medical College implemented a new curriculum in 1993, which will be phased in over a four-year period. Basic and clinical sciences are integrated into themes (primarily organ systems) stressing normal function in Year I and pathological function in Year II. All four years of school offer three themes that include clinical skills, ethical and health systems issues, and epidemiology. In every theme, students receive exposure to clinical presentations. These begin with the development of patient interviewing skills at the start of Year I, and by year's end have included clinical exposure in the ICU, the neonatal units, and the cardiac operating rooms. All first-year students spend an afternoon with a primary care giver at a staff model HMO. Basic science seminars reinforce the importance of the basic sciences in years III and IV. Emphasis is placed on primary care throughout the four years, with an increased emphasis on care in ambulatory settings in the clinical rotations of Year III. Year IV will emphasize specialty care in some required rotations. Elective rotations will also be available in Year IV at Albany Medical Center Hospital, other affiliated hospitals, and at other institutions in the United States and abroad. Senior students may plan with their advisors programs that provide opportunities to explore career possibilities as well as revisit basic science foundations of clinical medicine.

## REQUIREMENTS FOR ENTRANCE

Applicants for admission must have completed at least three years of study at an accredited college preferably in the United States or Canada. Most students admitted, however, will have earned the bachelor's degree.

Minimal course requirements for admission are:

|  | Sem./Qtr. hrs. |
| --- | --- |
| Biology or zoology (with lab) | 6/9 |
| Inorganic chemistry (with lab) | 6/9 |
| Organic chemistry (with lab) | 6/9 |
| General physics (with lab) | 6/9 |

Proficiency in oral and written English is required.

When achievement in the required science courses is less than optimum, the desirability of augmenting the minimum requirements with additional experience in the fields of chemistry, embryology, genetics, and mathematics should be considered. On the other hand, ideally a physician's education should also rest on a base of general knowledge that includes a broad liberal arts education. Accordingly, students who have majored in the arts or humanities are considered on an equal basis with those who have majored in the sciences, provided that these students have demonstrated good capability in the required science studies.

The MCAT is also required and must be taken no later than the fall one year prior to the intended date of matriculation.

## SELECTION FACTORS

In selecting students, emphasis is placed upon character, academic achievement, integrity, motivation, emotional stability, and social and intellectual suitability. The Albany Medical College is committed to the belief that educational opportunities should be available to all eligible persons without regard to race, creed, age, sex, religion, marital status, handicap, or national origin. Admission is not restricted to New York State residents. Although preference is usually given to U.S. citizens, the committee will from time to time admit outstanding applicants who are citizens of other countries.

For the 1995 entering class, all matriculants had a mean cumulative GPA of 3.5.

All applications are individually reviewed by members of the Committee on Admissions who are looking for qualities other than and in addition to the MCAT scores and GPA. If an interview is desired by the Committee on Admissions, the college will notify the candidate. Pertinent preapplication inquiries are welcome at any time.

## FINANCIAL AID

The college attempts to assist all students in every feasible manner by awarding scholarship and loan assistance as well as through guidance in employment. Eighty percent of the student body receive some scholarship and/or loan assistance. An announcement regarding application for financial assistance is distributed to all students by January 15 for the following academic year. Awards of scholarship and loan assistance are made in April by the Financial Aid Committee. Additional or new requests for financial assistance in the form of loans are accepted throughout the year. In the Albany Medical Center there are opportunities for part-time employment for students through a federally funded work-study program.

## INFORMATION FOR MINORITIES

The Office of Minority Affairs is responsible for developing and implementing programs that enhance educational opportunities for minorities to enter the medical school, graduate school, and the allied health professions. This office also coordinates academic, social, and cultural support services for matriculated minority students.

The Office of Minority Affairs coordinates two programs for minority high school students: the Science and Technology Entry Program (STEP), a health career awareness and science enrichment and readiness program for high school students; and the Minority High School Research Apprenticeship Program.

An endowed scholarship fund for minority medical students was established in 1986. Each year there are several merit scholarships, both full and partial, to be applied towards tuition. Both scholarships are managed by the Office of Minority Affairs.

The director of minority affairs is actively involved in the admissions process and reviews the applications of all minority candidates. More information may be obtained by contacting the Office of Minority Affairs; telephone (518) 262-5824.

Private Institution

## APPLICATION AND ACCEPTANCE POLICIES FOR 1997–98 FIRST-YEAR CLASS

*School participates in AMCAS. See Chapter 4.*

Filing of AMCAS application
 Earliest date: June 1, 1996
 Latest date: Nov. 15, 1996
School application fee to all applicants: $70
Oldest MCAT scores considered: 1992
Does not have Early Decision Program
Acceptance notice to regular applicants
 Earliest date: Oct. 15, 1996
 Latest date: Until class is filled
Applicant's response to acceptance offer
 Maximum time: 2 weeks
Requests for deferred entrance considered: Yes
Deposit to hold place in class (applied to tuition):
 $100, due with response to acceptance offer
Deposit refundable prior to: May 15, 1997
Estimated number of new entrants: 137
Starting date: Aug. 1997

## TUITION AND STUDENT FEES PER YEAR FOR 1995–96 FIRST-YEAR CLASS

Tuition               Student fees: None
 Resident: $24,074
 Nonresident: $25,346

## INFORMATION ON 1995–96 FIRST-YEAR CLASS

| Number of | In-State | Out-of-State | Total |
|---|---|---|---|
| Applicants | 2,496 | 7,596 | 10,092 |
| Applicants Interviewed | 284 | 570 | 854 |
| New Entrants* | 52 | 83 | 135 |

*63% took the MCAT; 70% had baccalaureate degrees.

(NOTE: Students applying through AMCAS must take the MCAT; students matriculating through Albany's accelerated program have not earned their baccalaureate degree.)

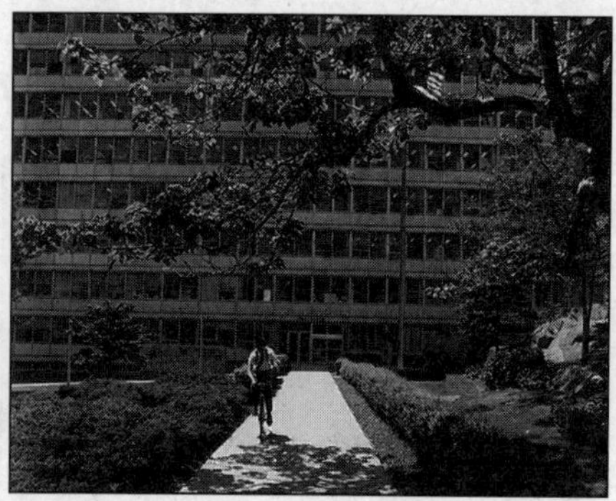

# Albert Einstein College of Medicine of Yeshiva University

**Bronx, New York**

Dr. Dominick P. Purpura, *Dean*
Noreen Kerrigan, *Assistant Dean for Student Admissions*
Lloyd Greenberg, *Financial Aid Officer*

## ADDRESS INQUIRIES TO:

Office of Admissions
Albert Einstein College of Medicine
of Yeshiva University
Jack and Pearl Resnick Campus
1300 Morris Park Avenue
Bronx, New York 10461
(718) 430-2106; 430-8825 (FAX)
E-Mail: admissions@aecom.yu.edu

## GENERAL INFORMATION

The Albert Einstein College of Medicine is a privately endowed, coeducational, and nondenominational institution situated on a 17-acre site in a residential area of the northeast Bronx. Clinical education takes place in affiliated acute care hospitals, long-term care and skilled nursing facilities, hospices, and neighborhood health centers that serve the health care needs of a very diverse population of patients in the boroughs of the Bronx, Queens, Manhattan, and Brooklyn. These institutions include two public hospitals, Jacobi Hospital and North Central Bronx Hospital, and five private voluntary hospitals, Beth Israel Medical Center, Montefiore Medical Center, Bronx Lebanon Hospital Center, Long Island Jewish Medical Center, and Catholic Medical Center. In addition to these clinical sites, there are extensive facilities devoted to biomedical research and teaching.

Apartments for students are located on and close to the campus, and a recreational sports center with a swimming pool is located on the grounds of the main apartment building complex.

## CURRICULUM

The first two years of the curriculum consist mainly of biomedical science courses, including an extensive interdisciplinary case based approach to the teaching of pathophysiology and pathology. The Introduction to Clinical Medicine course includes encounters with patients in a wide variety of clinical settings and small-group conferences under the guidance of faculty physicians. The preclerkship curriculum includes a substantial amount of unscheduled time, especially in the first year. A one-year period of clerkship rotations in the third year enables students to acquire clinical skills and knowledge while working with patients at various health care sites in inpatient and outpatient settings. The senior year provides extensive experience in ambulatory care as well as additional responsibilities for the care of hospitalized patients during a subinternship. Special senior elective opportunities include overseas exchange programs, international health fellowships, and a research program that leads to the M.D. degree with distinction in the student's research discipline. Evaluation of performance is on a pass/fail basis in Year 1, supplemented by honors in Year 2 and further supplemented by detailed narrative reports in clinical courses.

A fully funded M.D.-Ph.D. program is offered to students in the first year, several students may also be selected at the end of the second year. It is a requirement that all students pursue an in-depth study of an area of interest and prepare a written, referenced report of scholarly substance prior to graduation.

A generalist mentorship program has been established to meet the particular needs of students with career interests in generalist disciplines. Students with excellent backgrounds and interests in the sciences are encouraged to join the Biomedical Sciences Pathway.

Tutoring in most basic science courses is available, and individual counseling is provided to students in need of long-term assistance to assure retention.

## REQUIREMENTS FOR ENTRANCE

The MCAT and a minimum of three years of full-time undergraduate study are required; four years are preferred. The minimum course requirements are:

|  | *Sem. hrs.* |
|---|---|
| Biology (with lab) | 8 |
| General chemistry (with lab) | 8 |
| Organic chemistry (with lab) | 8 |
| Physics (with lab) | 8 |
| College mathematics | 6 |
| (May include statistics and computer science) | |
| English | 6 |

The undergraduate major is not an important selection factor, and the scholarly pursuit of a broad liberal arts education, including the study of humanities and social sciences, is strongly recommended.

Applicants should provide evidence of participation in intra- or extramural activities that serve to enhance one's communication and interpersonal skills. Such activities may include tutoring, counseling, and community service, as well as experience in the health care system.

## SELECTION FACTORS

Students are carefully selected on the basis of academic performance, letters of recommendations, MCAT scores, potential for professional achievement, and motivation and evidence of other personal qualities deemed essential for the study and practice of medicine. Letters of recommendation from commercial educational consultants will not be considered. Applicants are considered without regard to race, age, sex, religion, national origin, state of residence, or physical handicap. Students who do not gain admission are discouraged from reapplying the subsequent year or until such time as they can present new data to warrant a more favorable decision.

Foreign nationals may apply for admission; however, because they are ineligible for federal loan programs, it is their responsibility to secure private funding for tuition. The 1995 entering class represented 19 states, 68 undergraduate colleges, and is 47 percent female. Receipt of the application will be acknowledged, and the applicant will be requested to submit letters of recommendation and the college application fee. A decision regarding a formal interview is made upon receipt of all supporting documents. Interviews are required of all applicants under serious consideration.

## FINANCIAL AID

Every attempt is made to assist students and their families in meeting both their financial obligations to the college and the student's essential personal needs. Financial status is not a determinant in selecting among qualified applicants. Awards and loans from the college are available after all other means of financial assistance have been exhausted. Financial aid applications are available only after acceptance. Advice on financial assistance and applications are available from the Student Finance Office. About 50 percent of the students receive institutional loans and/or scholarships, and about 75 percent of them qualify for outside loans and/or grants.

The application fee may be waived upon written request from the financial aid officer of the undergraduate college. It may be waived also upon a written request from the applicant after a fee waiver from AMCAS has been granted.

## INFORMATION FOR MINORITIES

The College of Medicine is actively seeking and welcomes applications from minority students. Abundant opportunities exist for medical students to participate in special programs for high school and college students.

---

Private Institution

### APPLICATION AND ACCEPTANCE POLICIES FOR 1997–98 FIRST-YEAR CLASS

*School participates in AMCAS. See Chapter 4.*

Filing of AMCAS application
   Earliest date: June 1, 1996
   Latest date: Nov. 1, 1996
School application fee to all applicants: $75
Oldest MCAT scores considered: 1991
Does have Early Decision Program (EDP)
   EDP application period: June 1–Aug. 1, 1996
   EDP applicants notified by: Oct. 1, 1996
Acceptance notice to regular applicants
   Earliest date: Jan. 15, 1997
   Latest date: Until class is filled
Applicant's response to acceptance offer
   Maximum time: 2 weeks until May 1, 1997;
      1 week thereafter
Requests for deferred entrance considered: Yes
Deposit to hold place in class (applied to tuition):
   $100, due with response to acceptance offer
Deposit refundable prior to: June 1, 1997
Estimated number of new entrants: 180
Starting date: Aug. 1997

### TUITION AND STUDENT FEES PER YEAR FOR 1995–96 FIRST-YEAR CLASS

Tuition: $24,550          Student fees: $1,200

### INFORMATION ON 1995–96 FIRST-YEAR CLASS

| Number of | In-State | Out-of-State | Total |
|---|---|---|---|
| Applicants | 2,385 | 6,750 | 9,135 |
| Applicants Interviewed | 542 | 1,236 | 1,778 |
| New Entrants* | 85 | 95 | 180 |

*All took the MCAT; 99% had baccalaureate degrees.

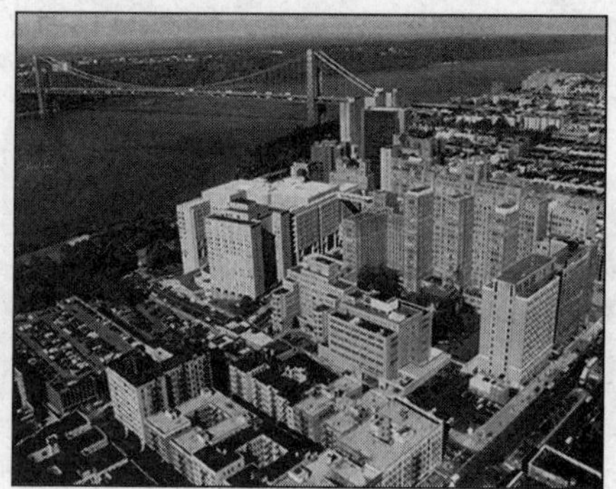

# Columbia University
# College of Physicians and Surgeons

**New York, New York**

Dr. Herbert Pardes, *Vice President for Health Sciences and Dean, Faculty of Medicine*
Dr. Andrew G. Frantz, *Chairman, Committee on Admissions*
Ellen Spilker, Director, *Office of Student Affairs (Financial Aid)*

## ADDRESS INQUIRIES TO:

Columbia University
College of Physicians and Surgeons
Admissions Office, Room 1-416
630 West 168th Street
New York, New York 10032
(212) 305-3595

## GENERAL INFORMATION

The College of Physicians and Surgeons originated in 1767 as the Medical Faculty of King's (later Columbia) College and was the first school to award an earned doctor of medicine degree in the American colonies. The college is now a part of the Columbia-Presbyterian Medical Center. Clinical teaching is provided at the Medical Center; Roosevelt-St. Luke's Hospital Center, and Harlem Hospital Center in Manhattan; Bassett Hospital in Cooperstown, New York; and Morristown Memorial Hospital and Overlook Hospital in New Jersey.

University housing is available for unmarried and married students.

## CURRICULUM

The first portion of the curriculum provides information and experiences considered essential for all physicians, regardless of their ultimate area of specialization. Teaching in small groups is emphasized. There are opportunities for patient contact in the first two years by elective courses as well as by regularly scheduled exercises. Students interested in research, aside from those enrolled in the M.D.-Ph.D. program, may pursue research projects in the interval between the first and second years as well as during the fourth year. The goals of the teaching program include the usual ones of providing the students with knowledge of and experience with the techniques that physicians are expected to master. In various courses and settings, instructors and students discuss the analysis of scientific evidence to equip students with some ability, beyond the use of statistical criteria, to evaluate the new developments certain to occur in the years after graduation. Also, the program is designed to inculcate the school's attitudes about patient care, which include the attitude that the patient is not simply a disease entity and is being improperly cared for if treated as one. The concept of the patient as a whole person is fostered by means of a variety of teaching experiences that attempt to instill a belief in the importance of developing a sensitivity to the total needs of a patient. Ethical problems are discussed in these teaching sessions. This aspect of the curriculum begins in the first year in an interdisciplinary course entitled the Introduction to Clinical Practice; it is taught with clinical faculty members serving as preceptors for relatively small groups of students. Further consideration of these topics occurs in a variety of settings in subsequent years.

In early July after the second year, students begin a full year of clerkships in which they participate in all of the clinical services. From July after the third year until graduation, the student follows an individually selected program of studies.

A great variety of elective courses is offered, including research electives and opportunities for study abroad. Courses also may be taken in other branches of the university. In cooperation with 14 of the university's departments and programs, an M.D.-Ph.D. program is offered for which a maximum of eight openings are usually available annually.

An M.D.-M.P.H. program also is offered in conjunction with our School of Public Health.

Courses are graded on the basis of honors, pass, and fail.

## REQUIREMENTS FOR ENTRANCE

The MCAT and a minimum of three years of full-time study in an accredited college are required; four years are recommended. The undergraduate program must include the following courses:

|  | *Years* |
|---|---|
| Biology | 1 |
| Mammalian biology preferred. | |
| General chemistry | 1 |
| Organic chemistry | 1 |
| Physics | 1 |
| English | 1 |

Applicants who have more than one of the required courses to complete are at a disadvantage in the competition for admission.

Admission is possible for all qualified applicants regardless of sex, race, age, religion, national origin, or handicap.

The area of undergraduate concentration is not an important selection factor.

## SELECTION FACTORS

Admission is offered to those applicants who have given evidence that they are qualified to complete all of the curriculum requirements of the college and have shown the greatest promise that they are likely to graduate as ethical, compassionate, and competent physicians. Competence implies, in part, mastery of the scientific basis of medicine. Competence also requires mastery of the art of medicine for which certain personal qualities and attitudes are essential. These qualities and attitudes are evaluated by several means: the tenor of letters of recommendation, the nature of extracurricular and summer activities (assuming choice was not restricted by financial need), the breadth of the undergraduate education, and the personal interview.

Each year some applicants are accepted who display extraordinary promise in regard to either the science or art of medicine, even though they do not meet, in optimal measure, all of the criteria described above.

## FINANCIAL AID

Financial aid is based solely on need and consists of scholarship awards and long-term loans. Accepted applicants, along with their parents, complete a financial aid questionnaire if aid is to be requested. An appropriately sized combination of scholarship money and loans is awarded in accordance with guidelines provided by the Financial Aid Office. Financial aid resources are equally available to the four classes.

The college cannot promise to meet fully the financial needs of students, although it makes every effort to do so. Its resources provide aid for a substantial segment of the student body, however. About 68 percent of the students currently receive financial aid.

## INFORMATION FOR MINORITIES

The college welcomes applications from qualified minority students. Members of minority groups constitute 20 percent of the Committee of Admissions. The evaluation it accords minority applicants is both experienced and, as with all applicants, highly individualized. Beyond three years of college and the required courses, the admissions criteria are, within limits, flexible for all applicants.

All students have the same educational program and equal access to resources for financial aid and tutorial assistance.

Private Institution

## APPLICATION AND ACCEPTANCE POLICIES FOR 1997–98 FIRST-YEAR CLASS

Filing of application
    Earliest date: June 15, 1996
    Latest date: Oct. 15, 1996
School application fee to all applicants: $65
Oldest MCAT scores considered: 1992
Does not have Early Decision Program
Acceptance notice to regular applicants
    Earliest date: Feb. 1, 1997
    Latest date: Varies
Applicant's response to acceptance offer
    Maximum time: 3 weeks
Requests for deferred entrance considered: Yes
Deposit to hold place in class: None
Estimated number of new entrants: 148
Starting date: Aug. 1997

## TUITION AND STUDENT FEES PER YEAR FOR 1995–96 FIRST-YEAR CLASS

Tuition: $23,740                Student fees: $1,597

## INFORMATION ON 1995–96 FIRST-YEAR CLASS

| Number of | In-State | Out-of-State | Total |
|---|---|---|---|
| Applicants | 1,009 | 3,257 | 4,266 |
| Applicants Interviewed | 328 | 1,126 | 1,454 |
| New Entrants* | 39 | 111 | 150 |

*All took the MCAT and had baccalaureate degrees.

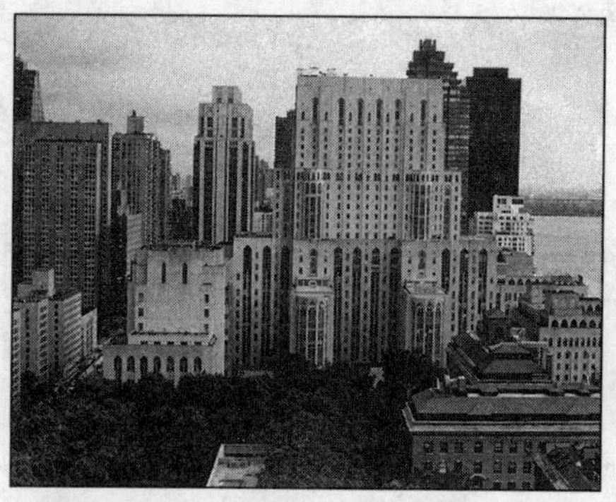

# Cornell University Medical College

**New York, New York**

Dr. Robert Michels, *Dean*
Dr. Gordon F. Fairclough, Jr., *Associate Dean and Chairman,*
*Committee on Admissions*
Joan M. May, *Assistant Dean for Financial Aid*

## ADDRESS INQUIRIES TO:

Office of Admissions
Cornell University Medical College
445 East 69th Street
New York, New York 10021
(212) 746-1067
Web Site: http://www.med.cornell.edu

## GENERAL INFORMATION

Cornell University Medical College was established in 1898. Although the university is situated in Ithaca, the Medical College was opened in New York City to take advantage of the facilities of a large urban area. Clinical instruction is carried on in the New York Hospital; Memorial Sloan-Kettering Cancer Center; the Hospital for Special Surgery; the New York Hospital Medical Center of Queens; the New York Methodist Hospital; the New York Community Hospital of Brooklyn; St. Barnabas Hospital; the Burke Rehabilitation Center in White Plains, New York; United Hospital Medical Center in Port Chester, New York; and the Tompkins Community Hospital in Ithaca, New York.

## CURRICULUM

Medical education at Cornell aims to develop individuals who not only recognize and are dedicated to the highest quality patient care, but also those who understand their responsibility for contributions through continuing personal scholarship. Many Cornell alumni pursue academic and research careers in addition to the clinical practice of medicine. The education process at Cornell has undergone a recent revision with the major goals of integrating the teaching of the basic and clinical sciences throughout the four years of study and emphasizing problem-solving in the context of scientific inquiry and clinical care.

Core basic science materials are presented during Years 1 and 2, and advanced basic science courses are offered during Years 3 and 4. Learning during the first two years occurs in the setting of problem-based tutorials, small group conferences, laboratories, lectures, and a journal club. Information is presented in a series of highly integrated, multi-disciplinary block courses: From Molecules to Cells, Genes and Development, Human Structure and Function, Host Defenses, Neuroscience and Behavior, and Human Organ System Dysfunction.

Clinical instruction begins in Year 1 with a full day-a-week course, Medicine, Patients, and Society I, during which the student acquires early clinical skills in an ambulatory setting, studies the doctor-patient relationship and socioeconomic, behavioral, and public health issues. This course continues as Medicine, Patients, and Society II in Year 2 with the student gaining experience in the physical examination of patients and clinical problem solving. In Year 3, the focus of Medicine, Patients, and Society III is on student experience with patients, clinical dilemmas, and multiculturalism. Clinical clerkships begin during the later third of Year 2 and include a new primary care clerkship which in conjunction with the Medicine, Patients, and Society sequence constitutes the central features of the primary care curriculum. The clinical clerkships include rotations in medicine, neurology, obstetrics and gynecology, pediatrics, psychiatry, and surgery. Year 4 provides the major time block for clinical electives. Performance is graded by an honors/pass/fail system during the basic science curriculum and an honors/high pass/pass/fail system during the core curriculum.

For students interested in teaching and research careers in the medical sciences, Cornell University Medical College offers a fully funded Tri-Institutional M.D.-Ph.D. Program which is coordinated with the Cornell University Graduate School of Medical Sciences, Memorial Sloan-Kettering Cancer Center, and Rockefeller University. Applicants interested in applying to this program should contact the Tri-Institutional M.D.-Ph.D. Program, 1300 York Avenue, Room D-115, or telephone (212) 746-6023.

## REQUIREMENTS FOR ENTRANCE

A minimum of three years in an accredited college and the MCAT are required; most students have completed four years of undergraduate work and hold a baccalaureate degree. The Committee on Admissions considers a strong foundation in the sciences a fundamental requirement but does not wish to establish rigid guidelines for admission. Therefore, Cornell requires satisfactory completion of at least 24 semester hours in science courses including biology or zoology, general chemistry, organic chemistry, and physics. In addition, six semester hours are required in English literature or composition. For nonscience majors, at least two terms of biology beyond the introductory course are suggested. Cornell regards a broad liberal arts education as fundamental for the making of a good physician. The Committee on Admissions will review and evaluate achievement in the humanities and social sciences.

All required premedical courses should be completed no later than the end of January of the year for which admission is sought.

The MCAT is viewed by the Committee on Admissions as evidence of minimal academic competence and as a standardized test which allows appropriate comparisons.

## SELECTION FACTORS

Students are selected for their leadership potential in various areas of medicine. There is an attempt to select the best qualified students from various academic, geographic, and social backgrounds. Maturity, stability, motivation, academic achievement, and other qualities are evaluated. Recent preparation for the study of medicine, particularly in the sciences, is preferred.

The fall 1995 entering class had the following characteristics: *sex,* 50 women; *mean science GPA,* 3.54; *average MCAT score,* 10.3 in each subtest; *minorities,* 24 students; *undergraduate major,* 65 percent in sciences.

Cornell University Medical College policy actively supports equality of education and employment opportunity and is committed to the maintenance of affirmative action programs, which will assure the continuation of such equality of opportunity.

Students who are unsuccessful in gaining acceptance to Cornell University Medical College are rarely successful on reapplication unless there has been substantial improvement in their qualifications.

## FINANCIAL AID

Admissions decisions are made without regard to financial need. Every effort is made to assist students to finance their medical education without incurring unreasonable debt. Substantial institutional grants and subsidized loans are available and are allocated according to need after an analysis of student and family resources. Fifty-five percent of the students receive Medical College support, and 80 percent receive grants or loans from some source. Since subsidized housing is available for all students at the Medical College, living costs and transportation expenses are reasonable. Support for community service, summer research, and international electives is available for all students. The application fee will be waived if it represents a hardship to the applicant.

## INFORMATION FOR MINORITIES

The Medical College makes a nationwide effort to enroll qualified minority group students.

Cornell conducts a research fellowship program for about 20 minority group premedical students during the summer between their junior and senior college years. The program

consists of research activities with faculty members of the medical center and brief course work in cardiovascular physiology which provides a preview of the basic science years of medical school. The participants are housed in the medical students' residence.

---

Private Institution

### APPLICATION AND ACCEPTANCE POLICIES FOR 1997–98 FIRST-YEAR CLASS

*School participates in AMCAS. See Chapter 4.*

Filing of AMCAS application
    Earliest date: June 1, 1996
    Latest date: Oct. 15, 1996
School application fee to all applicants: $65
Oldest MCAT scores considered: 1992
Does have Early Decision Program (EDP)
    EDP application period: June 1–Aug. 1, 1996
    EDP applicants notified by: Oct. 1, 1996
Acceptance notice to regular applicants
    Earliest date: Oct. 15, 1996
    Latest date: Until class is filled
Applicant's response to acceptance offer
    Maximum time: 2 weeks
Requests for deferred entrance considered: Yes
Deposit to hold place in class (applied to tuition):
    $100, due May 15, 1997
Deposit refundable prior to: May 15, 1997
Estimated number of new entrants: 101 (5 EDP)
Starting date: Aug. 1997

### TUITION AND STUDENT FEES PER YEAR FOR 1995–96 FIRST-YEAR CLASS

Tuition: $22,365      Student fees: $560

### INFORMATION ON 1995–96 FIRST-YEAR CLASS

| Number of | In-State | Out-of-State | Total |
|---|---|---|---|
| Applicants | 1,747 | 5,682 | 7,429 |
| Applicants Interviewed | 855 | 386 | 1,241 |
| New Entrants* | 61 | 40 | 101 |

*All took the MCAT and had baccalaureate degrees.

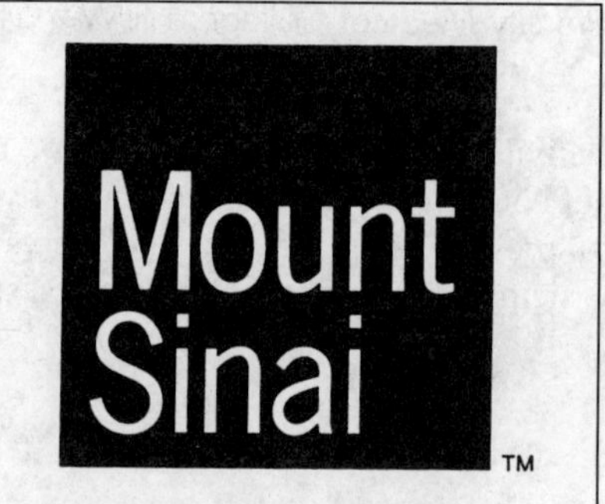

# Mount Sinai School of Medicine
## of the City University of New York

**New York, New York**

Dr. Nathan Kase, *Dean*
Dr. Alex Stagnaro-Green, *Dean for Student Affairs*
Jay A. Cohen, *Assistant Dean for Admissions and Student Affairs,
Director of Admissions and Financial Aid*

## ADDRESS INQUIRIES TO:

Director of Admissions
Mount Sinai School of Medicine
Annenberg Building, Room 5-04
One Gustave L. Levy Place-Box 1002
New York, New York 10029-6574
(212) 241-6696
Web Site: http://www.mssm.edu

## GENERAL INFORMATION

Mount Sinai School of Medicine, an integral part of the Mount Sinai Medical Center, is privately endowed, coeducational, and nondenominational. Developed from the 140-year tradition of patient care, professional education, and research of the Mount Sinai Hospital, it enrolled its first students in 1968 and is officially affiliated with the City University of New York.

The Medical Center's 22 buildings include a hospital, numerous research and service laboratories, teaching facilities, the Postgraduate School of Medicine, and the Graduate School of Biological Sciences.

The Mount Sinai Hospital, a 1,300-bed facility with a clinical research center, constitutes the basic resource for clinical training. The school is also affiliated with the Bronx Veterans Affairs Medical Center, City Hospital Center at Elmhurst, Englewood Hospital, Jewish Home and Hospital for the Aged, North General Hospital, Queens Hospital Center, and Staten Island University Hospital.

## CURRICULUM

The curriculum of the School of Medicine represents a philosophy balancing the educational needs of the physician and integrating quantitative biology with clinical medicine. Provision is made for close integration of preclinical and clinical sciences and instruction in social aspects of disease and medical care.

The framework of the curriculum in the first two years includes a period of instruction in the language and principles of the basic sciences, followed by integrated interdepartmental teaching of organ systems or clinical disciplines. A generalist physician initiative provides all students in the first two years with a continuity experience in primary care ambulatory medicine. The third year and part of the fourth year permit more intensive study of organ system diseases by means of rotation through various clinical disciplines. An ambulatory experience is an important component of all the clinical clerkships in the third year. In addition to the extensive facilities of the Mount Sinai Hospital, the other hospitals affiliated with the school are used for clinical teaching.

The Medical Scientist Training Program (MSTP) was developed for students interested in a career in medical research and academic medicine. This M.D.-Ph.D. program is funded by a training grant from the NIH as well as by other extramural and intramural awards. Students may apply for the combined program at the time of application for admission or during the second year of medical school.

A new master of science degree in community medicine is available, and is designed to produce a new generation of leaders in preventive medicine while providing advanced training in the population-based medical sciences. A master's program in bioethics, science, and society is also available for interested students. The core courses provide a framework for understanding the philosophical, social, and scientific background that underlie bioethical issues.

The objective of the School of Medicine is to provide a climate that will stimulate individual development in research and clinical skills, emphasize creativity, strengthen a desire to extend the learning process for the entire life cycle, and foster the dedication of medical knowledge for the benefit of all.

## REQUIREMENTS FOR ENTRANCE

A minimum of three years of college and the MCAT are required. Most students admitted have earned the bachelor's degree. The prospective student should have basic knowledge of the biological and physical sciences and mathematics, plus an appreciation of the social forces influencing man. Students majoring in nonscience disciplines who meet all admission requirements will be given consideration on an equal basis with those having specific scientific backgrounds.

Admission requirements include accredited college work in the following subjects:

|  | *Years* |
| --- | --- |
| Biology | 1 |
| Inorganic chemistry | 1 |
| Organic chemistry | 1 |
| Physics | 1 |

Mathematics . . . . . . . . . . . . . . . . . . . . . . . . . . . . . . . . . . . . 1
English . . . . . . . . . . . . . . . . . . . . . . . . . . . . . . . . . . . . . . . 1

## SELECTION FACTORS

The school is keenly interested in a total appraisal of a student's potential for a career in medicine. Excellence in scholarship, personal maturity, integrity, intellectual creativity, and motivation for medicine are important factors. The interview is given considerable weight; premedical advisory committee letters of recommendation and MCAT scores are criteria for evaluation. All applicants, regardless of race, creed, sex, age, handicap, or national origin, are given serious and thorough consideration by the Admissions Committee.

Accepted students for the 1995 entering class had the following characteristics: *mean GPA,* 3.5 (90 percent above 3.0); *sex,* 51 percent women. Distribution of undergraduate major reflects the distribution in the applicant pool.

## FINANCIAL AID

It is the policy of the school to provide as much financial assistance as possible to students who require such assistance in order to maintain attendance. Students who are accepted for admission are provided financial assistance applications on which they may document their request for financial aid. Applications are treated confidentially, and awards are made by a faculty committee on financial aid. Each applicant is considered on an individual basis so that the greatest support for the most needy students can be distributed.

Financial aid may be offered in the form of a scholarship, a loan, or both, in accordance with the requirements of the individual situation and the availability of funds in the various categories. Over 75 percent of the students receive financial assistance; 70 percent receive direct institutional support.

## INFORMATION FOR UNDERREPRESENTED MINORITY APPLICANTS

Strongly motivated students from underrepresented minority backgrounds are actively sought and encouraged to apply. A pre-entrance summer program is available for students who are accepted to the freshman class. Tutorial assistance is available for all students.

Private Institution

## APPLICATION AND ACCEPTANCE POLICIES FOR 1997–98 FIRST-YEAR CLASS

*School participates in AMCAS. See Chapter 4.*

Filing of AMCAS application
  Earliest date: June 1, 1996
  Latest date: Nov. 1, 1996
School application fee to all applicants: $100
Oldest MCAT scores considered: 1977
Does have Early Decision Program (EDP)
  EDP application period: June 1–Aug. 1, 1996
  EDP applicants notified by: Oct. 1, 1996
Acceptance notice to regular applicants
  Earliest date: Nov. 15, 1996
  Latest date: Varies
Applicant's response to acceptance offer
  Maximum time: 2 weeks
Requests for deferred entrance considered: Yes
Deposit to hold place in class: None
Estimated number of new entrants: 115 (5 EDP)
Starting date: Aug. 1997

## TUITION AND STUDENT FEES PER YEAR FOR 1995–96 FIRST-YEAR CLASS

Tuition: $21,000                Student fees: $825

## INFORMATION ON 1995–96 FIRST-YEAR CLASS

| Number of | In-State | Out-of-State | Total |
|---|---|---|---|
| Applicants | 1,747 | 3,671 | 5,418 |
| Applicants Interviewed | 439 | 448 | 887 |
| New Entrants* | 73 | 42 | 115 |

*All took the MCAT and had baccalaureate degrees.

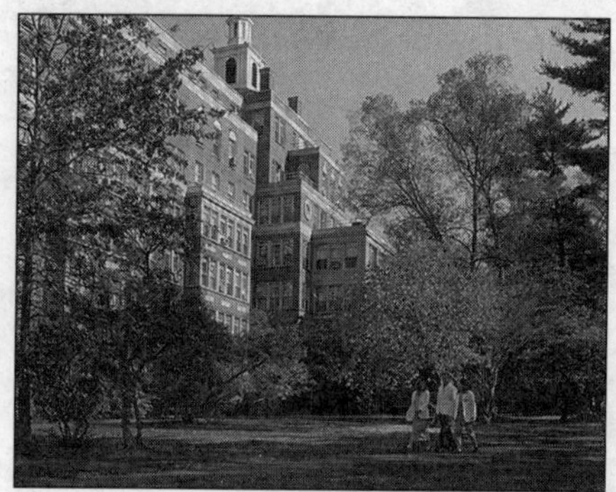

# New York Medical College

## Valhalla, New York


Dr. Ralph A. O'Connell, *Provost and Dean of the Medical College*
Dr. Fern Juster, *Associate Dean and Chair, Committee on Admissions*
Anthony M. Sozzo, *Associate Dean and Director of Student Financial Aid*


## ADDRESS INQUIRIES TO:

Office of Admissions
Sunshine Cottage
New York Medical College
Valhalla, New York 10595
(914) 993-4507; 993-4976 (FAX)

## GENERAL INFORMATION

Founded in 1860, the New York Medical College, is a private, not-for-profit university comprising the nation's third largest medical school and two graduate schools in health sciences and basic medical sciences. The college, about 25 miles from New York City, is located on a suburban campus in Westchester County, New York, which becomes home base for students in the first two years. The college is affiliated with 30 hospitals in the New York City metropolitan area, from which students select the sites for their clinical clerkships in years three and four. These affiliations include urban medical centers, small suburban hospitals and technologically advanced, regional tertiary care facilities. This vast network endows the university with diverse resources for teaching, learning, research, and patient care activities.

## CURRICULUM

The first two years of the M.D. program focus on developing a thorough understanding of the sciences basic to medicine—anatomy, biochemistry, physiology, microbiology, pathology, and pharmacology—through lectures, laboratory work, small group discussions, clinical case conferences, and direct patient contact. Clinical electives, as well as opportunities to pursue research interests in basic science and clinical departments are available during the summer following the first year.

The third year runs for a full calendar year, during which students complete clerkships in seven disciplines—medicine, neurology, surgery, pediatrics, psychiatry, obstetrics and gynecology, and the generalist clerkship. Superb resources are provided by the college's wide network of affiliated hospitals, which include two academic medical centers. The fourth year is composed of both required clinical rotations, taken at the college's affiliated hospitals, and electives which can be taken at medical institutions across the country and around the world.

Anticipating the need for more generalist physicians, a decade ago the college began exposing medical students to primary care training and mentors. This initiative continues today and includes the following programs:

Introduction to Primary Care—An innovative two-year selective which places first- and second-year students in the offices of generalist faculty. Students work closely with a physician preceptor, examining patients and focusing on topics such as health maintenance, ethics, and cultural perspectives of health care.

Generalist Clerkship—This one-month clerkship allows third-year students to work directly with primary care physicians in an outpatient setting that stresses continuity, preventive medicine, and the integration of the behavioral sciences in clinical practice.

Six-Year Program—Students in this program condense into six years the sequence of four years of medical school and three years of a residency in general internal medicine. They accomplish this by completing the fourth year of medical school at the same time they begin the first year of residency. Loans for the fourth year of medical school are forgiven for students who practice primary care for three years after completing the program.

## REQUIREMENTS FOR ENTRANCE

It is strongly recommended that the applicant successfully complete undergraduate college work leading to a baccalaureate degree from an accredited college of arts and sciences in the United States or Canada. All courses offered in satisfaction of the requirements for admission must be taken in or accepted as transfer credit by an accredited college in the United States or Canada and must be acceptable to that institution toward a baccalaureate degree in general arts or sciences. The Committee on Admissions has no preference for a major field of undergraduate study, but any college work submitted must include the specified credits below.

Each student's credentials must include:

|  | *Sem. hrs.* |
| --- | --- |
| Biology (with lab) | 8 |
| Inorganic chemistry (with lab) | 8 |
| Organic chemistry (with lab) | 8 |
| Physics (with lab) | 8 |
| English | 6 |

All candidates are required to take the MCAT.

## SELECTION FACTORS

Students are selected on the basis of motivation, character, intellectual curiosity, and academic excellence. The college strives to select students who have a strong sense of dedication to the service of others. In addition they must possess the requisite sensory, cognitive, motor, and organizational skills, including the ability to synthesize and apply knowledge necessary to complete the entire curriculum satisfactorily.

No persons shall be denied admission to any educational program or activity on the basis of any legally prohibited discrimination involving, but not limited to, such factors as race, creed, religion, national or ethnic origin, sex, age, or handicap.

## FINANCIAL AID

Approximately 85 percent of the student body receives some form of financial assistance. Financial aid is awarded on the basis of need; limited grants and scholarships are also available. The college provides information and services including debt management, loan counseling, information regarding outside sources of aid, and management of resources while attending the college. Students are discouraged from seeking outside employment during the academic year. All students will receive a financial aid packet of information upon acceptance to the college. For further information call the Office of Student Financial Planning at (914) 993-4491.

## INFORMATION FOR EDUCATIONALLY DISADVANTAGED

Strongly motivated students from educationally deprived backgrounds are actively sought and encouraged to apply. A pre-entrance summer program which provides an intensive review of basic science courses and an introduction to preclinical medicine is available to students.

Private Institution

## APPLICATION AND ACCEPTANCE POLICIES FOR 1997–98 FIRST-YEAR CLASS

*School participates in AMCAS. See Chapter 4.*

Filing of AMCAS application
    Earliest date: June 1, 1996
    Latest date: Dec. 1, 1996
School application fee to all applicants: $75
Oldest MCAT scores considered: 1993
Does have Early Decision Program (EDP)
    EDP application period: June 1–Aug. 1, 1996
    EDP applicants notified by: Oct. 1, 1996
Acceptance notice to regular applicants
    Earliest date: Oct. 15, 1996
    Latest date: Until class is filled
Applicant's response to acceptance offer
    Maximum time: 2 weeks
Requests for deferred entrance considered: Yes
Deposit to hold place in class (applied to tuition):
    $100, due May 15, 1997
Deposit refundable prior to: May 15, 1997
Estimated number of new entrants: 190 (10 EDP)
Starting date: Aug. 1997

## TUITION AND STUDENT FEES PER YEAR FOR 1995–96 FIRST-YEAR CLASS

Tuition: $25,150          Student fees: $465

## INFORMATION ON 1995–96 FIRST-YEAR CLASS

| Number of | In-State | Out-of-State | Total |
|---|---|---|---|
| Applicants | 2,581 | 9,708 | 12,289 |
| Applicants Interviewed | 348 | 1,065 | 1,413 |
| New Entrants* | 42 | 146 | 188 |

*All took the MCAT and had baccalaureate degrees.

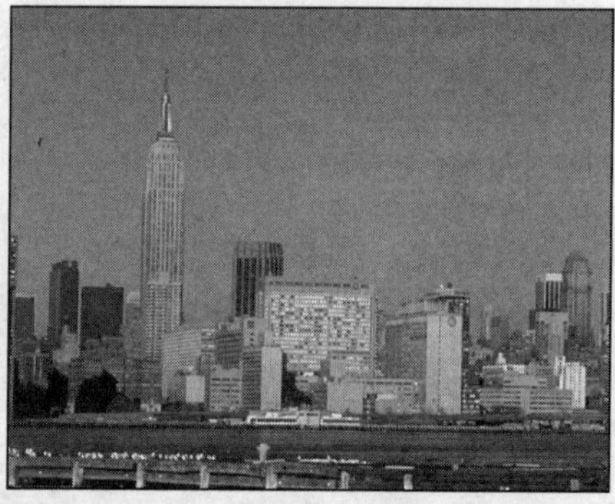

# New York University School of Medicine

## New York, New York


Dr. Saul J. Farber, *Dean*

Raymond J. Brienza, *Assistant Dean for Admissions and Director of Financial Aid*


## ADDRESS INQUIRIES TO:

Office of Admissions
New York University
School of Medicine
P.O. Box 1924
New York, New York 10016
(212) 263-5290

## GENERAL INFORMATION

The New York University School of Medicine was founded in 1841 when it admitted a class of 239 students to a four-month course of lectures conducted by six professors on the faculty. The medical school is a constituent of New York University (NYU), one of the oldest and largest private universities in the United States.

## CURRICULUM

Several changes in the curriculum have been implemented in the past few years. These innovations are designed to promote independent learning through an increase of small-group seminars, problem-solving exercises, and computer-assisted instruction. Study of the basic sciences provides students with the essential facts, concepts, and skills necessary to understand the scientific principles upon which clinical medicine is based. The basic science program is enriched by the honors program, the Hippocrates project and opportunities for independent study research. Study of the clinical sciences, which begins in the third year, promotes excellence in clinical and decision-making skills. Flexibility in the scheduling of required clerkships and electives throughout the third and fourth year permits students to design a course of study specific to their educational and career goals. A rich ambulatory care experience provides students with an understanding of the physician-patient relationship and underscores issues of disease prevention.

## REQUIREMENTS FOR ENTRANCE

The requirements for admission are as follows: the MCAT; a minimum of three years of college work; and the following courses plus an acceptable concentration in any of these fields, or in any other field, at the college level:

|  | *Sem. hrs.* |
| --- | --- |
| Biology (with lab) | 6 |
| Inorganic chemistry (with lab) | 6 |
| Organic chemistry (with lab) | 6 |
| General physics (with lab) | 6 |
| English | 6 |

Genetics and a course in embryology or developmental biology are recommended for students who select extra work in biology and have all options open to them as far as their college is concerned.

Biochemistry is recommended for all students.

It is strongly recommended that candidates complete their college work for the baccalaureate degree.

Applicants should take the MCAT in the spring of the year in which they are applying to medical school to achieve an earlier processing of their applications in the fall. In no case should the MCAT be taken later than August of the application year.

## SELECTION FACTORS

The selection process involves judging the applicant from several viewpoints, among them the following: excellence in course work at the college level; evaluation of the student by college instructors, premedical committees, and other similar mechanisms provided by the colleges; an interview at NYU; and the results of the MCAT. The Committee on Admissions does not computerize the candidate's profile in terms of MCAT scores and GPAs because qualitative considerations, such as college evaluation and interview impression, are also given great weight in the final evaluation. The Committee on Admissions does lend some weight to trends in the student's college progress. Students who may, for one reason or another, get off to a slow start in college and then show that they are capable of honors work in later years are given sympathetic consideration, regardless of GPAs. The medical school's student body is drawn mainly from the eastern seaboard—a reflection of the composition of the applicant pool. Applications from outside the region are welcome. NYU is a private institution and has no geographical or other quotas. It should be noted, however, that foreign nationals who do not hold a permanent resident visa have only a slight chance of being admitted.

Women have constituted from 33 to 42 percent of recent entering classes. The acceptance rates for men and women are approximately the same.

Only those students who on the basis of application data appear to merit serious consideration for admission are interviewed.

## FINANCIAL AID

The Financial Aid Office reviews all applications for financial assistance. The school's resources are drawn from scholarships and loan programs. Enrolled students and those students accepted for admission to the school are eligible to file applications for assistance. The School of Medicine participates in the Primary Care Loan and the Perkins Loan Program, which provide low-interest support for deserving students. Loans are also available through the New York Higher Education Assistance Corporation. New York State Tuition Assistance Program Awards are available to many residents of New York who are degree candidates.

Applicants requesting financial aid must file a financial aid profile through the College Scholarship Service. (See Part 1 for details.)

## INFORMATION FOR MINORITIES

Minorities are welcomed into the school. Every effort is made in the case of all candidates, including minorities, to reach some determination on motivation, character, and capacities of the candidate, regardless of such standard measures as test scores and college performance. Considerable reliance is placed on the evaluation of students by their college teachers. This is particularly important in terms of the candidate's motivation under adverse circumstances. It is possible to have application fees waived in cases of demonstrated need.

---

Private Institution

## APPLICATION AND ACCEPTANCE POLICIES FOR 1997–98 FIRST-YEAR CLASS

Filing of application
    Earliest date: Aug. 15, 1996
    Latest date: Dec. 1, 1996
School application fee to all applicants: $75
Oldest MCAT scores considered: 1993
Does not have Early Decision Program
Acceptance notice to regular applicants
    Earliest date: Dec. 20, 1996
    Latest date: Until class is filled
Applicant's response to acceptance offer
    Maximum time: 2 weeks
Requests for deferred entrance considered: Yes
Deposit to hold place in class (applied to tuition):
    $100, due with response to acceptance offer
Deposit refundable prior to: May 1, 1997
Estimated number of new entrants: 160
Starting date: Sept. 1997

## TUITION AND STUDENT FEES PER YEAR FOR 1995–96 FIRST-YEAR CLASS

Tuition: $20,900        Student fees: $3,720

## INFORMATION ON 1995–96 FIRST-YEAR CLASS

| Number of | In-State | Out-of-State | Total |
|---|---|---|---|
| Applicants | * | * | 4,445 |
| Applicants Interviewed | * | * | 981 |
| New Entrants† | 77 | 82 | 159 |

*Information not available.

†All took the MCAT and had baccalaureate degrees.

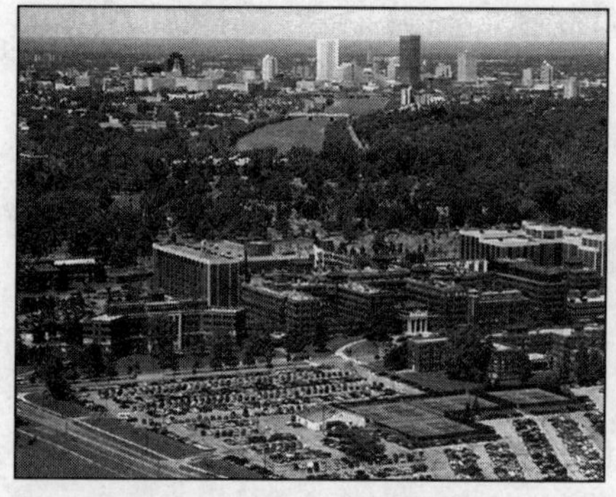

# University of Rochester
# School of Medicine and Dentistry

**Rochester, New York**

Dr. Lowell A. Goldsmith, *Dean*
Dr. Mary Lou Meyers, *Associate Dean for Admissions*
Barbara A. Rupp, *Director of Admissions*

## ADDRESS INQUIRIES TO:

Director of Admissions
University of Rochester
School of Medicine and Dentistry
Medical Center Box 601
Rochester, New York 14642
(617) 275-4539; 273-1016 (FAX)
E-Mail: admish@urmc.rochester.edu

## GENERAL INFORMATION

The School of Medicine and Dentistry was established in 1920 as an academic division of the University of Rochester, a privately endowed institution founded in 1850. The university was one of the first to combine a medical school and a teaching hospital within the same facility. The original medical center has been greatly expanded to include a modern medical education wing, many new research opportunities, and the new Strong Memorial Hospital. Clinical teaching also is conducted at affiliated hospitals within the community. Opportunities for independent work include summer and full-year fellowships and a wide selection of elective offerings. More than half of the students elect participation in research.

## CURRICULUM

During the first two years, the basic medical sciences are stressed, and students develop broad knowledge of human biology and behavior in health and illness. Programs include considerable interdisciplinary teaching and case- and problem-based learning. Developing skills in problem solving and gaining an appreciation of principles are emphasized. From the beginning, students at Rochester learn to interact with patients; examine the biological, psychological, and social dimensions of health and illness; and develop the qualities important to becoming informed, caring, and dedicated physicians. A tutorial system and broad elective programs are offered.

At the start of the third year, in a unique interdepartmental course entitled General Clerkship, students focus on the basic techniques of clinical medicine, including the interview, physical examination, and clinical laboratory methodology. Students complete basic departmental clerkships during the remainder of the third year. An enriched fourth year is devoted to advanced clinical work in emergency and ambulatory care,

selected medical specialties, and electives. Each student participates in a four- to six-week externship (subinternship) in one of the major clinical disciplines. In both the third and fourth years, programs provide balanced exposure to primary care and specialty experiences.

Individual tutoring and remedial work are available to all students in the school with special academic needs.

A variety of special programs are offered, reflecting the rich and diverse opportunities available to students. A strong M.D.-Ph.D. program and a year out research fellowship program are offered, reflecting the institution's commitment to research and the preparation of medical scientists and academicians. Opportunities to participate in volunteer service to the Rochester community and to experience medicine in other cultures through our international medicine program reflect the school's commitment to providing students the broadest possible educational experience.

## REQUIREMENTS FOR ENTRANCE

A minimum of three years of college is required, but almost all entering students have completed the baccalaureate degree. The MCAT is not required, but applicants who have taken or will take the test must submit a score report to the Admissions Committee.

Satisfactory completion of the following premedical course work is required:

|  | Sem. Hr. |
| --- | --- |
| Biology (with lab) | 6-8 |
| General or inorganic chemistry | 6-8 |
| Organic chemistry | 6-8 |

One semester of biochemistry may be substituted for a semester of organic chemistry. Within the two-year chemistry sequence, one year of laboratory is required.

| | |
| --- | --- |
| Physics (with lab) | 6-8 |
| Expository Writing | 6-8 |

May be met with writing, English, or nonscience courses that involve expository writing

| | |
| --- | --- |
| Humanities and/or social or behavioral sciences | 12-16 |

The requirements above are designed with the expectation that students will enter with a broad, liberal, and diversified education. In addition, courses in calculus and statistics, and experience in research, clinical practice, public health, or health policy issues are strongly recommended.

To further encourage diversity in one's undergraduate experience, Rochester favors the use of advanced placement credit as a means to take additional college courses that otherwise might not be possible to schedule. However, advanced placement credit may not be used to satisfy the biology, English, or nonscience requirements. Advanced placement courses may substitute for one semester of general chemistry and/or one semester of physics only.

## SELECTION FACTORS

Evaluation of applicants includes a careful examination of the entire academic record, letters of recommendation, and the candidate's personal statement. Candidates who show particular promise of achievement are invited for interviews.

Demonstrated excellence in a demanding academic program, including a high level of achievement in the natural sciences, is an absolute requirement for acceptance. Evidence of intrinsic intellectual drive and curiosity is highly valued since the program at Rochester emphasizes independent opportunities for individual students. Particular attention is given to achievements that demonstrate breadth and commitment. The school is characterized by an atmosphere in which students and faculty work closely together towards the attainment of knowledge and understanding and in which patients are treated with compassion and sensitivity. Students are sought who will contribute to this climate for learning.

Selections are made without regard to gender, sexual orientation, race, religion, national origin, age, or handicap. Well-qualified applicants from all parts of the United States are encouraged to apply. State residency is not a factor in selection.

All applicants must have completed at least two years of undergraduate college study in the United States, including all premedical requirements.

Applicants who have not been accepted may reapply in a subsequent year, but applicants who twice have been unsuccessful in gaining admission are discouraged from reapplying.

## FINANCIAL AID

The medical school offers scholarships and long-term loans to those students who demonstrate financial need. Decisions concerning admission are made independently of financial circumstances.

In 1993–94, over 80 percent of the enrolled students received financial assistance from either school or noninstitutional sources. Entering students applying for institutional financial aid are required to provide a FAFSA, an additional more detailed financial statement including parent information, and the School of Medicine's financial aid application. These are distributed to all interviewed applicants in early January.

## INFORMATION FOR UNDERREPRESENTED MINORITIES

The Office of Minority Affairs represents a serious commitment on the part of the University of Rochester School of Medicine and Dentistry to meet the urgent need for minority physicians in all aspects of the medical profession. An active recruitment program seeks applicants for both the M.D. and M.D.-Ph.D. programs.

The Summer Research Fellowship (SURF) Program is designed to provide minority undergraduates with a 9-week exposure to the research and clinical areas. Rising seniors in the program are urged to apply to medical or graduate school during this time. Early interviews, in addition to informational meetings with admissions, financial aid, and other pertinent areas, provide students with valuable information required for the medical school application process.

---

Private Institution

### APPLICATION AND ACCEPTANCE POLICIES FOR 1997–98 FIRST-YEAR CLASS

Filing of application
    Earliest date: June 15, 1996
    Latest date: Oct. 15, 1996
School application fee to all applicants: $65
Oldest MCAT scores considered: 1993
Does not have Early Decision Program
Acceptance notice to regular applicants
    Earliest date: Dec. 15, 1996
    Latest date: Until class is filled
Applicant's response to acceptance offer
    Maximum time: 2 weeks
Requests for deferred entrance considered: Yes
Deposit to hold place in class: None
Estimated number of new entrants: 100
Starting date: Aug. 1997

### TUITION AND STUDENT FEES PER YEAR FOR 1995–96 FIRST-YEAR CLASS

Tuition: $22,700      Student fees: $1,680

### INFORMATION ON 1995–96 FIRST-YEAR CLASS

| Number of | In-State | Out-of-State | Total |
|---|---|---|---|
| Applicants | 1,082 | 2,877 | 3,959 |
| Applicants Interviewed | 220 | 499 | 719 |
| New Entrants* | 35 | 64 | 99 |

*All had baccalaureate degrees; 85% took the MCAT.

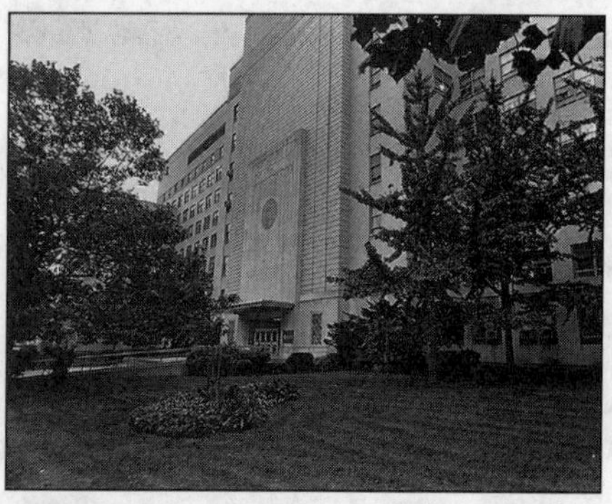

# State University of New York Health Science Center at Brooklyn College of Medicine

## Brooklyn, New York

Dr. Eugene B. Feigelson, *Dean*
Liliana Montano, *Director of Admissions*
Deborah Pointer, *Director of Financial Aid*

## ADDRESS INQUIRIES TO:

Director of Admissions
State University of New York
Health Science Center at Brooklyn
450 Clarkson Avenue-Box 60M
Brooklyn, New York 11203
(718) 270-2446

## GENERAL INFORMATION

The College of Medicine of the State University of New York Health Science Center at Brooklyn traces its roots to the founding in 1860 of the Long Island College Hospital, the first hospital-based medical school in the country. In 1950, the College of Medicine joined the State University of New York system and developed into a major center for health sciences. The University Hospital, a 376-bed teaching hospital, opened in 1966. In addition to its own hospital, the Health Science Center uses several major affiliated community hospitals in the clinical years. In 1992, the campus' new Health Science Education Building opened. It houses state of the art classrooms, laboratories, a 500-seat auditorium, and the Medical Research Library of Brooklyn.

## CURRICULUM

The first two years provide a comprehensive education in the basic sciences, employing a combination of lectures, small group experiences, and computer-assisted instruction. During the first year, attention is focused on the basic components of human biology and behavior, as well as on the essential aspects of physician-patient relationship. Using this foundation, the second-year student begins the study of human disease, its diagnosis, prevention, and treatment and is taught the techniques of medical interviewing and examination. The second-year curriculum is organized in an organ system approach with the following topic areas: cardiovascular, pulmonary, oncology, gastrointestinal, reproductive, and others. The emphasis is on the development of clinical reasoning and problem-solving skills. Clinical electives are available as early as the first year. All students are required to sit for Step 1 of the USMLE at the end of their second year. The third year is devoted to clerkships in the six clinical disciplines of medicine: obstetrics, gynecology, neurology, surgery, pediatrics, and psychiatry. The fourth year comprises an ambulatory care

rotation, a subinternship, and a minimum of 20 weeks of clinical electives.

The Problem-Based Learning Track offers an alternative to the first two years of the conventional curriculum. It incorporates tutorial sessions in which students are actively engaged in learning basic science material as they attempt to solve patient problems.

The Generalist Physician Track is for students committed to entering careers in primary care (internal medicine, pediatrics, or family practice). During the first two years, one afternoon per week, students participate in a clinic under the supervision of attending physicians from one of our affiliates, Lutheran Medical Center. In the third year, some of the required clerkships are completed at Lutheran Medical Center.

All courses are graded unsatisfactory, pass, high pass, and honors.

The College of Medicine and the School of Graduate Studies sponsor a combined M.D.- Ph.D. program designed for students who are interested in academic medicine involving a combination of research, teaching, and clinical activities.

A B.A. M.D. Honors program is offered in conjunction with Brooklyn College of the City University of New York. Information on special admission and matriculation criteria is available from the Office of Admissions at Brooklyn College.

## REQUIREMENTS FOR ENTRANCE

Applicants must have taken the new MCAT and completed a minimum of 90 semester credits of undergraduate work at an accredited college. Courses required for admission are:

*Semester Credits*

| | |
|---|---|
| General biology (with lab) | 8 |
| Inorganic chemistry (with lab) | 8 |
| Organic chemistry (with lab) | 8 |
| General physics (with lab) | 8 |
| English | 6 |

If freshman English is exempted, a more advanced course is required.

The remainder of the courses should be in the liberal arts curriculum and credited toward a bachelor's degree. At least one year of college mathematics, one of an advanced scientific subject, and a course in biochemistry are recommended. Students educated abroad must complete a minimum of one year of full-time college study in an accredited college or university in the United States or Canada.

Applicants are urged to take the MCAT in the spring of the year of application and to have completed the premedical requirements at the time of application.

## SELECTION FACTORS

The Committee on Admissions considers the total qualifications of each applicant without regard to sex, sexual orientation, race, color, creed, religion, national origin, age, or disability. Women and members of underrepresented minority groups are encouraged to apply. Decisions are based on a number of factors, including prior academic performance; completion of required courses; the potential for academic success including performance on the MCAT; communication skills, character, personal skills; demonstrated commitment to community-social service outreach activities; and motivation for medicine. Preference is given to qualified New York state residents. Reapplicants adhere to the same procedures, policies, and deadlines as first time applicants.

Admission to advanced standing is limited to U.S. citizens or permanent residents who are matriculated, in good standing, and in attendance as medical students in a College of Medicine in the U.S. Applications are accepted to the third-year class, and admissions preference is given to New York State residents.

## FINANCIAL AID

The College is committed to help students meet their educational expenses through various types of financial assistance. Aid is granted on the basis of need (determined in accordance with federal regulations); and for some scholarships, on academic achievement. The major portion of our assistance is derived from federal and state allocations: grants, scholarships, loans and/or college work study. Loans are the most common form of assistance. Financial aid application materials are sent to all accepted applicants and students' financial aid needs are reviewed annually.

## INFORMATION FOR MINORITIES

The SUNY Health Science Center maintains a tradition of commitment to the enrollment of historically underrepresented groups. The Office of Minority Affairs directs several programs targeted to furnish information and support to students from minority backgrounds. Operation Success is an eight-week elective summer enrichment program designed to provide first-year minority students with a head start on the first semester medical curriculum. Entering minority students are matched with a faculty mentor. The Daniel Hale Williams Society, the primary voice of minority students on campus, provides peer support.

Public Institution

## APPLICATION AND ACCEPTANCE POLICIES FOR 1997–98 FIRST-YEAR CLASS

*School participates in AMCAS. See Chapter 4.*

Filing of AMCAS application
   Earliest date: June 1, 1996
   Latest date: Dec. 15, 1996
School application fee to all applicants: $65
Oldest MCAT scores considered: 1994
Does have Early Decision Program (EDP)
   For New York state residents only
   EDP application period: June 1–Aug. 1, 1996
   EDP applicants notified by: Oct. 1, 1996
Acceptance notice to regular applicants
   Earliest date: Oct. 15, 1996
   Latest date: Until class is filled
Applicant's response to acceptance offer
   Maximum time: 2 weeks
Requests for deferred entrance considered: Yes
Deposit to hold place in class (applied to tuition):
   $100, due with response to acceptance offer;
   refundable upon written request prior to
   May 15, 1997
Estimated number of new entrants: 185 (20 EDP)
Starting date: Aug. 1997

## TUITION AND STUDENT FEES PER YEAR FOR 1995–96 FIRST-YEAR CLASS

Tuition                 Student fees: $220
   Resident: $10,840
   Nonresident: $21,940

## INFORMATION ON 1995–96 FIRST-YEAR CLASS

| Number of | In-State | Out-of-State | Total |
|---|---|---|---|
| Applicants | 2,818 | 3,323 | 6,141 |
| Applicants Interviewed | 709 | 87 | 796 |
| New Entrants* | 178 | 8 | 186 |

*All took the MCAT and had baccalaureate degrees.

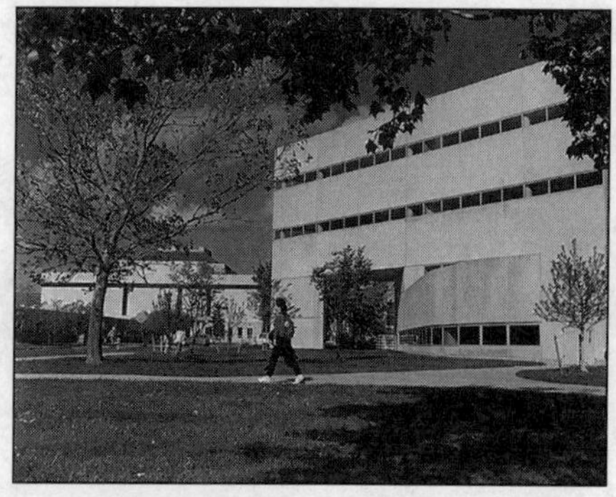

# University at Buffalo
# School of Medicine and Biomedical Sciences

**Buffalo, New York**

Dr. John Naughton, *Vice President for Clinical Affairs and Dean*
Dr. Thomas J. Guttuso, *Assistant Dean, Admissions*
Elias G. Eldayie, Director, *Student Finances and Records*

## ADDRESS INQUIRIES TO:

Office of Medical Admissions
University at Buffalo
35 CFS Building
Buffalo, New York 14214-3013
(716) 829-3466; 829-2798 (FAX)
E-Mail: jrosso@ubmedc.buffalo.edu

## GENERAL INFORMATION

The School of Medicine was founded by Millard Filmore and a group of physicians in 1846 and is celebrating its sesquicentennial this year. It was a privately supported school until the University of Buffalo joined the State University of New York (SUNY) system in 1962. The University at Buffalo has the most comprehensive campus in the SUNY system and was honored in 1989 with election to the Association of American Universities. The preclinical campus and library are located on the Main Street Campus at the northeastern corner of the city. The clinical education program is conducted in cooperation with nine area hospitals.

## CURRICULUM

The curriculum is designed to emphasize the relevance of medical education to the practice of primary care medicine, demonstrate the relevance of basic science to clinical practice, introduce patient contact and patient centered learning in the first year of medical school, and increase the experience in ambulatory care in the clinical years. Innovative new courses, including introduction to clinical medicine and interdisciplinary medicine, will be taught throughout the first two years and are designed to prepare students in the knowledge, skills, and attitudes required to successfully enter the clinical clerkships in the third year and provide the foundation for their medical careers. Ethics, the doctor-patient relationship, principles of health promotion, disease prevention, and promotion of self-learning and inquiry are emphasized, in addition to extensive education in the skills basic to medical practice and patient care. All students must take Step I of the USMLE upon completion of the basic science years. The clinical years include required clerkships in internal medicine, surgery, pediatrics, obstetrics and gynecology, psychiatry, neurology, family medicine, primary ambulatory care and surgical specialties. There is ample free time in the senior year for electives here or away. UB's goal is to prepare its graduates to enter and complete graduate education, qualify for licensure, provide excellence in medical care, and have the educational background for continued learning.

## REQUIREMENTS FOR ENTRANCE

The new MCAT is required and should be taken no later than the fall of the year preceding admission. A bachelor's degree from an approved college or university is desired. The following minimal premedical course requirements must be completed prior to enrollment:

|  | *Semesters* |
| --- | --- |
| Biology (with labs) | 2 |
| With not more than one semester of botany. | |
| Chemistry (with labs) | 3 |
| At least one semester must be organic. | |
| General physics | 2 |
| English | 2 |

The choice of undergraduate concentration is optional. The prerequisites for admission reflect the need for a basic preparation in the sciences and are meant to encourage the student to develop a foundation in the social sciences and the humanities.

Medical Scientist Training Program (MSTP) is a seven- to eight-year program designed for preparation for careers in biomedical sciences and combines the training for both the M.D. and Ph.D. degrees. Interested applicants should request an application from the MSTP Office, University at Buffalo, 27 Cary Hall, Buffalo, NY 14214; phone: 716-829-3236.

## EARLY ASSURANCE PROGRAM

Undergraduate sophomores can apply to this program if they have demonstrated a high level of academic competence by attaining around a 3.5 GPA in science and nonscience courses and have completed at least half of the premedical course requirements. Underrepresented minorities in medicine with a competitive record are especially encouraged to apply. Application deadline is February 1, 1997. Submission of SAT scores is required. Accepted candidates are not required to take the MCAT, are encouraged to pursue their intellectual interests in their remaining college years, and will commence their medical education in August 1999. Approximately 30 are accepted each year.

## SELECTION FACTORS

The Admissions Committee seeks to identify and select students who display favorable qualities deemed important for the pursuit of a career in medicine. In making its assessments and determinations, the committee relies on information contained in the application and in documents submitted in support of the applicant. Based on careful screening, applicants are invited to appear for an interview. Reapplications are treated no differently than initial applications. Rejected applicants should seek the advice and counsel of their premedical adviser.

Students are accepted without regard to race, sex, creed, national origin, age, or handicap. All applicants will receive the *Essential Functions of the Medical School Curriculum* including technical statndards after their application is reviewed. Preference is given to qualified residents of New York State. Out-of-state applicants should consider this carefully before applying. Applications are not accepted from foreign nationals. All applicants must have completed at least two full years or 60 credit hours of higher education in the United States or Canada. The present freshman class has an average GPA of 3.62 and an average MCAT of 9.8 with a composition of 47 percent female and 6 percent minority. Transfer students are accepted into the third year only with four seats available for Americans in a foreign school. Transfer from American schools are considered only under conditions of hardship.

## FINANCIAL AID

The FAFSA should be received at the Federal Student Aid Office (see Part 1) by May 15, 1997, for all students applying to the 1997 entering class. Forms received after the deadline are subject to funds available. Requests for financial aid are considered after admission, and awards are made based on the student's need as estimated by the university's Office of Financial Aid. In most financial aid requests, parental income information is required regardless of dependency status. All financial aid is need based. A limited number of scholarships based on academic merit and financial need are provided each year.

## INFORMATION FOR MINORITIES

A Summer Enrichment and Support Program is available to facilitate students' retention in medical school. The enrichment program, designed for first-year educationally and socio-economically disadvantaged students admitted to SUNY-Buffalo, offers histology; a preceptorship program; and learning skills development. The program begins June 1 and runs through July. Tutorial and counseling services are offered during the summer and throughout the academic year. The School of Medicine has a strong retention program; however, each student must meet the academic standards established by the faculty.

Public Institution

### APPLICATION AND ACCEPTANCE POLICIES FOR 1997–98 FIRST-YEAR CLASS

*School participates in AMCAS. See Chapter 4.*

Filing of AMCAS application
  Earliest date: June 1, 1996
  Latest date: Nov. 1, 1996
School application fee to all applicants: $65
Oldest MCAT scores considered: 1991
Does have Early Decision Program (EDP)
  EDP application period: June 1–Aug. 1, 1996
  EDP applicants notified by: Oct. 1, 1996
Acceptance notice to regular applicants
  Earliest date: Oct. 15, 1996
  Latest date: Until class is filled
Applicant's response to acceptance offer
  Maximum time: 2 weeks
Requests for deferred entrance considered: Yes
Deposit to hold place in class (applied to tuition):
  $100, due with response to acceptance offer
Deposit refundable prior to: May 1, 1997
Estimated number of new entrants: 135 (10 EDP)
Starting date: Aug. 1997

### TUITION AND STUDENT FEES PER YEAR FOR 1995–96 FIRST-YEAR CLASS

Tuition                    Student fees: $350
  Resident: $10,840
  Nonresident: $21,940

### INFORMATION ON 1995–96 FIRST-YEAR CLASS

| Number of | In-State | Out-of-State | Total |
|---|---|---|---|
| Applicants | 2,817 | 969 | 3,786 |
| Applicants Interviewed | 444 | 16 | 460 |
| New Entrants* | 133 | 2 | 135 |

*All took the MCAT and had baccalaureate degrees. This does not include EAP

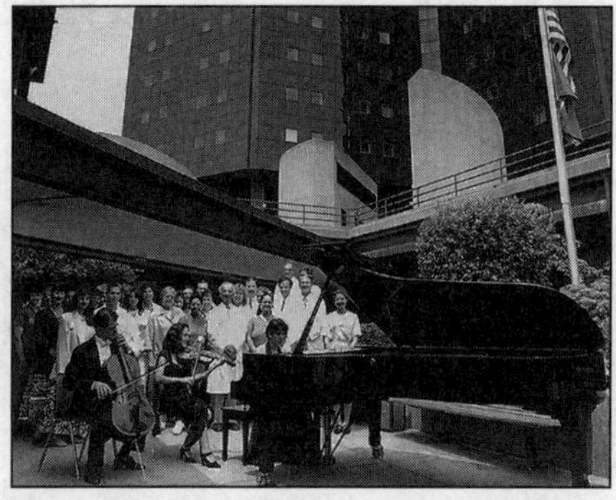

# SUNY at Stony Brook
# School of Medicine
# Health Sciences Center

**Stony Brook, New York**

Dr. Norman H. Edelman, *Dean and Vice President*
Debra Gillers, *Associate Dean and Director for Admissions*
Dr. Aldustus E. Jordan, *Associate Dean and Financial Aid Officer*

## ADDRESS INQUIRIES TO:

Committee on Admissions
Level 4, Room 147
Health Sciences Center
SUNY Stony Brook
School of Medicine
Stony Brook, New York 11794-8434
(516) 444-2113; 444-2202 (FAX)
E-Mail: admissions@dean.som.sunysb.edu

## GENERAL INFORMATION

SUNY Stony Brook School of Medicine accepted its first class in 1971. It is part of the SUNY-Stony Brook Health Sciences Center which includes the 540-bed University Hospital.

## CURRICULUM

The curriculum of the School of Medicine is designed to provide the opportunity for extensive training in the basic medical sciences and teaching in the clinical disciplines of medicine. The curriculum requires the acquisition and utilization of a variety of skills in basic and clinical sciences. The faculty has determined that a successful candidate for the M.D. degree must pass each unit of curriculum and that waiver of units of curriculum is offered only to those who because of prior experience are able to place out through examination. The grading system is honors/pass/fail.

The first year of the curriculum consists of integrated instruction in the basic sciences and introductions to clinical skills, human behavior, and preventive medicine. The second-year curriculum includes microbiology, pharmacology, and an interdisciplinary course in pathophysiology of the different organ systems. In both the first and second years, students participate in the introduction to clinical medicine and medicine in contemporary society courses.

On completion of the systems program, students move to a series of clinical clerkships in medicine, surgery, pediatrics, obstetrics and gynecology, psychiatry, and family medicine, where opportunities for problem solving and patient responsibility are presented. Clinical teaching in the introduction to clinical medicine course, in the systems program, and in the clinical clerkships takes place at the University Hospital and various clinical facilities affiliated with the School of Medicine. The clerkship program is followed by selectives and electives in the fourth year. The curriculum emphasizes social issues in medicine and bioethics at each level of medical training.

In addition, four-year programs leading to the M.D. with distinction in research, M.D. with distinction in humanities, and M.D. with distinction in primary care, and a six- to seven-year federally funded MSTP (M.D.-Ph.D. program) are available.

## REQUIREMENTS FOR ENTRANCE

In anticipation that both the spring and fall administrations of the MCAT will be offered in the state of New York and that official test scores will be forwarded to New York schools, candidates for admission to the 1997 entering class are required to take the MCAT no later than fall 1996 and have official scores sent to Stony Brook. Because of the rigorous competition, candidates are advised to submit applications early in the application period. All applications must be submitted through AMCAS. Prospective applicants should be aware that those who successfully applied to us in the past represent an exceptional, able, and diverse group.

Specific minimum course requirements are:

|  | Years |
|---|---|
| Biology (with lab) | 1 |
| Inorganic chemistry (with lab) | 1 |
| Organic chemistry (with lab) | 1 |
| Physics (with lab) | 1 |
| English | 1 |

This minimum of preparation should be completed prior to filing the application. The Committee on Admissions makes a careful examination of the candidate's preparation and promise for creative work in medicine, regardless of the area of concentration prior to medical school. A basic course in biochemistry is very helpful in preparing students for the first year of medical school; however, it is neither a requirement nor a criterion for admission. It is expected that each student admitted will be capable of completing the full curriculum of required courses and electives under the established policies.

## SELECTION FACTORS

Grades, MCAT scores, letters of evaluation, and extracurricular and work experiences are carefully examined.

Motivational and personal characteristics as indicated in the application, letters of evaluation, and a personal interview are also a major part of the admissions assessment. There is no discrimination in the admissions review and selection process on the basis of sex, race, religion, national origin, age, marital status, or handicap.

Students learn from each other as well as from their teachers, their textbooks, and their patients; therefore, the school attempts to acquire a class representative of a variety of backgrounds and academic interests. Indeed, given the demands on physicians in the twenty-first century, breadth of individual background is particularly important. SUNY-Stony Brook hopes to attract a significant representation of groups that have historically been underrepresented in medicine. Applicants from foreign schools must have completed at least one year in an American college or university. Residents of New York constitute the majority of the applicants and entrants; however, applications for the M.D.-Ph.D. program are encouraged from both in-state and out-of-state applicants.

Required supporting documentation includes official transcripts of all college work and a letter of official evaluation from the applicant's premedical adviser (or, when no adviser exists at the applicant's college, from two instructors, one of whom must be from science field). If there are other individuals who also may be in a position to provide important information, the school would be happy to receive letters from them. Personal interviews will be arranged at the initiative of the school for candidates who appear to be serious contenders for admission.

The school is committed to giving all applicants the individualized attention that they merit.

## FINANCIAL AID

SUNY Stony Brook participates in all financial aid programs available at the medical schools of the SUNY system. Financial aid and counseling are available through the Office of Student Affairs, as is assistance in securing housing and in meeting other personal needs. On-campus housing is available. Students are advised to have transportation available because there is no public transportation to the outlying clinical facilities.

## INFORMATION FOR MINORITIES

SUNY Stony Brook encourages applications from members of groups that have been historically underrepresented in medicine, and the school makes a detailed review of these applications.

Public Institution

## APPLICATION AND ACCEPTANCE POLICIES FOR 1997–98 FIRST-YEAR CLASS

*School participates in AMCAS. See Chapter 4.*

Filing of AMCAS application
    Earliest date: June 1, 1996
    Latest date: Nov. 15, 1996
School application fee to all applicants: $65
Oldest MCAT scores considered: 1992
Does have Early Decision Program (EDP)
    EDP applicaton period: June 1–Aug. 1, 1996
    EDP applicants notified by: Oct. 1, 1996
Acceptance notice to regular applicants
    Earliest date: Oct. 15, 1996
    Latest date: Until class is filled
Applicant's response to acceptance offer
    Maximum time: 15 days, unless otherwise specified
Requests for deferred entrance considered: Yes
Deposit to hold place in class: None
Deposit refundable prior to: May 15, 1997
Estimated number of new entrants: 100 (5 EDP)
Starting date: Aug. 1997

## TUITION AND STUDENT FEES PER YEAR FOR 1995–96 FIRST-YEAR CLASS

Tuition                           Student fees: $130
  Resident: $10,840
  Nonresident: $21,940

## INFORMATION ON 1995–96 FIRST-YEAR CLASS

| Number of | In-State | Out-of-State | Total |
|---|---|---|---|
| Applicants | 2,887 | 1,095 | 3,982 |
| Applicants Interviewed | * | * | 817 |
| New Entrants† | 92 | 8 | 100 |

*Data not available.

†All took the MCAT and had baccalaureate degrees.

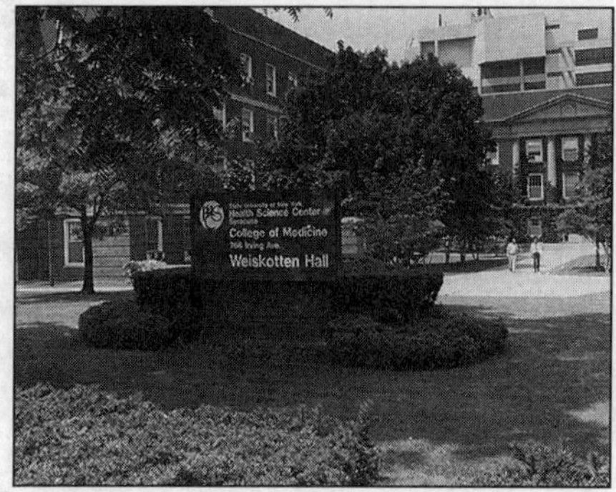

# State University of New York Health Science Center at Syracuse College of Medicine

## Syracuse, New York

Dr. Gregory Eastwood, *Dean, College of Medicine*
Ronald Wolk, *Interim Dean, Student Affairs and Academic Sciences*
Irvin Bodofsky, *Director of Financial Aid*

## ADDRESS INQUIRIES TO:

Admissions Committee
State University of New York
Health Science Center at Syracuse
College of Medicine
155 Elizabeth Blackwell Street
Syracuse, New York 13210
(315) 464-4570; 464-8867 (FAX)

## GENERAL INFORMATION

The Health Science Center at Syracuse's College of Medicine was established in 1834 as the Geneva Medical College. The college joined Syracuse University in 1872 and was transferred to the State University of New York (SUNY) in 1950 as the Upstate Medical Center. In 1986 its name was officially changed to the Health Science Center at Syracuse to reflect more accurately its broad and diverse mission in medical care and research, nursing, health professional training, and graduate education.

## CURRICULUM

The medical education program is designed in three phases. During the first phase, students directly explore the normal structure, function, and systemic processes of the human body. In the second phase, students develop an understanding of the nature and progression of disease, the interaction and response of the human host to microorganisms, the principles of human behavior, and pharmacology. Interviewing and counseling skills, physical diagnosis, ethics, law, and economic issues also are addressed throughout the second phase. During the third phase, the students apply the principles of basic science to clinical problem-solving. Clinical clerkships in pediatrics, medicine, surgery, obstetrics-gynecology, psychiatry, and radiology constitute the core of this phase. Clerkships in subspecialty services are required for all students. Thereafter, each student has the opportunity to attain their individual educational objectives during 26 weeks of available elective time.

The Health Science Center's clinical campus at Binghamton provides a core curriculum with programs in internal medicine, growth and development, perinatology, child and adolescent health, geriatrics, ambulatory surgery, neuropsychiatry, and primary care. A community orientation fosters a close working relationship between the campus and practicing physicians and other health care professionals.

A medical student research track is available, as are other research opportunities. Students who wish to develop skills in research may elect a special course of study. After selecting a project adviser, these students spend the first two summers as well as elective time on an independent research project.

Early assurance and deferred matriculation programs are available for qualified candidates. The M.D.-Ph.D. program is designed for those interested in investigating fundamental and applied issues of human health and disease. The central goal is to emphasize the best training in contemporary science in combination with the most practical experience in patient care. The Rural Medical Education program places students in rural communities for nine consecutive months of clinical and didactic education.

An extended program under which the first two academic phases are spread over three years is available upon request and approval.

A modified pass/fail grading system is used; however, students may earn honors for outstanding performance in their courses.

## REQUIREMENTS FOR ENTRANCE

Admissions preference is given to New York State residents. However, some out-of-state applicants are admitted each year. Applications are accepted from U.S. citizens and from permanent residents who have completed at least three years of college study (90 semester hours) in the United States or Canada in an accredited institution of higher education. International applicants and individuals from foreign schools must complete at least two years of study, which include all course requirements, in an accredited American or Canadian college or university prior to application and demonstrate competency in English composition and expression. Preference is also given to those applicants who have completed the courses required for admission at the time of application. Reapplicants are discouraged unless their qualifications have significantly improved.

The MCAT and satisfactory completion of the following courses are required:

*Sem. hrs.*

Chemistry . . . . . . . . . . . . . . . . . . . . . . . . . . . . . . . . . 8–12
  Inorganic (with lab) . . . . . . . . . . . . . . . . . . . . . . . . . . (6–8)

Organic (with lab) . . . . . . . . . . . . . . . . . . . . . . . . . (6–8)
Biology or zoology (with lab) . . . . . . . . . . . . . . . . . . . 6–8
Physics (with lab) . . . . . . . . . . . . . . . . . . . . . . . . . . . 6–8
English . . . . . . . . . . . . . . . . . . . . . . . . . . . . . . . . . . . 6

Choice of major should be determined by the student's chief interests. Achieving excellence in the basic sciences is essential; however, academic work in the humanities and social sciences is equally important, as are meaningful experiences in relating to people.

## SELECTION FACTORS

The Admissions Committee endeavors to take into consideration as much information as possible that delineates an applicant's total qualifications for the study and practice of medicine, without regard to race, creed, religion, national origin, age, sex, marital status, or degree of physical handicap. Several application forms are used in the medical school admission process. Each form collects information appropriate to the program an applicant may be seeking. Preadmission inquiries which relate to gender, age, ethnicity, veteran status, or other characteristics are collected for statistical purposes only. This information has no bearing on the selection process or final decisions regarding admission to the college.

Major factors in selection of applicants include: review of college records, which include scholastic aptitude and science aptitude; MCAT scores; letters of recommendation from premedical advisory committees; communication skills; character; motivation; and an evaluation of the personal interview.

## FINANCIAL AID

Accepted applicants are eligible to apply for financial aid to the Office of Admissions and Student Affairs. Financial need is determined by the ACT needs analysis system (see Part 1). The Financial Aids Committee generally makes awards in July. The major portion of financial aid for each student is in loans. Scholarships are not readily available except for those state residents who qualify for the Tuition Assistance Program Awards.

## INFORMATION FOR MINORITIES

The SUNY Health Science Center at Syracuse is committed to making student enrollment reflective of the diverse population in New York state. Underrepresented minorities and disadvantaged students are actively sought and are eligible for special assistance in the entry and retention programs of Project 90, which includes both a matriculation summer program and an extended curriculum. Premed counseling, application fee waivers, and off-campus interview programs are available. Program descriptions and further information can be obtained from either the Admissions Office or the Office of Multicultural Resources.

Public Institution

## APPLICATION AND ACCEPTANCE POLICIES FOR 1997–98 FIRST-YEAR CLASS

*School participates in AMCAS. See Chapter 4.*

Filing of AMCAS application
    Earliest date: June 1, 1996
    Latest date: Nov. 1, 1996
School application fee to all applicants: $60
Oldest MCAT scores considered: 1994
Does have Early Decision Program (EDP)
    EDP application period: June 1–Aug. 1, 1996
    EDP applicants notified by: Oct. 1, 1996
Acceptance notice to regular applicants
    Earliest date: Oct. 15, 1996
    Latest date: Varies
Applicant's response to acceptance offer
    Maximum time: 2 weeks
Requests for deferred entrance considered: Yes
Deposit to hold place in class: None
Estimated number of new entrants: 150 (5 EDP)
Starting date: Aug. 1997

## TUITION AND STUDENT FEES PER YEAR FOR 1995–96 FIRST-YEAR CLASS

Tuition               Student fees: $215
    Resident: $10,840
    Nonresident: $21,940

## INFORMATION ON 1995–96 FIRST-YEAR CLASS

| Number of | In-State | Out-of-State | Total |
|---|---|---|---|
| Applicants | 2,884 | 1,205 | 4,089 |
| Applicants Interviewed | 559 | 124 | 683 |
| New Entrants* | 141 | 7 | 148 |

*All took the MCAT and had baccalaureate degrees.

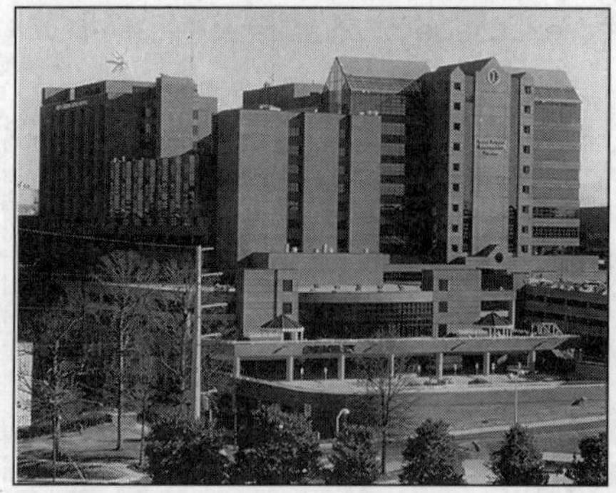

# Bowman Gray School of Medicine of Wake Forest University

## Winston-Salem, North Carolina

Dr. James N. Thompson, *Dean*
Dr. Lewis H. Nelson, III, *Associate Dean for Admissions*
Melissa Stevens, *Financial Aid Director*

## ADDRESS INQUIRIES TO:

Office of Medical School Admissions
Bowman Gray School of Medicine
of Wake Forest University
Medical Center Boulevard
Winston-Salem, North Carolina 27157-1090
(910) 716-4264; 716-5807 (FAX)
Web Site: http://www.is.bgsm.edu

## GENERAL INFORMATION

The School of Medicine was established in 1902 at Wake Forest, North Carolina, and of the existing 166 medical schools, it was one of 11 that required college preparation. Patient care, research, education, and community service remain the fourfold mission of the school as part of the Wake Forest University Medical Center.

The main teaching hospital of the medical school is the 806-bed North Carolina Baptist Hospitals, Inc. Affiliated institutions include the 896-bed Forsyth Memorial Hospital, Reynolds Health Center, and Northwest Area Health Education Center.

## CURRICULUM

The curriculum is organized to meet the seven stated goals of the undergraduate medial education program: self-directed learning and life-long learning skills, core biomedical science knowledge, clinical skills, problem solving/clinical reasoning skills, interviewing and communication skills, information management skills, and professional attitudes and behavior. Students elect to study in the lecture-based traditional curriculum or the problem-based parallel curriculum.

The traditional curriculum primarily utilizes a discipline-oriented approach to the study of the basic sciences. Small-group learning activities and clinical correlations are utilized within this curriculum. Morphology, including gross anatomy and histology, biochemistry, immunology, embryology, neuroscience, physiology, and aspects of community medicine are studied in the first year. Students begin the course, Foundations of clinical medicine (FCM), in the first semester of first-year and continue with this course throughout the first two years. Courses covering the spectrum of organ systems as well as population-specific courses (eg., pediatrics, geriatrics), are taught in the second year. Pharmacology, pathology, and radi-

ology topics are correlated with the clinical courses across the second year. Medical Microbiology is taught at the beginning of second year. Issues related to the practice of medicine are discussed within the course, medicine as a profession (MAPP), which extends across the first two years of the curriculum. The third year consists of required clerkships in medicine, surgery, pediatrics, psychiatry, obstetrics and gynecology, family medicine, neurology, and radiology/anesthesiology. The fourth year consists of 11 four week rotations: two in community medicine; four in basic clinical fields-medicine, surgery, pediatrics, or obstetrics-gynecology; and emergency medicine. The remainder are electives. Performance is evaluated on a zero-to-four scale.

Since 1987, part of the class is admitted to the parallel curriculum, which uses an integrated problem-based approach rather than the discipline-oriented approach of the traditional curriculum. Using the case-study method, small group tutorials led by faculty members address both basic and clinical sciences. Participation is voluntary, and the emphasis is on independent, self-directed learning to develop sound clinical reasoning and problem-solving skills. Students participate in the MAAP course with their traditional curriculum counterparts.

## EARLY ASSURANCE PROGRAM (EAP)

Well-qualified college students, who are residents of North Carolina, upon completion of the sophomore year, may apply for acceptance to the class entering two years later. Eligibility requires a GPA of 3.5, a science GPA of 3.5, and completion of half of the required prerequisites. The MCAT will not be required.

A student applies early in the junior year through the AMCAS process (November 1 deadline), asking consideration for the EAP. The applicant must agree to complete requisite courses, to continue academic excellence, to demonstrate high ethical conduct, and not to apply to any other medical school. Non-acceptance by the EAP does not influence future applications. The EAP should not be confused with the Early Decision Program.

## JOINT DEGREE PROGRAMS

The Bowman Gray School of Medicine offers two five-year joint degree programs. An M.D.-M.B.A. program is offered in conjunction with the Babcock Graduate School of

Wake Forest University, and an M.D.-M.S. (epidemiology) program is offered through the medical center.

The M.D.-M.B.A. program responds to the growing need for professionals trained in both medicine and management. The M.D.-M.S. program provides students with the knowledge and skills to conduct applied clinical research.

Applicants for either program must be accepted by separate admissions processes to the business or graduate school. The Babcock School requires the GMAT, and the graduate school requires the GRE.

Arrangements can be made for an M.D.-Ph.D. program.

## REQUIREMENTS FOR ENTRANCE

The MCAT is required except for EAP. The minimum requirement for admission is 90 semester hours of college work, although most candidates benefit from a well-rounded four-year college curriculum. Required courses should be completed by the time of application. Generally, prerequisites are:

|  | *Sem. hrs.* |
|---|---|
| General biology | 8 |
| General or inorganic chemistry | 8 |
| Organic chemistry | 8 |
| General physics | 8 |

## SELECTION FACTORS

Candidates are selected on the basis of the quality of their academic records, MCAT scores, and general qualifications. Although North Carolina residents compose the majority of the class (50 to 60 percent), nonresidents are given equal and careful consideration. There are no restrictions because of race, creed, sex, religion, age, physical disadvantages, marital status, or national origin. Early application is urged because of the large volume of applications.

The Committee on Admissions will evaluate each application. Applicants whose performance suggests they would have difficulty in handling the curriculum are notified. All other applicants are sent a supplemental application, which requires a $55 processing fee, and are asked to furnish letters of evaluation from their premedical advisory committees or from individuals. Only applicants who have completed files are considered for interviews. Candidates are invited for local interviews at the discretion of the Committee on Admissions. No regional interviews are conducted.

Students in the 1995 entering class represented 23 states and attended 47 colleges and universities. Some characteristics of the class were the following: *sex,* 41 percent women; *acceptance rate,* 7 percent of all applicants were interviewed and 35 percent of those were offered acceptance for 108 places.

## FINANCIAL AID

Financial aid is awarded to students on the basis of need and academic standing. All students duly enrolled and in good standing are eligible for loans. Special state and institutional funds are available for scholarships and loans to residents of North Carolina. Eighty-five percent of the student body receive financial assistance. Students are strongly discouraged from seeking part-time employment.

## INFORMATION FOR MINORITIES

The Office of Minority Affairs actively recruits minority students and has developed summer enrichment, academic reinforcement, tutorial, and counseling services for enrolled students. Address inquiries to the Office of Minority Affairs.

---

Private Institution

### APPLICATION AND ACCEPTANCE POLICIES FOR 1997–98 FIRST-YEAR CLASS

*School participates in AMCAS. See Chapter 4.*

Filing of AMCAS application
   Earliest date: June 1, 1996
   Latest date: Nov. 1, 1996
School application fee to all applicants: $55
Oldest MCAT scores considered: 1993
Does have Early Decision Program (EDP)
   EDP application period: June 1–Aug. 1, 1996
   EDP applicants notified by: Oct. 1, 1996
Acceptance notice to regular applicants
   Earliest date: Nov. 1, 1996
   Latest date: Until class is filled
Applicant's response to acceptance offer
   Maximum time: 2 weeks
Requests for deferred entrance considered: Yes
Deposit to hold place in class (applied to tuition):
   $100, due with response to acceptance offer
Deposit refundable prior to: May 15, 1997
Estimated number of new entrants: 108 (3 EDP)
Starting date: Aug. 1997

### TUITION AND STUDENT FEES PER YEAR FOR 1995–96 FIRST-YEAR CLASS

Tuition: $18,500

### INFORMATION ON 1995–96 FIRST-YEAR CLASS

| Number of | In-State | Out-of-State | Total |
|---|---|---|---|
| Applicants | 830 | 7,457 | 8,287 |
| Applicants Interviewed | 269 | 319 | 588 |
| New Entrants* | 60 | 48 | 108 |

*All had baccalaureate degrees; 99% took the MCAT.

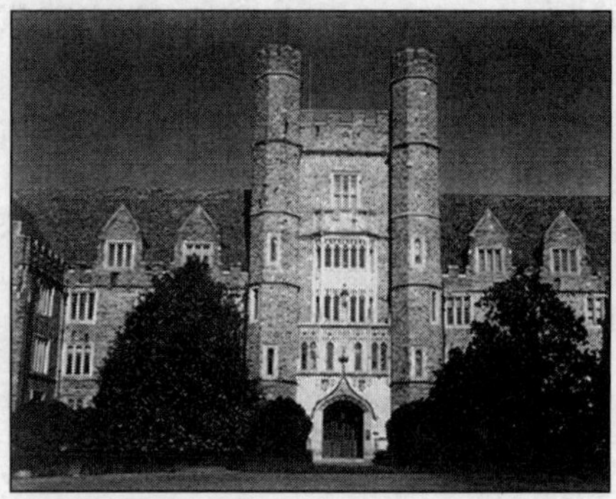

# Duke University School of Medicine

## Durham, North Carolina

Dr. Dan G. Blazer, *Dean, Medical Education*
Dr. Lois A. Pounds, *Associate Dean, Director of Admissions*
Nell Andrews, *Financial Aid Administrator*

## ADDRESS INQUIRIES TO:

Committee on Admissions
Duke University
School of Medicine
Duke University Medical Center
P.O. Box 3710
Durham, North Carolina 27710
(919) 684-2985; 684-8893 (FAX)

## GENERAL INFORMATION

The Duke University Medical Center is located on the campus of Duke University in Durham, North Carolina. A hospital was opened for patients in July 1930, and the first medical students were admitted in October of that year. The first doctor of medicine degrees were conferred in June 1932. Duke Hospital (1,000 beds) is supplemented by the Durham Veterans Administration Hospital (489 beds) for clinical teaching.

## CURRICULUM

The curriculum has been designed to provide the flexibility to encompass the rapid expansion of medical knowledge as well as the broad range of individual student interests and talents. First-year students receive instruction in the basic science principles of modern medicine. The second year is an introduction to the clinical sciences. The third and fourth years are elective; and with the guidance of an advisory dean and several senior faculty advisers, students design their programs to include half basic science and half clinical course work. In the third year each student may participate in a research project to learn not only how to do research, but how to critically evaluate the research of others. Having completed the required courses in the first and second years, students may explore relevant areas of basic science in more depth and complement their first-year acquisition of science knowledge. In the fourth year, clinical courses may be elected to enhance general medical education in more depth and breadth. Students graduate prepared to pursue careers in community practice, academic medicine, or public health and to contribute expertise in health policy and medical ethics issues.

The Medical Scientist Training Program is designed to provide both the M.D. and Ph.D. degrees over a six- to seven-year period of study. The first two years are spent in the medical school program, followed by a three- to four-year period of graduate study. Upon completion of the Ph.D. degree, the last year is spent in the clinical sciences. It is expected that candidates for this combined degree plan to have careers in academic medicine.

Other combined-degree programs include law (M.D.-J.D.), medical history (M.D.-M.A. and M.D.-Ph.D.), public policy sciences (M.D.-M.A.), and public health (M.D.- M.P.H.).

## REQUIREMENTS FOR ENTRANCE

The MCAT and three years of college are required. The spring MCAT is preferred and advantageous. A minimum of 90 semester hours of approved college credit is also required. Prerequisite courses must be taken within seven years before application. Course work must include:

| | *Years* |
|---|---|
| Biology | 1 |
| Inorganic chemistry | 1 |
| Organic chemistry | 1 |
| General physics | 1 |
| Calculus | 1 |
| English | 1 |

An introductory course in biochemistry is suggested during the senior year.

Premedical students should be aware of the importance of a well rounded general education as a preparation for the study of medicine and not limit themselves to scientific courses. The Committee on Admissions places more importance on the way applicants handle their undergraduate work than on the subject matter taken.

## SELECTION FACTORS

The selection of students is based upon the quality rather than the quantity of preparation and upon demonstrated evidence of personal attributes of intelligence, character, and general fitness for the study and practice of medicine. In considering an applicant, many sources of information may be consulted: curricular and extracurricular college record; fitness as reflected by carefully prepared, confidential appraisals by teachers who know the individual well; MCAT scores; and the applicant's showing in the interview which is held with members of the Committee on Admissions or one of its regional representatives.

Accepted students for the 1995 entering class had high GPAs and MCAT scores. Special consideration is given to residents of North Carolina. There were 46 women in the 1995 entering class. The Committee on Admissions does not discriminate on the basis of race, sex, sexual preference, creed, age, handicap, or national origin.

## FINANCIAL AID

The first $5,000 of need is met with the Stafford Student Loan (SSL). The remaining need is then met with half institutional grant and half institutional low-interest loan, in amounts up to total school-approved costs, depending on applicant's documented financial need. Each applicant obtains the full SSL before school loans are packaged. FAFSA and FAF serve as the basis for determining an applicant's resources (see Part 1). Part-time employment is discouraged. The financial circumstance of an applicant has no bearing on the admission process.

Seven Dean's Tuition Scholarships for minority students are awarded each year by the Scholarship Committee on the basis of candidates' academic credentials.

North Carolinians' need up to $11,750 is met with a special grant package followed by the package described above to meet additional need.

Financially needy, disadvantaged, and minority students selected for the North Carolina Board of Governors Medical Scholarship receive full tuition, fees, and a stipend.

Medical Scientist Training Program recipients receive full tuition, fees, and a stipend.

A wide variety of employment opportunities are available for the student's spouse at Duke University and its Medical Center and the nearby, rapidly expanding Research Triangle Park.

Approximately 75 percent of the student body receives financial assistance.

## INFORMATION FOR MINORITIES

Minority medical students have access to a dean/faculty/student group which supports freshman students and meets regularly to discuss common issues pertinent to minority student experience. Active recruitment is in place and an excellent advising program supports all students.

Private Institution

## APPLICATION AND ACCEPTANCE POLICIES FOR 1997–98 FIRST-YEAR CLASS

*School participates in AMCAS. See Chapter 4.*

Filing of AMCAS application
  Earliest date: June 1, 1996
  Latest date: Oct. 15, 1996
School application fee to all applicants: $55
Oldest MCAT scores considered: 1993
Does not have Early Decision Program
Acceptance notice to regular applicants
  Earliest date: Feb. 28, 1997
  Latest date: Until class is filled
Applicant's response to acceptance offer
  Maximum time: 3 weeks
Requests for deferred entrance considered: Yes
Deposit to hold place in class (applied to tuition):
  $100, due May 15, 1997; nonrefundable
Estimated number of new entrants: 100
Starting date: Aug. 1997

## TUITION AND STUDENT FEES PER YEAR FOR 1995–96 FIRST-YEAR CLASS

Tuition: $22,400          Student fees: $1,341

## INFORMATION ON 1995–96 FIRST-YEAR CLASS

| Number of | In-State | Out-of-State | Total |
|---|---|---|---|
| Applicants | 480 | 7,013 | 7,493 |
| Applicants Interviewed | * | * | 853 |
| New Entrants† | 32 | 69 | 101 |

*Data not available.

†All took the MCAT and had baccalaureate degrees.

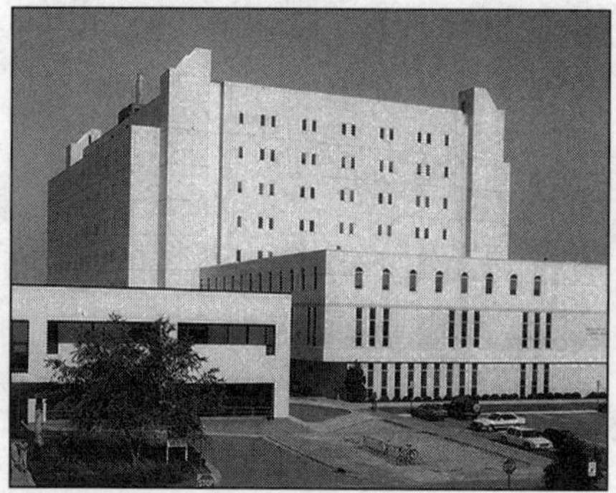

# East Carolina University School of Medicine

## Greenville, North Carolina

Dr. James A. Hallock, *Vice Chancellor for Health Sciences and Dean*
Dr. Dean H. Hayek, *Associate Dean for Admissions*
Vicki Ogden, *Director of Financial Aid and Student Services*

## ADDRESS INQUIRIES TO:

Associate Dean
Office of Admissions
East Carolina University
School of Medicine
Greenville, North Carolina 27858-4354
(919) 816-2202

## GENERAL INFORMATION

In 1972 East Carolina University enrolled students in the First-Year Program in Medical Education. The Board of Governors of the University of North Carolina system and the General Assembly of North Carolina authorized East Carolina University to expand the First-Year Program and establish a degree-granting School of Medicine. The School of Medicine enrolled the first class of students in August 1977.

The school's educational facilities are located on the 100-acre Health Sciences Center campus. Preclinical instruction is offered in the nine-story Brody Medical Sciences Building, which is contiguous to the Pitt County Memorial Hospital. Comprehensive clinical instruction is offered in the hospital (725 beds). The regional Leo W. Jenkins Cancer Center and magnetic resonance and other clinical settings, either adjacent to or near the Health Sciences Center, include the Child Development Evaluation Clinic, Mental Health Center, Alcoholic Rehabilitation Center, Rehabilitation Center, Area Health Education Center, and the Intensive/Intermediate Care Neonatal Unit. The three-fold mission of the school is recruitment and education of minority/disadvantaged students, primary care, and service.

Our generalist physician program was designed to amplify and complement activities to meet the school's major mission of the education of primary care physicians. The generalist program extends across the entire four-year curriculum and involves intensive contact with community physicians. Emphasis is placed on meeting the primary health care needs of those in rural and underserved areas. All students interested in primary care careers are given the opportunity to develop long-term mentor relationships with community-based family physicians, general pediatricians, and general internists.

## CURRICULUM

The first year of the four-year curriculum is devoted to the study of the anatomy and functions of the body through courses in gross and microscopic anatomy, biochemistry, physiology, microbiology/immunology, and genetics. Correlative clinical lectures in these as well as courses in psychosocial basis of medical practice, primary care conference, ethical and social issues in medicine, and clinical skills I. A primary care preceptorship is mandatory.

The second-year curriculum is directed toward clinical medicine. Courses include clinical skills II, pathogenic microbiology, pharmacology, pathology, and introduction to medicine. Also included in the second-year curriculum are courses in psychiatry, psychopathology and human sexuality, physical diagnosis and clinical assessment, primary care conference, life-style abuse, ethical and social issues in medicine, and a primary care preceptorship.

The third year is composed of six required clerkships: 8 weeks each in family medicine, obstetrics and gynecology, pediatrics, and psychiatry and 10 weeks each in internal medicine and surgery.

The fourth year is composed of 36 weeks of clerkships and both clinical and basic science electives. Students select an individualized curriculum after consulting with faculty advisers.

Student performance is evaluated by letter grade, and promotion to the next year's class is recommended to the dean by the Promotions Committee of the respective year.

## REQUIREMENTS FOR ENTRANCE

The MCAT and a minimum equivalent of three undergraduate years of preparation are required. Minimum course work requirements are:

|  | *Years* |
|---|---|
| General biology or zoology (with lab) | 1 |
| Inorganic chemistry (with lab) | 1 |
| Organic chemistry (with lab) | 1 |
| Physics (with lab) | 1 |
| English | 1 |

Additional courses in the humanities and social sciences and a second year of English are recommended.

## SELECTION FACTORS

Factors considered in the selection process encompass the social, personal, and intellectual development of each applicant. All available application data are evaluated: MCAT scores; academic performance; comments contained in letters of reference/recommendation; and the results of two personal interviews, conducted only at the medical school campus, with two members of the Admissions Committee.

The School of Medicine seeks competent students of diverse personalities and backgrounds, and all applicants are evaluated without regard to race, religion, sex, age, national origin, or handicap. First preference will be given to qualified residents of North Carolina.

Characteristics of the 1995 entering class of 72 students were: *mean GPA,* 3.34; *sex,* 35 women; *minorities,* 17 students. *MCAT scores* (mean and ranges): *VR*-8.6 (4–12); *PS*-7.8 (4–11); *WS*-P (K–S); *BS*-8.0 (3–11).

## FINANCIAL AID

Resources are available for loans and scholarships. The Financial Aid Office will make every effort to provide information and financial aid to those students who demonstrate need for financial assistance in order to meet the costs of their educational and living obligations. Awards are based on need as determined by confidential information supplied by the student. Merit awards are available.

Part-time employment is not permitted during the first two years and may be undertaken during the last two years only by permission of the dean. Sixty-five percent of the student body receive some financial assistance.

## INFORMATION FOR MINORITIES

Those members of minority groups, in particular those holding residence in North Carolina, are encouraged to apply. Minority representation on the Admissions Committee is significant, and the Academic Support and Counseling Center offers a wide range of services to students desiring assistance or guidance.

---

Public Institution

## APPLICATION AND ACCEPTANCE POLICIES FOR 1997–98 FIRST-YEAR CLASS

*School participates in AMCAS. See Chapter 4.*

Filing of AMCAS application
    Earliest date: June 1, 1996
    Latest date: Nov. 15, 1996
School application after screening: $35
Oldest MCAT scores considered: 1995
Does have Early Decision Program (EDP)
    For North Carolina residents only
    EDP application period: June 1–Aug. 1, 1996
    EDP applicants notified by: Oct. 1, 1996
Acceptance notice to regular applicants
    Earliest date: Oct. 15, 1996
    Latest date: Class matriculation date
Applicant's response to acceptance offer
    Maximum time: 3 weeks
Requests for deferred entrance considered: No
Deposit to hold place in class (applied to tuition):
    $100, due with response to acceptance offer
Deposit refundable prior to: May 15, 1997
Estimated number of new entrants: 72 (9 EDP)
Starting date: Aug. 1997

## TUITION AND STUDENT FEES PER YEAR FOR 1995–96 FIRST-YEAR CLASS

Tuition                 Student fees: $833
    Resident: $1,952
    Nonresident: $20,466

## INFORMATION ON 1995–96 FIRST-YEAR CLASS

| *Number of* | *In-State* | *Out-of-State* | *Total* |
|---|---|---|---|
| Applicants | 981 | 990 | 1,971 |
| Applicants Interviewed | 645 | 2 | 647 |
| New Entrants* | 72 | 0 | 72 |

*All took the MCAT and had baccalaureate degrees.

# University of North Carolina at Chapel Hill School of Medicine

**Chapel Hill, North Carolina**

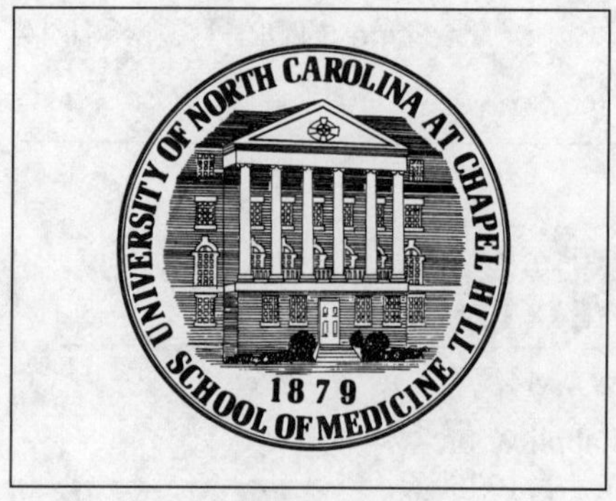

Dr. Michael A. Simmons, *Dean*

Dr. Elizabeth S. Mann, *Associate Dean, Commitee on Admissions*

## ADDRESS INQUIRIES TO:

Admissions Office
CB# 7000 MacNider Hall
University of North Carolina at Chapel Hill
School of Medicine
Chapel Hill, North Carolina 27599-7000
(919) 962-8331

## GENERAL INFORMATION

The School of Medicine of the University of North Carolina (UNC) at Chapel Hill was established in 1879 and expanded to a four-year school in 1952. Schools of dentistry, nursing, pharmacy, and public health are adjacent to the medical school on the university campus. Physical facilities include modern classrooms, multidisciplinary student laboratories, and a health sciences library with 247,000 print volumes, 4,400 audiovisual programs, 36,000 microform pieces, and current subscriptions to 4,590 periodicals. The University of North Carolina Hospitals, the Biological Sciences Center, and the Cancer Research Center are major on-campus teaching resources. Area health education centers throughout the state provide clinical experience in community settings.

## CURRICULUM

The curriculum emphasizes the application of science to the solution of clinical problems. Course committees composed of basic and clinical science faculty members are responsible for the courses of the first two years. Required clinical clerkships make up the third year. An additional year consisting primarily of clinical electives is required. It includes two required rotations in community primary care settings. Students may design individualized research projects under faculty direction. Combined-degree programs leading to M.D.-Ph.D. or M.D.-M.P.H. are offered. The honors/pass/fail grading system is used.

## REQUIREMENTS FOR ENTRANCE

Requirements for admission are under review and are subject to change. At this time a minimum of 96 semester hours of accredited college work and the MCAT are required. The test must be taken no later than the August before the student hopes to enter medical school.

Students are encouraged to pursue one or more scholarly interests in depth during the undergraduate years, but course work must demonstrate proficiency in the natural sciences. Course work in the humanities and social sciences, as well as advanced work in the sciences and mathematics, is valued. Proficiency in the use of the English language is essential. Specific course work must include:

|  | Sem. hrs. |
| --- | --- |
| Biology/zoology (with labs) | 8 |
| General chemistry including qualitative and quantitative analysis (with labs) | 8 |
| General physics (with lab) | 8 |
| Organic chemistry | 8 |
| English | 6 |

## SELECTION FACTORS

The Committee on Admissions evaluates the qualifications of all applicants to select those with the greatest potential for accomplishment in one of the many careers open to medical graduates. Preference is given to North Carolina residents. Among nonresident applicants, only those presenting truly superior credentials are competitive. The University of North Carolina does not discriminate on the basis of race, national origin, religion, sex, age, or handicap.

The AMCAS application is used for initial screening. Qualified North Carolina applicants and selected nonresidents are sent a supplementary application and are interviewed in Chapel Hill. In making its final selections from the group of qualified in-state applicants, the committee considers evidence of each candidate's motivation, maturity, leadership, and integrity and a variety of other personal qualifications and accomplishments in addition to the scholastic record. All information available about each applicant is considered without assigning priority to any single factor. No special admission tracks or quotas are applied among in-state applicants. The undergraduate major is not an important consideration, but excellence in the chosen field is expected. Previously rejected applicants are considered without prejudice.

Highly qualified resident and nonresident applicants are encouraged to consider application through the Early Decision Program.

## FINANCIAL AID

Scholarships and low-interest, long-term loans are available to students with financial need, determined through an evaluation by the Student Aid Committee of the total resources available to the student. Awards are based on information obtained from confidential applications submitted by the students. Fifty-four percent of the student body receive financial aid from funds controlled by the university. Financial need will not adversely affect a student's chances of admission, and no student once admitted should have to leave for personal financial need. Part-time employment is discouraged. A few scholarships are awarded for academic achievement and promise.

Minority and disadvantaged students admitted to the School of Medicine are eligible to participate in the Board of Governors' Medical Scholars Program. Those students who are selected receive annual stipends of $5,000 plus tuition and fees. Recipients must be residents of North Carolina who are enrolled in the School of Medicine on a full-time basis and who demonstrate financial need.

For additional information contact Clare Aselin at (919) 962-8335.

## INFORMATION FOR MINORITIES

Minority students are encouraged to apply, and there is an active recruitment program for minority students. The Medical Education Development Program is available to premedical and entering minority and disadvantaged students to acquaint them with the medical school curriculum and faculty and to assist them with learning skills development for medical school.

The Office of Academic and Student Programs provides academic counseling to students after they are admitted to medical school. Academic assistance is provided to students through tutorial programs, the Learning and Assessment Laboratory, and other resources within the university. Faculty members are available to assist students, and students are encouraged to see them for specific curricular problems. For students who have significant problems mastering the curriculum, a reduction in courses can be considered. A review program during the summer is provided for students with limited academic deficiencies. Students are reexamined at the end of the review period and promoted upon successfully passing the reexamination.

Public Institution

## APPLICATION AND ACCEPTANCE POLICIES FOR 1997–98 FIRST-YEAR CLASS

*School participates in AMCAS. See Chapter 4.*

Filing of AMCAS application
　Earliest date: June 1, 1996
　Latest date: Nov. 15, 1996
School application fee to all applicants: $55
Oldest MCAT scores considered: 1991
Does have Early Decision Program (EDP)
　EDP application period: June 1–Aug. 1, 1996
　ADP applicants notified by: Oct. 1, 1996
Acceptance notice to regular applicants
　Earliest date: Oct. 15, 1996
　Latest date: Until class is filled
Applicant's response to acceptance offer
　Maximum time: 3 weeks
Requests for deferred entrance considered: Yes
Deposit to hold place in class (applied to tuition):
　$100, due with response to acceptance offer
Deposit refundable prior to: May 15, 1997
Estimated number of new entrants: 160 (10 EDP)
Starting date: Aug. 1997

## TUITION AND STUDENT FEES PER YEAR FOR 1995–96 FIRST-YEAR CLASS

Tuition　　　　　　　　　　Student fees: $733
　Resident: $1,952
　Nonresident: $20,466

## INFORMATION ON 1995–96 FIRST-YEAR CLASS

| Number of | In-State | Out-of-State | Total |
|---|---|---|---|
| Applicants | 1,042 | 2,378 | 3,420 |
| Applicants Interviewed | 750 | 104 | 854 |
| New Entrants* | 143 | 17 | 160 |

*All took the MCAT and had baccalaureate degrees.

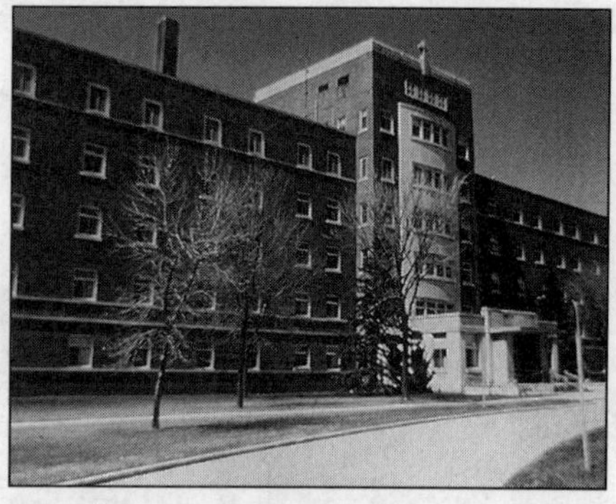

# University of North Dakota School of Medicine

**Grand Forks, North Dakota**

Dr. H. David Wilson, *Dean*
Judy L. DeMers, *Associate Dean, Student Affairs and Admissions*
Sandra K. Elshaug, *Financial Aid Administrator*

## ADDRESS INQUIRIES TO:

Secretary, Committee on Admissions
University of North Dakota
School of Medicine
501 North Columbia Road, Box 9037
Grand Forks, North Dakota 58202-9037
(701) 777-4221; 777-4942 (FAX)
E-Mail: judy.heit@medicine.und.nodak.edu

## GENERAL INFORMATION

The School of Medicine was established in 1905 as a basic science school offering the first two years of medical education. In 1973, legislative action created an expanded curriculum with the third year at the University of Minnesota or Mayo medical schools and the fourth year of elective clerkships on community campuses in North Dakota. In 1981, the legislature approved a full four-year medical school program within the state of North Dakota. The School of Medicine is university based but utilizes community physicians, clinics, and hospitals for the last two years of clinical education.

## CURRICULUM

The School of Medicine emphasizes the training of primary care physicians. The freshman and sophomore years are spent at the University of North Dakota (UND) in Grand Forks. The junior year of clinical clerkships is in the hospitals and clinics of either Bismarck or Fargo. The senior-year elective experiences are available in Bismarck, Fargo, Grand Forks, Minot, and 27 other communities in North Dakota.

The School of Medicine also offers accredited undergraduate degrees in the allied health fields of medical technology, cytotechnology, occupational therapy and sports medicine. A physician assistant program also is offered on a non-degree basis. Graduate degrees in anatomy, biochemistry, microbiology, pathology, physical therapy, physiology, and pharmacology also are offered. Information on these programs may be obtained from the UND undergraduate and graduate catalogs.

A student, additionally, may apply for a combined M.D.-Ph.D. program once accepted for admission to the School of Medicine.

The school utilizes a grading system of honors-satisfactory-unsatisfactory.

## REQUIREMENTS FOR ENTRANCE

The MCAT and the equivalent of three academic years or a minimum of 90 semester hours from an approved college are required for admission. Preference is given to applicants who will have completed four years of college prior to enrollment.

Course work must include the following:

| | Sem. hrs. |
|---|---|
| General biology or zoology | 8 |
| Inorganic and qualitative chemistry | 8 |
| Organic chemistry* | 8 |
| General physics | 8 |
| College algebra | 3 |
| Psychology or sociology | 3 |
| English composition and literature | 6 |

*A semester or quarter of biochemistry may be substituted for the final semester/quarter of organic chemistry.

It also is highly recommended that students be computer literate.

## SELECTION FACTORS

A student should have maintained a GPA of 3.0 or better (A=4.0) to be considered for admission. Selection is based upon the scholastic record, letters of recommendation, MCAT scores, and a personal interview. Interviews are conducted only at the medical school.

In addition to high academic achievement, selection is based on a number of factors, including the demonstration of such qualities as motivation and commitment to a medical career, empathy, compassion in interpersonal relationships, and problem solving.

Qualified North Dakota residents are given preference in admission. Almost all accepted students in recent classes have been residents of North Dakota. The only exceptions for non-North Dakota residents include a limited number of Minnesota residents or admission through either the Indians into Medicine (INMED) Program or through WICHE participation. Women are considered on the same basis as men.

The School of Medicine participates in the Professional Students Exchange Program administered by WICHE, under which legal residents of western states without a medical school may receive preference in admission. Certified WICHE students pay resident tuition. To be certified as eligible for this program, students must write to the WICHE certifying officer in their state of legal residence for the program application form. The number of students to be supported in each state in the field of medicine depends upon state appropriations. Addresses of state certifying officers are available from the Office of Student Affairs at the UND School of Medicine or from WICHE (see Part 1).

The fall 1995 entering class had the following profile: *GPA Mean:* overall undergraduate, 3.56; science, 3.52; GPA Range: overall undergraduate, 2.37–4.0; science, 2.40–4.0. The *mean MCAT scores* were as follows: *VR*-9.0; *PS*-8.7; *BS*-8.9. The *range of the MCAT variables* was 12 to 5. The *MCAT reading score* ranged from J to S with a median score of 0. *Gender,* 42 percent female; *minorities,* 9 students (16 percent) from under-represented minority groups; 7 INMED students.

It is the policy of the University of North Dakota that there shall be no discrimination against persons because of race, religion, sex, national origin, or handicap and that equal opportunity and access to facilities be available to all.

## FINANCIAL AID

The financial resources of applicants are not considered in the selection process. Immediately after acceptance into the School of Medicine, the applicant is sent all available financial aid information and may make application for financial aid.

The awarding of financial aid is based on documented need. Loans and a limited number of scholarships and prizes are available. Some awards and scholarships are based on scholarship as well as need. Approximately 85 percent of the students receive some form of financial aid. Students are discouraged from working. The financial aid office may be reached at (701) 777-2849.

## INFORMATION FOR MINORITIES

The INMED Program is a minority recruitment program for American Indian students. Up to seven qualified Native American students are admitted yearly through this program. State residency is not a consideration for admission through the INMED Program.

Public Institution

## APPLICATION AND ACCEPTANCE POLICIES FOR 1997–98 FIRST-YEAR CLASS

Earliest date: July 1, 1996
Latest date: Nov. 1, 1996
School application fee to all applicants: $35
Oldest MCAT scores considered: Fall 1993
Does not have Early Decision Program
Acceptance notice to regular applicants
    Earliest date: Dec. 15, 1996
    Latest date: Until class is filled
Applicant's response to acceptance offer
    Maximum time: 4 weeks
Requests for deferred entrance considered: Yes
Deposit to hold place in class (applied to tuition):
    $75, due with response to acceptance offer
Deposit refundable prior to: May 15, 1997
Estimated number of new entrants: 57
Starting date: Aug. 1997

## TUITION AND STUDENT FEES PER YEAR FOR 1995–96 FIRST-YEAR CLASS

Tuition                Student fees: $318
  Resident: $8,460
  Nonresident: $22,588
  Minnesota Residents: $9,411

## INFORMATION ON 1995–96 FIRST-YEAR CLASS

| *Number of* | *In-State* | *Out-of-State* | *Total* |
|---|---|---|---|
| Applicants | 145 | 177 | 322 |
| Applicants Interviewed | 98 | 50† | 148 |
| New Entrants* | 43 | 14† | 57 |

*All took the MCAT and had baccalaureate degrees.
†Includes INMED, MN, and WICHE applicants.

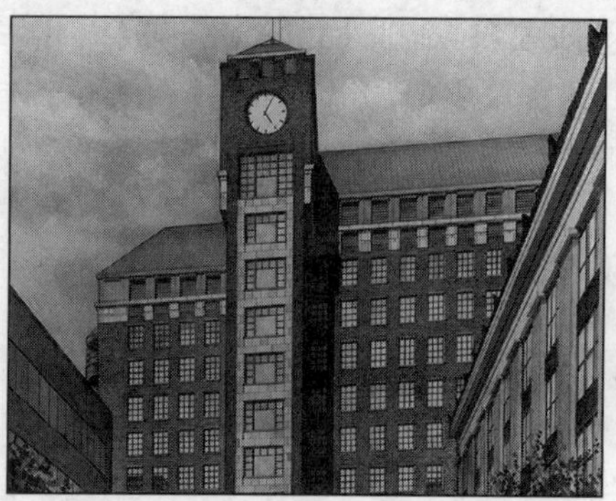

# Case Western Reserve University School of Medicine

**Cleveland, Ohio**

Dr. Nathan A. Berger, *Interim Dean, and*
*Interim Vice President for Medical Affairs*
Dr. Albert C. Kirby, *Associate Dean for Admissions and Student Affairs*
Wanda L. Rollins, *Manager of Financial Aid*

## ADDRESS INQUIRIES TO:

Associate Dean for Admissions and Student Affairs
Case Western Reserve University
School of Medicine
10900 Euclid Avenue
Cleveland, Ohio 44106-4920
(216) 368-3450; 368-4621 (FAX)

## GENERAL INFORMATION

The School of Medicine is located on the campus of Case Western Reserve University (CWRU), an independent and privately supported institution. Case Western Reserve is a comprehensive university with colleges of applied social sciences, dentistry, engineering, law, liberal arts, management, medicine, and nursing and a graduate school. The Ph.D. is available in 43 programs and the master's in 49. The university is one of over 90 cultural, educational, health, and service institutions in University Circle, a park-like area of 600 acres located five miles east of downtown Cleveland. Affiliated teaching hospitals are University Hospitals of Cleveland, MetroHealth Medical Center, MetroHealth St. Lukes Hospital, Veterans Affairs Cleveland Medical Center, and Mt. Sinai Medical Center, all in Cleveland and the Henry Ford Health System in Detroit, Michigan.

## CURRICULUM

The School of Medicine offers an atmosphere in which students are encouraged to take initiative and responsibility in self-education. The educational program has three components. The Core Academic Program occupies much of the first two years and features integrated teaching of the basic biomedical sciences with multidisciplinary faculty teams. Case-oriented clinical problem-solving is featured as a part of mastering the basic sciences. The Patient-Based Program begins in the first year with each student being responsible for a maternity patient in the family clinic. The program continues in the second year with physical diagnosis under the guidance of physician preceptors in a variety of outpatient settings. In the third year, students take hospital-based clerkships in internal medicine, obstetrics-gynecology, pediatrics, psychiatry, and surgery and a primary care clerkship in outpatient clinics. The Flexible Program is an electives program with over 180 course offerings, 160 research possibilities, and 20 areas of concentration in which students may focus their work. Student-initiated electives are encouraged. A significant fraction of time in the first two years is available for Flexible Program activity. The fourth year is devoted to clinical electives.

The basic science departments all offer Ph.D. programs. A Medical Scientist Training Program (combined M.D.-Ph.D.) is available.

## REQUIREMENTS FOR ENTRANCE

Only three years of college are required, but in practice few students without the baccalaureate degree have ever been admitted. All candidates are expected to take the MCAT. The quality of work done is much more important than the field in which the student has majored. Specific requirements are minimal and include:

*Biology:* A one-year course in modern biology which emphasizes biochemical and quantitative concepts. Courses in anatomy, botany, ecology, and taxonomy will not fulfill this requirement.

*Chemistry:* Two years of chemistry including organic. Courses with an organic/biological chemistry content are acceptable.

*Physics:* A one-year course in introductory physics.

*Demonstration of writing skills:* This can be met by a course in freshman expository writing; however, other courses with significant writing content are acceptable.

No other courses are required or recommended. Students should major in areas of their own choosing.

## SELECTION FACTORS

The Admissions Committee selects students without regard to age, national origin, race, religion, or sex. With respect to the handicapped, technical standards for admission are available on request. The School of Medicine deliberately seeks a heterogeneous student body and does not rely solely on grades and MCAT scores in the admission process. Over 20 states of residence and 70 to 80 undergraduate colleges are represented in each entering class.

Some characteristics of the 1995 entering class were: women, 44 percent; *minorities,* 16 percent; *age,* 11 percent over age 30; *residence,* 60 percent legal residents of Ohio;

*undergraduate major,* 60 percent in science; *average GPA,* 3.5; *average MCAT score,* 10.

## FINANCIAL AID

Financial aid is based on demonstrated need of the student. All applicants for aid must submit data for an analysis of need by GAPSFAS (see Part 1). This requires complete disclosure of resources available to the student from all sources. Approximately 75 percent of the students receive financial aid. Aid available from the school is a combination of loan and scholarship, with the proportions of each being dependent upon total need. Financial aid applications from the school are mailed in January, and awards are made June 1. Although the school's financial aid is generous, funds available from the school are limited and cannot meet full financial need in all cases. Students have to rely on other sources of support, including the Stafford Student Loan Program (formerly the Guaranteed Student Loan Program).

## INFORMATION FOR MINORITIES

A variety of support services for retention of all students are offered. Inquiries may be directed to the school's Office of Minority Programs.

Private Institution

## APPLICATION AND ACCEPTANCE POLICIES FOR 1997–98 FIRST-YEAR CLASS

*School participates in AMCAS. See Chapter 4.*

Filing of AMCAS application
    Earliest date: June 1, 1996
    Latest date: Oct. 15, 1996
School application fee to all applicants: $60
Oldest MCAT scores considered: 1993
Does have Early Decision Program (EDP)
    EDP application period: June 1–Aug. 1, 1996
    EDP applicants notified by: Oct. 1, 1996
Acceptance notice to regular applicants
    Earliest date: Oct. 15, 1996
    Latest date: Until class is filled
Applicant's response to acceptance offer
    Maximum time: 4 weeks
Requests for deferred entrance considered: Yes
Deposit to hold place in class: None
Estimated number of new entrants: 138 (30 EDP)
Starting date: Aug. 1997

## TUITION AND STUDENT FEES PER YEAR FOR 1995–96 FIRST-YEAR CLASS

Tuition: $23,100        Student fees: $790

## INFORMATION ON 1995–96 FIRST-YEAR CLASS

| Number of | In-State | Out-of-State | Total |
|---|---|---|---|
| Applicants | 1,162 | 6,540 | 7,702 |
| Applicants Interviewed | 411 | 448 | 859 |
| New Entrants* | 83 | 55 | 138 |

*All had baccalaureate degrees; 98% took the MCAT.

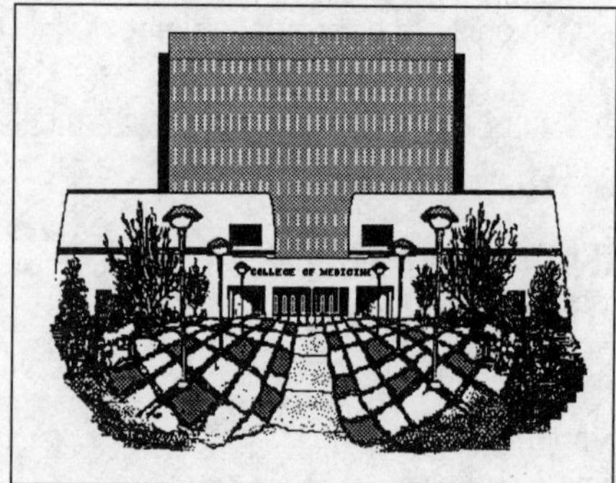

# University of Cincinnati College of Medicine

**Cincinnati, Ohio**


Dr. John J. Hutton, Jr., *Dean*
Dr. J. Robert Suriano, *Associate Dean for Student Affairs/Admissions*
Clarice P. Fooks, *Assistant Dean for Admissions*


## ADDRESS INQUIRIES TO:

Office of Student Affairs/Admissions
University of Cincinnati
College of Medicine
P.O. Box 670552
Cincinnati, Ohio 45267-0552
(513) 558-7314; 558-1165 (FAX)

## GENERAL INFORMATION

The University of Cincinnati Medical Center, which includes the Colleges of Medicine, Pharmacy, and Nursing and Health, is one of the leading academic health centers in the nation. A rich tradition in education, patient care, research, and community service is exemplified in the curriculum, unique learning opportunities, and student services. The College of Medicine provides both outstanding research facilities and superb clinical and teaching experiences. Graduates, ranked highly competitive by national residency program directors, chose careers in a broad range of specialty areas. Forty-seven percent of the 1995 graduating class chose a residency program in primary care.

Research opportunities for students are extensive. In Ohio, the College of Medicine is ranked first among all public medical schools in National Institute of Health research funding. In the nation, the college is ranked among the top third in outside research funding.

## CURRICULUM

During the first two years of the curriculum, students receive training in basic medical sciences. A clinical continuum containing interviewing, history-taking, ethics, bio-psychosocial issues, human sexuality, and preceptorships with a physician begins in the first year and continues into the second year with emphasis on physical diagnosis and clinical lectures. A multidisciplinary component in the second year includes problem-based learning and journal club seminars. In the summer between the first and second year, there are opportunities to obtain clinical and research experiences.

Third-year clerkships include 8-week rotations each in internal medicine, pediatrics, and surgery; 6-week rotations each in psychiatry and obstetrics-gynecology; a 4-week rotation in family medicine; a 2-week rotation in radiology; and 6 weeks of selectives.

The fourth-year requirements are an 8-week acting internship in internal medicine, a 4-week neuroscience selective, and 24 weeks of electives which must include a 4-week internal medicine elective, a 4-week outpatient elective, and a 4-week Area Health Education Center (AHEC) elective in an underserved rural or urban community. Portions of the elective time may be taken at other U.S. medical centers or abroad.

Evaluation of students is by an honors, high pass, pass, remediated pass and fail grading system. Students are required to take and pass Step 1 and Step 2 of the USMLE examinations. All students are required to pass Step 1 prior to promotion into Year III. *Summer Prematriculation Program.* The opportunity to apply for the summer prematriculation program is offered to all accepted students; however, enrollment is limited to 18–20 students. The program provides an introduction to the first year of medical school. A strong learning skills component is an integral part of the program. Student support services and study skills are also available throughout the curriculum for all students.

## REQUIREMENTS FOR ENTRANCE

The new revised MCAT and the completion of a minimum of 90 semester hours at an accredited four-year degree-granting institution of higher education are required. Over the past several years, 99 percent of all entering students have received a minimum of a bachelor's degree; however, a small number of students demonstrate a high level of academic achievement, maturity, and motivation by the end of their junior year to qualify for admission.

All undergraduate majors are considered of value. Applicants are encouraged to engage in a rigorous undergraduate program which enables them to acquire an understanding of the basic principles of the sciences fundamental to medicine and an appreciation of the psychosocial nature of man.

Applicants are expected to have the knowledge usually obtained in one-year courses in biology, chemistry, organic chemistry, physics and mathematics. In addition, the undergraduate program should provide the applicant with the understanding of the basic social, cultural, and behavioral factors that influence individuals, families, and communities. Regardless of the area of concentration, the applicant should have acquired effective learning, communication, and problem-solving skills.

Priority will be given to U.S. and Canadian citizens, permanent residents, and to foreign applicants eligible for federal financial aid. All matriculating students must meet the college's technical standards with or without reasonable accommodations.

## SELECTION FACTORS

Based on a preliminary review of the AMCAS information and the most current MCAT scores, applicants will be selected to receive the University of Cincinnati Secondary Application. Upon receipt of all information, the committee will notify candidates by postcard that their applications are complete.

All interviews are generated by the committee and are arranged at a mutually convenient time. Approximately 625 candidates will be invited to interview each year. Students invited to the college will interview with members of the committee, have lunch, meet with the director of financial aid, tour the medical center, and meet with faculty.

Notification of final decisions will be made on or near the 15th of each month. Prior to January, acceptances may be sent out on a weekly basis.

Offers of acceptance are based upon overall evaluation of grades, the MCAT, motivation, maturity, coping skills, leadership abilities, interpersonal skills, personal attitudes and values, and critical thinking skills. Students are admitted on the basis of individual qualifications, regardless of age, sex, sexual orientation, race, color, national origin, or physical or mental disabilities. Preference is given to first-time applicants and residents of Ohio.

## FINANCIAL AID

The college provides students with information about options for funding a medical education and counseling to help them make sound financial decisions. This counseling emphasizes budgeting, debt management, and financial planning.

Over 80 percent of enrolled students receive some type of financial assistance. A financial aid packet is mailed to accepted applicants in January. Students who wish to be considered for need-based funds administered by the college must submit the need access diskette.

Institutional resources provide scholarships and subsidized loans for students with financial need. The current level of indebtedness for graduates is below the national mean for all medical students. For further information, please contact the Financial Aid Office at (513) 558-6797.

## INFORMATION FOR MINORITIES AND NONTRADITIONAL STUDENTS

Members of underrepresented minority groups and nontraditional students are encouraged to apply. The college provides a strong supportive environment for all students and welcomes diversity in each entering class. A minority student brochure is available upon request.

## MEDICAL SCIENCE SCHOLARS PROGRAM

The college offers an integrated interdisciplinary program leading to the M.D.-Ph.D. combined degree. Full financial support is provided. Research focus areas include carcinogenesis, cardiovascular biology, developmental biology, environmental health, genetics, infectious diseases, neonatology and perinatology, and neuroscience. Students should request information directly from Terri Berning, administrative secretary, College of Medicine, University of Cincinnati, P.O. Box 670555, Cincinnati, Ohio 45267-0555; phone (513) 558-2380.

---

Public Institution

### APPLICATION AND ACCEPTANCE POLICIES FOR 1997–98 FIRST-YEAR CLASS

*School participates in AMCAS. See Chapter 4.*

Filing of AMCAS application
 Earliest date: June 1, 1996
 Latest date: Nov. 15, 1996
School application fee to all applicants: $25
Oldest MCAT scores considered: 1994
Does have Early Decision Program (EDP)
 EDP application period: June 1–Aug. 1, 1996
 EDP applicants notified by: Oct. 1, 1996
Acceptance notice to regular applicants
 Earliest date: Oct. 15, 1996
 Latest date: Until class is filled
Applicant's response to acceptance offer
 Maximum time: 2 weeks
Requests for deferred entrance considered: Yes
Deposit to hold place in class: None
Estimated number of new entrants: 160
Starting date: Aug. 1997

### TUITION AND STUDENT FEES PER YEAR FOR 1995–96 FIRST-YEAR CLASS

Tuition         Student fees: $504
 Resident: $10,533
 Nonresident: $18,861

### INFORMATION ON 1995–96 FIRST-YEAR CLASS

| Number of | In-State | Out-of-State | Total |
|---|---|---|---|
| Applicants | 1,489 | 3,730 | 5,219 |
| Applicants Interviewed | 444 | 181 | 625 |
| New Entrants* | 132 | 28 | 160 |

*All took the MCAT and had baccalaureate degrees.

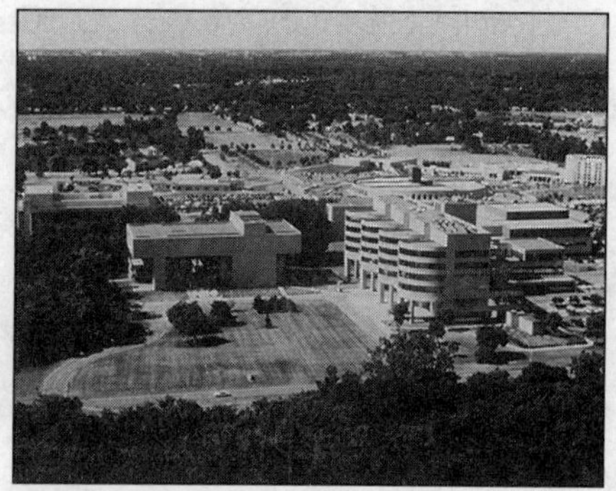

# Medical College of Ohio

## Toledo, Ohio

Dr. Richard F. Leighton, *Vice President for Academic Affairs and Dean, School of Medicine*

Dr. Barry L. Richardson, *Associate Dean for Admissions and Minority Affairs*

Deb Heineman, *Director of Student Financial Aid and Information Systems*

## ADDRESS INQUIRIES TO:

Admissions Office
Medical College of Ohio
P.O. Box 10008
Toledo, Ohio 43699
(419) 381-4229; 381-4005 (FAX)
Web Site: http://www.mco.edu

## GENERAL INFORMATION

The Medical College of Ohio graduated its first students in June 1972. The institutional mission statement focuses on the creation and maintenance of an academic environment that attracts the most highly qualified faculty and fosters the pursuit of excellence in health education, research, and service. The academic medical center is located on 475 acres in a residential/commercial area of south Toledo. The center has almost 400 faculty members and 1,100 volunteer faculty members. The faculty is dedicated to establishing a learning atmosphere through balanced teaching, research, and patient care.

The Medical College of Ohio has five endowed chairs and conducts biomedical research in many areas, including genetics of hypertension, autoregulation of blood pressure, genetics of carcinogenesis, mechanism of fungi formation, role of immunophilius in steroid action carcinogenesis and environmental microbiology.

In this medical school setting, the entering student is considered a graduate scholar by faculty members at all levels of seniority. The Medical College of Ohio seeks students who can grow intellectually and personally in this academic atmosphere.

In addition, clinical topics are presented during the second year in the three segments of the introduction to clinical medicine course—nutrition, medical ethics, and geriatrics. Substance use disorders are discussed during a course that spans both Years I and II. Topics in medical decision making are presented during the first quarter of the second year.

## CURRICULUM

The curriculum of the Medical College of Ohio is composed of a traditional four-year approach to medical education with an evolving emphasis on clinically oriented objectives and problem-based learning. The first year is devoted to anatomy, biochemistry, physiology, and behavioral sciences.

The second year follows with approximately seven months devoted to microbiology, pathology, and pharmacology. Introduction to primary care runs concurrently with the basic sciences throughout the first two years. This component includes basic science correlations and clinical preceptorships. Clinical contact and patient procedure experiences continue in the second year, culminating in the physical diagnosis course. Additionally during the first year, medical school students are trained to take a medical history and learn patient interviewing skills with an emphasis on identifying common high incidence disease processes. Students will be required to pass Step 1 of the USMLE for graduation.

The last two years of the curriculum are devoted to mandatory clerkships in internal medicine, surgery, pediatrics, obstetrics and gynecology, psychiatry, and family practice; neurology; and electives. All students are required to rotate through a clinical Area Health Education Center (AHEC) comprising 10 percent of their total clerkship time. Most components of the curriculum are evaluated on an honors, high pass, pass, fail system. The Medical College of Ohio also has an M.D.-Ph.D. and M.D.-M.S. program. Additionally, there is a FLEX program, which is a five-year curriculum for disadvantaged students.

During the clinical phase, each student is exposed to one or two months of internal medicine in generalist settings. One of these months is spent in an area health education center so that the student will see health care delivery in a rural setting. Additionally there is a four week exposure to family medicine.

The Medical College of Ohio School of Medicine offers a substantial amount of required generalist physician educational experiences and a wide variety of electives.

## REQUIREMENTS FOR ENTRANCE

The MCAT is required. A baccalaureate degree is strongly recommended.

Students must plan their educational sequence with due appreciation for the biologically oriented, psychologically sensitive task that they are undertaking for their life's work. The minimal premedical course requirements are:

|  | Years |
| --- | --- |
| Biology | 1 |
| Inorganic chemistry | 1 |
| Organic chemistry | 1 |
| Physics | 1 |

College mathematics . . . . . . . . . . . . . . . . . . . . . . . . . . . . 1
College English . . . . . . . . . . . . . . . . . . . . . . . . . . . . . . . 1

Additional biology courses are recommended.

A comprehensive command and understanding of the English language are essential.

Beyond these requirements, concentration in humanities, sciences, or other areas is viewed with equal favor. Close attention will be paid to the general scope of the applicant's academic background and to whether or not there is an adequate general understanding of the physical, biological, chemical, and social sciences and some reasonable sensitivity to the humanities.

## SELECTION FACTORS

In selecting applicants, the Medical College of Ohio looks more for evidence of general competence and capability than for specific areas of study. Students are admitted on the basis of individual qualifications, regardless of sex, religion, race, age, or handicap.

Students in the 1995 entering class had the following credentials: *mean science GPA,* 3.38; *mean total GPA,* 3.48; *mean MCAT scores,* VR-9.13, PS-9.17, BS-9.24; *sex,* 39 percent women; *minorities,* 14 percent; *undergraduate major,* 82 percent in science. Interviews are by invitation only. Reapplicants are not penalized. Preference is given to Ohio residents.

## FINANCIAL AID

Financial aid is awarded on the basis of demonstrated financial need according to federal methodology. Applicants for financial aid must file the FAFSA. Several scholarships are available on a competitive basis. These scholarships are funded by the Office of the Dean, the MCO Foundation, and the Associated Physicians of MCO.

## INFORMATION FOR MINORITIES

Members of racial minority groups are encouraged to apply. MCO has a longstanding summer prematriculation program, access to study management resources, and a five-year flexible curriculum (FLEX program) for disadvantaged students. Some scholarships are also available. For further information contact the Office of Minority Affairs.

---

Public Institution

## APPLICATION AND ACCEPTANCE POLICIES FOR 1997–98 FIRST-YEAR CLASS

*School participates in AMCAS. See Chapter 4.*

Filing of AMCAS application
   Earliest date: June 1, 1996
   Latest date: Nov. 1, 1996
School application fee to all applicants: $30
Oldest MCAT scores considered: 1994
Does have Early Decision Program (EDP)
   For Ohio residents only
   EDP application period: June 1–Aug. 1, 1996
   EDP applicants notified by: Oct. 1, 1996
Acceptance notice to regular applicants
   Earliest date: Oct. 15, 1996
   Latest date: Until class is filled
Applicant's response to acceptance offer
   Maximum time: 2 weeks
Requests for deferred entrance considered: Yes
Deposit to hold place in class: None
Deposit refundable prior to: May 15, 1997
Estimated number of new entrants: 140 (10 EDP)
Starting date: Aug. 1997

## TUITION AND STUDENT FEES PER YEAR FOR 1995–96 FIRST-YEAR CLASS

Tuition                  Student fees: $279
   Resident: $9,534
   Nonresident: $12,963

## INFORMATION ON 1995–96 FIRST-YEAR CLASS

| Number of | In-State | Out-of-State | Total |
|---|---|---|---|
| Applicants | 1,349 | 3,469 | 4,818 |
| Applicants Interviewed | 497 | 207 | 704 |
| New Entrants* | 116 | 19 | 135 |

*93% had baccalaureate degrees; 93% took the MCAT.

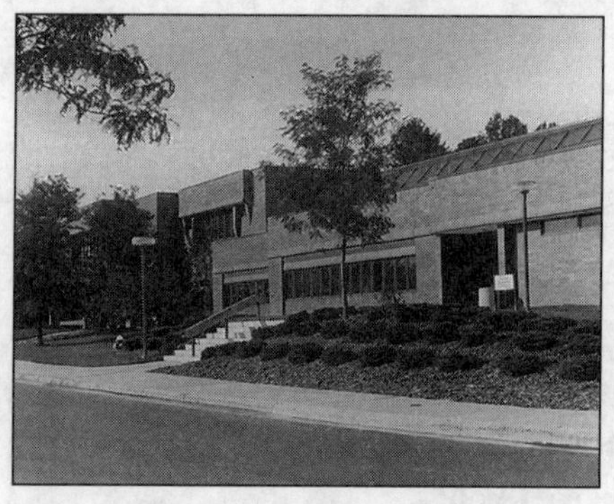

# Northeastern Ohio Universities College of Medicine

**Rootstown, Ohio**

Dr. Robert S. Blacklow, *President and Dean*
Dr. Bonnie Jones, *Associate Dean for Admissions and Educational Research*
Karen Berger, *Associate Director of Admissions*

## ADDRESS INQUIRIES TO:

Office of Admissions and Educational Research
Northeastern Ohio Universities
College of Medicine
P.O. Box 95
Rootstown, Ohio 44272-0095
(216) 325-2511; 325-8372 (FAX)
E-Mail: admit@neoucom.edu

## GENERAL INFORMATION

The Northeastern Ohio Universities College of Medicine (NEOUCOM) is a publicly supported medical school consisting of a basic medical sciences campus in Rootstown, three major public universities, and 18 community hospitals with over 6,500 teaching beds in the greater Akron, Canton, and Youngstown areas. The faculty numbers over 1,500.

## CURRICULUM

NEOUCOM offers primarily a combined B.S.-M.D. degree curriculum for honors level high school graduates who have not begun college study and, supplementarily, a four-year program leading to the M.D. degree.

B.S.-M.D. degree students spend their first two or three years at either the University of Akron, Kent State University, or Youngstown State University studying the sciences, mathematics, and the humanities while in the process of completing most or all of the required courses for the baccalaureate degree.

NEOUCOM's education of physicians is oriented to the practice of medicine at the community level. The freshman medical student concentrates on the basic medical sciences during the nine months spent on the Rootstown campus. During the sophomore year, students enroll in introduction to clinical medicine and organ system pathophysiology at ambulatory care teaching centers of the major associated teaching hospitals. They continue their clinical education through the core clerkships (internal medicine, surgery, pediatrics, psychiatry, obstetrics-gynecology, and family medicine) and a primary care preceptorship during the senior year at hospitals on the Akron, Canton, or Youngstown clinical campuses. The senior medical year includes electives and a specially designed course in the medical humanities as well as a community

health elective. All students are required to pass Step 1 and Step 2 of the USMLE. Course grading is on a pass/fail basis.

## REQUIREMENTS FOR ENTRANCE

Admission to the combined B.S.-M.D. degree program is restricted to students who have taken no college course work following high school graduation. Applicants should take the full science-oriented college preparatory sequence which their high school offers. The American College Test (ACT) or Scholastic Aptitude Test (SAT) must be taken, and the application deadline is December 31 of the year preceding anticipated entrance. Applications may be requested after September 1. Each year 105 students are chosen for the B.S.-M.D. degree program.

Persons who have completed the equivalent of at least three years of undergraduate study may be admitted to the M.D. degree program. These applicants are required to have completed at least one year each of university-level organic chemistry and physics. All students seeking direct entry into the M.D. degree program are required to take the MCAT no later than the fall prior to the year of anticipated enrollment. The number of spaces available for M.D. degree program candidates varies with the amount of attrition from Year II of the B.S.-M.D. degree program.

## SELECTION FACTORS

Applicants must demonstrate strong academic preparation as measured by GPAs and entrance examination scores. In addition, they must show appropriate personal characteristics and motivation for the practice of medicine. Selection interviews are by invitation only.

Admissions preference is given to Ohio residents. Typically, no more than 10 percent are non-Ohio residents; admissions criteria are more stringent for these candidates.

Applicants to the M.D. degree program who meet NEOUCOM's minimum academic criteria and who have taken the required course work are sent a supplementary application. Only those who complete supplementary applications are given full consideration by the Admissions Committee. Early submission of application materials is strongly encouraged, particularly through the Early Decision program if the applicant is competitive.

NEOUCOM does not discriminate on the basis of race, sex, creed, national origin, age, or handicap.

## FINANCIAL AID

Campus-based financial aid is awarded on the basis of demonstrated need. In general, students apply for this aid by completing the GAPSFAS application (see Part 1) and the NEOUCOM financial aid application and by submitting copies of federal income tax forms and financial aid transcripts. The awards are made through the Student Aid and Awards Committee after a thorough analysis of the student's financial situation.

Long-term federal educational loans are a major part of the aid program. A limited number of need-based scholarships of $1,000 each are available, as well as other limited scholarship funds for disadvantaged and/or medical minority students. About 75 percent of enrolled students receive some form of financial aid. Financial need is not a factor in admissions considerations.

## INFORMATION FOR MINORITIES

It is one of the goals of the Admissions Committee to seek out, recruit, and support qualified nontraditional applicants (members of medically underrepresented racial minorities and disadvantaged rural students). Students interested in further information should contact admissions or Dr. Kenneth Durgans, assistant to the president for minority affairs and affirmative action.

Public Institution

## APPLICATION AND ACCEPTANCE POLICIES FOR 1997–98 FIRST-YEAR CLASS

*School participates in AMCAS. See Chapter 4.*

Filing of AMCAS application
  Earliest date: June 1, 1996
  Latest date: Nov. 1, 1996
School application fee to all applicants: $30
Oldest MCAT scores considered: 1994
Does have Early Decision Program (EDP)
  EDP application period: June 1–Aug. 1, 1996
  EDP applicants notified by: Oct. 1, 1996
Acceptance notice to regular applicants
  Earliest date: Oct. 15, 1996
  Latest date: Until class is filled
Applicant's response to acceptance offer
  Maximum time: 2 weeks
Requests for deferred entrance considered: No
Deposit to hold place in class: None
Estimated number of new entrants: 15 (5 EDP)
Starting date: Aug. 1997

## TUITION AND STUDENT FEES PER YEAR FOR 1995–96 FIRST-YEAR CLASS

Tuition                              Student fees: $699
  Resident: $9,717
  Nonresident: $19,434

## INFORMATION ON 1995–96 FIRST-YEAR CLASS

| Number of | In-State | Out-of-State | Total |
|---|---|---|---|
| Applicants | 767 | 611 | 1,378 |
| Applicants Interviewed | 111 | 10 | 121 |
| New Entrants* | 24 | 1 | 25 |

NOTE: Figures do not include combined B.S.-M.D. degree program students.

*All took the MCAT and had baccalaureate degrees.

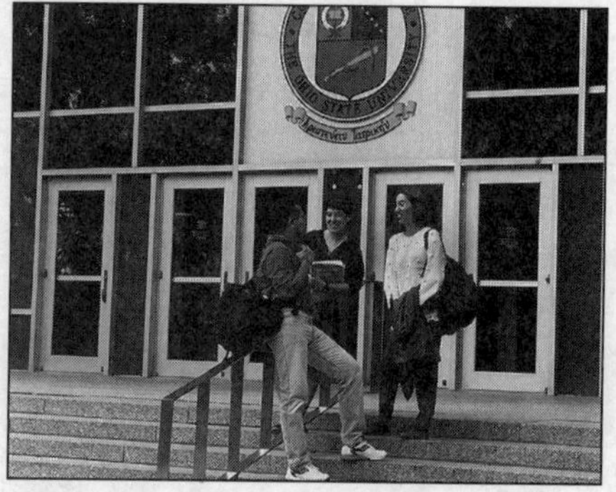

# Ohio State University College of Medicine

**Columbus, Ohio**

Dr. Bernadine P. Healy, *Dean, College of Medicine*
Dr. Judy Westman, *Chair, Admissions Committee*
Donna Cavell, *Financial Aid Officer*

## ADDRESS INQUIRIES TO:

Admissions Committee
270-A Meiling Hall
Ohio State University
College of Medicine
370 West Ninth Avenue
Columbus, Ohio 43210-1238
(614) 292-7137; 292-1544 (FAX)
E-Mail: admiss-med@osu.edu
Web Site: http://www.med.ohio-state.edu

## GENERAL INFORMATION

Established in 1914, the Ohio State University College of Medicine blends traditional medical education, innovative learning opportunities, and a strong reputation in the preparation of students for primary care and specialized residencies. As part of one of the largest public universities in the country, the College of Medicine provides an environment that encourages the research interests of students. Strong emphasis is placed on medical humanities and a biopsychosocial approach to patient care.

The College of Medicine is on the south edge of the main university campus, located in metropolitan Columbus. Medical center facilities include university hospitals, the Arthur James Cancer Hospital and Research Institute, and a network of outpatient facilities and affiliated small-town and rural hospitals and clinics. In addition, students can spend part of their clinical clerkships in other Columbus hospitals and at the Cleveland Clinic Foundation.

## CURRICULUM

Following an intensive initial 12-week course in anatomy, there are three different pre-clinical tracks for the first two years: a traditional lecture-discussion pathway; an independent study pathway; and a problem-based learning pathway. In all three pathways, the curriculum is interdisciplinary, using an organ systems approach, with an emphasis on providing a clinical context for learning.

The lecture-discussion pathway focuses on large-group presentations accomanpanied by tutorials and laboratories for selected topics. Lectures are held in the mornings, with afternoons used for tutorials and study.

In the independent study pathway (ISP) students use highly structured objectives, resource guides, and computer-based materials to read, review, and learn on their own. They proceed through the curriculum at their own pace within certain time limits. Faculty are available to coach students through difficult concepts and materials. Students who are successful in their first year in the ISP can request to spend their second year in the ISP at the Cleveland Clinic Foundation. It is possible to complete the independent study pathway program over a three-year period, an option that may interest non-traditional students with family obligations.

The problem-based learning pathway emphasizes student-centered, self-directed learning. Groups of seven students meet with a faculty facilitator two to three times per week. Students review cases and identify learning issues or areas they need to study. Students then work independently on learning issues before the next meeting, at which time the new information is discussed and refined.

All first-year students spend Wednesday in a medical humanities and behavioral sciences course. Some of the major components include the doctor-patient relationship, the physician's role in society, health care delivery, human development, human sexuality, and bioethics. Alternative medicine and the health care needs and issues of special populations are also presented and discussed. Emphasis is placed on small-group learning and discussion, including opportunities for electives on special topics. The first year also includes a longitudinal experience with a primary care physician in an outpatient setting.

During the second year, in addition to their science study, students take a physical examination course that includes preceptorships in both in-patient and out-patient settings. A more in-depth study of health care delivery systems, issues, and public health is also part of the second year.

The third year includes foundation clerkships in family medicine, general internal medicine, internal medicine, obstetrics and gynecology, pediatrics, psychiatry, and surgery. The fourth-year requirements include neuroscience and the differentiation of care selectives. The selectives are a series of four clerkships, each of which focuses on the care of patients at various stages of illness and wellness: the undifferentiated patient; the differentiated ambulatory patient; the patient with chronic care needs; and the acutely ill patient (subinternship). With the exception of the subinternship, all required clerkships include ambulatory experiences, with some done entirely in outpatient settings. Three electives and a month of vacation are also part of the fourth year.

## REQUIREMENTS FOR ENTRANCE

The MCAT and a bachelor's degree or certified eligibility for a degree in absentia are required. No specific undergraduate curriculum or major is required or preferred. A medical school candidate should follow an undergraduate program that is as broad and comprehensive as possible in order to prepare best for a career in a people-oriented profession in a changing society. Candidates are urged to take advantage of the undergraduate opportunity to study history, art, literature, creative writing, philosophy, social sciences, and communications skills.

The minimum course requirements are:

|  | *Years* |
|---|---|
| Biology | 1 |
| Inorganic chemistry (with lab) | 1 |
| Organic chemistry (with lab) | 1 |
| General physics | 1 |

Waiver of any requirement must be approved by the Admissions Committee.

## SELECTION FACTORS

First consideration is given to applicants who are Ohio residents and whose academic record and MCAT scores predict a high degree of academic accomplishment in medical school.

Successful candidates have had the follow ing general profile of characteristics: *GPA*, 3.5 (90 percent over 3.0); *residence*, about 80 percent from Ohio.

Applicants are carefully processed and reviewed by the staff and faculty members of the Admissions Committee to be certain that excellent candidates who do not fit a general profile are not overlooked.

Additional factors that lend significant weight in further consideration are undergraduate academic recommendations and personal information in the application itself. Further consideration by way of interview is by invitation; interviews are held on the campus. Nonacademic accomplishments and evidence of suitability for the study of medicine are carefully considered and account for a significant range in grades, MCAT scores, and other parameters of the admitted class.

## FINANCIAL AID

Scholarships and loans are awarded on the basis of need. All accepted candidates are mailed financial aid materials prior to entering to be considered with students already in school. Financial need is not a deterrent to acceptance, and no students are lost through inability to find sufficient resources for continuing their education.

Roessler Foundation Student Research Scholarships provide stipends for many students doing part-time and full-time research during their medical school career.

## INFORMATION FOR MINORITIES

Students whose previous educational and economic deprivation warrant special consideration are carefully evaluated and are offered special help in the acquisition of additional resources. Special programs, such as the MedPath Medical Careers Pathway, are provided to enhance students' educational development.

The Medpath Medical Careers Pathway is a five-quarter postbaccalaureate program aimed at developing the academic knowledge-base and skills of students prior to their entrance into medical school. The program is designed to increase the number of underrepresented minority students accepted into medical school.

---

Public Institution

### APPLICATION AND ACCEPTANCE POLICIES FOR 1997–98 FIRST-YEAR CLASS

*School participates in AMCAS. See Chapter 4.*

Filing of AMCAS application
 Earliest date: June 1, 1996
 Latest date: Nov. 1, 1996
School application fee to all applicants: $30
Oldest MCAT scores considered: 1994
Does have Early Decision Program (EDP)
 EDP application period: June 1–Aug. 1, 1996
 EDP applicants notified by: Oct. 1, 1996
Acceptance notice to regular applicants
 Earliest date: Oct. 7, 1996
 Latest date: Until class is filled
Applicant's response to acceptance offer
 Maximum time: 2 weeks
Requests for deferred entrance considered: Yes
Deposit to hold place in class: None
Estimated number of new entrants: 210 (15 EDP)
Starting date: Aug. 1997

### TUITION AND STUDENT FEES PER YEAR FOR 1995–96 FIRST-YEAR CLASS

Tuition                              Student fees: $234
 Resident: $9,174
 Nonresident: $26,460

### INFORMATION ON 1995–96 FIRST-YEAR CLASS

| *Number of* | *In-State* | *Out-of-State* | *Total* |
|---|---|---|---|
| Applicants | 1,376 | 4,535 | 5,911 |
| Applicants Interviewed | 435 | 243 | 678 |
| New Entrants* | 170 | 40 | 210 |

*All took the MCAT and had baccalaureate degrees.

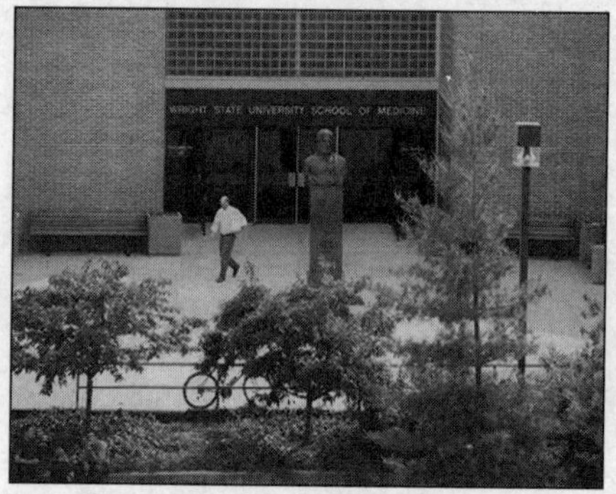

# Wright State University School of Medicine

**Dayton, Ohio**

Dr. Kim Goldenberg, *Dean*
Dr. Paul G. Carlson, *Associate Dean for Student Affairs/Admissions*
Jacqueline McMillan, *Financial Aid and Minority Affairs*

## ADDRESS INQUIRIES TO:

Office of Student Affairs/Admissions
Wright State University
School of Medicine
P.O. Box 1751
Dayton, Ohio 45401
(513) 873-2934; 873-3322 (FAX)

## GENERAL INFORMATION

The Wright State University School of Medicine was established in 1973 and enrolled its first class of students in 1976. It is located on the university campus in Fairborn, a suburb of Dayton. Clinical facilities associated with the medical school include seven major teaching hospitals with 3,823 patient beds. These hospitals emphasize and provide experience with modern scientific technology. A faculty of over 1,000 provides students with the opportunity for individualized attention. The school has a strong interest in preparing students for careers in primary care as family practitioners, general internists, and general pediatricians. The educational program emphasizes humanistic and compassionate care, outpatient experiences, health promotion and disease prevention, the provision of care to underserved populations, and cultural diversity.

## CURRICULUM

The primary objective of the educational program is to educate physicians to provide comprehensive care to patients and their families. During the first two years, the scientific basis of medicine is introduced with fundamental concepts in anatomy, physiology, biometrics, biochemistry, microbiology, immunology, pathology, and pharmacology. The behavorial sciences, medical humanities, and an introduction to clinical medicine course provide an early opportunity to interact with patients and understand the importance of health promotion and disease prevention. Throughout the first two years, patient interviewing and physical examination are taught along with the basic sciences. A unique feature of the curriculum is a two-week elective period following each quarter providing complementary opportunities in clinical areas. The last two years include required clerkships in family medicine, internal medicine, obstetrics-gynecology, pediatrics, psychiatry, surgery, emergency medicine, clinical neuroscience, and orthopedics. The fourth year includes six months devoted to electives, as

well as a student-administered senior seminar enrichment program focusing on timely topics in the practice of medicine. Emphasized throughout the curriculum are problem-based learning, clinical pharmacology, computers in medicine, geriatrics, humanistic medicine, and health promotion and disease prevention. In addition to the four year medical school curriculum, a biomedical sciences Ph.D. program is also available to interested students. Both letter grades and honors/pass/fail are utilized in the grading system.

## REQUIREMENTS FOR ENTRANCE

The MCAT and three years (90 semester hours or 135 quarter hours) of collegiate preparation in an approved college or university in the United States or Canada are required. Applicants must be U.S. citizens or possess a permanent resident visa. Applicants are expected to present the equivalent of the usual premedical preparation. Course work must include:

|  | *Years* |
| --- | --- |
| Biology | 1 |
| Chemistry | 2 |
| Must include organic chemistry. | |
| Physics | 1 |
| College mathematics | 1 |
| English | 1 |

While a basic understanding of the physical and biological sciences is important to a medical education, a broad appreciation of individuals and their social, cultural, and artistic efforts is equally necessary. Each applicant's credentials for admission will be individually reviewed and evaluated. The MCAT should be taken in the spring of the year in which the application is filed and no more than three years prior to making application. Only those MCAT scores available at the time of review will be considered by the Admissions Committee.

## SELECTION FACTORS

It is the philosophy of the School of Medicine to seek a student body of diverse social, ethnic, and educational backgrounds. Women, minority students, and applicants from rural Ohio are particularly encouraged to apply. However, applicants are admitted solely on the basis of individual qualifications without regard to race, gender, creed, national origin, age, or handicap. Dedication to human concerns, intellectual capacity, and personal maturity in the applicant are of greater

180

importance to the Admissions Committee than specific areas of preprofessional preparation. The Admissions Committee, which is broadly based, also seeks positive evidence of motivation, selflessness, and human empathy in the prospective medical student. The committee carefully reviews the completed application, the academic record, MCAT performance, letters of recommendation, and the results of a personal interview (by invitation only) in making its final selection. Ohio residents are given preference, but a small number of nonresidents are accepted. Disadvantaged and minority applicants are encouraged to apply regardless of state of residence.

Upon receipt of the AMCAS application, the applicant will be invited to submit a supplementary application and letters of evaluation. After review of all submitted material, applicants will be invited for interviews.

## FINANCIAL AID

Financial aid in the form of scholarships, grants, loans, and various work opportunities is available to assist students in financial need. The Office of Student Affairs/Admissions offers financial counseling services and assists students in obtaining needed support. An emergency loan fund for students in good academic standing is also available through this office. The financial status of applicants has no effect whatever on their acceptance to the School of Medicine.

## INFORMATION FOR MINORITIES

The Wright State University School of Medicine and its faculty have a stated policy of providing educational opportunities to students from minority groups or disadvantaged backgrounds. The school is in the top 15 percent of the U.S. medical schools in the enrollment of students from underrepresented minority groups. Special support services that meet the needs of minority students include a prematriculation program, a mentoring program in which students are paired with minority physicians in the community, a big brother/big sister program, tutoring, board preparation courses, and assistance in development of skills in critical thinking and learning. The admissions process gives careful consideration to minority applicants. Both resident and nonresident minority students are strongly encouraged to apply.

Public Institution

## APPLICATION AND ACCEPTANCE POLICIES FOR 1997–98 FIRST-YEAR CLASS

*School participates in AMCAS. See Chapter 4.*

Filing of AMCAS application
  Earliest date: June 1, 1996
  Latest date: Nov. 15, 1996
School application fee to all applicants: $30
Oldest MCAT scores considered: 1993
Does have Early Decision Program (EDP)
  EDP application period: June 1–Aug. 1, 1996
  EDP applicants notified by: Oct. 1, 1996
Acceptance notice to regular applicants
  Earliest date: Oct. 15, 1996
  Latest date: Until class is filled
Applicant's response to acceptance offer
  Maximum time: 3 weeks
Requests for deferred entrance considered: Yes
Deposit to hold place in class: None
Estimated number of new entrants: 90 (10 EDP)
Starting date: Aug. 1997

## TUITION AND STUDENT FEES PER YEAR FOR 1995–96 FIRST-YEAR CLASS

Tuition             Student fees: $672
  Resident: $12,244
  Nonresident: $17,332

## INFORMATION ON 1995–96 FIRST-YEAR CLASS

| Number of | In-State | Out-of-State | Total |
|---|---|---|---|
| Applicants | 1,341 | 2,332 | 3,673 |
| Applicants Interviewed | 392 | 45 | 437 |
| New Entrants* | 78 | 12 | 90 |

*All took the MCAT and had baccalaureate degrees.

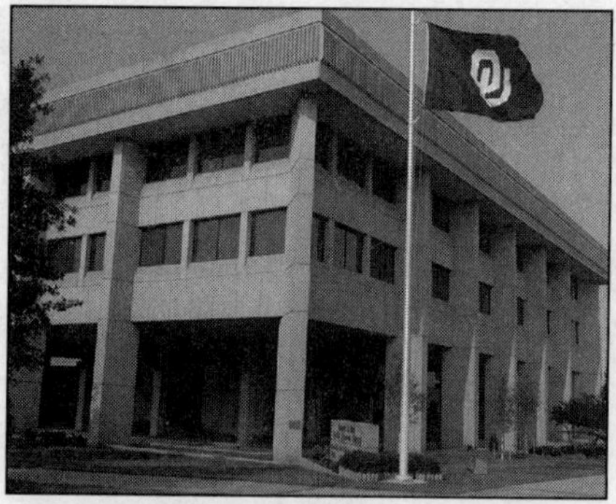

# University of Oklahoma College of Medicine

**Oklahoma City, Oklahoma**


Dr. Douglas W. Voth, *Executive Dean*
Dotty Shaw Killam, *Assistant Director for Admissions*
Jan Osborne, *Associate Director, Financial Aids*


## ADDRESS INQUIRIES TO:


Dotty Shaw Killam
University of Oklahoma
College of Medicine
P.O. Box 26901
Oklahoma City, Oklahoma 73190
(405) 271-2331; 271-3032 (FAX)
E-Mail: Dotty-Shaw@uokhsc.edu
Web Site: http://www.uokhsc.edu


## GENERAL INFORMATION

The University of Oklahoma College of Medicine offers students a quality education with added advantages. Access to modern patient care facilities and an aggressive research program are provided at a reasonable cost with a proven record of first choice residency placement.

Students gain experience in a variety of settings. The college is part of a modern health sciences complex that serves as the state's principal education and research facility for physicians, dentists, nurses, biomedical scientists, pharmacists, public health administrators, and a wide range of allied health professionals. The mission of the Health Sciences Center on behalf of the people of Oklahoma is three-fold: teaching, research, and community service.

Seven colleges—medicine, dentistry, nursing, pharmacy, public health, allied health, and the graduate college—educate more than 3,000 graduate and undergraduate students through programs offering degrees at several levels from baccalaureate through doctorate. The College of Medicine offers programs in Oklahoma City and Tulsa. The Health Sciences Center in Oklahoma City is part of a 200-acre complex of 17 public and private institutions known as the Oklahoma Health Center.

## CURRICULUM

The four-year curriculum consists of two years of study in the basic sciences and two in the clinical sciences. Letter grades are awarded for all course work on a course-hour basis rather than a credit-hour basis.

There are 17 required courses in the basic science portion of the curriculum. They account for 1,973 hours of instruction or 35 percent of the total. First-year courses provide a strong basic science foundation, and second-year classes form a bridge leading directly into the clinical portion of the curriculum. A significant feature of this portion of the curriculum is early exposure to patients through the continuum courses: principles of clinical medicine I and II. The bioethical and legal issues in medicine course is also offered.

The clinical program provides training at two sites. "The Tulsa Option" offers third- and fourth-year students the opportunity to complete their clinical training in the setting of a community-based educational program. Approximately 25 percent of the class will complete their education in several community hospitals in the Tulsa area. The clinical curriculum consists of 3,654 hours of instruction representing 65 percent of the total curriculum. A unique feature of the fourth year is a required rural preceptorship experience under the guidance of a physician in an Oklahoma community of less than 10,000 people.

## REQUIREMENTS FOR ENTRANCE

The MCAT is required and should be taken the spring of the year in which the application is filed. Applicants who have completed only 90 semester hours of college work may be considered; however, the college discourages such applications except from students who have demonstrated personal and intellectual maturity.

The following courses are required:

|  | *Semesters* |
|---|---|
| General zoology or general biology (with lab) | 1 |
| Cell biology, embryology, histology, genetics, or comparative vertebrate anatomy | 1 |
| Inorganic (general) chemistry | 2 |
| Organic chemistry | 2 |
| General physics | 2 |
| English | 3 |
| Psychology, sociology, anthropology, philosophy, humanities, or foreign language (any combination) | 3 |

Additional course work in the social sciences is suggested.

Pass/fail grading, advanced placement, and CLEP courses are accepted. It is encouraged that higher courses be taken for a grade.

No particular major is given preference; however, the applicant must provide evidence of their capability of understanding and utilizing scientific methods.

The University of Oklahoma has an October 15 deadline for applications to be submitted to AMCAS. A request for supplemental information is sent upon notification from AMCAS of a candidate's interest. The supplemental information consists of a filing fee, a pre-medical advisory committee letter of recommendation, plus an additional faculty recommendation, or three faculty letters. Applicants must have a complete file by November 1.

## SELECTION FACTORS

Acceptance into the College of Medicine is based on GPA, MCAT scores, letters of evaluation from faculty and premedical committees, and personal interviews conducted on campus by members of the Admissions Board. Emphasis is placed on noncognitive evaluations, including health care experience, commitment, maturity, leadership, community service, and altruism.

Currently nonresidents can represent 15 percent of the student body. The University of Oklahoma encourages applications from nonresidents.

In the 1995 entering class there were 63 women, and the mean GPA of the class was 3.57.

The University of Oklahoma College of Medicine does not discriminate on the basis of race, sex, creed, national origin, age, or handicap.

## FINANCIAL AID

The College of Medicine offers a number of financial assistance opportunities in addition to the federally sponsored programs. The most prominent scholarships are the Regents' Scholarship Fee Waiver, the Oklahoma Rural Medical Education Loan Scholarship Fund designed for residents wishing to practice in rural communities, and the Oklahoma Tuition Aid Grant. The loan funds established by the Shepherd Foundation, Inc., and the Lew Wentz Foundation, along with over 20 other scholarships, also aid many students annually. Additional support for underrepresented students is available through the State Regents for Higher Education, the Ungerman Trust, the Belknap, Culpeper, Maurer and Reid-Winnie scholarships.

About 94 percent of all students receive some form of assistance through the Office of Financial Aid.

## INFORMATION FOR UNDERREPRESENTED MINORITIES

The shortage of trained minority medical personnel in Oklahoma has created a need for innovative solutions to this problem. The University of Oklahoma has a strong commitment to identify, recruit, and educate qualified underrepresented minorities (African Americans, Native Americans, and all Hispanics). Applications are strongly encouraged from these ethnic groups as well as from any candidate with a disadvantaged background. Special consideration is given to each application.

*The Native American Center of Exellence.* A federally funded Native American Center of Excellence Consortium has been established in the colleges of dentistry and medicine to recruit more Native Americans into the colleges, to develop curriculum components related to Native American health issues, to recruit Native American faculty, and to stimulate research activities related to Native American health issues.

---

Public Institution

### APPLICATION AND ACCEPTANCE POLICIES FOR 1997–98 FIRST-YEAR CLASS

*School participates in AMCAS. See Chapter 4.*

Filing of AMCAS application
 Earliest date: June 1, 1996
 Latest date: Oct. 15, 1996
School application fee to all applicants: $50
Oldest MCAT scores considered: 1992
Does not have Early Decision Program
Acceptance notice to regular applicants
 Earliest date: Dec. 1, 1996
 Latest date: Until class is filled
Applicant's response to acceptance offer
 Maximum time: 2 weeks
Requests for deferred entrance considered: Yes
Deposit to hold place in class (applied to tuition):
 $100, due with response to acceptance offer
Deposit refundable prior to: May 15, 1997
Estimated number of new entrants: 150
Starting date: Aug. 1997

### TUITION AND STUDENT FEES PER YEAR FOR 1995–96 FIRST-YEAR CLASS

Tuition                 Student fees: $325
 Resident: $7,550
 Nonresident: $18,658

### INFORMATION ON 1995–96 FIRST-YEAR CLASS

| Number of | In-State | Out-of-State | Total |
| --- | --- | --- | --- |
| Applicants | 477 | 1,224 | 1,701 |
| Applicants Interviewed | 315 | 57 | 372 |
| New Entrants* | 132 | 17 | 149 |

*All took the MCAT; 95% had baccalaureate degrees.

---

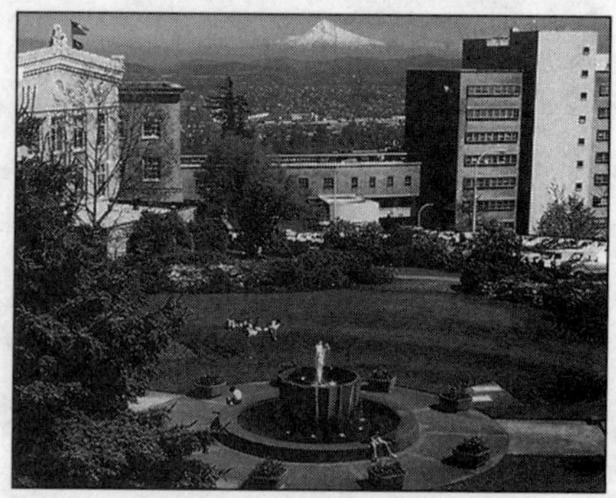

# Oregon Health Sciences University
# School of Medicine

**Portland, Oregon**

Dr. Edward Keenan, *Associate Dean, Medical Education*
Vicki Fields, *Administrative Director, Education and Student Affairs*
Debbie Melton, *Admissions Officer*

## ADDRESS INQUIRIES TO:

Office of Education and Student Affairs, L102
Oregon Health Sciences University
3181 S.W. Sam Jackson Park Road
Portland, Oregon 97201
(503) 494-2998; 494-3400 (FAX)

## GENERAL INFORMATION

The University of Oregon Medical School was established by charter from the Board of Regents of the University of Oregon in 1887. The name was changed in November 1974 when the School of Medicine and the schools of nursing and dentistry reorganized under the University of Oregon Health Sciences Center; in 1981 it was renamed Oregon Health Sciences University (OHSU). The OHSU occupies a 101-acre site in Sam Jackson Park overlooking the city but within one and a half miles of the business center. Campus physical facilities include basic science, research, and laboratory buildings; two hospital units with a licensed capacity of 509 beds; an outpatient clinic; Crippled Children's Division; Child Development and Rehabilitation Center; a hearing and speech center; a library and auditorium; and a student activities building. The School of Medicine is affiliated with the 563-bed Veterans Administration Hospital. A residence hall is provided on the campus, and apartment rentals are available in the area.

The School of Medicine provides educational programs for medical students, nurses, graduate students in basic medical sciences, and residents and interns as well as programs for radiologic technologists, medical technologists, and dietitians. An extensive postgraduate program exists.

## CURRICULUM

The first two years of the curriculum are primarily devoted to the sciences basic to medicine focusing initially on the normal structure and function of the human body and continuing with the study of the pathological basis of disease and its treatment. Principles of Clinical Medicine is presented concurrently during the first and second years to develop fundamental knowledge and skills in patient interviewing and physical diagnosis. The socioeconomic, behavioral, and population health issues are also introduced during this period. Clinical clerkship experiences undertaken at University Hospital and Clinics as well as affiliate hospitals in the Portland area constitute the third and fourth years of the curriculum. During the clinical phase of the curriculum, a six-week community health experience is required and opportunities to pursue elective courses in clinical and basic sciences.

The OHSU M.D.-Ph.D. Combined-Degree Program provides an opportunity for students to experience the rewards of research while pursuing a medical education. The School of Medicine has a vigorous research program funded by grants totalling about 27.8 million dollars per year. Ph.D. degrees may be obtained in the following basic science departments: biochemistry and molecular biology, cell biology and anatomy, molecular and medical genetics, medical psychology, microbiology and immunology, pharmacology, and physiology. Research training is also available through the School of Medicine in the Vollum Institute for Advanced Biomedical Research, the Veterans Administration Medical Center, the Oregon Regional Primate Research Center, the Shriner's Hospital for Crippled Children, and the Neurological Sciences Institute of Good Samaritan Hospital and Medical Center.

The combined-degree program is designed for superior students with a strong basic science background. Successful applicants must show a potential for excellent performance in both the M.D. and Ph.D. programs and a firm commitment toward a career in academic medicine. Prior research experience is advantageous. Applicants from all parts of the United States are given equal consideration.

## REQUIREMENTS FOR ENTRANCE

To receive serious consideration by the Admissions Committee, all applicants must meet the following requirements.

A bachelor of arts or bachelor of science degree, or its equivalent, from an accredited college or university is required prior to matriculation to medical school. No particular major is preferred, but a broad educational background is encouraged.

The following are prescribed as the minimum acceptable college level courses for admission. Note: One academic year is equivalent to two semesters or three quarters.

*Chemistry*—two academic years of chemistry (with lab) to include general chemistry (with lab) and organic chemistry (with lab). An introductory course in biochemistry is advantageous. Courses in advanced chemistry are recommended for applicants considering special medical programs with emphasis in the basic sciences (e.g., M.D.-Ph.D. Combined Degree Program).

*Biology*—one academic year of general biology. A course in basic genetics is advantageous. Advanced courses in molecular biology are recommended for applicants considering the M.D.-Ph.D. Program.

*Physics*—one academic year of general physics (with lab).

College mathematics—one college level math course (semester/quarter) such as algebra, calculus, etc.

*Humanities, Social Sciences, and English*—one academic year of humanities, one academic year of social sciences, and one academic year of English to include at least one course in composition.

MCAT test scores from 1994 or later will be accepted.

## SELECTION FACTORS

In evaluating candidates, attention is given to the entire academic record, the results of the MCAT, college recommendations by the premedical committee or individuals of the college faculty, and personal interviews with representatives of the Admissions Committee. Under certain circumstances the interview may be waived. Preference is given to residents of Oregon, underrepresented minorities, residents from western states having no medical schools (certified WICHE residents), M.D.-Ph.D. and M.D.-M.P.H. candidates, and applicants with superior achievements, such as academics, related experiences, etc. All applicants including M.D.-Ph.D. and underrepresented ethnic minorities must have citizenship or resident alien status in the United States. Each applicant is considered on the basis of qualifications without regard to race, creed, age, disability, marital status, national origin, or sex.

The mean GPA was 3.6 for the 1995 entering class.

## FINANCIAL AID

About 90 scholarships of approximately $500 to $3,000 each are available.

Loan funds have been established to help worthy students in need of financial aid. Both short-term and long-term loans are available at reasonable interest rates.

Public Institution

## APPLICATION AND ACCEPTANCE POLICIES FOR 1997–98 FIRST-YEAR CLASS

*School participates in AMCAS. See Chapter 4.*

Filing of AMCAS application
Earliest date: June 1, 1996
Latest date: Oct. 15, 1996
School application fee to all applicants: $60
Oldest MCAT scores considered: 1994
Does not have Early Decision Program
Acceptance notice to regular applicants
Earliest date: Nov. 1, 1997
Latest date: Until class is filled
Applicant's response to acceptance offer
Maximum time: 2 weeks
Requests for deferred entrance considered: No
Deposit to hold place in class: None
Estimated number of new entrants: 96
Starting date: Sept. 1997

## TUITION AND STUDENT FEES PER YEAR FOR 1995–96 FIRST-YEAR CLASS

Tuition                 Student fees: $2,997
  Resident: $13,466
  Nonresident: $28,339

## INFORMATION ON 1995–96 FIRST-YEAR CLASS

| Number of | In-State | Out-of-State | Total |
|---|---|---|---|
| Applicants | 394 | 1,689 | 2,083 |
| Applicants Interviewed | 225 | 136 | 361 |
| New Entrants* | 73 | 23 | 96 |

*All took the MCAT and had baccalaureate degrees.

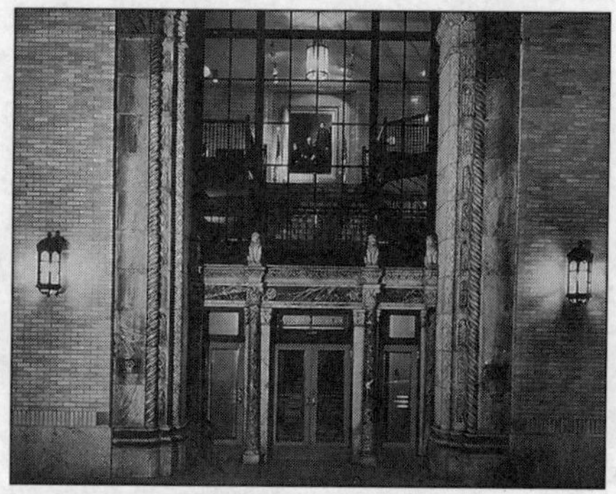

# Jefferson Medical College of Thomas Jefferson University

## Philadelphia, Pennsylvania

Dr. Joseph S. Gonnella, *Senior Vice President and Dean*
Dr. Benjamin Bacharach, *Associate Dean for Admissions*
Dr. Raelynn Cooter, *Director of Student Financial Aid*

## ADDRESS INQUIRIES TO:

Associate Dean for Admissions
Jefferson Medical College
of Thomas Jefferson University
1025 Walnut Street
Philadelphia, Pennsylvania 19107
(215) 955-6983; 923-6939 (FAX)

## GENERAL INFORMATION

As one of the oldest institutions of higher education in the nation, Thomas Jefferson University has, since its founding as the Jefferson Medical College in 1824, emphasized the attainment of clinical excellence in its educational programs. A recent significant expansion of the research programs has created a better balanced institutional mission and has enhanced the clinical instruction at Thomas Jefferson University Hospital and 18 affiliated federal and community hospitals.

## CURRICULUM

The goals of the curriculum at Jefferson Medical College are to provide learning experiences which will enable students to acquire basic knowledge and skills as well as to develop the proper habits and attitudes needed by all physicians. The curriculum also allows students to pursue some of their special interests early in their medical training.

The first two years of instruction will encompass both a departmental and systems approach. The first-year curriculum includes anatomy, biochemistry and molecular biology, ethics, nutrition, biostatistics, histology, physiology, neuroscience, life cycle, genetics, and introduction to clinical medicine. The curriculum in the second year includes microbiology and immunology, pathology, pharmacology, introduction to clinical medicine, and medicine and society.

The clinical program consists of two 42-week phases. Phase I covers required clerkships, including family medicine, general surgery, internal medicine, pediatrics, psychiatry, and obstetrics and gynecology. Advanced basic science, rehabilitation medicine, the medical and surgical subspecialties and inpatient and outpatient subinternships in medicine or surgery are usually included in the second clinical phase. Courses in the basic sciences are given numerical grades.

Jefferson Medical College and the Pennsylvania State University select highly qualified high school seniors to earn both the B.S. and M.D. degrees in six years. The Medical Scholars Program involving the University of Delaware and Jefferson Medical College allows highly qualified students a coordinated program of education for the baccalaureate and medical degrees. Physician Shortage Area Program serves to recruit selected students who agree to practice family medicine in physician shortage areas (especially in rural communities of Pennsylvania). Residents of the state of Delaware are admitted to Jefferson Medical College through a program involving the Delaware Institute of Medical Education and Research. There are two M.D.-Ph.D. programs for students interested in research and academic medicine, as well as an M.D.-M.B.A. and M.D.-M.H.A. progam. Opportunities in basic science research and in clinical research are also available to students.

## REQUIREMENTS FOR ENTRANCE

A minimum of three years (90 semester hours or equivalent) in an accredited college or university and the MCAT are required. A baccalaureate degree is preferred. It is recommended that, regardless of major, each student acquire a baccalaureate education which includes broad study in the natural and social sciences and in the humanities. The undergraduate program should include a strong preparation in the sciences and mathematics basic to medical school studies. Courses taken to meet the basic requirements should be rigorous and, in general, comparable to courses accepted for concentration in these disciplines.

Course work must include:

|  | *Years* |
| --- | --- |
| General biology (with lab) | 1 |
| Inorganic chemistry (with lab) | 1 |
| Organic chemistry (with lab) | 1 |
| General physics (with lab) | 1 |

In individual cases, specific requirements may be waived at the discretion of the admissions committee.

Students may take additional upper level science courses out of interest or to fulfill requirements of their major.

If advanced placement credits in required subjects are submitted, additional courses in similar subjects are encouraged.

All academic requirements must be completed prior to the date of matriculation. A personal on-site inverview (by invitation) is a requirement for admission.

Students are advised to take the MCAT in the spring of the year of application.

## SELECTION FACTORS

Jefferson, in accordance with local, state, and federal law, is committed to providing equal educational and employment opportunities for all persons, without regard to race, color, national and ethnic origin, religion, sexual orientation, age, handicap or veteran's status. Jefferson complies with all relevant ordinances and state and federal statutes in the administration of its educational and employment policies and is an affirmative action employer. The selection of students is made after careful consideration of many factors, including the college attended, the academic record, the letters of recommendation, the MCAT scores, and the interview results of the Committee on Admissions and their opinion of the applicant's personal qualities, motivation, interpersonal skills, and achievement in nonacademic areas. Jefferson Medical College traditionally has given special consideration to offspring of faculty and alumni, minority applicants, applicants to Jefferson's special programs and, in the past, residents of Pennsylvania. Qualified foreign students are encouraged to apply. Foreign applicants must have a degree from an accredited U.S. or Canadian college or university.

The 223 members of the 1995 entering class came from 91 different undergraduate schools, 26 different states and 1 foreign country (Hong Kong). A profile of the matriculated students includes the following: *mean science* GPA, 3.4; *mean MCAT score,* 9.9; *sex,* 43 percent women; *mean age,* 24 (range 18–38).

Each year several applicants are accepted who display extraordinary personal qualities and promise in regard to medicine, even though they do not meet all of the criteria described above.

## FINANCIAL AID

Financial aid awards are based on need determined by a confidential analysis of information that is provided by the student and the student's family to the designated needs analysis service. If need is established, the student is directed to obtain a federally subsidized Stafford loan. If need exists beyond this program, Jefferson will try to meet a portion of this need from loan and grant funds. Applications for financial aid are available after December 18 from the Office of Student Financial Aid. Completed financial aid applications for the next academic year must be submitted before April 1 or within two weeks of the date of acceptance. Seventy percent of the 1994 entering class received financial assistance.

## INFORMATION FOR MINORITIES

Applications from qualified members of racial minority groups are encouraged.

Private Institution

### APPLICATION AND ACCEPTANCE POLICIES FOR 1997–98 FIRST-YEAR CLASS

*School participates in AMCAS. See Chapter 4.*

Filing of AMCAS application
    Earliest date: June 1, 1996
    Latest date: Nov. 15, 1996
School application fee to all applicants: $65
Oldest MCAT scores considered: 1994
Does have Early Decision Program (EDP)
    EDP application period: June 1–Aug. 1, 1996
    EDP applicants notified by: Oct. 1, 1996
Acceptance notice to regular applicants
    Earliest date: Oct. 15, 1996
    Latest date: Until class is filled
Applicant's response to acceptance offer
    Maximum time: 2 weeks
Requests for deferred entrance considered: Yes
Deposit to hold place in class (applied to tuition):
    $100, due with response to acceptance offer
Deposit refundable prior to: May 15, 1997
Estimated number of new entrants: 223 (20 EDP)
Starting date: Aug. 1997

### TUITION AND STUDENT FEES PER YEAR FOR 1995–96 FIRST-YEAR CLASS

Tuition: $24,500          Student fees: None

### INFORMATION ON 1995–96 FIRST-YEAR CLASS

| Number of | In-State | Out-of-State | Total |
| --- | --- | --- | --- |
| Applicants | 1,407 | 10,287 | 11,694 |
| Applicants Interviewed | * | * | 935 |
| New Entrants† | 92 | 131 | 223 |

*Data not available.

†All took the MCAT; 87% had baccalaureate degrees; 32 students are in the Penn State-Jefferson Accelerated Program.

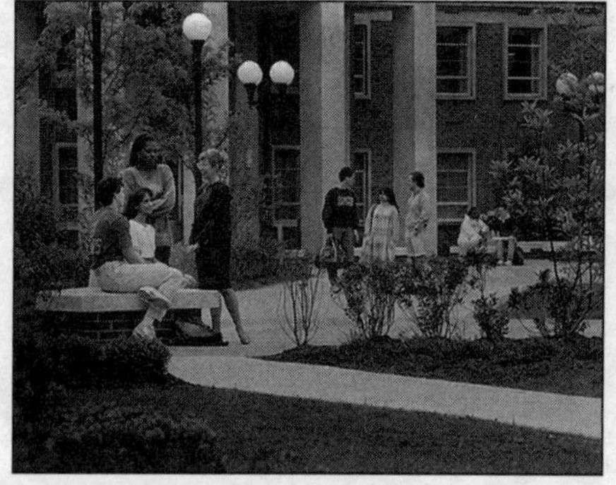

# Medical College of Pennsylvania and Hahnemann University School of Medicine

## Philadelphia, Pennsylvania

Dr. Leonard L. Ross, *Provost and Dean*
Dr. Andrew B. Beasley, *Associate Dean for Student Affairs (Admissions)*
Larry Buss, *Director of Financial Planning*

## ADDRESS INQUIRIES TO:

Admissions Office
Medical College of Pennsylvania
and Hahnemann University
School of Medicine
2900 Queen Lane Avenue
Philadelphia, Pennsylvania 19129
(215) 991-8202; 843-1766 (FAX)

## GENERAL INFORMATION

The Medical College of Pennsylvania (MCP) was founded in 1850 as the first medical school in the nation for women. Coeducational since 1969, the college continues to live up to its rich history, actively seeking students with diverse backgrounds and experiences. Hahnemann University, a private nondenominational institution, was founded in 1848. These two institutions have come together, melding their rich histories and many resources to provide diversity, strength, and excellence in medical education. The medical school has a supportive environment that fosters a spirit of teamwork and personal interaction. It draws on its strengths as the academic medical anchor in a multihospital system.

The Medical College of Pennsylvania and Hahnemann University School of Medicine is a member of Allegheny Health Education and Research Foundation (AHERF). Medical students have the opportunity for clinical training in the extensive, statewide network of hospitals of the AHERF system and at a large number of affiliated hospitals and clinics. In 1992 the college opened a new education and research facility on a 15-acre site. This facility is the home of the first and second years of medical education.

## CURRICULUM

The curriculum is designed to provide a thorough knowledge of the basic sciences with attention to the correlation of such material with the clinical sciences. This is provided by means of curricular and other programs, which include the introduction of clinical skills training in the first year. The basic clinical clerkships are offered in the third year and include experiences in all the major disciplines of medical practice. The fourth year includes a balance of four-week-long required and elective clinical experiences arranged by students with their advisors to be consistent with general medical train-ing and the student's ultimate career goals. The curriculum is monitored by both faculty and students, and appropriate modifications are made to achieve the overall educational objective.

The Medical College of Pennsylvania and Hahnemann University School of Medicine offers the Program for Integrated Learning, a problem-based curriculum track, to a number of interested students accepted into the entering class. Students accepted into this track learn the preclinical sciences in a small-group, interactive process using case descriptions to provide the context for acquisition of preclinical science knowledge. Students in this program learn clinical problem-solving, communication, and small-group and independent learning skills in this process. Students work with faculty facilitators in small groups and interact with resource faculty representing their respective scientific disciplines.

The Medical College of Pennsylvania and Hahnemann University School of Medicine has joint accelerated programs with Lehigh University and Villanova University in which qualified students can earn the baccalaureate and M.D. degrees in six to seven years. It offers standard eight-year programs in conjunction with Chatham College, Colby-Sawyer College, Duquesne University, Gannon University, Muhlenberg College, Rosemont College, Wells College, West Chester University, and Wilkes University for early assurance of medical school admission to qualified high school seniors. Postbaccalaureate early admissions programs exist with Bryn Mawr College, the University of Pennsylvania, Goucher College, Columbia University, Duquesne University, West Chester University, and Bennington College. Combined M.D.-Ph.D. programs are available for qualified students.

## REQUIREMENTS FOR ENTRANCE

The MCAT and a minimum of 90 semester hours from an accredited college are required. The baccalaureate degree is highly desirable. To expedite the processing of applications, the MCAT and the required course work should be completed prior to the time of application.

The required courses are:

*Semesters*

Inorganic chemistry (with lab) . . . . . . . . . . . . . . . . . . . . . . 2
Organic chemistry (with lab) . . . . . . . . . . . . . . . . . . . . . . 2
Biology (with lab) . . . . . . . . . . . . . . . . . . . . . . . . . . . . . . 2

Physics (with lab) . . . . . . . . . . . . . . . . . . . . . . . . . . . . . . . 2
English . . . . . . . . . . . . . . . . . . . . . . . . . . . . . . . . . . . . . . . . 2

Biochemistry should not be counted in this total but may be taken in addition.

## SELECTION FACTORS

In accord with the historical commitment of this institution, applications from women, students brought up in small towns or rural areas, those who come from Pennsylvania, students interested in a career as a generalist physician, and underrepresented minorities are particularly encouraged.

Matriculated students had an average GPA of 3.50 and MCAT scores at or above the 75th percentile level. In addition to academic criteria, the interview, which is conducted by a faculty member, is used in selecting our students.

Administrative regulations relative to the application of Public Law 93-380 (Family Educational Rights and Privacy Act) shall govern.

The medical school reserves the right to change, without notice, degree requirements, curriculum, courses, teaching personnel, rules, regulations, tuition, fees and any other information published herein.

The medical school actively supports equality of educational opportunity. The school does not discriminate on the basis of race, color, national origin, gender, sexual preference, age, religion, creed or handicap in admission or access to, or treatment or employment in, its programs and activities. The compliance coordinator in the Office of Student Affairs is the senior associate dean.

All students must be able to meet the technical standards of the medical school.

## STUDENT FINANCIAL PLANNING

In addition to the Federal Stafford Student Loan Program, the Primary Care Loan Program, other federally funded aid programs, and assistance in obtaining money from foundation sources, the Office of Financial Planning has at its disposal limited private grant and loan funds. A College Work-Study Program for qualified students is also available. All money allocated by the school is awarded on the basis of financial need. Information and applications are available from the Office of Student Financial Planning.

## INFORMATION FOR UNDERREPRESENTED MINORITIES

Applications are actively encouraged from students of minority and disadvantaged backgrounds.

Private Institution

## APPLICATION AND ACCEPTANCE POLICIES FOR 1997–98 FIRST-YEAR CLASS

*School participates in AMCAS. See Chapter 4.*

Filing of AMCAS application
 Earliest date: June 1, 1996
 Latest date: Dec. 1, 1996
School application fee to all applicants: $55
Oldest MCAT scores considered: 1994
Does have Early Decision Program (EDP)
 EDP application period: June 1–Aug. 1, 1996
 EDP applicants notified by: Oct. 1, 1996
Acceptance notice to regular applicants
 Earliest date: Oct. 15, 1996
 Latest date: Until class is filled
Applicant's response to acceptance offer
 Maximum time: 3 weeks
Requests for deferred entrance considered: Yes
Deposit to hold place in class (applied to tuition):
 $100, due with response to acceptance offer
Deposit refundable prior to: May 15, 1997
Estimated number of new entrants: 250 (12 EDP)
Starting date: Aug. 1997

## TUITION AND STUDENT FEES PER YEAR FOR 1995–96 FIRST-YEAR CLASS

Tuition: $22,500          Student fees: $500

## INFORMATION ON 1995–96 FIRST-YEAR CLASS

| Number of | In-State | Out-of-State | Total |
|---|---|---|---|
| Applicants | 1,442 | 12,160 | 13,602 |
| Applicants Interviewed | 420 | 803 | 1,223 |
| New Entrants* | 135 | 105 | 240 |

*98% took the MCAT; 96% had baccalaureate degrees.

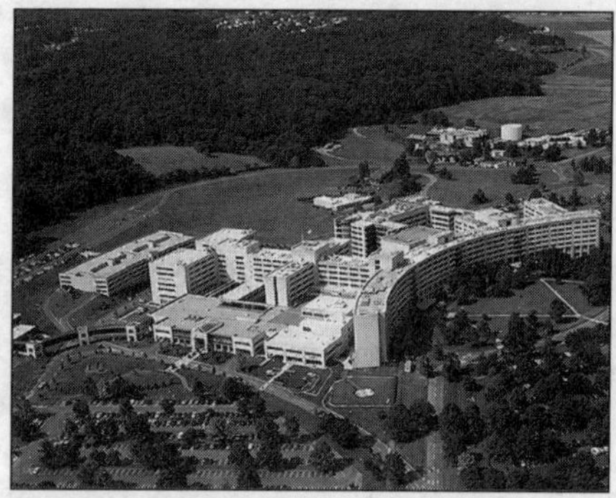

# Pennsylvania State University College of Medicine

**Hershey, Pennsylvania**

Dr. C. McCollister Evarts, *Senior Vice President for Health Affairs and Dean*
Dr. Dwight Davis, *Assistant Dean for Admissions*
Jill B. Wagner, *Admissions Representative*

## ADDRESS INQUIRIES TO:

Office of Student Affairs
Pennsylvania State University
College of Medicine
P.O. Box 850
Hershey, Pennsylvania 17033
(717) 531-8755; 531-6225 (FAX)
Web Site: http://www.hmc.psu.edu/

## GENERAL INFORMATION

The Pennsylvania State University College of Medicine was founded in 1964 through a $50 million gift from the Milton S. Hershey Foundation for the establishment of a medical school and teaching hospital at the Milton S. Hershey Medical Center. Additional construction funds were received from the U.S. Public Health Service, and the College of Medicine enrolled its first class in September 1967.

The 550-acre campus contains a medical sciences building, including a cancer research wing; a 504-bed hospital; a children's hospital; a biomedical research building; student-housestaff apartments; a fitness center complete with gym, racquetball and squash courts, and a variety of exercise equipment; a magnetic resonance imaging building; and a heliport for LIFE LION, an aeromedical service. The University Physicians Center, which provides a variety of outpatient services, allows students to learn in an office setting.

To accommodate growth in academic and clinical programs, Pennsylvania State University College of Medicine is in the midst of a $200 million expansion. Construction was completed on the seven-story hospital addition and the east addition in 1991. The seven-story Biomedical Research Building was completed in the spring of 1993. Construction of an expansion to the University Physicians Center was completed in the fall of 1993.

The George T. Harrell Library has 125,000 volumes and receives over 1,800 periodicals.

## CURRICULUM

Instruction in the first year is organized around the basic science core curriculum with an integrated approach to the teaching of organ systems and correlations between scientific principles and patient material. The first-year courses include microscopic anatomy, embryology, biological chemistry, gross anatomy, physician-patient interaction, molecular and human genetics, physiology, neurobiology, physical diagnosis, behavioral science, radiobiology, and clinical correlations. Elective course time is provided for humanities.

A track in problem-based learning is available for first- and second-year volunteer students. Problem-based learning is offered as an alternative educational method for students who wish to work in smaller groups with faculty tutors. The learning objectives for students in the PBL track will be similar to those for students in the "traditional track." The second year consists of an interdisciplinary organ system approach to clinical science and pathology integrated with microbiology, pharmacology, and physical diagnosis. Required also in the second year are longitudinal courses in behavioral science and psychiatry with particular emphasis on preventive medicine and organized systems of health care delivery.

The third year consists of required clinical clerkship experiences distributed among medicine, obstetrics and gynecology, surgery, pediatrics, psychiatry, primary care, and family and community medicine. The fourth year contains both selective and elective periods, with students selecting basic science or clinical science electives consistent with their educational and career plans. A final requirement is the completion of an original clinical or basic science study before graduation (medical student research).

There is an honors, high pass, pass, fail grading system.

## REQUIREMENTS FOR ENTRANCE

The MCAT and three years of college are required for admission. The baccalaureate degree is highly desirable.

The following subjects are considered by the Medical Student Selection Committee to be required:

|  | *Years* |
|---|---|
| Biology | 1 |
| Inorganic chemistry | 1 |
| Organic chemistry | 1 |
| Physics | 1 |
| Mathematics | 1 |
| Humanities | 1/2 |
| Behavioral Science | 1/2 |

Other recommended courses are calculus, statistics, psychology, sociology, radiobiology, genetics, and anthropology.

Students should be exposed to a broad background in the humanities and social sciences. Studies that develop verbal competence and enlarge perspectives and capacities for critical, historical, and moral judgments are especially encouraged.

Students are urged to take the MCAT in the spring of the year they expect to apply. Taking the MCAT in the fall will delay consideration of the application. It is recommended that basic science courses be completed before applying.

## SELECTION FACTORS

Applicants must show evidence of superior undergraduate achievement and outstanding personal characteristics. Each application is considered individually; a decision is reached after thorough evaluation of the applicant's academic record, letters of assessment, MCAT scores, and personal interview. Since the practice of medicine requires a lifelong devotion to self-education, emphasis is placed on the excellence of the individual scholar no matter what the student's previous area of study. An important consideration is the student's understanding of the relationship between the sciences and liberal arts.

Applicants are considered without regard to sex, race, religion, sexual orientation, or national origin. Students with an interest in primary care are encouraged to apply.

Some characteristics of accepted students in the 1995 entering class were: *average GPA,* 3.61; *sex,* 45 percent women; 33 percent minority.

## FINANCIAL AID

All financial aid is granted to students on the basis of need as determined by a federally approved needs analysis document. A student is considered for all funds available through the College of Medicine including federal as well as institutional funds when a needs analysis document is filed. Approximately 85 percent of the student body receive financial assistance from some source; 60 percent receive funds from school sources. Students' financial needs are reviewed annually, and awards for each year reflect the financial situation of students and their families for that year. Awards are usually distributed throughout the entire year (fall and spring semesters). All funds disbursed by the school, including Federal Work-Study Program funds, are described in detail in the school catalog. Specific inquiries should be addressed to the Office of Student Affairs.

## INFORMATION FOR MINORITIES

Applications from minority group students are encouraged. Faculty members, with student support, are active in the recruitment of minority students.

Private Institution

## APPLICATION AND ACCEPTANCE POLICIES FOR 1997–98 FIRST-YEAR CLASS

*School participates in AMCAS. See Chapter 4.*

Filing of AMCAS application
  Earliest date: June 1, 1996
  Latest date: Nov. 15, 1996
School application fee to all applicants: $40
Oldest MCAT scores considered: 1994
Does have Early Decision Program (EDP)
  EDP application period: June 1–Aug. 1, 1996
  EDP applicants notified by: Oct. 1, 1996
Acceptance notice to regular applicants
  Earliest date: Oct. 1, 1996
  Latest date: Until class is filled
Applicant's response to acceptance offer
  Maximum time: 2 weeks
Requests for deferred entrance considered: Yes
Deposit to hold place in class (applied to tuition):
  $100, due May 15, 1997
Deposit refundable prior to: May 15, 1997
Estimated number of new entrants: 120 (2 EDP)
Starting date: Aug. 1997

## TUITION AND STUDENT FEES PER YEAR FOR 1995–96 FIRST-YEAR CLASS

Tuition                 Student fees: $1,048
  Resident: $15,708
  Nonresident: $22,615

## INFORMATION ON 1995–96 FIRST-YEAR CLASS

| Number of | In-State | Out-of-State | Total |
|---|---|---|---|
| Applicants | 1,385 | 5,900 | 7,285 |
| Applicants Interviewed | * | * | 636 |
| New Entrants† | 57 | 62 | 119 |

*Data not available.

†All took the MCAT and had baccalaureate degrees.

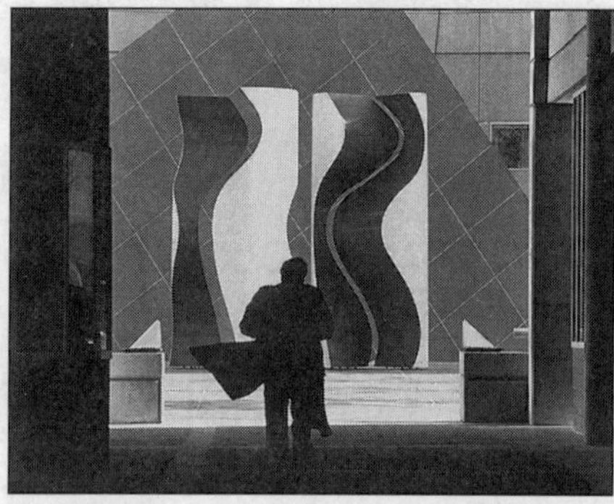

# University of Pennsylvania School of Medicine

**Philadelphia, Pennsylvania**

Dr. William N. Kelley, *CEO and Dean*
Dr. Gail Morrison, *Vice Dean for Education*
Gaye W. Sheffler, *Director of Admissions and Financial Aid*

## ADDRESS INQUIRIES TO:

Director of Admissions and Financial Aid
Edward J. Stemmler Hall, Suite 100
University of Pennsylvania
School of Medicine
Philadelphia, Pennsylvania 19104-6056
(215) 898-8001; 573-6645 (FAX)
Web Site: http://www.med.upenn.edu

## GENERAL INFORMATION

The School of Medicine, the first in the United States, was founded in 1765 and is a private, nondenominational school located on the urban campus of the University of Pennsylvania.

As part of the one university concept, medical students participate throughout their enrollment as members of the university as well as the School of Medicine community. In their clinical years, medical students receive their education mostly in the Hospital of the University of Pennsylvania and the Children's Hospital of Philadelphia, immediately adjacent to the school, and in the local, formally affiliated Graduate and Veterans's Administration of Philadelphia hospitals and Presbyterian Medical Center of Philadelphia. Student housing, both on and off campus, is plentiful.

## CURRICULUM

The curriculum is designed to prepare students for a variety of careers in medicine. It stresses understanding concepts, emphasizes techniques of problem-solving, and facilitates independent study. The curriculum is divided into three stages: Stage I, the 10-month first year, emphasizing basic science; Stage II, the first six months of the second year, emphasizing the pathophysiology of disease and introduction to clinical medicine; and Stage III, the remainder of the curriculum, emphasizing clinical medicine. Clinical teaching, including bedside teaching, is introduced early in the first year. Approximately half of the clinical curriculum is elective. Curricular topics such as health and public nutrition, bioethics, and preventive medicine are integrated throughout the curriculum. An honors/pass/fail system is used for grading in the basic sciences, with honors/high pass/pass/fail for clinical courses.

Numerous opportunities are available to augment medical studies with expanded study experiences, which may (1) further the development of an existing scholarly interest, (2) add desired specialized skills and knowledge to those gained through the general curriculum, and (3) permit the exploration of potential interests in research, academic medicine, and other career options for physicians.

The special experiences range in length from two-month summer research programs to several additional years, which may be undertaken by students working toward both the M.D. and Ph.D. degrees. Opportunities exist for involvement in a full-year expanded study experience, which may involve basic science or clinical research, or study and special projects in other schools of the university. The School of Medicine is addressing society's need for generalist physicians and has established a department of family practice and community medicine. All medical students take a primary care clerkship which provides training in an ambulatory care setting in either family practice, general medicine, or general pediatrics. The University of Pennsylvania Health System has established a growing network of primary care physicians who serve as mentors and role models to students. Students who are interested in primary care careers that include responsibilities as community leaders can add to their qualifications through combined-degree programs offering master's degrees in business/health care economics, government administration, clinical epidemiology, and education.

## REQUIREMENTS FOR ENTRANCE

The MCAT and a baccalaureate degree from an accredited U.S. college or university are required. Students with degrees from foreign institutions must have completed one year of course work in the sciences in a U.S. college or university.

Students are encouraged to obtain a broad education in the liberal arts while undertaking preparation in the sciences which is appropriately rigorous. Science courses should include laboratory experience, which enables students to become active participants in problem solving.

Because the content of courses varies among different educational institutions, the School of Medicine does not have specific course requirements. Students are expected to acquire appropriate competence in English and communication, biology, chemistry, physics, and mathematics. The school has developed general outlines of the requisite knowledge and skills in these disciplines, which are available upon request from the Office of Admissions.

In addition, students should carry out additional work in accordance with their own interests and curiosity. They should attempt to develop, through their formal course work and other educational experiences, an appreciation of the basic social, cultural, and behavioral factors that influence both individuals and communities in their approach to health and disease.

## SELECTION FACTORS

The School of Medicine will emphasize those qualities of motivation, intellect, and character essential to the physician. Consideration also will be given to special features of background and experience which may contribute to a candidate's potential for a medical career. Applicants should give evidence of their capacity to deal effectively with other people, organize their own activities, set priorities, accept responsibility, and function under stress.

While the Committee on Admissions has no preference regarding the area of concentration, applicants are expected to have approached their chosen field in scholarly fashion and to have demonstrated excellence in whatever courses of study they have pursued.

In evaluating candidates, the Committee on Admissions reviews the academic record, recommendations from college premedical evaluation committees, scores on the MCAT, quality of and commitment to extracurricular activities, and strength of personal qualifications. Interviews are required for admission and are arranged by invitation of the Committee on Admissions. Applicants from all sections of the country are invited to apply, although some preference is given to Pennsylvania residents.

In recent years, applicants granted admission have had a mean GPA of 3.6 and mean MCAT scores in the 10–11 range.

The class entering in September 1995 was composed of 39 percent *women;* 27 percent *Pennsylvania residents;* 25 percent *nonwhite ethnic groups,* 19 percent *underrepresented minorities;* and 36 percent *nonscience majors.*

The University of Pennsylvania does not discriminate on the basis of race, sex, sexual preference, age, religion, national or ethnic origin, or physical handicap.

## FINANCIAL AID

Grant and loan assistance is available for students who qualify on the basis of need and who are U.S. citizens or U.S. permanent residents. Over 75 percent of the student body receive financial assistance from some source. Approximately one-third of the students received school scholarship and loan funds. The ability of students to pay for their medical education does not affect the decision on their applications for admission.

## INFORMATION FOR MINORITIES

Minority students are encouraged to apply. Detailed information and statistics on minority applicants, acceptances, and enrollment are available in the *Information for Minority Applicants* brochure which can be obtained by writing to the Office of Minority Affairs, Suite 100, Stemmler Hall.

---

Private Institution

### APPLICATION AND ACCEPTANCE POLICIES FOR 1997–98 FIRST-YEAR CLASS

*School participates in AMCAS. See Chapter 4.*

Filing of AMCAS application
   Earliest date: June 1, 1996
   Latest date: Nov. 1, 1996
School application fee to all applicants: $55
Oldest MCAT scores considered: 1991
Does not have Early Decision Program
Acceptance notice to regular applicants
   Earliest date: Feb. 1997
   Latest date: Until class is filled
Applicant's response to acceptance offer
   Maximum time: 2 weeks
Requests for deferred entrance considered: Yes
Deposit to hold place in class (applied to tuition):
   $100, due with response to acceptance offer
Deposit refundable prior to: May 15, 1997
Estimated number of new entrants: 150
Starting date: Aug. 1997

### TUITION AND STUDENT FEES PER YEAR FOR 1995–96 FIRST-YEAR CLASS

Tuition: $24,530       Student fees: $1,183

### INFORMATION ON 1995–96 FIRST-YEAR CLASS

| Number of | In-State | Out-of-State | Total |
|---|---|---|---|
| Applicants | 1,004 | 7,923 | 8,927 |
| Applicants Interviewed | 152 | 931 | 1,083 |
| New Entrants* | 41 | 110 | 151 |

*All took the MCAT; 99% had baccalaureate degrees.

University of Pittsburgh

*School of Medicine*

# University of Pittsburgh School of Medicine

**Pittsburgh, Pennsylvania**

Dr. George K. Michalopoulos, *Associate Vice Chancellor, Health Sciences and Interim Dean*
Dr. Edward I. Curtiss, *Associate Dean of Admissions*
Linda A. Berardi-Demo, *Director of Admissions*

## ADDRESS INQUIRIES TO:

Office of Admissions
518 Scaife Hall
University of Pittsburgh
School of Medicine
Pittsburgh, Pennsylvania 15261
(412) 648-9891; 648-8768 (FAX)
E-Mail: admissions@fsl.dean-med.pitt.edu
Web Site: http://www.omed.pitt.edu/~omed/homepage2.html

## GENERAL INFORMATION

The Western Pennsylvania Medical College, chartered in 1886, became associated with the University of Pittsburgh in 1908. The School of Medicine is located in the Oakland district of Pittsburgh in the Alan Magee Scaife Hall of the Health Professions. The University of Pittsburgh Medical Center (UPMC) encompasses the School of Medicine, Montefiore University Hospital, Presbyterian University Hospital, Western Psychiatric Institute and Clinic, and the Pittsburgh Cancer Institute. The University of Pittsburgh Medical Center coordinates its activities with other university-affiliated hospitals and facilities, including Children's Hospital of Pittsburgh, Magee-Womens Hospital, and the Veterans Affairs Medical Centers.

## CURRICULUM

The School of Medicine has initiated extensive curricular revisions which were implemented in the fall of 1992. The goal-oriented, integrated, and centrally governed new curriculum emphasizes general principles and encourages student self-learning based on actual clinical cases. In the first two years, the curriculum employs a multi-disciplinary approach organized by organ systems (such as the heart, lungs, and kidneys) rather than by individual disciplines (e.g., physiology and biochemistry). It emphasizes problem-solving skills and learning in smaller groups. The curriculum mainstreams social, cultural, and ethical issues and introduces the student to clinical medicine during the first year. The final several weeks of the second year are devoted to an Integrated Case Studies course. This course emphasizes data acquisition, problem-solving, and communication skills. It is intended to help the student actively review the material presented during the first two years and serves as a bridge to the patient-care responsibilities assumed in the third-year clinical clerkships. In the third year of medical school, all students have required rotations in family medicine, internal medicine, obstetrics-gynecology, pediatrics, psychiatry, surgery, as well as ambulatory subspecialties. Some students rotate through anesthesia during the third year, while others take it during the fourth year. All fourth-year students rotate through both neurology and diagnostic imaging clerkships. Some students have one elective scheduled during the third year, and all students have extensive elective time during the fourth year.

In addition to the curricular offerings, there are opportunities for students to interact with community physicians through the Western Pennsylvania Health Preceptorship Program.

An honors/pass/fail system is used for grading.

The M.D.-Ph.D. Program of the University of Pittsburgh and Carnegie Mellon University offers exceptionally talented students the opportunity to undertake a physician-scientist training program tailored to their specific research interests. Over a period of seven or eight years, these individuals meet the degree requirements of both a graduate school and the medical school. Information may be obtained from the M.D.-Ph.D. office in 526 Scaife Hall. The telephone number is (412) 648-2324.

## REQUIREMENTS FOR ENTRANCE

The faculty of the School of Medicine consider currently enrolled students and graduates of accredited collegiate institutions for admission. Only under exceptional circumstances are students accepted to the School of Medicine with fewer than 120 hours of undergraduate work. The MCAT is required.

Specific minimum admission requirements include:

*Years*

Biology, exclusive of botany (with lab) . . . . . . . . . . . . . . . . 1
General or inorganic chemistry (with lab) . . . . . . . . . . . . . . 1
Organic chemistry (with lab) . . . . . . . . . . . . . . . . . . . . . . . . 1
Physics (with lab) . . . . . . . . . . . . . . . . . . . . . . . . . . . . . . . . . 1
English . . . . . . . . . . . . . . . . . . . . . . . . . . . . . . . . . . . . . . . . . 1

English courses must engender effective writing skills as well as familiarity with the great works of literature. A strong background in mathematics is highly recommended. Studies in social and behavioral sciences and humanities are strongly encouraged.

Acceptance of course requirements taken at foreign universities is determined on an individual basis at the discretion of the dean of admissions.

Applicants should have completed most premedical requirements to receive serious consideration. All requirements must be met prior to matriculation.

## SELECTION FACTORS

Applicants are chosen on the basis of intellect, integrity, maturity, and the ability to interact sensitively with people. In the competitive evaluation of applicants, consideration is given to the past academic record; evaluations of college pre-professional committees; letters of recommendation, preferably from faculty members with whom the student has interacted in scholarly pursuits; extracurricular activities; and personal interviews. No one is accepted without an interview. Interviews are conducted at the medical school campus with few exceptions. All applicants are considered without regard to race, color, religion, ethnicity, national origin, age, sex, sexual orientation, marital, veteran, or handicap status. Foreign nationals must have permanent resident visas and have completed at least one full year of undergraduate education in the United States, preferably the premedical requirements. Some preference is given to Pennsylvania residents since the university is a state-related school. For the entering class of 1995, matriculated students had an average science GPA of 3.59 and a mean MCAT of 10.5.

The School of Medicine is committed to increasing the number of underrepresented minority students (African American, Mexican American, Mainland Puerto Rican, and Native American) in medicine, and thus actively recruits and strongly encourages applications from minority students. The school hosts pre-medical summer enrichment programs, as well as a prematriculation program for admitted students. Following admission, a broad range of support services are available to ensure retention. Specific information on the services provided to minority applicants can be obtained by contacting the Office of Student Affairs/Minority Programs at (412) 648-8987.

## FINANCIAL AID

All loans and scholarships are awarded on the basis of financial need as documented by the FAFSA. Students demonstrating financial need are expected to obtain the first $8,500 from the Federal Stafford Student Loan.

---

Private Institution

### APPLICATION AND ACCEPTANCE POLICIES FOR 1997–98 FIRST-YEAR CLASS

*School participates in AMCAS. See Chapter 4.*

Filing of AMCAS application
Earliest date: June 1, 1996
Latest date: Nov. 1, 1996
School application fee to all applicants: $60
Oldest MCAT scores considered: 1993
Does have Early Decision Program (EDP)
EDP application period: June 1–Aug. 1, 1996
EDP applicants notified by: Oct. 1, 1996
Acceptance notice to regular applicants
Earliest date: Oct. 15, 1996
Latest date: Until class is filled
Applicant's response to acceptance offer
Maximum time: 2 weeks
Requests for deferred entrance considered: Yes
Deposit to hold place in class: $100 (nonrefundable, which must reach our office between May 16–24, 1997).
Estimated number of new entrants: 140 (4 EDP)
Starting date: Aug. 1997

### TUITION AND STUDENT FEES PER YEAR FOR 1995–96 FIRST-YEAR CLASS

Tuition          Student fees: $415
Resident: $18,170
Nonresident: $24,300

### INFORMATION ON 1995–96 FIRST-YEAR CLASS

| Number of | In-State | Out-of-State | Total |
|---|---|---|---|
| Applicants | 1,233 | 5,454 | 6,687 |
| Applicants Interviewed | 259 | 591 | 850 |
| New Entrants* | 84 | 55 | 139 |

*All took the MCAT and had baccalaureate degrees.

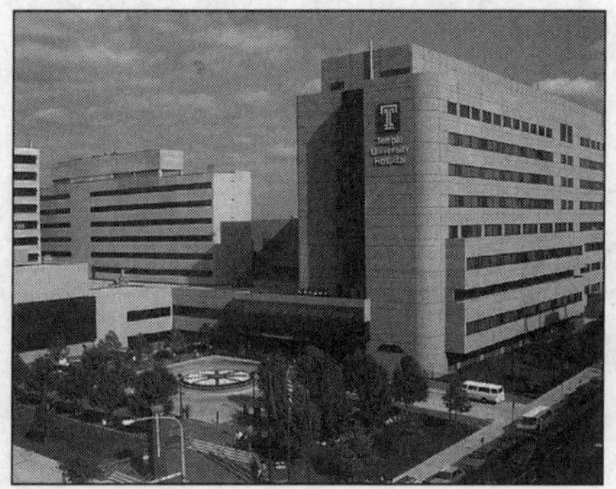

# Temple University
# School of Medicine

## Philadelphia, Pennsylvania

Dr. Richard Kozera, *Acting Dean*
Dr. Ronald F. Tuma, *Assistant Dean for Admissions*
Dr. Moses L. Williams, *Director of Admissions*

## ADDRESS INQUIRIES TO:

Admissions Office
Suite 305, Student Faculty Center
Temple University
School of Medicine
Broad and Ontario Streets
Philadelphia, Pennsylvania 19140
(215) 707-3656; 707-6932 (FAX)

## GENERAL INFORMATION

The Temple University School of Medicine opened as a college of Temple University in 1901. The School of Medicine shares a campus with Temple Hospital, other health-related schools of the university, and the Student/Faculty Center. Clinical experience and instruction are given at the new Temple University Hospital, St. Christopher's Hospital for Children, Albert Einstein Medical Center (Northern Division), and 23 other affiliated hospitals, both in Philadelphia and other Pennsylvania cities.

## CURRICULUM

The curriculum is designed to prepare students for graduate medical education by providing them with a background of basic factual knowledge and concepts, a command of the language of biomedical science, a mastery of the skills necessary for clinical problem-solving and therapy, and a habit of continued self-education.

In the first two years, although primary emphasis is on the basic sciences taught in large measure in a small-group format, attention is also given to the clinical application of this material. In addition, courses on clinical medicine and primary care concepts prepare the students to assume initial clinical responsibilities. The third year includes clerkships in family practice, internal medicine, obstetrics-gynecology, pediatrics, psychiatry, and surgery which provide experience in clinical diagnosis, problem solving, therapeutic planning, and patient relationships. In the fourth year, four weeks are devoted to oncology and to disorders of individual organ systems. There are required rotations in emergency medicine, neuroscience, a surgical specialty, and a subinternship and 20 weeks of individually planned electives which permit students to explore career choice, correct deficits, and expand clinical knowledge.

There is an honors/high pass/pass/conditional/fail grading system.

An M.D.-Ph.D. program is available.

## REQUIREMENTS FOR ENTRANCE

The MCAT and a minimum of 90 semester hours in an accredited college or university are required for admission. Applicants need not major in science, and a strong background and preparation in the humanities with particular emphasis on expository writing are essential. Students who have not completed the baccalaureate degree but who have demonstrated exceptional academic capability and evidence of unusual maturity may apply. The undergraduate program must include:

*Sem. hrs.*

Biology (with lab) . . . . . . . . . . . . . . . . . . . . . . . . . . . . . . . 8
Inorganic chemistry (with lab) . . . . . . . . . . . . . . . . . . . . . . 8
Organic chemistry (with lab) . . . . . . . . . . . . . . . . . . . . . . 8
General physics (with lab) . . . . . . . . . . . . . . . . . . . . . . . . 8
Humanities . . . . . . . . . . . . . . . . . . . . . . . . . . . . . . . . . . . 6

Applicants are asked to have recommendations from their undergraduate premedical committee or faculty in two of the following three subjects: biology, chemistry, and physics.

It is suggested that the MCAT be taken in the spring of the calendar year of application and that all courses required for medical school be completed by the time of application.

## SELECTION FACTORS

A variety of objective and subjective factors are considered in making decisions. Among these are the academic record and the college attended, MCAT scores, recommendations from faculty, extracurricular activities, and work experience. Those candidates who are to be given very serious consideration are invited for personal interviews with a member of the Admissions Committee.

As a state-related school, Temple shows preference to residents of Pennsylvania; however, a significant percentage of matriculants may be residents of other states. Nonresidents with a particular interest in Temple and strong credentials are encouraged to apply.

Temple University School of Medicine does not discriminate on the basis of race, sex, creed, national origin, age, or handicap.

Selected characteristics of the 1994 entering class are as follows: *average science GPA,* 3.4; *average MCAT: sciences,* 10; *sex,* 41 percent women; *minorities,* 20 percent (about 16 percent African American).

## FINANCIAL AID

With the exception of a restricted number of scholarships, all financial aid is in the form of loans and is based solely on need. Need is established by the use of a national standard financial aid application through GAPSFAS which details financial resources of students (or their families) and balances them against a standard budget plus special need factors. A modicum of relatively low cost financial aid comes from Temple University based moneys as part of the federal programs for the Health Professions Student Loan and the Perkins Loan. The initial source of assistance for most students will be the Stafford Student Loan Program; in fact, all eligible students are expected to secure the first $7,500 of aid from this source. For many students, the primary source of funds is the Health Education Assistance Loan (HEAL) Program. Other sources of assistance may come from medical societies, fraternal organizations, church groups, and, in the case of minority students, from the National Medical Fellowships, Inc. In selected instances students have applied to the scholarship programs of the Armed Forces and the National Health Service Corps. Approximately 80 percent of the students receive financial aid.

## INFORMATION FOR MINORITIES

An active program, Recruitment, Admission, and Retention (RAR), meets the special needs of minority applicants. RAR provides exceptional resources for professional academic guidance and personal counseling. Participation in the Summer Educational Reinforcement Activity is encouraged for accepted minority students and others.

Private Institution

## APPLICATION AND ACCEPTANCE POLICIES FOR 1997–98 FIRST-YEAR CLASS

*School participates in AMCAS. See Chapter 4.*

Filing of AMCAS application
  Earliest date: June 1, 1996
  Latest date: Dec. 1, 1996
School application fee to all applicants: $55
Oldest MCAT scores considered: 1994
Does have Early Decision Program (EDP)
  EDP application period: June 1–Aug. 1, 1996
  EDP applicants notified by: Oct. 1, 1996
Acceptance notice to regular applicants
  Earliest date: Oct. 15, 1996
  Latest date: Aug. 15, 1997
Applicant's response to acceptance offer
  Maximum time: 2 weeks
Requests for deferred entrance considered: Yes
Deposit to hold place in class (applied to tuition):
  $100, due with response to acceptance offer
Deposit refundable prior to: May 15, 1997
Estimated number of new entrants: 180 (4 EDP)
Starting date: Aug. 1997

## TUITION AND STUDENT FEES PER YEAR FOR 1995–96 FIRST-YEAR CLASS

Tuition                                    Student fees: $358
  Resident: $19,416
  Nonresident: $24,555

## INFORMATION ON 1995–96 FIRST-YEAR CLASS

| Number of | In-State | Out-of-State | Total |
|---|---|---|---|
| Applicants | 1,409 | 7,375 | 8,784 |
| Applicants Interviewed | 420 | 544 | 964 |
| New Entrants* | 107 | 80 | 187 |

*All took the MCAT and had baccalaureate degrees.

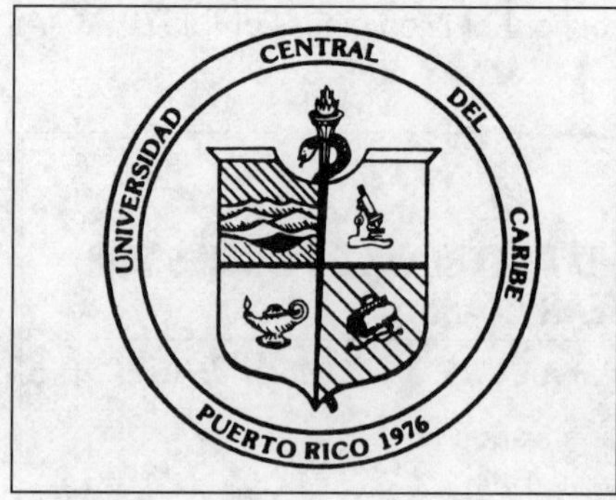

# Universidad Central del Caribe
# School of Medicine

**Bayamón, Puerto Rico**

Dr. Raúl A. Marcial-Rojas, *President*
Dr. Julia Bonilla, *Dean of Medicine*

## ADDRESS INQUIRIES TO:

Office of Admissions
Universidad Central del Caribe
School of Medicine
Ramón Ruíz Arnau University Hospital
Call Box 60-327
Bayamón, Puerto Rico 00960-6032
(809) 740-1611 Ext. 210; 269-7550 (FAX)

## GENERAL INFORMATION

The Universidad Central del Caribe School of Medicine was founded in 1976 as a nonprofit private institution chartered under the laws of the Commonwealth of Puerto Rico. The new building for the basic sciences, library, animal house, and central administration was inaugurated in 1990 adjacent to Dr. Ramón Ruíz Arnau University Hospital, which serves as the principal teaching hospital. The school facilities are located in a 56-acre academic health center in the city of Bayamón.

## CURRICULUM

The stated educational goal of the medical school is to develop an individual who is oriented toward the provision of primary health care. In line with this goal, the medical school experience emphasizes community health, family medicine, and primary medical care aspects of internal medicine, surgery, pediatrics, obstetrics and gynecology, and psychiatry.

The medical curriculum is organized in two years of preclinical and two years of clinical experiences. Clinical correlations are included in the basic sciences courses. Introduction to clinical medicine, offered in the second year, has as its foundation the biopsychosocial model. This is a problem-based course structured around prevalent problems encountered in primary care. The third-year learning experience evolves around the required clerkships in internal medicine, pediatrics, obstetrics-gynecology, general surgery, and family and community medicine. The latter takes place in the ambulatory setting. During the fourth year, students enroll in the surgical subspecialties and psychiatry clerkships. Sixteen weeks of electives are provided.

Individual student evaluation in all requisite basic science and clinical science courses is based on letter grade and pass/fail systems. Student evaluation in all elective courses is based on an honors/pass/fail system.

## REQUIREMENTS FOR ENTRANCE

The MCAT and a minimum of 90 credits of satisfactory work in an accredited undergraduate institution are required. A baccalaureate degree is highly recommended. All premedical course requirements must either be completed or be in progress prior to consideration for admission.

Required premedical courses and minimum required credits are:

|  | Sem. hrs. |
|---|---|
| General biology or zoology | 8 |
| General chemistry | 8 |
| Organic chemistry | 8 |
| General physics | 8 |
| College mathematics | 6 |
| English | 6 |
| Spanish | 6 |
| Behavioral/Social sciences/Humanities | 6 |

The applicant must demonstrate proficiency in both Spanish and English. Teaching in basic sciences and clinical sciences is conducted mainly in Spanish.

A strong background and preparation in the humanities and behavioral sciences is highly encouraged so that the applicant may obtain a well-rounded undergraduate education. This background should provide the applicant with a broad cultural foundation, and it will allow our institution to produce physicians with a humanistic approach to the practice of the profession. As long as students fulfill the basic requirements for admission, they may obtain a baccalaureate degree in any field of learning.

Applicants are strongly urged to take the MCAT in the spring prior to application and to have completed the required courses by the time of application since applications are not reviewed by the Admissions Committee until the MCAT scores and grades are available. Taking the fall MCAT or having required courses in process may delay consideration of an application, thus reducing the applicant's chances of acceptance.

## SELECTION FACTORS

The selection of candidates for admission is made exclusively by the Admissions Committee. The admission process does not discriminate against any individual on the basis of sex, age, race, religion, economic status, political ideology, or national origin. Major factors considered in the selection of candidates for admission include undergraduate academic record, general GPA and science GPA, performance in all areas of the MCAT, results of a personal interview, and letters of recommendation. A personal interview is required prior to consideration for admission. All interviews are arranged by the Office of Admissions and are conducted at the medical school facilities in Bayamón. Rejected applicants are given the opportunity to reapply for admission.

For the 1995 entering class the mean undergraduate general GPA was 3.12, and 47 percent of the entering students were women.

## FINANCIAL AID

The Office of the Dean for Student Affairs provides financial aid counseling to all prospective students. Incoming freshmen qualify for application to all pertinent federal and commonwealth scholarship and loan programs. Economic status of the applicant is not a consideration during the selection of candidates for admission.

Private Institution

## APPLICATION AND ACCEPTANCE POLICIES FOR 1997–98 FIRST-YEAR CLASS

*School participates in AMCAS. See Chapter 4.*

Filing of AMCAS application
   Earliest date: June 1, 1996
   Latest date: Dec. 15, 1996
School application fee to all applicants: $50
Oldest MCAT scores considered: 1995
Does have Early Decision Program (EDP)
   EDP application period: June 1–Aug. 1, 1996
   EDP applicants notified by: Oct. 1, 1996
Acceptance notice to regular applicants
   Earliest date: Feb. 1997
   Latest date: Varies
Applicant's response to acceptance offer
   Maximum time: 10 days
Requests for deferred entrance considered: No
   Deposit to hold place in class: $100, due with
   response to acceptance offer; nonrefundable
Estimated number of new entrants: 60 (10 EDP)
Starting date: Aug. 1997

## TUITION AND STUDENT FEES PER YEAR FOR 1995–96 FIRST-YEAR CLASS

Tuition                             Student fees: $789
   Resident: $17,800
   Nonresident: $24,000

## INFORMATION ON 1995–96 FIRST-YEAR CLASS

| Number of | In-State | Out-of-State | Total |
|---|---|---|---|
| Applicants | 435 | 644 | 1,079 |
| Applicants Interviewed | 185 | 17 | 202 |
| New Entrants* | 51 | 9 | 60 |

*All took the MCAT; 97% had baccalaureate degrees.

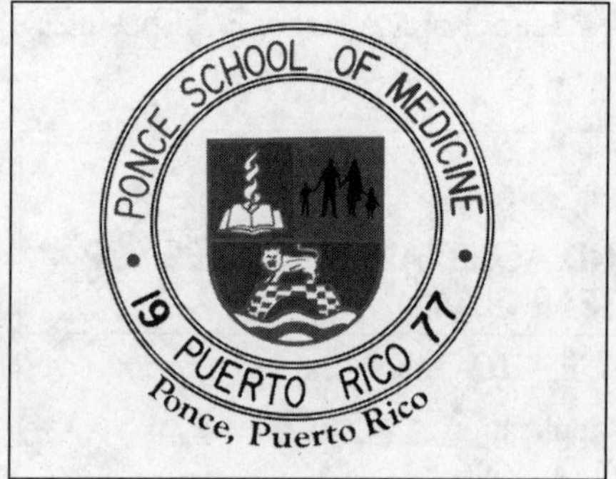

# Ponce School of Medicine

**Ponce, Puerto Rico**

Dr. Jaime Rivera Dueño, *President and Dean*
Dr. Carmen M. Mercado, *Assistant Dean for Admissions*
Sixta Gaud, *Financial Aid Director*

## ADDRESS INQUIRIES TO:

Admissions Office
Ponce School of Medicine
P.O. Box 7004
Ponce, Puerto Rico 00732
(809) 840-2511; 844-3685 (FAX)

## GENERAL INFORMATION

The Ponce School of Medicine of the Ponce Medical School Foundation, Inc., formerly Catholic University of Puerto Rico School of Medicine, took over the operations on July 1, 1980, under the government of a board of trustees. The school graduated its first class in June 1981.

Clinical training is offered at the following facilities in Ponce: Damas Hospital, a private institution with 356 beds; La Playa Diagnostic Center, which serves as the main training area for community and family practice; Ponce District Hospital with 550 beds; Dr. Pila Hospital with 160 beds; and St. Luke's Hospital with 160 beds. Clinical training is also offered at the Concepción Hospital with 188 beds, located in San Germán, and at Yauco Regional Hospital with 140 beds.

## CURRICULUM

The medical program's basic objective is to provide the Commonwealth of Puerto Rico, especially the southern region of the island, with ethically motivated, professionally competent primary care physicians. The curriculum provides students with an early experience in family and community health needs. During the first two years the basic medical sciences are thoroughly emphasized. Clinical experience takes precedence during the third and fourth years. The correlation between the basic and clinical sciences is achieved in a multidisciplinary program. Throughout the four-year program, great emphasis is placed on the students' contact with patients and their families, as a complement to the students' academic-hospital experience.

Every academic semester contains, in addition to the regular curricula, a series of supplementary seminars dealing with the ethical and social components of medical practice and with additional specific subjects that are incidental and relevant to the profession. The program seeks to develop well balanced, mature general practitioners, equally well qualified in the professional and ethical aspects of medicine.

Students' work is graded according to an honors/pass/fail/incomplete/extended system.

## REQUIREMENTS FOR ENTRANCE

The MCAT and a minimum of three years (90 semester hours) of accredited college work are required. Accredited courses should include the following minimum requirements:

|  | Sem. hrs. |
|---|---|
| Biology | 8 |
| Inorganic chemistry | 8 |
| Organic chemistry | 8 |
| Physics | 8 |
| College mathematics or trigonometry | 6 |
| Humanities* | 6 |
| English | 12 |
| Spanish | 12 |

*Course work must be in sociology, psychology, political science, economics, or anthropology.

Academic requirements should be met not later than during the academic year immediately preceding the applicant's anticipated entrance to the school. Applicants are required to submit written evaluations from three faculty members of the institution where they have recently studied or one from their premedical advisory committee.

## SELECTION FACTORS

Selection of applicants is made by the Admissions Committee on the basis of academic achievement, MCAT scores, evaluation letters, and personal interviews. The interviews are used to determine the motivation and character of the applicants. Only those who pass a preliminary screening, based on MCAT scores and college grades, are interviewed. Careful consideration is given to all applicants regardless of racial or ethnic background, religious affiliation, sex, or national origin. Residents of Puerto Rico are given preference, although a limited number of applicants who live in the United States may be accepted. Candidates who do not have at least a functional knowledge of both English and Spanish are not encouraged to apply, since instruction is given in both languages.

The 1995 entering class had the following profile: *average GPA,* 3.30 (85 percent above 3.0); *sex,* 45 percent female; *residence,* 77 percent from Puerto Rico, 23 percent from the continental United States; *undergraduate major,* 68 percent in biology and general science.

## FINANCIAL AID

Most of the regular opportunities are locally available, including loans through banking institutions. The Student Financial Aid Office offers individual advice and assistance depending on need and existing possibilities properly verified and certified.

About 86.6 percent of the 1995 entrants received financial aid. Students are informed about opportunities for financial assistance prior to acceptance to the School of Medicine.

Private Institution

## APPLICATION AND ACCEPTANCE POLICIES FOR 1997–98 FIRST-YEAR CLASS

*School participates in AMCAS. See Chapter 4.*

Filing of AMCAS application
   Earliest date: June 1, 1996
   Latest date: Dec. 15, 1996
School application fee to all applicants: $50
Oldest MCAT scores considered: 1995
Does have Early Decision Program (EDP)
   EDP application period: June 1–Aug. 1, 1996
   EDP applicants notified by: Oct, 1, 1996
Acceptance notice to regular applicants
   Earliest date: Oct. 15, 1996
   Latest date: Until class is filled
Applicant's response to acceptance offer
   Maximum time: 4 weeks
Requests for deferred entrance considered: No
Deposit to hold place in class (applied to tuition):
   $1,000, due with response to acceptance offer
Estimated number of new entrants: 60 (5 EDP)
Starting date: July 1997

## TUITION AND STUDENT FEES PER YEAR FOR 1995–96 FIRST-YEAR CLASS

Tuition                         Student fees: $1,813
   Resident: $16,973
   Nonresident: $25,304

## INFORMATION ON 1995–96 FIRST-YEAR CLASS

| Number of | In-State | Out-of-State | Total |
|---|---|---|---|
| Applicants | 368 | 606 | 974 |
| Applicants Interviewed | 178 | 30 | 208 |
| New Entrants* | 46 | 14 | 60 |

*All took the MCAT; 82% had baccalaureate degrees.

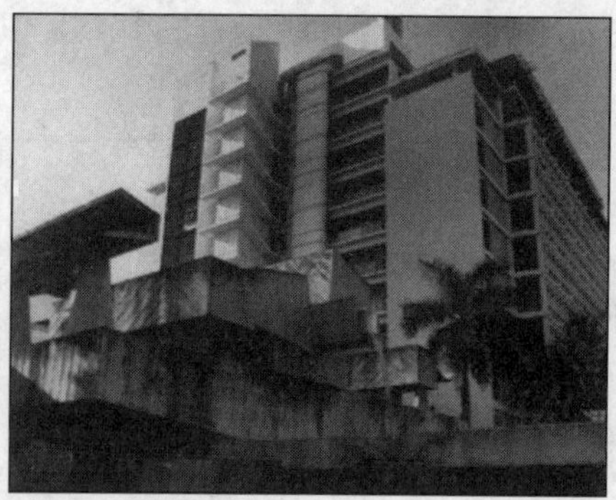

# University of Puerto Rico
# School of Medicine

**San Juan, Puerto Rico**

Dr. Angel Roman-Franco, *Acting Dean*
Rita Aponte-Rodriguez, *Director of Admissions*
Lourdes Pont, *Director, Financial Aid Office*

## ADDRESS INQUIRIES TO:

Central Admissions Office
School of Medicine
Medical Sciences Campus
University of Puerto Rico
P.O. Box 365067
San Juan, Puerto Rico 00936-5067
(787) 758-2525, Ext. 5213; 282-7117 (FAX)
E-Mail: R_APONTE@RCMAD.UPR.CLU.EDU

## GENERAL INFORMATION

The University of Puerto Rico School of Medicine was established in 1949. The chief teaching institution is the University District Hospital. The affiliated hospitals of the Puerto Rico Medical Center and the Hospital Consortium, which include the main health care facilities in other cities, serve the medical school for teaching purposes. Besides the School of Medicine, the Medical Sciences Campus provides space for the School of Dentistry, the College of Allied Health Professions, the Faculty of Biosocial Sciences and Graduate School of Public Health, the School of Nursing, and the School of Pharmacy. Its location, adjacent to the University District Hospital, permits integration of basic and clinical departments and an improved utilization of all Medical Sciences Campus resources.

## CURRICULUM

The new curriculum has been designed to last four academic years. The first two include the fundamentals of biological, behavioral, and clinical sciences and are mostly handled by the basic sciences departments. Part of the sophomore year is dedicated to pathophysiology, physical diagnosis, and basic clerkship, which are offered by a multidisciplinary faculty. Small-group sessions utilizing the problem-based learning approach are introduced at the beginning of the medical studies. Human behavior, environmental factors, and public health teaching is integrated into the curriculum. The third year is primarily dedicated to clinical experiences, and the fourth year is spent in required clinical experiences and elective courses. The use of diverse educational techniques, increased use of educational technology, and diversification of teaching exercises are emphasized. Through the Hispanic Center of Excellence, the curriculum has been focused toward more primary care exposure. Support services, counseling, tutorials, and other services are provided to students to assist in retention. Students are graded on a letter grade system in all four years.

## REQUIREMENTS FOR ENTRANCE

The MCAT and a minimum of 90 semester hours of accredited college work, which must be completed no later than the academic year (not summer session) preceding admission, are required. The MCAT should not be taken later than August of the year before admission. Fluency in Spanish and English is required. College work must include the following courses:

|  | Sem. hrs. |
|---|---|
| Biology | 8 |
| General chemistry (with lab) | 8 |
| Organic chemistry (with lab) | 8 |
| Physics (with lab) | 8 |
| English | 12 |
| Spanish | 12 |
| Behavioral and social sciences | 6 |

Course work must be in sociology, psychology, political sciences, economics, or anthropology.

The School of Medicine accepts CLEP and advanced placement examinations toward the fulfillment of admission requirements if credits are granted for having passed the exams and are clearly indicated on the undergraduate college transcripts as having been accepted by that college.

Since the preclinical courses in the School of Medicine are largely scientific in nature, it is to the student's advantage to obtain a well-rounded undergraduate education.

## SELECTION FACTORS

In selecting students the Admissions Committee considers the candidate's academic record, MCAT scores, recommendations of instructors, attitudinal and other personality factors assessed in personal interviews, extracurricular activities, and any other pertinent information. Personal interviews are conducted only by invitation from the Admissions Committee to those students with high numerical ranks according to a formula approved by the Academic Senate. This personal interview is conducted only on the site of the medical school, or the affiliated hsopitals at the Puerto Rico Medical Center. The formula gives equal weight to academic indices and MCAT socres, with somewhat less weight being given to ratings derived from evaluations by premedical committees and interviewers. Rejected applicants are given the opportunity to reapply for admission. Applicants, without exception, must submit all application material and supporting credentials by December 1 of the year preceding the school year for which they request admission.

The School of Medicine accepts transfer applications into the third-year class from candidates who are presently enrolled and have satisfactorily completed the first two years of the medical curriculum at a LCME-accredited medical school. Promotion into the third year must be recommneded by the original school. Besides having completed all the same requirements for admissions into the first year class, they must pass Step I of the USMLE. Deadline to submit application and supporting documents is May 1 of the same year of admission.

The School of Medicine has the policy of giving equal opportunity for education and training in the practice of the health professions without regard to race, creed, sex, national origin, age, or handicap. Since the school is mainly supported by the Commonwealth of Puerto Rico, preference is given to U.S. citizens who are legal residents of Puerto Rico.

Accepted students for the 1995 class had the following credentials: *mean GPA,* 3.48 (range 2.70–3.98; 93 percent above 3.0); *mean science grade index,* 3.38 (range 2.62–4.00; 83 percent above 3.00); *mean and range MCAT scores,* VR-7 (3–12), PS-7 (5–12), WS-L/M (J–T), BS-8 (5–13); *sex,* 48 percent female; *residence,* 99 percent from Puerto Rico; *overall acceptance rate,* 984 applications were received, and 130 offers of acceptance were made to obtain a class of 115 freshmen.

## FINANCIAL AID

Financial aid is available to students in all four years. More than 50 percent of the students receive some kind of financial aid from the Medical Sciences Campus at some time during their four years of study. Awards are made by the Committee on Scholarships and Loans on the basis of confidential applications submitted by the students. Financial need is the major criterion. Applicants who require scholarship assistance may make application in conjunction with the application for admission or at any time before April 30, but financial need will not influence the selection process. Forms are available from the Financial Aid Office of the Office of the Dean for Student Affairs at the Medical Sciences Campus upon request.

Public Institution

## APPLICATION AND ACCEPTANCE POLICIES FOR 1997–98 FIRST-YEAR CLASS

*School participates in AMCAS. See Chapter 4.*

Filing of AMCAS application
  Earliest date: June 1, 1996
  Latest date: Dec. 1, 1996
School application fee to all applicants: $15
Oldest MCAT scores considered: 1994
Does not have Early Decision Program
Acceptance notice to regular applicants
  Earliest date: Dec. 15, 1996
  Latest date: March 15, 1997
Applicant's response to acceptance offer
  Maximum time: 15 days
Requests for deferred entrance considered: Yes
Deposit to hold place in class (applied to tuition):
  $100, due with response to acceptance offer;
  nonrefundable
Estimated number of new entrants: 115
Starting date: Aug. 1997

## TUITION AND STUDENT FEES PER YEAR FOR 1995–96 FIRST-YEAR CLASS

Tuition                              Student fees: $580
  Resident: $5,500
  Nonresident: $10,500; Pays according to a
    standardized fee scale (U.S. mainland and
    foreign residents)

## INFORMATION ON 1995–96 FIRST-YEAR CLASS

| Number of | In-State | Out-of-State | Total |
|---|---|---|---|
| Applicants | 365 | 619 | 984 |
| Applicants Interviewed | 151 | 5 | 156 |
| New Entrants* | 114 | 1 | 115 |

*All took the MCAT; 80% had baccalaureate degrees.

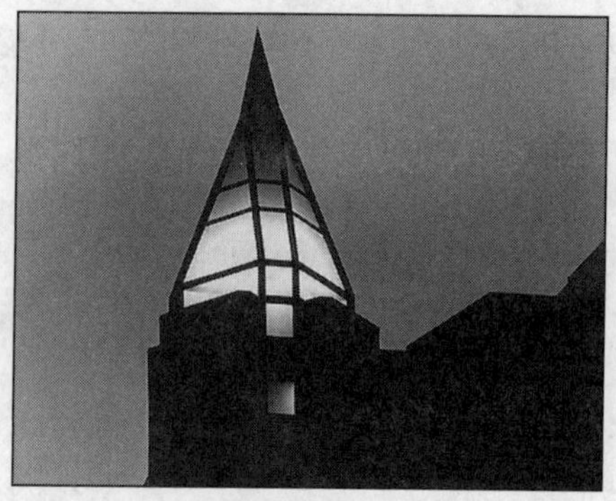

# Brown University
# School of Medicine

## Providence, Rhode Island

Dr. Donald J. Marsh, *Dean of Medicine and Biological Sciences*
Dr. Stephen R. Smith, *Associate Dean for Medical Education*
Kathleen A. Massone, *Director of Admissions and Financial Aid*

## ADDRESS INQUIRIES TO:

Office of Admissions and Financial Aid
Brown University
School of Medicine
97 Waterman St., Box GA 212
Providence, Rhode Island 02912-9706
(401) 863-2149; 863-2660 (FAX)
E-Mail: MedSchool_Admissions@brown.edu
Web Site: http://www.brown.edu

## GENERAL INFORMATION

**Important Note.** *The Brown University program is an eight-year continuum of college and medical school (Program in Liberal Medical Education) which offers admission to high school seniors (see Chapter 9). However, limited spaces are available for admission into the first year of medical school. Please read carefully the information provided below regarding eligibility for admission before requesting an application.*

## GENERAL INFORMATION

Brown University, founded in 1764, is the seventh oldest college in America and the third oldest in New England. In 1963 a Master of Medical Science Program, a six-year course of study emphasizing the basic sciences and encompassing the four years of premedical education and the first two years of medical school, was inaugurated. A program in medicine leading to the M.D. degree was accredited in 1975 as a four-year medical school. In 1981 the trustees of Dartmouth College and the Corporation of Brown University approved the Brown-Dartmouth Medical Program to which 15 medical students are admitted jointly. Students spend the first two years at Dartmouth Medical School and transfer to the Brown University School of Medicine for the last two years.

Entry into the first year of the Brown University School of Medicine is available only to applicants applying to the M.D.-Ph.D. program; to students enrolled in post-baccalaureate premedical study at Brown University, Bryn Mawr College, or Columbia University; to students enrolled in the Early Identification Program at Providence College, Tougaloo College, Rhode Island College, or the University of Rhode Island; and to undergraduate and graduate students at Brown University. The traditional avenue of medical school admission is limited because the majority of first-year entrants are from the eight-year continuum program. The Brown-Dartmouth Medical Program enrolls 15 students each year for the first two years of medical study at Dartmouth and the last two years at Brown. Students who are interested in this program should apply through Dartmouth Medical School. (See Dartmouth Medical School entry for further information.) Students attending any school accredited by the Liaison Committee on Medical Education and Rhode Island residents attending foreign medical schools accredited by the W.H.O. may apply for advanced standing admission into the School of Medicine.

## CURRICULUM

The School of Medicine is based on Brown's campus and in the university's affiliated hospitals (Bradley, Butler, Memorial, Miriam, Rhode Island, Roger Williams, Women and Infants, and Veterans Administration hospitals).

The first year is devoted to courses in human morphology, mammalian physiology, human histology, social and behavioral sciences, medical microbiology, biochemical pharmacology, general pathology, molecular and regulatory biochemistry and neurosciences.

The second-year curriculum consists of pathophysiology, neurosciences, systemic pathology, organ system pharmacology, and introductory courses in psychiatry and physical diagnosis.

Students in the third and fourth years are required to satisfactorily complete 48 weeks of clinical clerkships and 32 weeks of electives. The clinical clerkships include internal medicine (12 weeks), surgery (12 weeks), psychiatry (6 weeks), obstetrics and gynecology (6 weeks), pediatrics (6 weeks), family medicine (6 weeks), and community health which is integrated into the clerkships in medicine and family medicine. A four-week advanced clinical clerkship (subinternship) is also required as is an ambulatory longitudinal clerkship elective (one-half day per week for six months).

The graduate programs offered to M.D.-Ph.D. candidates are artificial organs, biomaterials, and cellular technology; ecology and evolutionary biology; epidemiology and gerontology; molecular biology, cell biology, and biochemistry; neuroscience; and pathobiology.

## REQUIREMENTS FOR ENTRANCE

The MCAT is required only if the applicant is applying to the Brown-Dartmouth Program. Students admitted to the School of Medicine are expected to attain competence in the sciences basic to medicine sufficient for adequate preparation for medical school. Although the majority of students demonstrate competence through course work, such preparation may also be demonstrated through individualized study, research, or work experience. The following areas of study are recommended as guidelines to be used in selecting courses:

*Semesters*

| | |
|---|---|
| Biology | 2 |
| Biochemistry | 1 |
| Calculus | 1 |
| Probability and statistics | 1 |
| General chemistry | 2 |
| Organic chemistry | 1 |
| Physics | 2 |
| Social and behavioral sciences | 2 |

## SELECTION FACTORS

Candidates are selected on the basis of academic achievement, faculty evaluations, evidence of maturity, motivation, leadership, intergrity, and compassion. Candidates must also present a 3.0 minimum grade point average (on a 4.0 scale).

In addition, applicants must be capable of meeting the competency requirements expected of all graduates, with reasonable accommodation. These requirements are sent to applicants following their acceptance.

Applicants are assessed without regard to race, religion, national or ethnic origin, sexual preference, age, or physical handicap. Applications from medically underrepresented minority groups and Rhode Island residents are especially encouraged.

## FINANCIAL AID

The School of Medicine makes every effort to assist students in meeting the cost of their medical education through a combination of low-interest loans, scholarships, and interest subsidies on unsubsidized loans. Approximately 65 percent of the students receive some type of financial assistance. Employment during the school year is strongly discouraged. Financial aid may be awarded to foreign national students on a limited basis. M.D.-Ph.D. students are eligible for a graduate fellowship (tuition and stipend) during the Ph.D. portion of their studies and a full tuition scholarship during the last two years of medical school following successful completion of Ph.D. work.

## INFORMATION FOR MINORITIES

Brown University particularly invites applications from individuals who are members of ethnic and racial groups traditionally underrepresented in American medicine. Established in 1981, the Office of Minority Affairs (OMA) has as its primary objective the recruitment, retention, and graduation of minority students. The OMA provides academic and personal counseling, workshops on test-taking approaches, information and guidance on special prizes and scholarship awards, and a program which links minority students with minority alumni/ae. In addition, the OMA offers an exchange program with Tougaloo College in Mississippi and a summer research program to help undergraduate minority students gain research experience in the biological and medical sciences.

---

Private Institution

### APPLICATION AND ACCEPTANCE POLICIES FOR 1997–98 FIRST-YEAR CLASS

Filing of application
  Earliest date: Aug. 15, 1996
  Latest date: March 1, 1997
        (Jan 1, 1997—M.D.-Ph.D. applicants)
School application fee to all applicants: $60
Oldest MCAT scores considered: 1987
        (for M.D.-Ph.D. applicants only)
Does not have Early Decision Program
Acceptance notice to regular applicants
  Earliest date: Mar. 15, 1997
  Latest date: April 15, 1997
Applicant's response to acceptance offer
  Maximum time: 3 weeks
Requests for deferred entrance considered: Yes
Deposit to hold place in class: None
Estimated number of new entrants: 68
Starting date: Sept. 9, 1997

### TUITION AND STUDENT FEES PER YEAR FOR 1995–96 FIRST-YEAR CLASS

Tuition: $23,840          Student fees: $1,603

### INFORMATION ON 1995–96 FIRST-YEAR CLASS

The first-year class is composed primarily of students enrolled in the eight-year continuum. Refer to the General Information section on the previous page and Chapter 9 for application statistics and more information.

NOTE: All new entrants had baccalaureate degrees and 39% took the MCAT.

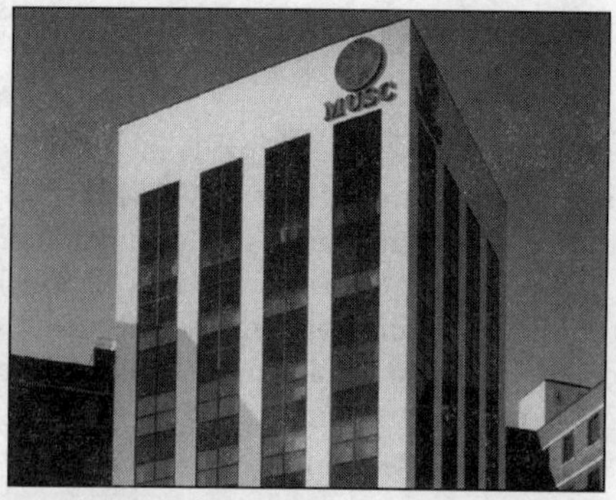

# Medical University of South Carolina
# College of Medicine

## Charleston, South Carolina

Dr. Layton McCurdy, *Dean*
Dr. Joanne Conroy, *Assistant Dean for Admissions*
Steven B. Martin, *Admissions Director*

## ADDRESS INQUIRIES TO:

Office of Enrollment Services
Medical University of South Carolina
171 Ashley Avenue
Charleston, South Carolina 29425
(803) 792-3281; 792-3764 (FAX)
E-Mail: martinst@musc.edu
Web Site: http://www2.musc.edu

## GENERAL INFORMATION

The College of Medicine of the Medical University of South Carolina (MUSC) was founded in Charleston in 1824 and is the South's oldest medical school. Its major clinical facilities comprise the MUSC Medical Center, which consists of the Medical University Hospital, the Children's Hospital, the Storm Eye Institute, the Psychiatric Institute, and the newly opened Hollings Cancer Center. The adjacent Veterans' Administration Hospital and Charleston Memorial Hospital, along with consortium and community hospitals in Greenville, Spartanburg, Columbia, and Florence, supply additional facilities for clinical teaching.

In addition to the classical basic science and clinical departments, there is a Department of Family Medicine which conducts a model program in the clinical area.

## CURRICULUM

The goal of the College of Medicine is to produce a caring and competent physician capable of choosing any postgraduate career. The curriculum during the first two years addresses four major objectives: provision of basic science concepts; acquisition of problem-solving strategies; development of skills which permit the performance of an adequate history and physical examination; and an introduction to the role of the physician in society. During these years emphasis is placed on small-group instruction.

The junior year consists of seven core clerkships. The clinical core consists of eight weeks each of internal medicine, obstetrics-gynecology, pediatrics, psychiatry, and surgery, as well as four weeks each of family medicine and neurology. In addition, all students take a block of 40 hours of clinical nutrition. During these experiences, emphasis is placed on the development of clinical, interpersonal, and professional competence.

During the senior year, students take a minimum of seven 4-week rotations. The student is required to take a clinical externship (in general medicine, pediatrics, or surgery) and one month each of ambulatory surgery and internal medicine. The remaining four blocks are elective and, depending on previous academic performance, can be taken at approved sites throughout the state and country.

The two-year parallel curriculum or problem-based learning program is a method of teaching and learning which emphasizes reflective critical thinking and sound clinical reasoning. The content emphasis is on the basic sciences, as in the traditional curriculum; however, the methodology of learning is self-directed study with small-group interaction. Learning groups, composed of six students and two faculty members, are encouraged to use multiple learning resources—textbooks, journals, videotapes, computer data bases, and other faculty members to investigate learning issues. This program is open to all accepted applicants at the time of acceptance to the College of Medicine, and selection is made on a random basis.

The College of Graduate Studies and the College of Medicine offer a combined program leading to both the M.D. and Ph.D. degrees. The purpose of this combined program is to provide competence in medicine plus detailed knowledge and research training in one of the related sciences without sacrificing the customary requirements for either degree. A student interested in the combined program must apply simultaneously to the College of Medicine and the College of Graduate Studies.

## REQUIREMENTS FOR ENTRANCE

The MCAT and a minimum of three years of college (90 semester hours) are required. Preference is given to applicants who have completed four years of college and earned a baccalaureate degree. There are no specific course requirements. Students are advised to construct courses of study that are intellectually interesting and challenging for them individually. Any education that engenders curiosity and enthusiasm for learning is desirable. Students who choose to major in a science should select a broad range of studies outside the sciences as well.

An Early Assurance Program is available to academically excellent residents of South Carolina. Application may be made after the freshman year but before December 1 preceding the junior year in college. Selection criteria are based on pre-college Scholastic Aptitude Test (SAT) scores and college GPA. Approximately 10 percent of the incoming class will be selected through this program. Successful candidates are encouraged to obtain as broad a college education as possible.

## SELECTION FACTORS

Selection is based on a total evaluation of the student. Objectively derived data allow the College of Medicine to set a lower limit of academic performance in college (MCAT scores and GPA). Acceptance into medical school from the selection pool is based on evaluation of noncognitive traits and personal characteristics that are desirable in future physicians. These traits include emotional stability, integrity, intellectual honesty, enthusiasm, brightness, and genuine concern for others. Nonresident applications are considered, but superior credentials are necessary for acceptance. Application through the Early Decision Program is encouraged, and early decision is granted to students across the entire spectrum of acceptable candidates. The school does not discriminate on the basis of race, creed, national origin, sex, age, or handicap in its admission, employment, and educational activities and programs.

## FINANCIAL AID

Scholarship funds, including some state scholarships, are available to entering freshmen. The James B. Edwards Scholars Program provides full tuition, fees, and living expenses for the entire medical education of a few select entering freshmen. Loan programs are also available.

## INFORMATION ON MINORITIES

Minority students are strongly encouraged to apply, and there is an active recruitment program for minorities. The Postbaccalaureate Reapplication Education Program (PREP) is an integrative, individually tailored course of undergraduate study prescribed for underprepared but promising South Carolina students who seek admission to MUSC. The full-time, twelve-month curriculum may include undergraduate courses in the areas of biology, physics, chemistry, and mathematics, a learning strategies course, human gross anatomy, and a course in critical thinking/reasoning skills. Minority applicants who apply to the College of Medicine but do not meet the minimum academic requirements for interview automatically will be considered for the PREP.

The Office of Diversity provides counseling and support services; academic assistance is provided to students through tutorial programs, test taking skills, training, and the like.

---

Public Institution

## APPLICATION AND ACCEPTANCE POLICIES FOR 1997–98 FIRST-YEAR CLASS

*School participates in AMCAS. See Chapter 4.*

Filing of AMCAS application
   Earliest date: June 1, 1996
   Latest date: Dec. 1, 1996
School application fee to all applicants: $45
Oldest MCAT scores considered: 1992
Does have Early Decision Program (EDP)
   EDP application period: June 1–Aug. 1996
   EDP applicants notified by: Oct. 1, 1996
Acceptance notice to regular applicants
   Earliest date: Oct. 15, 1996
   Latest date: Until class is filled
Applicant's response to acceptance offer
   Maximum time: 2 weeks
Requests for deferred entrance considered: Yes
Deposit to hold place in class: None
   A $145 matriculation fee is due with response to acceptance offer; refundable prior to May 15, 1997
Estimated number of new entrants: 135 (15 EDP)
Starting date: Aug. 1997

## TUITION AND STUDENT FEES PER YEAR FOR 1995–96 FIRST-YEAR CLASS

Tuition                 Student fees: $2,796
   Resident: $6,496
   Nonresident: $17,416

## INFORMATION ON 1995–96 FIRST-YEAR CLASS

| Number of | In-State | Out-of-State | Total |
|---|---|---|---|
| Applicants | 498 | 2,919 | 3,417 |
| Applicants Interviewed | 309 | 84 | 393 |
| New Entrants* | 126 | 12 | 138 |

*All had baccalaureate degrees; 75% took the MCAT (students entering through the Early Assurance Program are not required to take the MCAT).

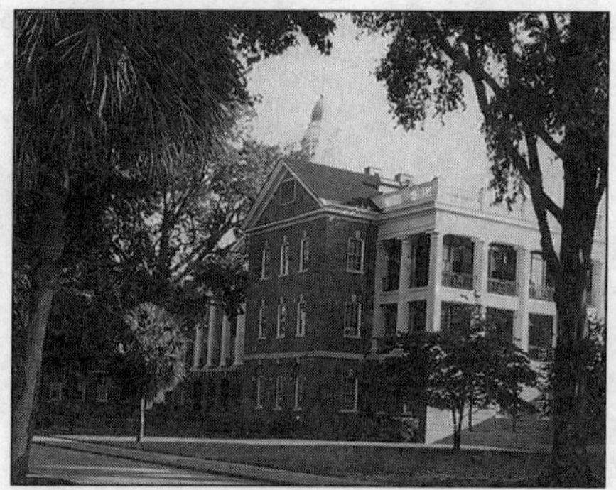

# University of South Carolina School of Medicine

## Columbia, South Carolina

Dr. Larry R. Faulkner, *Vice President for Medical Affairs and Dean*
Dr. Robert F. Sabalis, *Associate Dean for Student Programs*
Peggy Lynch, *Financial Aid Coordinator*

## ADDRESS INQUIRIES TO:

Associate Dean for Student Programs
University of South Carolina
School of Medicine
Columbia, South Carolina 29208
(803) 733-3325; 733-3328 (FAX)
Web Site: http://www.med.sc.edu

## GENERAL INFORMATION

The University of South Carolina School of Medicine was established in 1974 by the South Carolina General Assembly in conjunction with the Veterans Administration. The charter class matriculated in 1977 and graduated in 1981. Initially housed on the main campus of the University of South Carolina, the School of Medicine moved its administrative and faculty offices, teaching and research laboratories, and first- and second-year educational facilities in 1983 to completely renovated historic buildings on a 93-acre campus adjacent to the Dorn Veterans Hospital. The 85,000-volume medical library is accessible to medical students on a 24-hour-a-day basis.

Clinical instruction is provided in a variety of area hospitals which provide an ample number of teaching beds and extensive outpatient facilities. These include the 611-bed Richland Memorial Hospital, the major regional medical center; the 233-bed William S. Hall Psychiatric Institute, the teaching and research division of the South Carolina Department of Mental Health; the 460-bed Dorn Veterans Hospital; and the 410-bed Moncrief Army Hospital, a short-term general hospital located at Fort Jackson, the regional army training center. In addition, core clinical training can be pursued at the Greenville Memorial Hospital while elective opportunities are available throughout South Carolina at community hospitals affiliated with the Area Health Education Consortium (AHEC), other medical centers, and abroad.

## CURRICULUM

The School of Medicine offers a program of study designed to provide education and training in the art and science of medicine and to prepare students for a wide variety of medical career choices. Each of the first two years of the regular four-year medical program consists of two academic semesters composed of both basic science and clinically relevant course-

work in which students are exposed to patients in various inpatient, outpatient, community, and rural settings. The correlation between basic and clinical science information in the first two years is emphasized by means of an interdisciplinary, four-semester Introduction to Clinical Practice continuum.

The third year consists of required clinical clerkships in medicine, surgery, pediatrics, obstetrics-gynecology, family medicine, and psychiatry. The fourth year is devoted to advanced clinical work, both required and elective, during which students have the opportunity to strengthen their clinical skills and pursue individual academic interests and career goals in preparation for the lifelong study in medicine.

A six- to seven-year combined M.D.-Ph.D. program in biomedical sciences is available to students interested in careers in academic medicine and medical research. A combined M.D.-M.P.H. program is being developed.

## REQUIREMENTS FOR ENTRANCE

The MCAT and the equivalent of three years of undergraduate work are required. Strong preference is given to those applicants who will have earned their baccalaureate degrees prior to matriculation. Specific minimum course work requirements are:

|  | Sem. hrs. |
|---|---|
| General biology or zoology (with lab) | 8 |
| Inorganic chemistry (with lab) | 8 |
| Organic chemistry (with lab) | 8 |
| General physics (with lab) | 8 |
| College mathematics | 6 |
| A minimum of college algebra is required; calculus is recommended. | |
| English composition and literature | 6 |

The science and mathematics requirements must be acceptable for continued study by departmental majors.

With the exception of these specific courses, applicants are encouraged to pursue their personal educational interests without regard to any major field of study. Quality of course work rather than the field in which it is taken is the most important consideration.

Applicants are strongly urged to take the MCAT by the fall of the year of application. Applicants enrolled in advanced degree programs must complete their degrees prior to matriculation.

## SELECTION FACTORS

The selection process involves the comparative evaluation and review of all available application data, including MCAT scores, undergraduate academic performance, comments contained in letters of recommendation, and the results of personal interviews with members of the Admissions Committee. The opportunity for admission is greatest for legal residents of South Carolina. Competitive nonresidents must have superior credentials. The ultimate selection of a student is based upon a total and comparative appraisal of the applicant's suitability for the successful practice of medicine.

The AMCAS application is used for preliminary screening. After this initial review, the Admissions Committee may request the applicant to submit additional material for the final application, such as letters of recommendation, personal essay, and a photograph, as well as extend an invitation for personal interviews at the medical campus in Columbia. Each applicant is evaluated on the basis of individual qualifications without regard to age, race, creed, national origin, sex, or handicap.

## FINANCIAL AID

The School of Medicine participates in all federally funded loan and scholarship programs. Additionally, there is a School of Medicine-sponsored low-interest loan program available to students with proven need. Over 84 percent of enrolled students receive financial assistance in the form of scholarships, loans, and/or grants. The Office of Student Services makes every effort to provide information and assistance to help students meet their financial obligations. Ultimate responsibility for arranging the financing of his/her medical education must rest with the student. Students seeking part-time employment during medical school should have the prior approval of the associate dean for student programs.

## INFORMATION FOR MINORITIES

The associate dean for student programs actively encourages applications from members of minority groups. Applications from minority candidates for admission are reviewed individually by minority members of the Admission Committee.

Public Institution

### APPLICATION AND ACCEPTANCE POLICIES FOR 1997–98 FIRST-YEAR CLASS

*School participates in AMCAS. See Chapter 4.*

Filing of AMCAS application
  Earliest date: June 1, 1996
  Latest date: Dec. 1, 1996
School application fee to all applicants: $20
Oldest MCAT scores considered: 1994
Does have Early Decision Program (EDP)
  EDP application period: June 1–Aug. 1, 1996
  EDP applicants notified by: Oct. 1, 1996
Acceptance notice to regular applicants
  Earliest date: Oct. 15, 1996
  Latest date: Until class is filled
Applicant's response to acceptance offer
  Maximum time: 2 weeks
Requests for deferred entrance considered: Yes
Deposit to hold place in class (applied to tuition):
  $100, due with response to acceptance offer
Deposit refundable prior to: May 15, 1997
Estimated number of new entrants: 72 (12 EDP)
Starting date: Aug. 1997

### TUITION AND STUDENT FEES PER YEAR FOR 1995–96 FIRST-YEAR CLASS

Tuition                           Student fees: $25
  Resident: $7,290
  Nonresident: $18,620

### INFORMATION ON 1995–96 FIRST-YEAR CLASS

| Number of | In-State | Out-of-State | Total |
|---|---|---|---|
| Applicants | 398 | 1,480 | 1,878 |
| Applicants Interviewed | 210 | 139 | 349 |
| New Entrants* | 64 | 8 | 72 |

*All took the MCAT and had baccalaureate degrees.

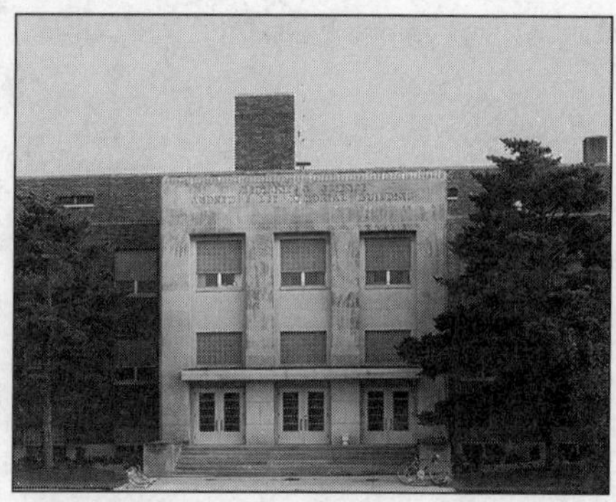

# University of South Dakota School of Medicine

## Vermillion, South Dakota

Dr. Robert C. Talley, *Dean*
Dr. Gerald J. Yutrzenka, *Director of Admissions*
Catherine Leiser, *Administrative Assistant II*

## ADDRESS INQUIRIES TO:

Office of Student Affairs, Room 105
University of South Dakota
School of Medicine
414 East Clark Street
Vermillion, South Dakota 57069-2390
(605) 677-5233; 677-5109 (FAX)

## GENERAL INFORMATION

The School of Medicine was established in 1907 as a two-year school for the basic medical sciences and has been in continuous operation since that time. The school was physically expanded in 1960 and again in 1969 and houses modern teaching facilities, research laboratories, and the medical library, including the Health Resource Library for South Dakota.

In 1974 a degree-granting program was funded by the state legislature. The first junior class of 40 students entered in May 1975 at two clinical training centers, one in Yankton and the other in Sioux Falls. Both centers are within 60 minutes of Vermillion. A clinical training center in Rapid City has been added, and the junior class has been expanded to 50 students. The primary objective of the medical school is the training of family practice physicians for South Dakota.

## CURRICULUM

A thorough knowledge of the basic medical sciences is emphasized during the first two years. An understanding of these basic concepts provides fundamental knowledge of the human body and hence a rational approach to the diagnosis and treatment of disease. Second-year students are also introduced to patients in the affiliated hospitals. The junior year consists of six major clerkships—family medicine, internal medicine, surgery, obstetrics-gynecology, psychiatry, and pediatrics. Four-week clerkships in emergency medicine, family medicine, and several surgery specialties are required in the senior year with a variety of other clerkships available on an elective basis. Each medical student finishing the first two years at the School of Medicine is required to spend the last four weeks of the sophomore year with a preceptor who is a primary care practicing physician in a South Dakota community.

Student progress is recorded each semester using the conventional letter grading system (A, B, C, D, F). Students must pass both Step 1 and Step 2 of the USMLE prior to graduation.

## REQUIREMENTS FOR ENTRANCE

The MCAT and at least three years of college are required. The baccalaureate degree is very desirable. Each applicant must have completed at least 64 semester hours from an accredited college to be considered for admission and have completed at least 90 semester hours to be admitted. At matriculation, a baccalaureate degree from an accredited undergraduate institution is preferred. The following courses are required, although specific courses may be waived under extenuating circumstances:

*Years*

General biology or zoology (with lab) . . . . . . . . . . . . . . . . . 1
General chemistry (with lab) . . . . . . . . . . . . . . . . . . . . . . 1
Organic chemistry (with lab) or
 second semester biochemistry . . . . . . . . . . . . . . . . . . . . . 1
General physics (with lab) . . . . . . . . . . . . . . . . . . . . . . . 1
College mathematics . . . . . . . . . . . . . . . . . . . . . . . . . . 1
 Analytical geometry and calculus are preferred.

All science courses should involve extensive lab work. Chemistry courses should include qualitative analysis and the study of aliphatic and aromatic compounds.

Additional courses in genetics, embryology, and computer science are recommended.

All required courses should be the same courses taken by majors in each area. Applicants are encouraged to arrange their premedical studies around an undergraduate major. Students are free to choose a major since there is no discrimination on the basis of field of study. Students are encouraged to obtain a broad background in the natural and social sciences and in the humanities, and they should develop good oral and written communication skills. In the case of courses waived by examination or by advanced placement, it is expected that students will enroll in advanced courses that would be more stimulating and challenging.

The MCAT should be taken no later than the fall of the year of application to avoid delay of consideration. No application is reviewed until the AMCAS application, letters of recommendation, and supplementary application have been received.

## SELECTION FACTORS

Applicants are chosen on the basis of intellect, character, and motivation. Information about the applicant considered by the Committee on Admissions includes: academic achievement as indicated by all of the student's scholastic records; retentiveness and ability to perform under pressure as reflected by MCAT scores; curiosity, learning habits, and fitness for a career in medicine as viewed by the applicant's former instructors; and assessments of personal factors of the applicant as determined by interviews conducted by the Committee on Admissions.

Accepted applicants for the 1995 entering class had the following credentials: *science GPA,* 3.53; *nonscience GPA,* 3.63; *total/overall GPA,* 3.58; *gender,* 43 percent women; *undergraduate major,* 80 percent in science and 20 percent in nonscience. *MCAT scores* (mean): *VR*-9.0; *PS*-8.3; *BS*-8.8.

The school does not discriminate on the basis of race, gender, creed, national origin, age, or disability. Preference is shown to legal residents of South Dakota, nonresidents with ties to South Dakota, and Native Americans, especially those affiliated with federally-recognized tribes in the region.

## FINANCIAL AID

Economic status plays no role in the admissions process. Low-interest loans are available to students on the basis of demonstrated financial need. Applications from freshman medical students for this financial aid are considered only after fall classes begin. Students are discouraged from seeking outside employment during academic periods. Approximately 88 percent of the student body receive financial aid.

Public Institution

## APPLICATION AND ACCEPTANCE POLICIES FOR 1997–98 FIRST-YEAR CLASS

*School participates in AMCAS. See Chapter 4.*

Filing of AMCAS application
  Earliest date: June 1, 1996
  Latest date: Nov. 15, 1996
School application fee to all applicants: $15
Oldest MCAT scores considered: 1994
Does not have Early Decision Program
Acceptance notice to regular applicants
  Earliest date: Dec. 23, 1996
  Latest date: Until class is filled
Applicant's response to acceptance offer
  Maximum time: 2 weeks
Requests for deferred entrance considered: Yes
Deposit to hold place in class (applied to tuition):
  $100, due with response to acceptance offer
Deposit refundable prior to: June 1, 1997
Estimated number of new entrants: 50
Starting date: Aug. 1997

## TUITION AND STUDENT FEES PER YEAR FOR 1995–96 FIRST-YEAR CLASS

Tuition             Student fees: $2,841
  Resident: $8,841
  Nonresident: $19,687

## INFORMATION ON 1995–96 FIRST-YEAR CLASS

| Number of | In-State | Out-of-State | Total |
|---|---|---|---|
| Applicants | 115 | 1,135 | 1,250 |
| Applicants Interviewed | 115 | 55 | 170 |
| New Entrants* | 40 | 10 | 50 |

*All took the MCAT and had baccalaureate degrees.

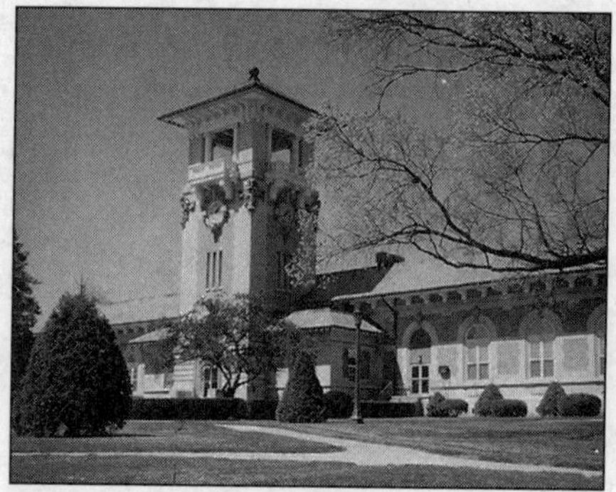

# East Tennessee State University
# James H. Quillen College of Medicine

**Johnson City, Tennessee**

Dr. Paul E. Stanton, Jr., *Vice President for Health Affairs and Dean*
Edwin D. Taylor, *Assistant Dean for Admissions and Records*

## ADDRESS INQUIRIES TO:

Assistant Dean for Admissions and Records
East Tennessee State University
James H. Quillen College of Medicine
P.O. Box 70580
Johnson City, Tennessee 37614-0580
(423) 929-6221; 929-6616 (FAX)
E-Mail: etsu.east-tenn-st.edu

## GENERAL INFORMATION

The ETSU College of Medicine opened its doors to its first class of 24 students in 1978. Emphasizing primary care medicine, the medical school has continued to develop, improve, and expand each year.

The school is located in Tennessee's fourth largest metropolitan area (population 1.2 million) and on the campus of the state's fourth largest university (enrollment 12,000 plus). It is supported by modern and convenient medical centers and clinics throughout the Tri-Cities, as well as hospitals and clinics located in small, rural communities like Rogersville and Mountain City, Tn. To enhance training in primary care medicine, ETSU successfully competed for and received a sizable grant from the W.K. Kellogg Foundation under their Community Partnership Program. This provided the opportunity to plan and execute an innovative interdisciplinary curriculum for training primary care physicians—the Rural Primary Care Track.

The school enrolls one class of 60 new students in August of each year. Residency training programs are available in family medicine, internal medicine, surgery, psychiatry, pediatrics, pathology, and OB-GYN. Accelerated residency training programs in family medicine and internal medicine are also available.

## CURRICULUM

The Quillen College of Medicine offers a traditional four-year medical program with the basic sciences being taught the first two years and intensive clinical application occurring throughout the last two years. The Rural Primary Care Track was designed to promote exposure to and training in rural locations and leads to an unrestricted M.D. degree. Over 60 percent of Quillen College of Medicine graduates have initially chosen residency training in primary care.

The curriculum includes a wide range of well-presented educational experiences, varied patient populations and hospitals, a small class size, and a highly diversified, caring faculty. Patient contact comes early in the curriculum and continues throughout. Flexibility is attained by allowing students to decelerate a portion of the curriculum for elective courses including research and advanced clinical studies.

Student input is a key component in curricular change, along with the rapidly changing body of knowledge and the needs of the profession. The goals of the curriculum are to prepare students to be well grounded in the sciences and art of medicine, capable practitioners of their profession, and self-directed, life-long learners.

## REQUIREMENTS FOR ENTRANCE

The MCAT and a minimum of 90 semester hours of credit, applicable toward a B.A. or B.S. degree at a regionally accredited institution, is the minimum requirement, although most selected students complete the entire four years. Specific required courses are:

| | Sem. hrs. |
|---|---|
| Biology (with lab) | 8 |
| General or inorganic chemistry (with lab) | 8 |
| Organic chemistry (with lab) | 8 |
| Physics (with lab) | 8 |
| Communications skills courses | 9 |

Applicants are urged to follow their personal interests in developing their premedical courses of study with the exception of the courses noted above. Preference is not given to any undergraduate major, but a broadly based education which prepares the student to be a self-directed life-long learner is suggested. CLEP credit in any of the required premedical courses is acceptable, provided that one or more advanced courses in the same area are successfully completed later.

The acquisition of important skills is further suggested, such as the ability to read with speed, comprehension and retention; the ability to understand concepts and draw logical conclusions; the ability to adapt; the ability to communicate effectively; and the ability to apply knowledge effectively.

Most courses and clerkships are graded on the standard A, B, C system with P/F grades used where appropriate. Flexibility in the curriculum is allowed for those with research interest or those seeking the masters or Ph.D. in biomedical science or other programs.

## SELECTION FACTORS

Admission to the College of Medicine is based upon a competitive selection process involving those applicants who meet the minimum requirements for admissions consideration. The responsibility of the Admissions Committee is to select those students who give the promise of being not merely satisfactory medical students but also capable, responsible physicians of high ethical standards. The Admissions Committee screens applicants on the basis of academic achievement, MCAT scores, letters of recommendation, pertinent extracurricular research and work experiences, and evidence of nonscholastic accomplishments.

After a general screening, the Admissions Committee may request supplementary information and a personal interview with the applicant. Interviews are held only on the campus and are at the applicant's expense.

Admission preferences are for residents of the state of Tennessee who are U.S. citizens, veterans of U.S. military service, and students with baccalaureate degrees prior to enrollment. Marginally qualified nonresidents should not apply.

Some characteristics of the students accepted for the 1995 entering class were: *mean GPA,* 3.4; *mean MCAT score,* (*VR*–9.3, *PS*–9.0, *BI*–9.1); *sex,* 50 percent women; *minorities,* 10 percent.

## FINANCIAL AID

The need for student financial assistance is not a consideration in the selection process. Scholarships, grants, and loans are available for students who demonstrate need as defined by a federal needs analysis and who meet the specific criteria set forth by the various agencies.

Further information may be obtained by writing directly to the medical school director for financial aid.

## INFORMATION FOR MINORITIES

The College of Medicine actively seeks applicants of both sexes and members of minority groups. A limited number of state grants are available for black matriculants who are state residents. Support services are available to matriculants to assist in the timely completion of the medical curriculum. ETSU does not discriminate on the basis of race, sex, creed, national origin, age, or handicap. The university is an equal opportunity/affirmative action employer.

Public Institution

## APPLICATION AND ACCEPTANCE POLICIES FOR 1997–98 FIRST-YEAR CLASS

*School participates in AMCAS. See Chapter 4.*

Filing of AMCAS application
　Earliest date: June 1, 1996
　Latest date: Dec. 1, 1996
School application fee to all applicants: $25
Oldest MCAT scores considered: 1994
Does have Early Decision Program (EDP)
　EDP application period: June 1–Aug. 1, 1996
　EDP applicants notified by: Oct. 1, 1996
Acceptance notice to regular applicants
　Earliest date: Oct, 15, 1996
　Latest date: Until class is filled
Applicant's response to acceptance offer
　Maximum time: 14 days
Requests for deferred entrance considered: Yes
Deposit to hold place in class (applied to tuition):
　$100, due with response to acceptance offer
Deposit refundable prior to: May 15, 1997
Estimated number of new entrants: 60 (8 EDP)
Starting date: Aug. 1997

## TUITION AND STUDENT FEES PER YEAR FOR 1995–96 FIRST-YEAR CLASS

| Tuition | Student fees: $408 |
|---|---|
| Resident: $8,750 | |
| Nonresident: $15,468 | |

## INFORMATION ON 1995–96 FIRST-YEAR CLASS

| Number of | In-State | Out-of-State | Total |
|---|---|---|---|
| Applicants | 637 | 1,453 | 2,090 |
| Applicants Interviewed | 222 | 86 | 308 |
| New Entrants* | 54 | 6 | 60 |

*All took the MCAT; 97% had baccalaureate degrees.

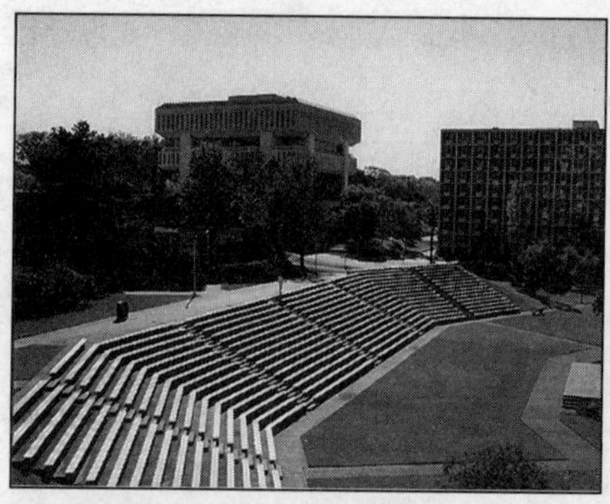

# Meharry Medical College
# School of Medicine

**Nashville, Tennessee**

Dr. John E. Arradondo, *Dean*
Sharon W. Hurt, *Director, Admissions and Records*
George J. McCarter, *Director, Student Financial Aid*

## ADDRESS INQUIRIES TO:

Director, Admissions and Records
Meharry Medical College
1005 D. B. Todd Boulevard
Nashville, Tennessee 37208
(615) 327-6223; 327-6228 (FAX)

## GENERAL INFORMATION

Meharry Medical College was founded in 1876 as the Medical Department of Central Tennessee College and became an independent institution in 1915. Meharry includes the schools of medicine, dentistry, graduate studies and research, and allied health.

Basic science instruction and research is carried out in the Harold D. West Basic Sciences Center. Clinical teaching facilities include the George W. Hubbard Hospital and the Community Mental Health Center. In addition, clinical instruction is carried out at the Murfreesboro Veterans Administration Hospital and a number of affiliated hospitals and clinics.

The provision of primary care, particularly in medically underserved areas, is a special emphasis, as is biomedical research into areas of concern to underserved populations.

## CURRICULUM

The curriculum consists of two parts: the preclinical and the clinical years. The preclinical years begin with anatomy, biochemistry, physiology, and behavioral sciences during the freshman year; they conclude with pharmacology, microbiology, pathology, physical diagnosis, introduction to clinical medicine, behavioral sciences, and medical genetics during the sophomore year.

The clinical years are treated in two distinctive units. The third-year students complete six 8-week blocks in internal medicine, surgery, pediatrics, obstetrics-gynecology, and psychiatry/family and preventive medicine. The fourth-year students take three 4-week blocks of surgery, Area Health Education Center, and radiology; two 4-week blocks in internal medicine; and three 4-week blocks of guided electives.

Internally and externally derived examinations are used in a variety of ways to evaluate students' performance. A letter grading system (A, B, C, E, F) is used.

## REQUIREMENTS FOR ENTRANCE

The MCAT is required. The baccalaureate degree is desirable; however, three years of college work is acceptable. Premedical work must include:

|  | Sem./Qtr. hrs |
|---|---|
| General biology or zoology (with lab) | 8/12 |
| General chemistry (with lab) | 8/12 |
| Organic chemistry (with lab) | 8/12 |
| General physics (with lab) | 8/12 |
| English (composition and literature) | 6/9 |

All premedical education must be taken at an approved college in the United States, including the courses listed as requirements for admission.

Applicants are urged to take the MCAT in the spring of the year of application to permit earlier consideration of their applications.

## SELECTION FACTORS

Applicants are selected on a competitive basis with regard to cognitive and noncognitive skills which denote probable success in medical school. Performance in the basic science prerequisite subjects (general biology, inorganic chemistry, organic chemistry, and physics) and MCAT scores form the basis for screening for the interview process in which the noncognitive aspects of the applicant are assessed. Meharry accepts students from all parts of the country, with preferential consideration given to equally qualified applicants from states that contract to subsidize the education of their citizens at Meharry. While special empathy is held for minority and disadvantaged applicants of all origins, Meharry Medical College seeks to attract a wide demographic, cultural, and educational population to reflect the caliber of social interchange in which the eventual practice of medicine will occur.

Early Decision Program applicants must have their complete application on file by August 1 for consideration.

Meharry Medical College does not discriminate on the basis of race, sex, creed, national origin, age, or handicap.

## FINANCIAL AID

Financial aid awards are based on analyses of student needs and academic achievement. The limited financial aid program includes scholarships, grants-in-aid, loans, and fellowships.

214

Because of fluctuation in federal and private support for financial aid programs, the types and amounts of awards are revised and adjusted on a continuing basis. Therefore, it is necessary for applicants to plan their financial program as carefully as their academic program.

## INFORMATION FOR MINORITIES

For over 118 years, Meharry has produced a large percentage of the minority health professionals in the United States and abroad. Of the 1994 entering class, 52 percent were women and 86 percent were minority students.

Private Institution

## APPLICATION AND ACCEPTANCE POLICIES FOR 1997–98 FIRST-YEAR CLASS

*School participates in AMCAS. See Chapter 4.*

Filing of AMCAS application
    Earliest date: June 1, 1996
    Latest date: Dec. 15, 1996
School application fee to all applicants: $25
Oldest MCAT scores considered: 1994
Does have Early Decision Program (EDP)
    EDP application period: June 1–Aug. 1, 1996
    EDP applicants notified by: Oct. 1, 1996
Acceptance notice to regular applicants
    Earliest date: Oct. 15, 1996
    Latest date: Varies
Applicant's response to acceptance offer
    Maximum time: 3 weeks
Requests for deferred entrance considered: Yes
Deposit to hold place in class (applied to tuition):
    $100, due with response to acceptance offer;
    nonrefundable
Estimated number of new entrants: 80 (6 EDP)
Starting date: June 1997

## TUITION AND STUDENT FEES PER YEAR FOR 1995–96 FIRST-YEAR CLASS

Tuition: $16,500            Student fees: $1,896

## INFORMATION ON 1995–96 FIRST-YEAR CLASS

| Number of | In-State | Out-of-State | Total |
|---|---|---|---|
| Applicants | 268 | 5,280 | 5,548 |
| Applicants Interviewed | 32 | 393 | 425 |
| New Entrants* | 9 | 71 | 80 |

*All took the MCAT; 84% had baccalaureate degrees.

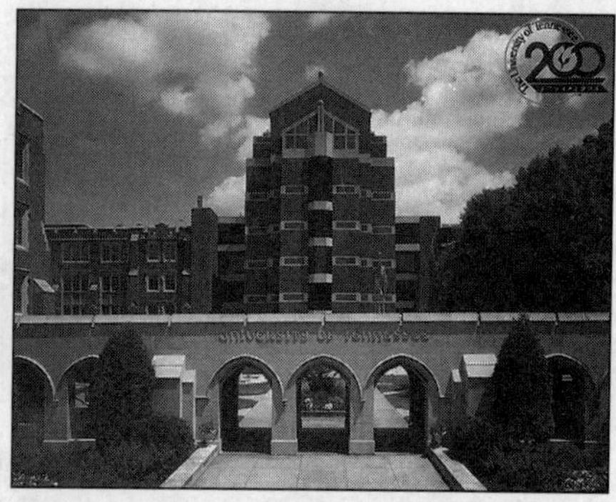

# University of Tennessee, Memphis College of Medicine

**Memphis, Tennessee**

Dr. Robert L. Summitt, *Dean*
Dr. Hershel P. Wall, *Associate Dean for Admissions and Students*
E. Nelson Strother, Jr., *Assistant Dean for Admission and Student Affairs*

## ADDRESS INQUIRIES TO:

University of Tennessee, Memphis
College of Medicine
790 Madison Avenue
Memphis, Tennessee 38163-2166
(901) 448-5559
Web Site: http://utmgopher.utmem.edu/utm.html

## GENERAL INFORMATION

Founded in 1851, the College of Medicine, the colleges of dentistry, pharmacy, nursing, allied health, and the College of Graduate Health Sciences comprise the University of Tennessee, Memphis. Within the 41-acre campus, there are over 6,000 patient beds and 15 hospitals and clinics affiliated with the University of Tennessee College of Medicine, including the University of Tennessee William F. Bowld Hospital, St. Jude Children's Hospital, LeBonheur Children's Hospital, Veterans Administration Hospital, Baptist Memorial Hospital, Regional Medical Center, LePasses Rehabilitation Center, and Campbell Clinic.

## CURRICULUM

The course of study at the University of Tennessee College of Medicine is designed to develop knowledge, skills, and attitudes appropriate to all doctors of medicine. It is sufficiently broad to allow the graduates to enter any graduate training programs designed for primary care specialties, medical and surgical specialties, or research and academic pursuits.

The medical curriculum is a 45-month program consisting of two major components: (1) biomedical science and (2) clinical clerkships and electives. The biomedical science portion of the curriculum includes, during the first year, courses such as gross anatomy, histology, biochemistry, fundamentals of cellular and molecular biology, medical genetics, physiology, preventive medicine, neuroanatomy, and behavorial science. The second year includes microbiology, pharmacology, neurosciences, pathology, pathophysiology, nutrition, and introduction to clinical skills. Students may elect to take three years for the biomedical science portion of the curriculum (optional expanded academic program). Application may be made at matriculation or in the first academic year.

The clerkship and the elective portion of the curriculum consist of 20 months of required and elective experiences. In general, students proceed from the biomedical sciences portion of the curriculum to the junior year of clerkship rotations. Selected clerkships and electives may be taken in Chattanooga, Knoxville, Jackson, and Nashville. Junior year clerkships include rotations in medicine, surgery, pediatrics, obstetrics-gynecology, psychiatry, and family medicine. The senior year consists of one-month required clerkships in neurology, ambulatory medicine, surgical subspecialties, junior internship (medicine), junior internship (any third-year clerkship discipline), and three months of electives.

All students enrolled in the College of Medicine are required to pass both Step 1 and Step 2 of the USMLE examinations as candidates.

## REQUIREMENTS FOR ENTRANCE

A minimum of 90 semester hours and the MCAT are required. However, with rare exception, the completion of an undergraduate degree will be necessary in order to meet educational expectations. The Committee on Admissions is particularly impressed by students whose education has provided a broad range of intellectual experience, including opportunities for analytical thinking and independent study. Furthermore, prospective candidates are strongly encouraged to major in their area of greatest interest; there is no requirement that a student major in the sciences. Regardless of choice of major, applicants are encouraged to pursue a course of study that achieves balance between both science and nonscience coursework. The required courses are:

*Sem. hrs.*

| | |
|---|---|
| Biology (with lab) | 8 |
| Inorganic chemistry (with lab) | 8 |
| Organic chemistry (with lab) | 8 |
| General physics (with lab) | 8 |
| English composition and literature | 6 |
| Electives | 52 |

## SELECTION FACTORS

The criteria the Committee on Admissions uses in the selection process are the academic record, MCAT scores, preprofessional evaluations, and personal interviews. The required personal interviews by members of the Committee on Admissions provide the candidates with an opportunity to review their curriculum and extracurricular activities. More importantly, the interviewers gain insights into the character of the applicants as well as how they have formulated individual plans for the study and practice of medicine.

Applicants must be citizens or permanent residents of the United States at the time of application. Applications are accepted from a nine-state region consisting of Tennessee and its contiguous states (Mississippi, Arkansas, Missouri, Kentucky, Virginia, North Carolina, Georgia, and Alabama). In addition, children of University of Tennessee alumni may apply regardless of their state of residence. Since priority is given to qualified Tennesseans, out-of-state applicants must possess superior qualifications to be considered by the Committee on Admissions.

Some characteristics of the 1995 entering class were the following: *mean GPA,* 3.5; *mean MCAT scores, VR*-9, *PS*-9, *WS*-0, *BS*-9.

## FINANCIAL AID

Various loan funds and scholarships are available for students who have demonstrated financial need. The College Scholarship Service is utilized in the determination of need. (See Chapter 6 for details.) Information packets concerning all available financial assistance are mailed to accepted students. The various academic scholarships are competitive and include a full tuition stipend awarded for each of the four years in school. Loans and scholarships are used in combination whenever possible. Part-time employment during the first two years is discouraged. The University of Tennessee, Memphis College of Medicine, offers conditional grants to 15 students in each entering class who agree to practice in a designated underserved area in the state after completion of residency training. Residencies must be completed in family medicine, general internal medicine, general pediatrics, medicine/pediatrics or obstetrics-gynecology. The conditional grant covers tuition, fees, and also provides additional funding for living expenses. The grant carries a year-for-year service obligation.

## INFORMATION FOR MINORITIES

The University of Tennessee College of Medicine seeks applications from members of minority groups underrepresented in medicine. The Committee on Admissions evaluates nonacademic as well as academic factors in the selection process, with consideration being given to the unique backgrounds and problems of minority and disadvantaged applicants. Academic support and retention programs are provided for students from minority and/or disadvantaged backgrounds. Scholarships are available to black students who are Tennessee residents and residents of contiguous states.

Public Institution

## APPLICATION AND ACCEPTANCE POLICIES FOR 1997–98 FIRST-YEAR CLASS

*School participates in AMCAS. See Chapter 4.*

Filing of AMCAS application
    Earliest date: June 1, 1996
    Latest date: Nov. 15, 1996
School application fee to all applicants: $25
Oldest MCAT scores considered: 1992
Does not have Early Decision Program
Acceptance notice to regular applicants
    Earliest date: Oct. 15, 1996
    Latest date: April 1, 1997
Applicant's response to acceptance offer
    Maximum time: 2 weeks
Requests for deferred entrance considered: Yes
Deposit to hold place in class (applied to tuition):
    $100, due with response to acceptance offer
Deposit refundable prior to: May 15, 1997
Estimated number of new entrants: 165
Starting date: Aug. 1997

## TUITION AND STUDENT FEES PER YEAR FOR 1995–96 FIRST-YEAR CLASS

Tuition                          Student fees: $858
    Resident: $8,690
    Nonresident: $16,120

## INFORMATION ON 1995–96 FIRST-YEAR CLASS

| Number of | In-State | Out-of-State | Total |
|---|---|---|---|
| Applicants | 723 | 1,614 | 2,337 |
| Applicants Interviewed | 334 | 62 | 396 |
| New Entrants* | 155 | 10 | 165 |

*All took the MCAT; 98% had baccalaureate degrees.

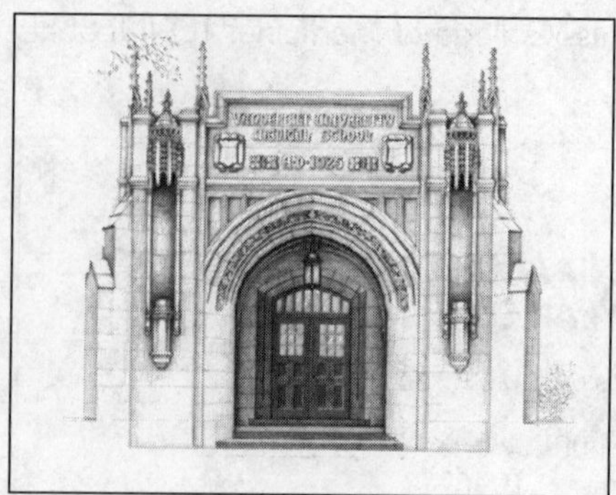

# Vanderbilt University School of Medicine

## Nashville, Tennessee


Dr. John E. Chapman, *Dean*
Dr. John N. Lukens, *Chairman, Committee for Admissions*
Vicky L. Cagle, *Director of Financial Aid*


## ADDRESS INQUIRIES TO:

Office of Admissions
209 Light Hall
Vanderbilt University
School of Medicine
Nashville, Tennessee 37232-0685
(615) 322-2145; 343-8397 (FAX)
E-Mail: medsch.admis@mcmail.vanderbilt.edu
Web Site: http://vumclib.mc.vanderbilt.edu/medschool

## GENERAL INFORMATION

Vanderbilt University School of Medicine is located on the campus of Vanderbilt University. The Vanderbilt University Medical Center and affiliated hospitals provide a total of over 5,000 beds for diversified, comprehensive clinical experience. These hospitals share common goals of education, research, patient care, and community service. Participation in fundamental and clinical research is encouraged.

## CURRICULUM

Medical education at Vanderbilt is oriented toward promoting the intellectual development of students and equipping them with the disciplined approach, knowledge, and skills required of both a physician and scientist. The curriculum provides the student with a fundamental knowledge of basic medical principles, but flexibility is stressed. Changes in curriculum content and teaching methods continually evolve from Vanderbilt's focus upon new ways to assist students in their preparation for a lifetime of learning. While sufficient structure is maintained for adequate guidance, the curriculum offers a productive blend of required and elective courses throughout all four years of the program.

Vanderbilt encourages students to develop their full intellectual talents and places great emphasis upon acquiring a sympathetic understanding of the behavior of the human being in health and sickness. The school's education is comprehensive, encompassing the entire span of medicine. In addition to providing a thorough basic education, the curriculum is designed to emphasize the relationship of emotional, social, and environmental factors to medical disorders.

To provide a well balanced exposure to both clinical and research experiences, Vanderbilt allows students wide latitude in their learning process and encourages self-motivation.

Research experience is part of the required curriculum for first-year students and is also available during the elective and summer periods. The Vanderbilt Medical Scientist Training Program in the Biomedical Sciences allows the student to engage in research and study in a basic discipline while pursuing studies toward the M.D. degree. For interested select students, this combined M.D.-Ph.D. program broadens the scope of training so that graduates may choose to assume positions of responsibility and leadership as investigators and medical educators.

The School of Medicine is organized to ensure opportunity for excellence by providing unusual opportunities for close association with the faculty.

## REQUIREMENTS FOR ENTRANCE

The MCAT is required. A bachelor's degree is recommended, and most successful candidates have earned the bachelor's degree by the time they enroll in the medical school. Required courses are:

|  | Sem. hrs. |
|---|---|
| Biology and/or zoology (with 2 hrs. of lab) | 8 |
| Not more than half may be in botany. | |
| Inorganic chemistry (with 2 hrs. of lab) | 8 |
| Organic chemistry (with 2 hrs. of lab) | 8 |
| Must cover aliphatic and aromatic compounds. | |
| Physics (with 2 hrs. of lab) | 8 |
| English and composition | 6 |

No preference is given to any one college major. Besides meeting the specific requirements, students should devote their time to strengthening their educational foundation of fundamental knowledge and broadening their cultural background. Vanderbilt considers for transfer and admission at advanced standing only applications from students in good standing at an LCME affiliated medical school. Applicants are eligible for transfer after the second year only. As the attrition rate is less than one percent, the opportunities for transfer are limited.

## SELECTION FACTORS

Applications are invited without regard to race, sex, creed, national origin, or state of residence. Applicants must possess sufficient intellectual ability, emotional stability, and sensory and motor functions to meet the academic requirements of the school of medicine, without fundamental alteration in the nature of this program. Applications are reviewed in two stages. The initial review is made from material provided through AMCAS. Competitive strength of credentials reflecting preparation for medical studies, motivation, personal qualities, and educational background, as these relate to career promise in medicine, is evaluated by the Admissions Committee and determines the recipients of final applications. Applicants receiving favorable initial review are invited to file a final application, which requires a $50 application fee, except in demonstrated circumstances of serious financial hardship. These applicants are interviewed by a faculty member or a regional representative of the committee.

## FINANCIAL AID

Limited scholarships, fellowships, loans, and other financial aid are available. Most scholarships, awards, and all loans are given on the basis of demonstrated financial need. The G. Canby Robinson Scholars Program uses a combination of academic excellence and financial need as the basis for selection of scholars.

Students selected for medical study at Vanderbilt should give careful attention to financial planning and are expected to utilize their own financial resources to the fullest extent possible. Financial aid will be heavily related to available federal programs.

The telephone number for the financial aid office is (615) 343-6310.

## INFORMATION FOR MINORITIES

Vanderbilt invites applicants from a broad spectrum of student backgrounds to submit an application for admission. Applications are sought from members of groups presently not adequately represented in medicine who feel a commitment to helping resolve the special problems of health care delivery to minority and underprivileged groups.

---

Private Institution

## APPLICATION AND ACCEPTANCE POLICIES FOR 1997–98 FIRST-YEAR CLASS

*School participates in AMCAS. See Chapter 4.*

Filing of AMCAS application
    Earliest date: June 1, 1996
    Latest date: Oct. 15, 1996
School application fee to all applicants: $50
Oldest MCAT scores considered: 1994
Does have Early Decision Program (EDP)
    EDP application period: June 1–Aug. 1, 1996
    EDP applicants notified by: Oct. 1, 1996
Acceptance notice to regular applicants
    Earliest date: Oct. 15, 1996
    Latest date: Until class is filled
Applicant's response to acceptance offer
    Maximum time: 2 weeks
Requests for deferred entrance considered: Yes
Deposit to hold place in class: None
Estimated number of new entrants: 104 (5 EDP)
Starting date: Aug. 1997

## TUITION AND STUDENT FEES PER YEAR FOR 1995–96 FIRST-YEAR CLASS

Tuition: $20,000          Student fees: $1,202

## INFORMATION ON 1995–96 FIRST-YEAR CLASS

| Number of | In-State | Out-of-State | Total |
|---|---|---|---|
| Applicants | 332 | 6,556 | 6,888 |
| Applicants Interviewed | 51 | 715 | 766 |
| New Entrants* | 9 | 94 | 103 |

*All had baccalaureate degrees; 96% took the MCAT.

# Baylor College of Medicine

## Houston, Texas

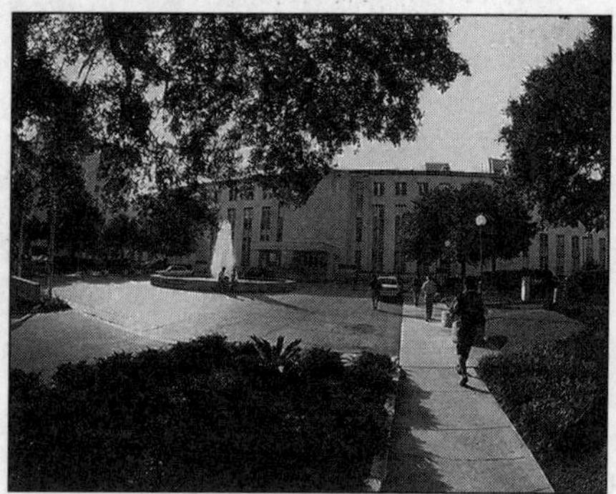

Dr. Ralph D. Feigin, *President*
Dr. Major Bradshaw, *Dean of Medical Education*
Dr. L. Leighton Hill, *Assistant Dean*

## ADDRESS INQUIRIES TO:

Office of Admissions
Baylor College of Medicine
One Baylor Plaza
Houston, Texas 77030
(713) 798-4842
E-Mail: melody@bcm.tmc.edu
Web Site: http://www.bcm.tmc.edu/bcm-educational.html

## GENERAL INFORMATION

Baylor College of Medicine is a private, nonsectarian institution governed by an independent Board of Trustees of community leaders. Baylor College of Medicine is the academic center around which the 356-acre Texas Medical Center was developed. The Baylor faculty currently is composed of 1,470 full-time members and another 2,261 on a part-time and voluntary basis. Facilities include teaching and research buildings and eight affiliated teaching hospitals (including private, city-county, and Veterans Administration hospitals) which together have approximately 5,000 beds. The Texas Medical Center is located in a university, residential and park area in the southwest section of Houston.

## CURRICULUM

The goal of the Baylor College of Medicine is to provide a firm foundation in the basic and clinical medical sciences which will enable students to pursue whatever type of professional activity they desire as physicians and upon which they may build during the remainder of their professional life. The college maintains a four-year curriculum but provides: (1) a significant amount of time in elective courses or clerkships; (2) flexibility in planning the sequence of clinical activities; (3) an option to take basic science electives during the clinical years; and (4) the opportunity to do research or to apply for a combined M.D.-Ph.D. program. The basic sciences are taught in slightly more than one and one-half years. Study and vacation periods are scheduled between each of these blocks. There are 68 weeks of required clinical clerkships and 20 weeks of elective experience. Approximately 300 discrete electives are available at Baylor. Others are available in the Texas Medical Center.

## REQUIREMENTS FOR ENTRANCE

The new MCAT (1991) is required. Applicants are strongly advised to take the MCAT in the spring of the year of application and to have their science course requirements completed at the time of application.

The baccalaureate degree is highly desirable. In recent years very few students matriculated without a baccalaureate degree. Applicants must have satisfactorily completed a minimum of 90 undergraduate semester hours (or an equivalent number of quarter hours) at a fully accredited college or university in the United States prior to enrollment. Courses must include:

|  | *Years* |
|---|---|
| General biology (with lab) | 1 |
| General chemistry (with lab) | 1 |
| Organic chemistry (with lab) | 1 |
| General physics (with lab) | 1 |
| English | 1 |

## SELECTION FACTORS

All applicants offered places in the class are interviewed on the Baylor College of Medicine campus. The Admissions Committee selects for interview applicants whose files are complete and who are considered to be competitive for admission. All information available is utilized in the selection process. In evaluating the applicant's academic record, attention is paid to course selections, academic challenge imposed by the student's curriculum, and the extent to which extracurricular activities and employment may have limited the applicant's opportunity for high academic achievement.

Intellectual ability and academic achievement alone are not sufficient to support the development of the ideal physician. To work effectively in a profession dependent upon interpersonal relationships, physicians should possess those traits of personality and character which permit them to communicate effectively with warmth and compassion.

There are 168 students in each first-year class; approximately 70 percent are residents of Texas.

Requests for deferred entrance (delayed matriculation) from accepted students will be considered but are not encouraged. Such requests must be in writing and will be reviewed on an individual basis.

Students matriculating in 1995 had the following credentials: *mean GPA,* 3.7; *average MCAT scores* for the subsets were in the 11 range; *sex,* 39 percent women; *undergraduate major,* 79 percent in sciences, with the remainder from a variety of fields.

Baylor College of Medicine does not discriminate on the basis of race, sex, creed, national origin, age, or handicap.

## FINANCIAL AID

Financial need is not a factor in the selection of students. All aid is based on financial need. Aid funds are provided by private donors, the Board of Trustees, and various state and federal loan and scholarship programs. Employment for spouses and part-time employment for students is available. Students are encouraged to seek out all available sources of financial assistance prior to enrollment as funds are limited. Financial aid information is sent to all accepted applicants upon request. A financial aid officer is available for consultation with students and parents.

## INFORMATION FOR MINORITIES

Baylor College of Medicine encourages applications from members of groups not adequately represented in medicine.

Minority students comprise a substantial portion of the student body, and there are minority members on the Admissions Committee.

Private Institution

## APPLICATION AND ACCEPTANCE POLICIES FOR 1997–98 FIRST-YEAR CLASS

Filing of application
  Earliest date: June 1, 1996
  Latest date: Nov. 1, 1996
School application fee to all applicants: $35
Oldest MCAT scores considered: 1991
Does have Early Decision Program (EDP)
  EDP application period: June 1–Aug. 1, 1996
  EDP applicants notified by: Oct. 1, 1996
Acceptance notice to regular applicants
  Earliest date: Oct. 15, 1996
  Latest date: Until class is filled
Applicant's response to acceptance offer
  Maximum time: 2 weeks
Requests for deferred entrance considered: Yes
Deposit to hold place in class (applied to tuition):
  $300, due May 1, 1997; nonrefundable
Estimated number of new entrants: 168 (5 EDP)
Starting date: Aug. 1997

## TUITION AND STUDENT FEES PER YEAR FOR 1995–96 FIRST-YEAR CLASS

Tuition                               Student fees: $1,559
  Resident: $6,550
  Nonresident: $19,650

## INFORMATION ON 1995–96 FIRST-YEAR CLASS

| Number of | In-State | Out-of-State | Total |
|---|---|---|---|
| Applicants | 1,473 | 1,750 | 3,223 |
| Applicants Interviewed | 506 | 182 | 688 |
| New Entrants* | 127 | 41 | 168 |

*All had baccalaureate degrees.

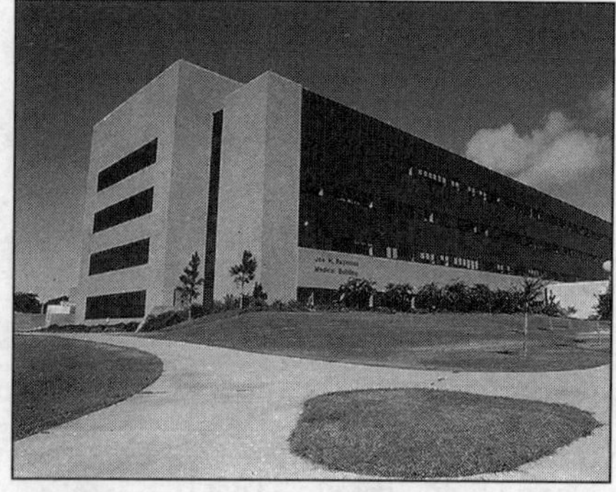

# Texas A&M University Health Science Center College of Medicine

## College Station, Texas

Dr. Elvin E. Smith, *Interim Dean*
Filomeno G. Maldonado, *Director of Admissons*

## ADDRESS INQUIRIES TO:

Associate Dean for Student Affairs
and Admissions
Texas A&M University Health Science Center
College of Medicine
College Station, Texas 77843-1114
(409) 845-7744; 847-8663 (FAX)
E-Mail: MED-STU-AFF@TAMU.EDU
Web Site: http://thunder.tamu.edu

## GENERAL INFORMATION

Established in 1971, Texas A&M University College of Medicine is part of the Texas A&M University Health Science Center. The College of Medicine's administrative offices and basic science campus are located in College Station on the campus of Texas A&M University. Texas A&M University, whose research budget is among the top five in the nation, is a comprehensive land, sea and space grant university with a total enrollment of 43,256 undergraduate students and 7,741 graduate and professional students. The clinical campus in Temple, Texas consists of the Olin E. Teague Veterans' Center, the Scott and White Clinic and Hospital, and Darnall Army Community Hospital at nearby Ft. Hood. These comprehensive facilities provide 1,714 teaching beds and aggregate annual outpatient visits in excess of 1.5 million. The college has 818 faculty members.

The College of Medicine is chartered to grant the degrees of doctor of medicine, master of science, and doctor of philosophy.

## CURRICULUM

The primary goal of the curriculum is to produce undifferentiated physicians of the highest caliber. A second principal mission is the systematic utilization of the vast intellectual and technological resources available within other disciplines of the parent university in collaborative research and instructional programs.

The College of Medicine offers a four-year program leading to the M.D. degree. The first two years are taught on the Texas A&M University campus in College Station and include, besides the traditional basic science disciplines, instruction in behavioral science, humanities in medicine, community medicine and leadership in medicine. Although the faculty is organized along disciplinary lines, courses are scheduled to assure a high degree of integration of subject matter across disciplines. Correlation of the basic sciences with clinical medicine is achieved from the start, with clinical correlation experiences in all courses and regularly scheduled sessions for clinical instruction and practice in both years one and two.

The third- and fourth-year clinical programs, conducted predominantly on the Temple campus at the Scott and White Clinic and Hospital and the Olin E. Teague Veterans' Center, consist of traditional clerkships and a mixed rotation of ambulatory care experiences. In addition, each student spends a minimum of six weeks in an approved family medicine clerkship in a nonurban location.

Electives are available in both basic and clinical sciences. A standardized letter grading system (A, B, C, F) is utilized.

Selected students may participate in the combined M.D.-Ph.D. program or enroll in other graduate programs concurrently with studies toward the M.D. degree.

## REQUIREMENTS FOR ENTRANCE

The MCAT and 60 semester hours of appropriate undergraduate study from an accredited U.S. institution are required. Students may apply during their sophomore year. Required courses are:

|  | *Years* |
| --- | --- |
| General biology (with lab) | 1 |
| Additional advanced biological science | ½ |
| Inorganic chemistry (with lab) | 1 |
| Organic chemistry (with lab) | 1 |
| General physics (with lab) | 1 |
| Calculus | ½ |
| English | 1 |

Applicants are urged to take the MCAT in the spring of the year of application. Early application is encouraged. Only U.S. citizens or applicants with permanent visas are considered for admission.

## SELECTION FACTORS

Academic ability, as evidenced by grades in college courses and performance on standardized tests such as the MCAT, is an important selection criterion. Equally important are personal traits such as interpersonal and communication skills, maturity, motivation, personal integrity and compassion. It is also important for applicants to have some knowledge of the demands and rewards of the profession they are asking to enter. All available information is utilized in the admissions process. Competitive candidates are invited for personal interviews. Enrollment of individuals who are residents of states other than Texas is limited to 10 percent and nonresidents must have exceptional credentials.

Admission to Texas A&M University Health Science Center College of Medicine is open to qualified individuals regardless of race, color, religion, sex, age, national origin, or educationally unrelated handicaps.

Some characteristics of the 1995 entering class were: *mean GPA,* 3.65; *mean MCAT,* 9.6; *gender,* 38 percent women; *underrepresented minorities,* 9.4 percent; *residents,* 98 percent Texas residents; *undergraduate major,* 89 percent in sciences and the remainder were non-science degrees varying from English to Public Health Policy.

## FINANCIAL AID

Scholarship and loan funds are available to students with financial need from local, state, and national sources. Financial needs of the applicant are not a consideration in the admission process, and after acceptance, every effort is made to assist students in meeting their financial requirements. Approximately 90 percent of the students currently in the program are receiving some form of financial aid. For further information, contact Ty Newton, director of student financial aid.

## INFORMATION FOR DISADVANTAGED AND MINORITY APPLICANTS

The College of Medicine is committed to identifying and recruiting qualified students from minority and disadvantaged backgrounds. As part of its commitment to this effort, the College of Medicine administers several programs for disadvantaged students. The Bridge to Medicine summer program is open to students from minority and disadvantaged backgrounds who have completed the requirements for medical school. It offers college students an intensive academic program to reinforce their knowledge of the basic sciences and prepare them for the MCAT. In addition, the Office of Minority Access to Medical Careers facilitates the adjustment and the retention of disadvantaged and underrepresented minority students attending the Texas A&M University Health Science Center College of Medicine.

Public Institution

## APPLICATION AND ACCEPTANCE POLICIES FOR 1997–98 FIRST-YEAR CLASS

Filing of application
  Earliest date: May 1, 1996
  Latest date: Nov. 1, 1996
School application fee to all applicants: $45
Oldest MCAT scores considered: 1992
Does not have Early Decision Program
Acceptance notice to regular applicants
  Earliest date: Nov. 15, 1996
  Latest date: Until class is filled
Applicant's response to acceptance offer
  Maximum time: 2 weeks
Requests for deferred entrance considered: Yes
Deposit to hold place in class: None
Estimated number of new entrants: 64
Starting date: Aug. 1997

## TUITION AND STUDENT FEES PER YEAR FOR 1995–96 FIRST-YEAR CLASS

Tuition                Student fees: $1,400
  Resident: $6,550
  Nonresident: $19,650

## INFORMATION ON 1995–96 FIRST-YEAR CLASS

| Number of | In-State | Out-of-State | Total |
|---|---|---|---|
| Applicants | 1,382 | 137 | 1,519 |
| Applicants Interviewed | 476 | 11 | 487 |
| New Entrants* | 63 | 1 | 64 |

*All took the MCAT; 97% had baccalaureate degrees.

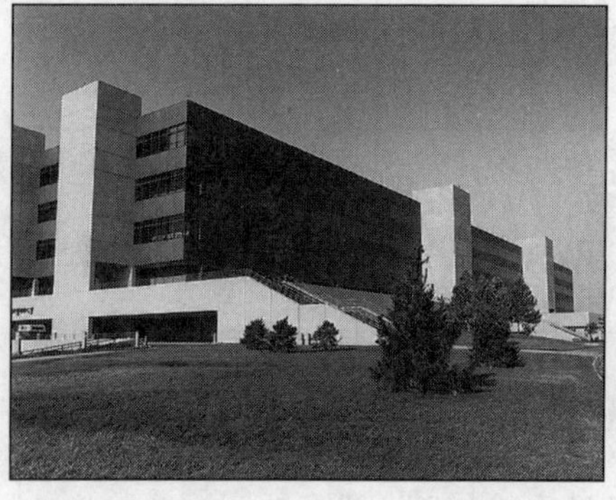

# Texas Tech University Health Sciences Center School of Medicine

**Lubbock, Texas**

Dr. Bernhard T. Mittemeyer, *Interim Dean*
Dr. James A. Chappell, *Associate Dean, Education*
E. Earl Hudgins, *Director, Student Financial Aid*

## ADDRESS INQUIRIES TO:

Office of Admissions
Texas Tech University
Health Sciences Center
School of Medicine
Lubbock, Texas 79430
(806) 743-2297

## GENERAL INFORMATION

Texas Tech University School of Medicine, established in 1969, is part of the Texas Tech University Health Sciences Center, which also includes schools of nursing and allied health. The Health Sciences Center is headquartered on the Lubbock campus of Texas Tech University, which has an enrollment of 24,000 students. As a regional medical school committed to developing opportunities for medical education in the 135,000 square miles of West Texas, the school has regional academic health centers in Amarillo, El Paso, and Odessa. All medical students spend the first two years at the Lubbock campus; junior and senior students receive their clinical training in Lubbock, Amarillo, and El Paso. At each academic health center the primary teaching hospital is located in close proximity to the medical school facility. Affiliations with the primary teaching hospital and other community hospitals provide over 2,900 beds for clinical teaching. The medical school has 314 full-time faculty members and over 775 volunteer clinical faculty members.

## CURRICULUM

The four-year curriculum provides a broad introduction to medical knowledge while developing the student's analytical, problem-solving skills. The first two years are divided into four terms, the first four of which are concerned with basic sciences. Introduction to clinical material begins early in the second year with the introduction to patient assessment course which integrates pathophysiology and physical diagnosis. The clinical curriculum includes clerkships in family medicine, internal medicine, neurology, obstetrics-gynecology, pediatrics, psychiatry, and surgery. It also includes experience with family medicine in the community setting. The electives program consists of five electives chosen by the students in consultation with their advisers.

Research opportunities are available in the summer following the first year and through the Research Honors Program in which the student devotes a full year to research between the second and third years. "Research Honors" is granted upon the successful completion of this program. An integrated M.D.-Ph.D. program providing stipends and tuition scholarships to especially qualified candidates is also available. Students are graded on a numerical system and must maintain a numerical average of 75 for promotion and graduation.

## REQUIREMENTS FOR ENTRANCE

At least three years of study (90 semester hours) in a U.S. or Canadian accredited college or university are required. The completion of four years of college and a B.S. or B.A. degree are highly desirable before entrance into medical school. Students applying without a baccalaureate degree are likely to be accepted only if they have academic records superior to those of students accepted with the baccalaureate degree. They must also exhibit definite evidence of maturity.

Specific course requirements have been kept at a minimum to permit maximum flexibility in the selection of well rounded students. The required courses are:

|  | *Hours* |
| --- | --- |
| Biology or zoology (with lab) | 16 |
| Inorganic chemistry (with lab) | 8 |
| Organic chemistry (with lab) | 8 |
| Physics (with lab) | 8 |
| English | 6 |

The MCAT is also a requirement for admission. It is recommended that students take the MCAT in the spring of the year in which application will be made.

## SELECTION FACTORS

Applications are invited from qualified residents of the state of Texas and the neighboring counties of New Mexico and Oklahoma which comprise the service area of the school. Only U.S. citizens or applicants with permanent resident visas are considered. Application forms and procedural information may be obtained directly from the Office of Admissions.

The Admissions Committee carefully reviews the applications of all individuals meeting the entrance requirements. Although evidence of high intellectual ability and a record of strong academic achievement are essential for success in the study of medicine, the committee recognizes that these are not the only qualities necessary for the development of a physician. Compassion, motivation, the ability to communicate with people, maturity, and personal integrity are additional qualities which the committee deems important. There is no discrimination on the basis of race, sex, creed, national origin, age, or handicap.

Personal interviews are offered to those candidates deemed competitive for admission. Interviews are conducted only at the Lubbock campus.

Students in the 1995 entering class had the following credentials: *mean GPA,* 3.52 (does not include decelerated students, AIMS); 24 percent *women;* 15 percent *Hispanic/ Mexican American,* 10 percent *Asian;* 80 percent *science majors;* 99 percent Texas *residents.*

## FINANCIAL AID

Financial aid is available for students who demonstrate need. Applications for financial assistance are processed after an applicant has been accepted. Detailed information on the available programs can be obtained from the director of student financial aid. Over 65 percent of the student body receive some type of financial assistance. Employment other than during the summer is discouraged.

## INFORMATION FOR MINORITIES

The School of Medicine encourages qualified minority candidates to apply. Minority students constitute a significant part of the student body, and there are always minority representatives on the Admissions Committee. An expanded 2½-year basic science curriculum is limited to four selected minority students who are not competitive in the regular admission process (AIMS).

---

Public Institution

### APPLICATION AND ACCEPTANCE POLICIES FOR 1997–98 FIRST-YEAR CLASS

Filing of application
    Earliest date: June 15, 1996
    Latest date: Nov. 1, 1996
School application fee to all applicants: $40
Oldest MCAT scores considered: 1992
Does have Early Decision Program (EDP)
    EDP application period: June 15–Aug. 1, 1996
    EDP applicants notified by: Oct. 1, 1996
Acceptance notice to regular applicants
    Earliest date: Oct. 15, 1996
    Latest date: Until class is filled
Applicant's response to acceptance offer
    Maximum time: 2 weeks
Requests for deferred entrance considered: Yes
Deposit to hold place in class (applied to tuition):
    $100, due April 1, 1997
Deposit refundable prior to: May 15, 1997
Estimated number of new entrants: 120 (3 EDP)
Starting date: Aug. 1997

### TUITION AND STUDENT FEES PER YEAR FOR 1995–96 FIRST-YEAR CLASS

Tuition                      Student fees: $1,101
  Resident: $6,550
  Nonresident: $19,650

### INFORMATION ON 1995–96 FIRST-YEAR CLASS

| Number of | In-State | Out-of-State | Total |
|---|---|---|---|
| Applicants | 1,579 | 17 | 1,596 |
| Applicants Interviewed | 355 | 2 | 357 |
| New Entrants* | 115 | 1 | 116† |

*All took the MCAT; 98% had baccalaureate degrees.

†Includes four from decelerated program (AIMS).

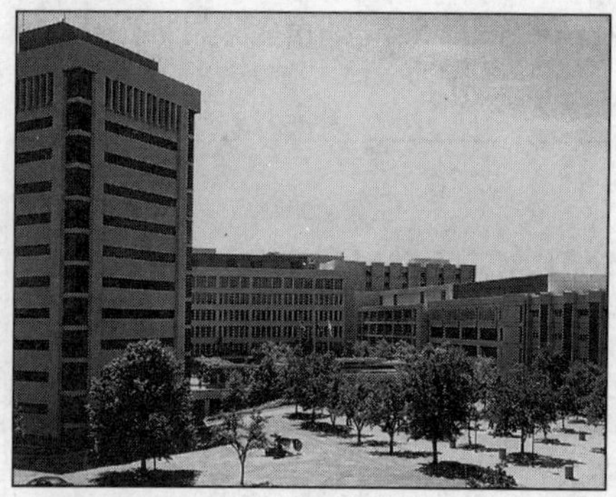

# University of Texas
# Southwestern Medical Center at Dallas
# Southwestern Medical School

## Dallas, Texas

Dr. William B. Neaves, *Dean, UT Southwestern Medical School*
Dr. Barbara C. Waller, *Associate Dean for Student Affairs*
Charles L. Kettlewell, *Registrar and Director of Student Financial Aid*

## ADDRESS INQUIRIES TO:

Office of the Registrar
University of Texas
Southwestern Medical Center at Dallas
5323 Harry Hines Boulevard
Dallas, Texas 75235-9096
(214) 648-2670; 648-3289 (FAX)
Web Site: http://www.swmed.edu

## GENERAL INFORMATION

Southwestern Medical School is a part of the University of Texas Southwestern Medical Center at Dallas, which also includes the Southwestern Graduate School of Biomedical Sciences and the Southwestern Allied Health Sciences School. The purpose of the program at Southwestern is to produce physicians who will be inspired to maintain lifelong medical scholarship and who will apply the knowledge gained in a responsible and sympathetic way to the care of patients.

The faculty and staff are keenly aware of the responsibility of the institution to serve the people not only in producing physicians of excellence and humanity but also in acquiring new knowledge.

## CURRICULUM

Southwestern Medical School has a four-year curriculum based on departmental as well as interdisciplinary teaching. The purpose of the first two years is to provide a strong background in the basic sciences as well as an introduction to clinical medicine.

The first-year curriculum is designed to begin the study of the normal human body and its processes at the molecular and cellular levels. Biochemistry, anatomy, and genetics are presented concurrently for the first portion of the year, building together the concepts of macromolecular and cellular interactions within tissues. The spring term is composed of courses in physiology and neurosciences, cell biology, and human behavior. At the completion of the first year, a vertical course in human reproduction and endocrinology provides an overall synthesis, based on the previous course work. A year-long, problem-based introduction to clinical medicine course introduces first-year students to taking histories from standardized patients along with content in ethics, human behavior, and prevention.

The second year begins a study of disease processes and provides insight into how man may interfere with those processes therapeutically. The material is presented in a block fashion similar to that of the freshman year. The year begins with microbiology and immunology and concludes with pharmacology. Extending throughout most of the year are pathology and introduction to clinical medicine, which serve to correlate the basic sciences with clinical medicine. Contact with patients begins early in the second year with history-taking and physical examination as well as visits to outpatient clinics. The basic concepts of psychiatry are presented over the first two years in a series of conferences and lectures.

The third and fourth years provide intense clinical experiences involving the student in direct inpatient and outpatient care. The junior year is composed of 12 weeks of internal medicine, 6 weeks each of psychiatry and obstetrics, 8 weeks each of surgery and pediatrics, and 4 weeks of family practice. The fourth year provides a series of one-month clinical rotations; required months in neurology, subinternship in internal medicine, and an intensive care unit or ambulatory care rotation; three selectives from the departments of obstetrics-gynecology, surgery, pediatrics, or family practice; and at least two months of electives.

## REQUIREMENTS FOR ENTRANCE

The MCAT and three years (90 semester hours) of accredited college work are required. Minimum course requirements are:

|  | *Years* |
|---|---|
| Biology | 2 |
|   One year must include lab. | |
| Inorganic chemistry (with lab) | 1 |
| Organic chemistry (with lab) | 1 |
| Physics (with lab) | 1 |
| Calculus | ½ |
| English | 1 |

Although some students with only 90 semester hours credit are admitted each year, preference is given to applicants who have earned the B.S. or B.A. degree.

Sound preparation in basic science is essential, but a broad background in the humanities and an understanding of people and their problems are equally necessary. Applicants are urged to take the MCAT in the spring of the year of application and to complete required course work before applying if possible. A grade average of C must be maintained in each required subject.

It should be noted that application forms and procedural information should be obtained from the University of Texas System Medical and Dental Application Center listed below.

## SELECTION FACTORS

Applicants are selected on the basis of demonstrated intellectual ability as evidenced by the academic record, performance on the MCAT, evaluation by the faculty of the undergraduate institution attended (preprofessional committee evaluation when available), and letters of recommendation when they reflect experience in the health or scientific fields. Ninety percent of the class must be residents of Texas by state law. The minimum credentials for nonresidents are more stringent than those for Texas residents.

Early application is strongly advised. A personal on-campus interview is required. Invitations for interviews are extended from early September until mid-December.

## FINANCIAL AID

Most of the financial aid available is obtained through federal and state loan programs. A limited number of scholarships from private sources are available. To date, no student has discontinued school for financial reasons.

## INFORMATION FOR MINORITIES

The Admissions Committee at Southwestern Medical School recognizes the need for increased numbers of physicians from racial minorities and encourages applications from Texas residents who are members of these groups.

---

Public Institution

## APPLICATION AND ACCEPTANCE POLICIES FOR 1997–98 FIRST-YEAR CLASS

Application must be made through the
   University of Texas System Medical and
   Dental Application Center, Suite 620,
   702 Colorado, Austin, Texas 78701
Filing of application
   Earliest date: April 15, 1996
   Latest date: Oct. 15, 1996
School application fee: None
Application Center fees
   Resident: $45 for application to one school plus
      $5 for each additional school applied to in the
      University of Texas system
   Nonresident: $80 for application to one school plus
      $10 for each additional school applied to in the
      University of Texas system
Oldest MCAT scores considered: 1993
Does not have Early Decision Program
Acceptance notice to regular applicants
   Earliest date: Jan. 15, 1997
   Latest date: Until class is filled
Applicant's response to acceptance offer
   Maximum time: 2 weeks
Requests for deferred entrance considered: Yes
Deposit to hold place in class: None
Estimated number of new entrants: 200
Starting date: Aug. 1997

## TUITION AND STUDENT FEES PER YEAR FOR 1995–96 FIRST-YEAR CLASS

Tuition                    Student fees: $696
   Resident: $6,550
   Nonresident*: $19,650

## INFORMATION ON 1995–96 FIRST-YEAR CLASS

| Number of | In-State | Out-of-State | Total |
| --- | --- | --- | --- |
| Applicants | 2,521 | 833 | 3,354 |
| Applicants Interviewed | 644 | 129 | 773 |
| New Entrants† | 176 | 23 | 199 |

*Nonresidents are eligible to pay resident tuition on receipt of a competitive academic scholarship worth at least $1,000 per year.

†All took the MCAT; 98% had baccalaureate degrees.

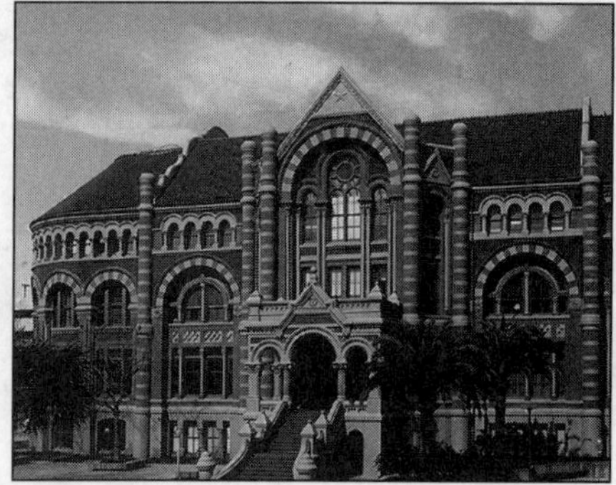

# University of Texas Medical School at Galveston

**Galveston, Texas**

Dr. George M. Bernier, Jr., *Dean of Medicine*
Dr. Billy R. Ballard, *Associate Dean for Student Affairs* and
  *Director of Medical School Admissions*
Betty Hazelbaker, *Director, Office of Fiscal Planning Management*

## ADDRESS INQUIRIES TO:

Office of Admissions
G-210, Ashbel Smith Building
University of Texas Medical Branch at Galveston
School of Medicine
Galveston, Texas 77555-1317
(409) 772-3517; 772-5753 (FAX)
E-Mail: pow.vpaa.utmb.edu
Web Site: http://www.utmb.edu

## GENERAL INFORMATION

The University of Texas Medical Branch at Galveston was established in 1881 and graduated its first class in 1892. It is a state-owned medical center with the Medical Branch hospitals under direct supervision and administrative control of the staff. Medical Branch hospitals have over 1,200 hospital beds located on the immediate campus. The Shriners Burn Institute, the Marine Biomedical Institute, and the Institute for the Medical Humanities also serve as teaching and research facilities.

## CURRICULUM

The medical curriculum is an integrated program which begins clinical training immediately upon matriculation. The curriculum is divided into the basic science core and clinical medicine. The basic science core is divided into four 16-week terms and completed with 10 weeks of introduction to clinical medicine. Clinical medicine is divided into 50 weeks of required core experience (clerkships) and 36 weeks of elective experience. The third year has an extensive ambulatory patient care experience, as well as the traditional in-patient care experience. In addition, a problem-based curriculum is offered to 24 students each year. Each student is assigned a faculty adviser to assist in developing individualized experience in clinical medicine. Electives may be taken either on campus or at other institutions with approval of the faculty adviser. Electives may be taken in foreign countries upon the approval of the associate dean for academic affairs. The elective experiences are flexible and can be designed to meet individual career goals. The grading system for the first three academic years is A, B, C, F for all core courses and pass/fail for elective courses.

Patient contact is initiated in the first week of medical school in the Introduction to Patient Evaluation (IPE) and the Community Continuity Experience (CCE) courses. Patient interviewing and physical examination techniques are initiated by IPE and put into practice in the CCE. These courses extend through the first two years of medical school. The courses are directed by generalists, with major participation from primary care disciplines (family medicine, general internal medicine, and pediatrics). Each of the primary care clerkships features experiences in ambulatory office-based patient care. These departments also offer clinical electives both for preclinical and fourth-year students, as well as career advisors and generalist-based student interest groups.

## REQUIREMENTS FOR ENTRANCE

The MCAT and a minimum of 90 semester hours of college work including specific courses are required. The baccalaureate degree is highly desirable. Course work is acceptable only if completed at U.S. colleges and universities with accreditation from one of the regional accrediting agencies.

Applicants are encouraged to take the MCAT in the spring of the year of application. Results from the MCAT taken in the spring of the year of anticipated matriculation will not be received in time to be considered. Applicants are encouraged to complete the required courses and/or take the MCAT by the time they submit an application.

The required courses are:

|  | *Years* |
| --- | --- |
| Biology | 2 |
| One year must include lab. | |
| Inorganic chemistry (with lab) | 1 |
| Organic chemistry (with lab) | 1 |
| General physics (with lab) | 1 |
| Calculus | ½ |
| English | 1 |

Science courses should be equivalent to course work required for college science majors. A broad background in the humanities is encouraged.

## SELECTION FACTORS

All information available is utilized in the selection process. The most significant factors are intellect, achievement, character, interpersonal skills, and motivation. In evaluating candidates, consideration is given to the total academic record, the results of aptitude and achievement tests, college preprofessional committee evaluations, and the personal interview. Only those applicants whose personal qualifications, academic records, aptitude and achievement test scores, and preprofessional evaluations are considered sufficiently competitive and are invited for personal interviews. Only U.S. citizens or applicants with permanent visas are considered. Preference is given to legal residents of Texas. Up to 10 percent of the class may be filled with residents of other states.

Accepted applicants for the 1995 entering class had the following credentials: *average GPA,* 3.5; *residence,* 94 percent from Texas.

## FINANCIAL AID

Long-term, low-interest loans and short-term loans of varying interest rates are available to students with financial need. A number of scholarships funded by private donors are available. Most of these are based on need; some are based on academic achievement. A number of scholarships are available to minority students. Considerable individual attention is provided to students to help them with their fiscal planning, with debt management, and with exploring the various funding options. Applications for financial assistance are provided to students who have been accepted for admission and have indicated that they will attend the University of Texas Medical School at Galveston. There are no fixed deadlines. Inquiries must be directed to the Office of Student Fiscal Planning and Management.

## INFORMATION FOR MINORITIES

The University of Texas Medical Branch at Galveston is committed to increasing the number of minority students in medicine. Each minority applicant is reviewed by experienced members of the Committee on Admissions with particular emphasis on the applicant's potential. Both cognitive and noncognitive qualifications are considered. There are no quotas, and all applicants are considered on the basis of individual achievement and promise. Following admission, a broad range of support services are available to assist students in completing the medical curriculum. Specific information about the services provided to minority applicants can be obtained by contacting the Office of Student Services. The University of Texas Medical Branch does not discriminate on the basis of race, sex, creed, national origin, age, or handicap.

Public Institution

## APPLICATION AND ACCEPTANCE POLICIES FOR 1997–98 FIRST-YEAR CLASS

Application must be made through the
   University of Texas System Medical and
   Dental Application Center, Suite 620,
   702 Colorado, Austin, Texas 78701
Filing of application
   Earliest date: April 15, 1996
   Latest date: Oct. 15, 1996
School application fee: None
Application Center fees
   Resident: $45 for application to one school plus
      $5 for each additional school applied to in the
      University of Texas system
   Nonresident: $80 for application to one school plus
      $10 for each additional school applied to in the
      University of Texas system
Oldest MCAT scores considered: 1993
Does not have Early Decision Program
Acceptance notice to regular applicants
   Earliest date: Jan. 15, 1997
   Latest date: Until class is filled
Applicant's response to acceptance offer
   Maximum time: 2 weeks
Requests for deferred entrance considered: Yes
Deposit to hold place in class: None
Estimated number of new entrants: 200
Starting date: Aug. 1997

## TUITION AND STUDENT FEES PER YEAR FOR 1995–96 FIRST-YEAR CLASS

Tuition                 Student fees: $427
   Resident: $6,550
   Nonresident: $19,650

## INFORMATION ON 1995–96 FIRST-YEAR CLASS

| *Number of* | *In-State* | *Out-of-State* | *Total* |
|---|---|---|---|
| Applicants | 2,601 | 615 | 3,216 |
| Applicants Interviewed | 1,184 | 163 | 1,347 |
| New Entrants* | 191 | 9 | 200 |

*All took the MCAT; 99% has baccalaureate degrees.

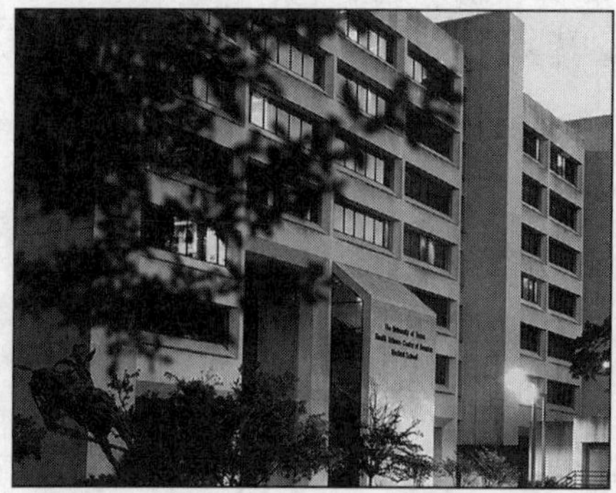

# University of Texas
# Houston Medical School

**Houston, Texas**

Dr. Cheves McC. Smythe, *Dean Pro Tem*
Dr. Albert E. Gunn, *Associate Dean for Admissions*
Sondra M. Ives, *Director of Admissions Services and Alumni Affairs*

## ADDRESS INQUIRIES TO:

Office of Admissions-Room G-024
University of Texas—
Houston Medical School
P.O. Box 20708
Houston, Texas 77225
(713) 792-4711; 794-4238 (FAX)
Web Site: http://www@www.med.uth.tmc.edu

## GENERAL INFORMATION

The University of Texas—Houston Medical School was authorized in May 1969 by the Texas Legislature. The Medical School is part of the University of Texas system.

The Medical School is located in the Texas Medical Center in Houston in order to take advantage of the many other medical institutions in the area. The major teaching hospital is Hermann Hospital, a 650-bed general medical and surgical hospital. Other affiliated hospitals include the University of Texas, M.D. Anderson Cancer Center, St. Joseph Hospital, San Jose Clinic, Southwest Memorial Hospital, and the Lyndon Baines Johnson Hospital, a facility of the Harris County Hospital District.

## CURRICULUM

In September 1977 a four-year educational program was begun. The first two academic years are divided into four semesters. Two months of vacation time are provided for first-year students between the first and second academic years. The initial four semesters are devoted to preparing the student for the specific clerkship experiences that comprise the third academic year. During the first two academic years the student becomes familiar with the basic and applied biomedical sciences. As the student progresses from a study of the morphology of the human body and the fundamentals of molecular and cellular biology to that of the normal and abnormal structure and function of the various organ systems, the techniques of interviewing, history-taking, and performance of physical and mental status examinations are introduced. Appropriate material from the behavioral sciences is presented concomitantly, as are opportunities to become familiar with the realities and problems of human medicine and family practice.

After completion of this educational sequence, the student progresses through a series of clinical clerkships in the major clinical disciplines for the next 12 months. In the remaining year, there are 3 months of required clerkships, 5 periods of electives, and one period reserved for additional instruction in medical jurisprudence and clinical epidemiology. In consultation with faculty, each student devises an educational sequence that relates specifically to ultimate career goals and postgraduate educational plans.

Problem-based learning is extensively employed in achieving the school's educational objectives.

## REQUIREMENTS FOR ENTRANCE

Students must take the MCAT and complete at least 90 undergraduate credit hours at a U.S. or Canadian university. A baccalaureate degree is highly desirable. The specific premedical credits listed below are required.

|  | Sem. hrs. |
|---|---|
| Biology | 14 |
| One year must include lab. | |
| Inorganic chemistry (with lab) | 8 |
| Organic chemistry (with lab) | 8 |
| Physics (with lab) | 8 |
| Calculus | 3 |
| English | 6 |

While the applicant should demonstrate aptitude for and achievement in the basic sciences, it is essential that an in-depth experience in some area of the humanities be obtained. Liberal arts majors are encouraged.

Applicants should take the MCAT in the spring of the year of application.

## SELECTION FACTORS

Applicants are selected on the basis of motivation and potential for service. Academic ability is evaluated to insure those who are accepted can complete medical studies. Emphasis is given to students who have a broad education and who display intellectual interest. A command of the language with ability to write and speak well is essential. The applicant's academic record is evaluated with special attention to the subjects taken and the demonstration of a broadly based comprehensive educational experience. The overall philosophy is that knowledge is an end in itself; while vocational type curricula are not ruled out, liberal arts are preferred. Universities with core curricula generally provide the type of diversity sought in subject distribution. Significant attention is given to humanitarian endeavors, achievement in a non-academic field of activity, and specific interest by the applicant in the University of Texas—Houston Medical School. Applicants are invited for personal interviews based on the factors above referenced. In the interview, which is an important element in the selection process, applicants are expected to cogently discuss their motivation and experiences that led them to a medical career. It is also anticipated they will discuss their intellectual interests and generally demonstrate their suitability to enter a learned profession. Admission decisions are made in light of the school's mission, with preference given to Texas residents. The University of Texas—Houston Medical School does not discriminate on the basis of race, sex, creed, national origin, age, or handicap.

Accepted students for the 1995 entering class had the following credentials: *mean GPA,* 3.44; *sex,* 55 percent women; *residence,* 90 percent from Texas.

## FINANCIAL AID

Scholarship and loan funds are available to students with financial need from local, state, federal, and national sources. Financial independence is not a criterion for admission as indicated by the fact that 60 percent of the students enrolled at present have received financial aid.

Public Institution

## APPLICATION AND ACCEPTANCE POLICIES FOR 1997–98 FIRST-YEAR CLASS

Application must be made through the
  University of Texas System Medical and
  Dental Application Center, Suite 620,
  702 Colorado, Austin, Texas 78701
Filing of application
  Earliest date: June 15, 1996
  Latest date: Oct. 15, 1996
School application fee: None
Application Center fees
  Resident: $45 for application to one school plus
    $5 for each additional school applied to in the
    University of Texas system
  Nonresident: $80 for application to one school plus
    $10 for each additional school applied to in the
    University of Texas system
Oldest MCAT scores considered: 1991
Does not have Early Decision Program
Acceptance notice to regular applicants
  Earliest date: Jan. 15, 1997
  Latest date: Until class is filled
Applicant's response to acceptance offer
  Maximum time: 2 weeks
Requests for deferred entrance considered: No
Deposit to hold place in class: None
Estimated number of new entrants: 200
Starting date: Aug. 1997

## TUITION AND STUDENT FEES PER YEAR FOR 1995–96 FIRST-YEAR CLASS

Tuition                 Student fees: $250
  Resident: $6,550
  Nonresident: $19,650

## INFORMATION ON 1995–96 FIRST-YEAR CLASS

| Number of | In-State | Out-of-State | Total |
|---|---|---|---|
| Applicants | 2,618 | 745 | 3,363 |
| Applicants Interviewed | 1,047 | 52 | 1,099 |
| New Entrants* | 184 | 16 | 200 |

*All took the MCAT; 99% had baccalaureate degrees.

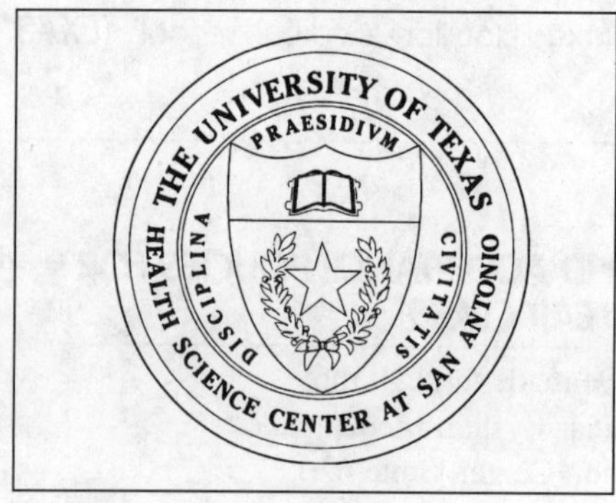

# University of Texas
# Medical School at San Antonio

## San Antonio, Texas


Dr. James J. Young, *Dean*
Dr. Carlos Pestana, *Associate Dean for Academic Affairs*
Dr. Leonard E. Lawrence, *Associate Dean for Student Affairs*


## ADDRESS INQUIRIES TO:

Medical School Admissions
Registrar's Office
University of Texas
Health Science Center at San Antonio
7703 Floyd Curl Drive
San Antonio, Texas 78284-7701
(210) 567-2665; 567-2685 (FAX)

## GENERAL INFORMATION

The University of Texas Medical School at San Antonio was created by the Texas Legislature in 1959 as a four-year school of medicine. In late 1972 the Medical School and its fellow institutions, the Dental School, and the Graduate School of Biomedical Sciences were designated the University of Texas Health Science Center at San Antonio. Clinical instruction is carried out at the University Hospital, Brady-Green Community Health Center, Audie Murphy Veterans Hospital, and affiliate hospitals which include Wilford Hall USAF Hospital, Brooke Army Hospital, the Aerospace Medical Division of USAF, Baptist Memorial Hospital System, and Santa Rosa Medical Center.

## CURRICULUM

A four-year curriculum is offered. The first year consists of 800 contact hours, which are devoted primarily to the traditional basic sciences. The first year also includes an introductory course in physical diagnosis. The second academic year contains about 750 contact hours, of which over 275 are devoted to the basic sciences of pathology and pharmacology. The remaining hours in the second year are devoted to introductory clinical topics in the areas of advanced physical diagnosis, medicine, surgery, obstetrics and gynecology, pediatrics, and psychiatry, as well as medical humanities. The third academic year is spent entirely in the clinical setting in eight consecutive assignments of six weeks each in family practice, medicine, the medical specialties, surgery, the surgical specialties, obstetrics and gynecology, psychiatry, and pediatrics. The senior year includes a didactic period of two months, with the rest of the academic year consisting of elective courses. Some time is also available to the students for interviews for postgraduate training or for vacation. A letter grading system is used.

## REQUIREMENTS FOR ENTRANCE

The MCAT and the equivalent of three academic years (90 semester hours) are required for admission. Courses specifically required (with a grade of C or better) are:

|  | Sem. Hrs. |
|---|---|
| Biology | 14 |
| One year must include lab. | |
| Inorganic chemistry (with lab) | 8 |
| Organic chemistry (with lab) | 8 |
| General physics (with lab) | 8 |
| Calculus | 3 |
| English | 6 |

Science courses should be equivalent to course work as required for college science majors. Candidates are desired who have a broad humanities background.

## SELECTION FACTORS

Ranking of applicants is done with consideration for GPA, MCAT scores, evaluation by premedical advisers, the candidate's potential relative to society's health care needs, and judgment by the Committee on Admissions of the candidate's academic achievements not reflected by grades, nonacademic achievements, and integrity, maturity, and motivation. No person shall be excluded from participation in, denied the benefits of, or subject to discrimination under any program or activity sponsored or conducted by the University of Texas system on the basis of age, race, national origin, religion, or sex. Although legal residents of Texas are preferred, up to 10 percent of entrants may be nonresidents if their credentials are especially outstanding.

Accepted students for the 1995 entering class had the following credentials: *mean GPA,* 3.38; *sex,* 43 percent women; *residence,* 5 percent nonresidents; *overall acceptance rate,* 281 acceptances were offered to obtain a class of 201 first-year students.

Application forms and any procedural information should be obtained from the University of Texas System Medical and Dental Application Center listed below. This center processes all applications to each medical school in the University of Texas system.

Questions related to completeness of an application or other information should be directed to the Office of Student Services at the Health Science Center.

## FINANCIAL AID

Financial assistance for students in need is available in the form of loans and a limited number of scholarships. Student employment, though not encouraged, is permissible provided a satisfactory level of achievement is maintained. Part-time student employment opportunities are available at the Health Science Center as well as in the hospitals located in close proximity. Financial considerations do not influence admission decisions, although the school recognizes that many families are unable to bear the full cost of medical education. Accepted applicants can obtain complete information regarding financial assistance from the financial aid administrator in the Office of Student Services.

## AFFIRMATIVE ACTION

The Medical School is committed to the recruitment, retention, and graduation of qualified minority applicants. In the selection of these individuals, preference is given to Texas residents. Both the Office of the Medical Dean and the Health Science Center's Office of Student Services through the coordinator of special programs are involved in the process of screening, monitoring, counseling, and advocacy for minority students. More specific information may be obtained from the Office of the Associate Dean for Student Affairs.

---

Public Institution

## APPLICATION AND ACCEPTANCE POLICIES FOR 1997–98 FIRST-YEAR CLASS

Application must be made through the
 University of Texas System Medical and
 Dental Application Center, Suite 620,
 702 Colorado, Austin, Texas 78701
Filing of application
 Earliest date: April 15, 1996
 Latest date: Oct. 15, 1996
School application fee: None
Application Center fees
 Resident: $45 for application to one school plus
  $5 for each additional school applied to in the
  University of Texas system
 Nonresident: $80 for application to one school plus
  $10 for each additional school applied to in the
  University of Texas system
Oldest MCAT scores considered: 1992
Does not have Early Decision Program
Acceptance notice to regular applicants
 Earliest date: Jan. 15, 1997
 Latest date: Until class is filled
Applicant's response to acceptance offer
 Maximum time: 14 days
Requests for deferred entrance considered: No
Deposit to hold place in class: None
Estimated number of new entrants: 200
Starting date: Aug. 1997

## TUITION AND STUDENT FEES PER YEAR FOR 1995–96 FIRST-YEAR CLASS

Tuition                    Student fees: $375
 Resident: $6,550
 Nonresident: $19,650

## INFORMATION ON 1995–96 FIRST-YEAR CLASS

| Number of | In-State | Out-of-State | Total |
|---|---|---|---|
| Applicants | 2,722 | 553 | 3,275 |
| Applicants Interviewed | 871 | 130 | 1,001 |
| New Entrants* | 191 | 10 | 201 |

*All took the MCAT; 89% had baccalaureate degrees.

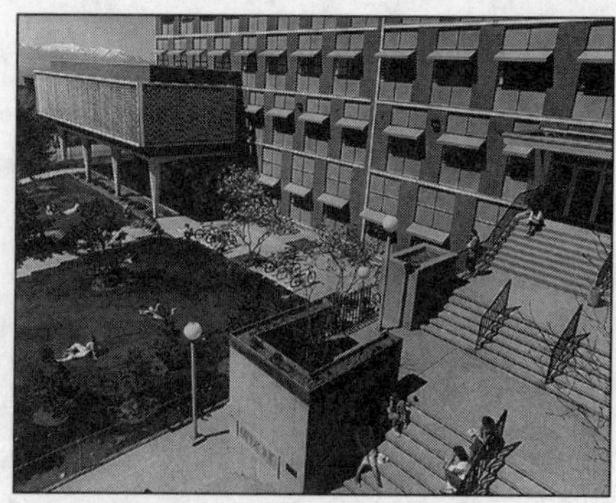

# University of Utah
# School of Medicine

**Salt Lake City, Utah**

Dr. Walter J. Stevens, *Dean*
Dr. Victoria E. Judd, *Assistant Dean, Admissions*
Rita Litsas, *Director, Medical Education and Financial* Aid

## ADDRESS INQUIRIES TO:

Millie M. Peterson
Director, Medical School Admissions
University of Utah
School of Medicine
50 North Medical Drive
Salt Lake City, Utah 84132
(801) 581-7498; 585-3300 (FAX)
E-Mail: Mylonakis@deans.med.utah.edu

## GENERAL INFORMATION

The School of Medicine was founded as a two-year school in 1905 and expanded to a four-year program in 1943. It is one of the 17 colleges of the University of Utah. The medical school is a component of the Utah Health Sciences Center, which also includes schools of pharmacy, nursing, health, a health sciences library, a Howard Hughes medical institute, Eccles Program for Human Molecular Biology and Genetics, Utah Genome Center, Utah Cancer Center, several other centers for special studies, the Moran Eye Center, and the University of Utah Hospital.

## CURRICULUM

The undergraduate medical curriculum is a mixture of required and elective courses. This design allows each student to acquire a knowledge basic to medical science while being able to pursue individual interests. The first two years of medical school offer basic sciences, physical diagnosis, organ system teaching, and a choice of electives. Six clerkships are required during the third year. The fourth year consists of a two-week neurology clerkship, a two-week medical ethics course, and electives.

Students are evaluated on an honors/pass/fail system, and opportunities for honor classes and independent study are provided. Students are represented on all college committees. Students receive guidance and assistance from offices of student affairs, minority affairs, and student advising and counseling.

Beginning with the 1994–95 academic year, the School of Medicine will have a combined M.D.-Ph.D. program. Applicants will be considered, after acceptance into medical school, on the basis of their credentials and undergraduate research experience. The school is looking for individuals interested in an academic career in medicine for these positions.

## REQUIREMENTS FOR ENTRANCE

The MCAT is required and must be taken within four years of application. The Admissions Committee is eager to admit students with a broad perspective of life. The school believes that the true physican not only is skilled in medicine and the allied sciences but also is a person of culture and broad intelligence.

The applicant must have subject matter competence in the following courses:

|  | *Years* |
| --- | --- |
| Chemistry (with lab) | 2 |
| Must include inorganic and organic chemistry and course work in qualitative and quantitative analysis. | |
| General physics (with lab) | 1 |
| Heat, light, electricity, and magnetism. | |
| English composition and/or basic communication | 1 |

Two college-level courses in biology, including cell biology and college-level courses in humanities and the social sciences, are required.

With the exception of advanced placement credit for general chemistry at a level of 4 or 5, CLEP, advanced placement, or home study credit will not be accepted for completion of required course work. These courses must be taken at a college or university in the United States.

Completion of four years of college work and a bachelor's degree are desirable before entering the School of Medicine. Rarely, the committee accepts an unusual applicant after only three years of college.

Only those students who have completed most of the undergraduate training in a U.S. or Canadian school will be considered.

## SELECTION FACTORS

Students are considered on the basis on scholarship, extracurricular activities including volunteer work, research and community work, letters or recommendation and assessment of personality, character, maturity, and motivation. The School of Medicine is state-assisted and a majority of the admissions are Utah residents. The University of Utah is an accredited WICHE school and the medical school has special arrangements with the state of Idaho to provide six positions for certified residents of this state. Competition for the few remaining nonresident positions is very keen. Nonresident applicants (excluding Idaho and Wyoming residents and those who qualify to apply under the affirmative action program for underrepresented minority students) are required to apply through the Early Decision Program. Nonresidents with background or ties to Utah may petition to have their application considered during the regular process. There is no discrimination because of age, race, creed, sex, or sexual orientation, and the selection process is conducted by the same committee for all applicants. The University of Utah provides reasonable accommodation to the known disabilities of applicants.

Applications should be filed no later than October 15 through AMCAS. The Admissions Committee will notify eligible candidates concerning interview appointments. Final selections are made by majority vote of the committee.

No more than four consecutive applications will be accepted from any one candidate. Transfer positions are available only when the total number of students in all four classes drops below the allotted 400 and either the second or third year is below 100.

## FINANCIAL AID

A very limited number of scholarships is awarded each year. Some loan funds are available to students on a long-term, low-interest basis. All awards are based on the student's need as determined by the university's Financial Aids Office. Because of fluctuation in federal support for financial aid programs, it is difficult to determine how much aid the school will be able to continue to give. It should be stressed, therefore, that most students will need to find outside resources for the majority of their financial support. It is necessary for applicants to plan their financial program as carefully as their academic program.

## INFORMATION FOR MINORITIES

The School of Medicine is committed to the selection and retention of qualified applicants from underrepresented minorities, particularly if they are Utah residents. The school recognizes these groups are not adequately represented in medicine.

Once admitted, those whose academic preparation is marginal are recommended to take appropriate supplemental course work, which may include a special basic sciences enrichment course in the summer prior to the regular medical school curriculum. Academic support programs are available to give students a maximum opportunity to succeed in their academic work and professional training. The school will also provide as much financial aid as possible through loans and grants. The Office of Minority Affairs is available to counsel and assist students and to acquaint them with the community.

Public Institution

## APPLICATION AND ACCEPTANCE POLICIES FOR 1997–98 FIRST-YEAR CLASS

*School participates in AMCAS. See Chapter 4.*

Filing of AMCAS application
    Earliest date: June 1, 1996
    Latest date: Oct. 15, 1996
School application fee to all applicants: $50
Oldest MCAT scores considered: 1993
Does have Early Decision Program (EDP)
    Nonresidents must apply through EDP
    EDP application period: June 1–Aug. 1, 1996
    EDP applicants notified by: Oct. 1, 1996
Acceptance notice to regular applicants
    Earliest date: Oct. 15, 1996
    Latest date: Until class is filled
Applicant's response to acceptance offer
    Maximum time: 2 weeks
Requests for deferred entrance considered: No
Deposit to hold place in class (applied to tuition):
    $100, due with response to acceptance offer
Deposit refundable prior to: May 15, 1997
Estimated number of new entrants: 100 (10 EDP)
Starting date: Sept. 1997

## TUITION AND STUDENT FEES PER YEAR FOR 1995–96 FIRST-YEAR CLASS

Tuition                          Student fees: $435
    Resident: $6,927
    Nonresident: $14,760

## INFORMATION ON 1995–96 FIRST-YEAR CLASS

| Number of | In-State | Out-of-State | Total |
|---|---|---|---|
| Applicants | 436 | 973 | 1,409 |
| Applicants Interviewed | 298 | 144 | 442 |
| New Entrants* | 75 | 25 | 100 |

*All took the MCAT and had baccalaureate degrees.

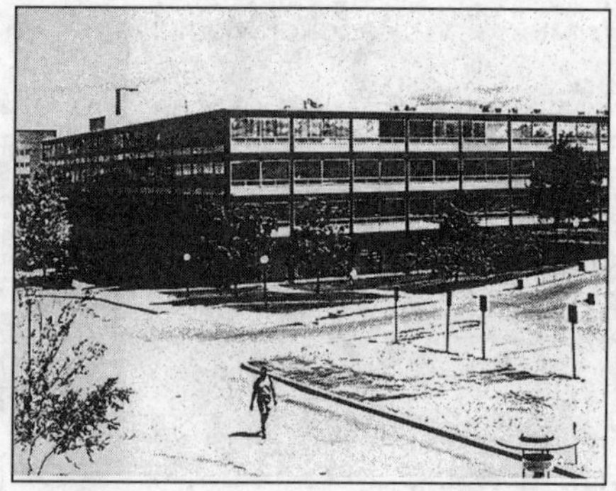

# University of Vermont College of Medicine

## Burlington, Vermont

Dr. John Frymoyer, *Dean*
Dr. Cathleen J. Gleeson, *Director of Admissions*
Deborah Altemus, *Financial Aid Officer*

## ADDRESS INQUIRIES TO:

Admissions Office
C-225 Given Building
University of Vermont
College of Medicine
Burlington, Vermont 05405
(802) 656-2154

## GENERAL INFORMATION

The University of Vermont College of Medicine is located on the eastern shore of Lake Champlain in the city of Burlington, Vermont, a community of about 38,000 people. Established in 1822, it is the seventh oldest medical school in the United States. The College of Medicine recognizes the need for primary care physicians, clinical specialists, and research scientists. Our curriculum provides a general professional education in both basic and clinical sciences, followed by a period structured to meet each student's individual goals.

Our principal teaching hospital is Fletcher Allen Health Care's Medical Center Hospital of Vermont Campus, a 500-bed hospital adjacent to the College of Medicine. The hospital provides community care for Burlington and the surrounding communities and tertiary referral care for patients from the entire state of Vermont and from the northern Adirondack region of New York State.

## CURRICULUM

The College of Medicine is committed to preparing students to become excellent practicing physicians, teachers, and scientific investigators.

The curriculum is divided into three phases. The first phase consists of 1½ years of instruction in the basic sciences. A clinical course called doctoring skills, which prepares the student for the study of medicine by the study of patients, is presented throughout this portion of the curriculum. The second phase, 12 months in length, is devoted to the clinical sciences of medicine. These two segments are designed to provide students with a broad general professional education. The final phase of the curriculum, the Senior Selective Program, extends through the 1½ years prior to graduation. This program enables students to select a course of study and experience best suited to their career objectives. Twelve months of

this final period are available for electives Fletcher Allen Health Care, elsewhere in the United States, or abroad.

We use an honors/pass/fail method of grading, coupled with individual narrative evaluations of performance in clinical rotations.

During the Basic Science Core, a parallel program called the Vermont Generalist Curriculum helps students translate classroom learning into clinical practice—especially primary care practice.

The Vermont Generalist Curriculum consists of three courses. The Physician in Society explores the human issues of being a physician as well as the ethical, social, cultural, and psychological factors affecting health and illness. Doctoring Skills provides training in physical examination, interviewing patients, and technical skills such as drawing blood and starting intravenous lines. Beginning in the second semester, a yearlong course called Doctoring in Vermont places each student in the primary care office of a generalist physician from family practice, internal medicine, or pediatrics for four hours every other week. Doctoring in Vermont also involves a community studies project that provides an understanding of a community health issue such as caring for the homeless.

## REQUIREMENTS FOR ENTRANCE

The MCAT is required and must be taken by August of the application year. Applicants must have completed at least three years of undergraduate study in an accredited college or university in the United States or Canada; the baccalaureate degree is highly desirable. In order to ensure serious consideration, applicants are urged to take the MCAT in the spring of the year of application and to have their basic premedical requirements completed at the time of application. The undergraduate program must include the following course work:

*Years/Credit Hours*

Biology or zoology (with lab) . . . . . . . . . . . . . . . . . . . . . . 1/8
General chemistry (with lab) . . . . . . . . . . . . . . . . . . . . . . 1/8
Organic chemistry (with lab) . . . . . . . . . . . . . . . . . . . . . . 1/8
General physics (with lab) . . . . . . . . . . . . . . . . . . . . . . . 1/8

Secondary school advanced placement courses will be recognized only if credit for them appears on the college transcript.

## SELECTION FACTORS

The Committee on Admissions seeks a heterogeneous student body. We look for evidence of the promise of excellence accompanied by genuine concern for the welfare of others. Effective interpersonal skills are considered especially important. Significant experience in health care or other direct human services, either as an employee or as a volunteer, is expected of all applicants. The University of Vermont does not discriminate on the basis of race, color, sex, sexual orientation, religion, age, handicap, national origin, or Vietnam Veteran status.

Selection of an applicant for admission is based upon the past pattern of academic performance plus an assessment of the applicant's fitness for the study and practice of medicine in terms of aptitude, interests, experience, motivation, attitudes, and maturity. Letters of recommendation and a personal interview form an important part of the application process. The interview is required and is by invitation. We do not offer off-campus interviews.

Preference for admission is given to qualified residents of Vermont and states which have contractual arrangements with the university (currently Maine). However, significant numbers of openings remain for qualified residents of other states. Members of minority groups are encouraged to apply for admission.

Transfer Students—The unique structure of the curriculum, and the minimal student attrition generally precludes accepting transfer students. However, students wishing to explore the possibility of transferring may request an application which outlines requirements for transfer. Students who transfer generally complete two years of school elsewhere and then enroll at the beginning or middle of the second year at the University of Vermont. Transfer applications are available after January 1. Decisions may be delayed until August.

The 1995 entering class had the following characteristics: *mean GPA,* 3.3; *mean MCAT,* 9.0; *sex,* 41 percent female; 59 percent male; *residence,* 30 from Vermont, 12 from Maine, 51 from other states; *undergraduate major,* 68 percent in the natural or biological sciences; *overall acceptance rate:* 8,647 applications received, 523 applicants interviewed, 151 acceptances offered to obtain a class of 93 students.

Because of the November 1 deadline, early application is recommended. Extensions are not granted.

## FINANCIAL AID

Financial aid funds are limited and are primarily in the form of loans. Funds are distributed according to relative need. Entering students are considered for awards on the same basis as those already enrolled. An applicant's financial status has no bearing on admission determination.

Public Institution

### APPLICATION AND ACCEPTANCE POLICIES FOR 1997–98 FIRST-YEAR CLASS

*School participates in AMCAS. See Chapter 4.*

Filing of AMCAS application
  Earliest date: June 1, 1996
  Latest date: Nov. 1, 1996
School application fee to all applicants: $70
Oldest MCAT scores considered: 1993
Does have Early Decision Program (EDP)
  EDP application period: June 1–Aug. 1, 1996
  EDP applicants notified by: Oct. 1, 1996
Acceptance notice to regular applicants
  Earliest date: Dec. 1996
  Latest date: Until class is filled
Applicant's response to acceptance offer
  Maximum time: 2 weeks
Requests for deferred entrance considered: Yes
Deposit to hold place in class (applied to tuition):
  $100, due with response to acceptance offer
Deposit refundable prior to: May 15, 1997
Estimated number of new entrants: 93 (15 EDP)
Starting date: Aug. 1997

### TUITION AND STUDENT FEES PER YEAR FOR 1995–96 FIRST-YEAR CLASS

Tuition                    Student fees: $535
  Resident: $14,150
  Nonresident: $26,650

### INFORMATION ON 1995–96 FIRST-YEAR CLASS

| Number of | In-State | Out-of-State | Total |
|---|---|---|---|
| Applicants | 86 | 8,561 | 8,647 |
| Applicants Interviewed | 60 | 463 | 523 |
| New Entrants* | 30 | 63 | 93 |

*All took the MCAT and had baccalaureate degrees.

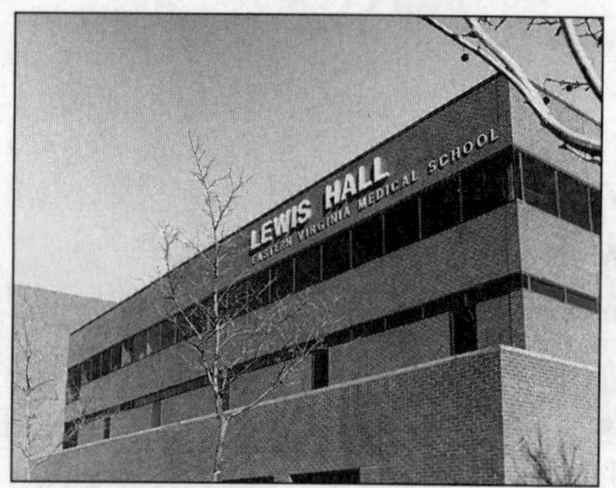

# Eastern Virginia Medical School of the Medical College of Hampton Roads

## Norfolk, Virginia


Dr. Jock R. Wheeler, *Dean/Provost*
Dr. Robert M. McCombs, *Associate Dean for Admissions and Student Affairs*
Susan L. Castora, *Coordinator of Admissions*


## ADDRESS INQUIRIES TO:

Office of Admissions
Eastern Virginia Medical School
721 Fairfax Avenue
Norfolk, Virginia 23507-2000
(804) 446-5812; 446-5817 (FAX)
Gopher Site: gopher://picard.evms.edu/1

## GENERAL INFORMATION

The Eastern Virginia Medical School (EVMS) is a community-based institution established in 1973 in response to the desire of the Hampton Roads community to improve the quality of health care throughout the eastern area of Virginia by creating an academic health center. Because of its history, the mission of EVMS is deeply rooted in educating and training primary care physicians, although interest in medical research and academic medicine is also encouraged. EVMS has committed as its top priority the implementation of a comprehensive institutional effort to revitalize its initial mission to produce primary care physicians through a series of innovative interventions established through its Center for Generalist Medicine.

With its affiliation with over 33 community-based health care facilities across the Hampton Roads area, EVMS leads the region in providing health care for more than one-quarter of the Virginia population and an important segment of the neighboring North Carolina community. EVMS is highly committed to providing a community-based education focusing on community health needs which will better equip students with the experiences most relevant to practicing medicine in the twenty-first century. Two hundred and eighty-three full-time faculty and 900 community faculty offer a diversity of resources to provide students with access to a broad range of clinical experiences and methods for the delivery of medical care.

## CURRICULUM

Throughout the first two years beginning with week one, students are introduced to early exposure to patients through a one-on-one longitudinal mentorship with a generalist physician in practice. Extensive coordination among basic sciences and generalist disciplines assures a carefully integrated generalist curriculum, required to understand the pathological, physical, and biopsychosocial aspects of health and well-being. Weekly small-group problem-solving sessions, facilitated by basic scientists and role model clinical scholars, introduce students to self-directed, clinically correlated learning. Areas covered include an array of topics related to clinical skills development, including medical interviewing, doctor-patient relationships, and medical ethics. In sum, through mentorship relationships with excellent role models, students learn accurate medical history-taking and physician examination skills and apply basic science knowledge to clinical medicine.

A substantial part of all clinical clerkships focus on ambulatory care in community-based sites in balance with basic inpatient care experiences. In addition to the required clerkships in family medicine, internal medicine, pediatrics, obstetrics and gynecology, psychiatry, and surgery are rotations in substance abuse, geriatrics, surgical subspecialties, and basic sciences. For those interested in generalist medicine, electives are offered in special populations, rural health care, and an elective honors track in generalist medicine. For those interested in research or subspecialty care, at least six months are available in elective opportunities. The Jones Institute for Reproductive Medicine, the Diabetes Center, and the Center for Pediatric Research are but a few of the excellent resources to enhance skills in research.

Extensive evaluation of clinical skills is a central component of the education process through the use of standardized patients. Students are expected to successfully pass the requirements of commencement objectives upon which progressive learning is based. Overall, students are graded as an honors, high pass, pass, or fail.

## REQUIREMENTS FOR ENTRANCE

The MCAT and a minimum of 100 college semester hours at an accredited American or Canadian college or university are required. Course work must include the following subjects:

|  | *Years* |
|---|---|
| Biology (with lab) | 1 |
| General chemistry (with lab) | 1 |
| Organic chemistry (with lab) | 1 |
| Physics (with lab) | 1 |

Applicants are expected to have grades of C or better in all required courses. Credits earned through advanced placement programs or CLEP are acceptable. Applicants may enhance their chances of acceptance by taking graduate course work in a natural science. In recent years, students matriculating at EVMS have had a mean GPA of 3.32 and have averaged 9 in each subject area of the MCAT.

## SELECTION FACTORS

EVMS does not discriminate on the basis of sex, race, creed, age, national origin, marital status, or handicap. For each applicant, the Admissions Committee considers the entire academic record, including science and overall GPA, MCAT scores, exposure to the medical field, maturity, character, and motivation. The application fee will be waived if a fee waiver is granted by AMCAS. Foreign nationals without permanent visas cannot be considered.

Preference is given to legal residents of Virginia. In addition, recognizing the goals set by the Virginia legislature, EVMS is seeking persons with personal and background traits, which indicate a high potential for becoming a family physician, general pediatrician, general internist, or a general obstetrician.

## FINANCIAL AID

The ability of a student to provide for the costs of education is not a factor in the admissions selection process. Students may fully meet the costs of medical school at EVMS, providing they meet all federal criteria, meet citizenship requirements, are credit worthy, and maintain satisfactory academic progress. Over 90 percent of the student body receives financial assistance. Scholarships are limited and loans constitute the majority of aid received. For those interested in a primary care obligation there are numerous federal and state scholarships available. Virginia residents also benefit from the state-funded Tuition Assistance Grant Program (TAGP), which provides annual grants of approximately $1,500.

Applicants for financial assistance must file the cost free FAFSA and other additional required forms. For additional details and assistance in financial planning, please contact the Office of Financial Aid at (804) 446-5813.

## INFORMATION FOR MINORITIES

Minority students are encouraged to apply. Every effort is made to evaluate these applicants giving due consideration to variances in educational and socioeconomic backgrounds. Academic scholarships are available each year for black students. EVMS has college-endorsed student organizations and faculty liaison committees that actively address minority concerns. Information is available from the minority affairs counselor, assistant dean for minority affairs.

Private Institution

## APPLICATION AND ACCEPTANCE POLICIES FOR 1997–98 FIRST-YEAR CLASS

*School participates in AMCAS. See Chapter 4.*

Filing of AMCAS application
  Earliest date: June 1, 1996
  Latest date: Nov. 15, 1996
School application fee to all applicants: $80
Oldest MCAT scores considered: 1994
Does have Early Decision Program (EDP)
  EDP application period: June 1–Aug. 1, 1996
  EDP applicants notified by: Oct. 1, 1996
Acceptance notice to regular applicants
  Earliest date: Oct. 15, 1996
  Latest date: Until class is filled
Applicant's response to acceptance offer
  Maximum time: 2 weeks
Requests for deferred entrance considered: Yes
Deposit to hold place in class (applied to tuition):
  $200, due with response to acceptance offer
Deposit refundable prior to: May 15, 1997
Estimated number of new entrants: 100 (15 EDP)
Starting date: Aug. 1997

## TUITION AND STUDENT FEES PER YEAR FOR 1995–96 FIRST-YEAR CLASS

Tuition                                    Student fees: $1,283
  Resident: $13,000
  Nonresident: $23,000

## INFORMATION ON 1995–96 FIRST-YEAR CLASS

| Number of | In-State | Out-of-State | Total |
|---|---|---|---|
| Applicants | 1,075 | 6,279 | 7,354 |
| Applicants Interviewed | 298 | 264 | 562 |
| New Entrants* | 77 | 24 | 101 |

*All had baccalaureate degrees; 96% took the MCAT.

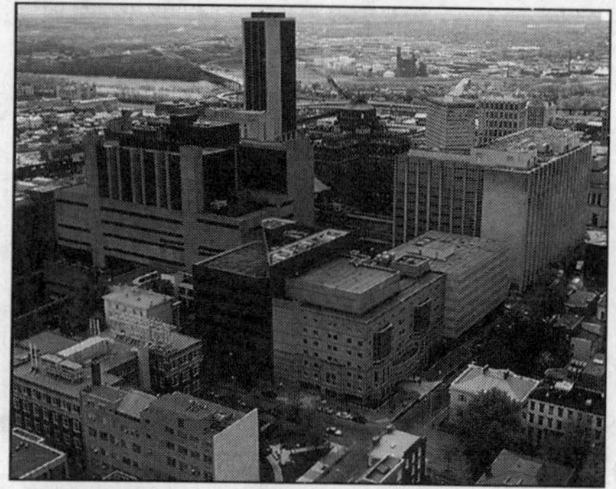

# Virginia Commonwealth University
# Medical College of Virginia School of Medicine

## Richmond, Virginia

Dr. Hermes A. Kontos, *Dean*
Cynthia M. Heldberg, *Assistant Dean for Admissions*
Marc T. Vernon, *Director of Financial Aid*

## ADDRESS INQUIRIES TO:

Medical School Admissions
Virginia Commonwealth University
Medical College of Virginia
MCV Station, Box 980565
Richmond, Virginia 23298-0565
(804) 828-9629; 828-7628 (FAX)
Web Site: http://www.vcu.edu

## GENERAL INFORMATION

The School of Medicine, which has been in continuous operation since 1838, is the founding institution of the Medical College of Virginia, Health Sciences Division of Virginia Commonwealth University. The health science campus includes not only the school of medicine but also the only school of dentistry in the state plus schools of nursing, pharmacy, basic science, and allied health professions. The vitality of MCV's research programs is reflected in the caliber of its faculty, the success of its patient care programs, and the level of research funding generated. Since the mid-1970s, federally-funded research has shown a straight line growth rate, due in part to the MCV Clinical Research Center, a program funded by the federal government since 1961. With 1,000 hospital beds at the main campus, the largest emergency room, and the largest neonatal intensive care unit in the state, plus 800 beds at one of the newest VA hospitals in the South, the Medical College of Virginia is the fourth largest university-owned medical center in the United States and affords its students an unparalleled clinical experience. The campus is located near the financial and governmental areas of downtown Richmond, the capital of Virginia and one of the South's most historic and cosmopolitan cities.

## CURRICULUM

The first year is spent studying normal structure and function in a mixture of discipline and organ system courses. Among the discipline courses, there is a coordination in the teaching of physiology and organ biochemistry. The second year emphasizes pathogenesis of disease and its manifestations and is taught in an organ system manner. Pathogenesis, pathology, pharmacology, and the major manifestations and principles of management are discussed in each of the major body systems.

There is a longitudinal experience in clinical medicine for first- and second-year students. Students spend two afternoons per month in a small group learning the fundamentals of clinical medicine. This is supplemented by a clinical experience in the office of a primary care physician two afternoons per month.

In the third year, the clinical rotations are at the University and Veterans Administration Hospitals, with ambulatory care rotations at nonuniversity primary care sites. A Learning Resource Center housed within the University Hospital supplements the information needs of students, housestaff, and faculty.

During the fourth year, the student may choose from a wide variety of electives both at the university and throughout the United States. Additionally there are elective programs serving the first and second years.

## REQUIREMENTS FOR ENTRANCE

The MCAT is required. A demonstrated competence in basic science is essential, although a science major is not required. Each matriculant must have at least 90 semester hours or equivalent in an accredited college. Courses must include:

|  | *Semesters* |
|---|---|
| Biology (with lab) | 2 |
| General chemistry (with lab) | 2 |
| Organic chemistry (with lab) | 2 |
| General physics (with lab) | 2 |
| College mathematics | 2 |
| English | 2 |

Applicants are urged to take the MCAT in the spring of the year of application and no later than the fall of that year. Early Decision Program applicants must have MCAT scores available when applying. The school has a guaranteed admissions program with Virginia Commonwealth University's undergraduate honors program. High school seniors who have 1200 or better on their SAT's and a GPA of 3.5 may apply. They must complete the usual pre-med requirements, all honors program requirements, and maintain a 3.5 GPA throughout their undergraduate years.

## SELECTION FACTORS

Applicants are selected on the basis of their potential as prospective physicians as well as students of medicine. Attributes of character, personality factors, and academic skills are considered along with academic performance, GPA, MCAT scores, letters of recommendation, and personal interviews at the School of Medicine.

The school gives preference to bona fide residents of the Commonwealth of Virginia and does not discriminate on the basis of age, race, sex, creed, national origin, or handicap. Foreign nationals must be permanent residents at the time of application.

The 1995 entering class of 174 students had the following credentials: *undergraduate major,* 25 percent in arts or humanities, 74 percent in sciences; *degrees,* 13 percent with graduate degrees, including 4 doctorate degrees; *residence,* 71.3 percent Virginia residents; *minorities,* 9.2 percent black; *sex,* 42.5 percent women; *overall undergraduate GPA,* 3.45; *MCAT average score,* 9.6. Qualified applicants with a sincere interest in the Medical College of Virginia are encouraged to apply through the Early Decision Program. Each year approximately 14 percent of the class is selected in this manner.

The uniform acceptance date is October 15 with additional selections in December and February. Applicants who have been rejected in previous years should demonstrate significant improvement in their academic credentials before reapplying.

## FINANCIAL AID

Assistance to students in meeting the cost of their medical education is available in the form of loans, scholarships, College Work-Study Program, and financial counseling offered by the Financial Aid Office of the Medical College of Virginia. The FAFSA is used in awarding need-based aid (see Part 1). Parent information should be included on this form to be considered for Health and Human Services Programs.

The university's Financial Aid Department administers all major federal aid programs and coordinates with the School of Medicine in the administration of state, private, and institutional scholarships and loans. The Financial Aid Department makes a written response to every student request. Application forms and aid fact sheets are available in mid-January of each year. Applications for aid may be made prior to notification of acceptance by the School of Medicine. Applicants are encouraged to seek all resources available to them and apply as early as feasible to maximize the possibility of obtaining funding.

Information may be obtained from the following address: Financial Aid Office, Medical College of Virginia, School of Medicine, Box 565-MCV Station, Richmond, Virginia 23298; the location is 12th and Broad Streets in Richmond.

Public Institution

## APPLICATION AND ACCEPTANCE POLICIES FOR 1997–98 FIRST-YEAR CLASS

*School participates in AMCAS. See Chapter 4.*

Filing of AMCAS application
 Earliest date: June 1, 1996
 Latest date: Nov. 15, 1996
School application fee to all applicants: $75
Oldest MCAT scores considered: 1993
Does have Early Decision Program (EDP)
 EDP application period: June 1–Aug. 1, 1996
 EDP applicants notified by: Oct. 1, 1996
Acceptance notice to regular applicants
 Earliest date: Oct. 15, 1996
 Latest date: Until class is filled
Applicant's response to acceptance offer
 Maximum time: 2 weeks
Requests for deferred entrance considered: Yes
Deposit to hold place in class (applied to tuition):
 $100, due with response to acceptance offer
Deposit refundable prior to: May 15, 1997
Estimated number of new entrants: 174 (30 EDP)
Starting date: Aug. 1997

## TUITION AND STUDENT FEES PER YEAR FOR 1995–96 FIRST-YEAR CLASS

Tuition                    Student fees: $1,008
 Resident: $9,552
 Nonresident: $23,317

## INFORMATION ON 1995–96 FIRST-YEAR CLASS

| *Number of* | *In-State* | *Out-of-State* | *Total* |
|---|---|---|---|
| Applicants | 1,183 | 4,114 | 5,297 |
| Applicants Interviewed | 432 | 427 | 859 |
| New Entrants* | 124 | 50 | 174 |

*All had baccalaureate degrees; 94% took the MCAT.

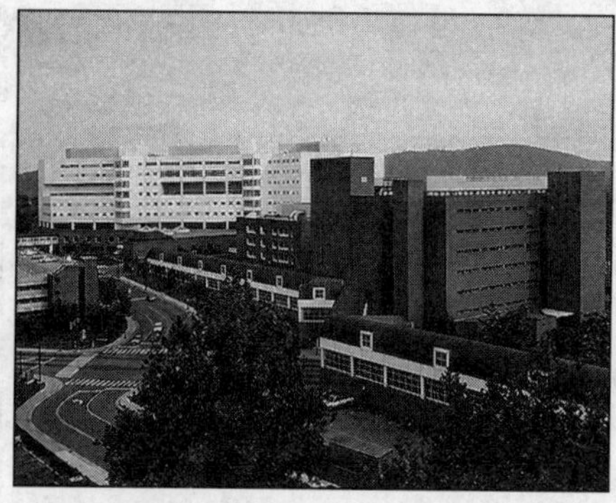

# University of Virginia School of Medicine

## Charlottesville, Virginia

Dr. Robert M. Carey, *Dean*
Dr. B. C. Sturgill, *Associate Dean of Admission*
Beth A. Bailey, *Director of Admissions*

## ADDRESS INQUIRIES TO:

Medical School Admissions Office, Box 235
University of Virginia
School of Medicine
Charlottesville, Virginia 22908
(804) 924-5571; 982-2586 (FAX)
Web Site: http://www.med.virginia.edu/home.html

## GENERAL INFORMATION

Authorized by Thomas Jefferson, the University of Virginia School of Medicine was opened for instruction in 1825, making it one of the oldest medical schools in the South.

Both the School of Medicine and the University of Virginia Hospital are located on the grounds of the University of Virginia in Charlottesville. The University of Virginia Medical Center has 757 beds, consisting of the new hospital (582 beds and 31 bassinets), the Kluge Children's Rehabilitation Center (30 beds), nearby Blue Ridge Hospital (114 beds), and a primary care center.

## CURRICULUM

Courses in the first year focus on the basic and clinical sciences that are requisite to understanding physical and psychological aspects of human health. The second-year curriculum focuses on disease and is coordinated with the problem-oriented Introduction to Clinical Medicine course.

The remainder of the curriculum consists of 12 months of required clinical clerkships and 8 months of elective opportunities. During the clerkships, the learning experience focuses on the social, ethical, and biomedical factors required for excellence in patient care. Teaching occurs primarily at the bedside; small tutorial seminars, lectures, and group discussions are also conducted. In addition to the clinical clerkships at the University of Virginia Hospital, all students can expect to have part of their clerkship experience at an affiliated hospital under the direction of full-time faculty members.

Students selected for the newly instituted Generalist Scholars Program receive enhanced training in disease prevention, health promotion, subtance abuse, family therapy, clinical epidemiology, and office procedural skills. The elective program of the fourth year offers students the opportunity to pursue widely their own interests and abilities and to sample diverse training experiences in medical centers from Alaska to South America. Students may choose from a variety of electives, including clinical experiences, graduate courses, and research activities. A summer elective program in family medicine is offered to a limited number of entering students.

Many opportunities exist for students who are interested in medical research. Prominent among these opportunities are the Summer Research Program and the Medical Scientist Training Program (MSTP). The MSTP is an accelerated program which leads to combined M.D. and Ph.D. degrees and which utilizes the facilities of both the School of Medicine and the Graduate School of Arts and Sciences. It is designed specifically to prepare a limited number of highly qualified men and women for careers in both research and clinical medicine. Information about this program is included in the supplementary application materials sent to each medical school applicant.

## REQUIREMENTS FOR ENTRANCE

The MCAT is required and must be taken no later than the fall of the year of application and no earlier than spring of 1994. The minimum undergraduate college requirement for admission is 90 semester hours of graded course work in a U.S. or Canadian school; however, it is unusual to accept students who will not have received the baccalaureate degree by the time of enrollment. Without exception the following courses are required:

|  | *Years* |
| --- | --- |
| Biology (with lab) | 1 |
| General chemistry (with lab) | 1 |
| Organic chemistry (with lab) | 1 |
| General physics (with lab) | 1 |

Ordinarily, these courses are considered invalid if at the time of matriculation more than seven years have elapsed since their completion, but the committee will consider appropriate requests for a waiver of this rule.

Other than these courses, the college curriculum for the premedical student should be planned in accord with individual interests and aptitudes to gain as broad an educational background as possible.

Advanced placement credit is acceptable if such credit is indicated on the undergraduate college transcripts as having been accepted by the college toward fulfillment of requirements for the bachelor's degree. Students are expected to pursue advanced courses if advanced placement credit was awarded for any of the required science courses (including laboratory work).

## SELECTION FACTORS

Preference is given to residents of Virginia. Applications from well qualified nonresidents are welcomed, but early application is advised. Foreign nationals should have baccalaureate degrees from American or Canadian colleges or universities; reapplicants should show significant improvement in their applications. The Committee on Admissions does not discriminate on the basis of race, gender, sexual preference, creed, national origin, age, or handicap.

In addition to numerical criteria, such factors as extracurricular activities, difficulty of curriculum and trends of performance, work and volunteer experience, diversity of interests, enthusiasm and communication skills as revealed in the application, recommendations, and the interview influence committee decisions. The Admissions Committee does not grant regional interviews or interviews by applicant request.

The class entering in 1995 had a mean GPA of 3.54 and mean MCAT scores in the 85th percentile.

## FINANCIAL AID

In addition to loans from the standard federal programs (see Part 1), school-funded scholarships and loans are available to students who demonstrate need via analysis of the family's financial situation by the College Scholarship Service (CSS). Parental financial information is required of all applicants for school-funded aid. Approximately 80 percent of the student body receive financial aid. Student employment is not encouraged. Financial aid applications should be requested by January 1. For more information, contact Catherine Anas, director of financial aid.

## INFORMATION FOR MINORITY STUDENTS

This institution is committed to increasing the representation of minority physicians in medicine. To this end, we welcome applications from competitive out-of-state and in-state minority students. Structures in place to facilitate preparation and success of students include: (1) content based MCAT program; (2) pre-matriculation academic advancement summer program for those accepted into the School of Medicine; (3) extensive tutorial and other academic support programs upon admission; and (4) need-based financial assistance. Early completion of application for admission is strongly recommended. The Admissions Committee includes minority members, and a team of committed faculty and administrators provides support at all levels for minority students.

Public Institution

## APPLICATION AND ACCEPTANCE POLICIES FOR 1997–98 FIRST-YEAR CLASS

*School participates in AMCAS. See Chapter 4.*

Filing of AMCAS application
    Earliest date: June 1, 1996
    Latest date: Nov. 1, 1996
School application fee to all applicants: $50
Oldest MCAT scores considered: 1994
Does not have Early Decision Program
Acceptance notice to regular applicants
    Earliest date: Oct. 15, 1996
    Latest date: Until class is filled
Applicant's response to acceptance offer
    Maximum time: 3 weeks
Requests for deferred entrance considered: Yes
Deposit to hold place in class: None
Estimated number of new entrants: 139
Starting date: Aug. 1997

## TUITION AND STUDENT FEES PER YEAR FOR 1995–96 FIRST-YEAR CLASS

Tuition                    Student fees: $922
    Resident: $8,484
    Nonresident: $20,458

## INFORMATION ON 1995–96 FIRST-YEAR CLASS

| Number of | In-State | Out-of-State | Total |
|---|---|---|---|
| Applicants | 1,041 | 4,395 | 5,436 |
| Applicants Interviewed | 239 | 240 | 479 |
| New Entrants* | 98 | 41 | 139 |

*All took the MCAT and had baccalaureate degrees.

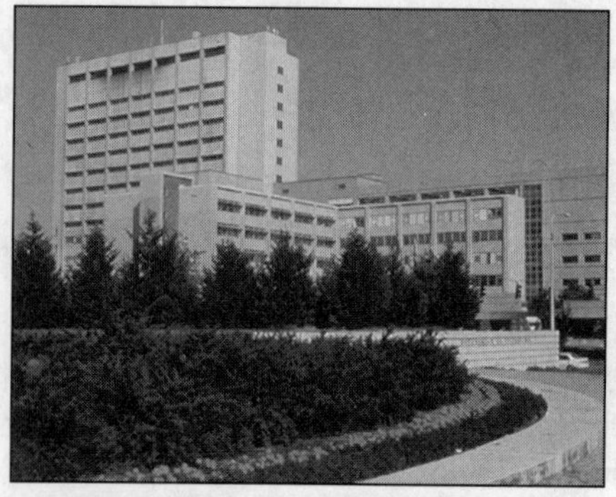

# University of Washington School of Medicine

**Seattle, Washington**

Dr. Philip J. Fialkow, *Dean*
Dr. Werner E. Samson, *Assistant Dean for Admissions*
Patricia T. Fero, *Admissions Officer*

## ADDRESS INQUIRIES TO:

Admissions Office
Health Sciences Center A-300, Box 356340
University of Washington
Seattle, Washington 98195-6340
(206) 543-7212
E-Mail: patf@u.washington.edu

## GENERAL INFORMATION

The University of Washington School of Medicine was established in 1945. For complete information about policies, procedures, and programs, candidates are referred to the current University of Washington School of Medicine Bulletin, available from the school.

## CURRICULUM

The first two years of the curriculum are identified as the basic organ system curriculum. It consists of three phases or groups of courses: pre-organ system courses; organ systems taught by basic and clinical disciplines; and introduction to clinical medicine and health care. The academic demands of the basic curriculum are scaled so that most students will be able to take elective courses.

The clinical curriculum is pursued predominantly in the third and fourth years. It includes three elements: prescribed clerkships to be completed by all students in medicine, obstetrics-gynecology, pediatrics, psychiatry, and surgery; a clinical selective series requiring a minimum number of credits in three clinical areas (family medicine, rehabilitation medicine/chronic care, and emergency care/trauma); and clinical clerkships elected by the student. The Independent Study in Medical Science requirement enables students to gain an understanding of the philosophy and methods of science as they relate to their chosen field of medicine.

One aspect of the curriculum is the WAMI program of decentralized medical education (see Chapter 4). All students enrolled at the University of Washington School of Medicine may receive as part of this program a portion of training at sites away from the University of Washington campus. Offers of acceptance, therefore, are conditional upon agreement to participate in the WAMI program.

## REQUIREMENTS FOR ENTRANCE

The MCAT taken in the spring of 1994 or thereafter is required. This exam must be taken no later than the autumn of the year before possible matriculation. Under exceptional circumstances, the GRE may be considered during the admissions process; however, if accepted, the applicant will be required to take the MCAT prior to matriculation. The following course requirements must be completed before matriculation:

|  | *Sem. hrs.* |
| --- | --- |
| Biology | 8 |
| Chemistry | 12 |

(May be satisfied by taking any combination of inorganic, organic, biochemistry, or molecular biology courses)

| | |
| --- | --- |
| Physics | 4 |
| Other science | 8 |

(May be satisfied by taking other courses in any of the above categories)

Proficiency in English, basic mathematics, and information technologies is also required. An understanding of the basic concepts underlying biochemistry and/or molecular biology is strongly encouraged.

Under exceptional circumstances, certain course requirements may be waived for individuals with unusual achievements and academic promise.

A minimum of three years of college is required; however, 99 to 100 percent of entrants in recent years have fulfilled requirements for a bachelor's degree. No major is preferred, but a broad educational background is encouraged.

Applicants who are seriously considered will be requested to submit supplemental information, one part of which will be a premedical committee evaluation or three individual letters submitted from instructors who have taught the candidate in a collegiate course (a mixture of evaluations from the sciences and humanities is recommended). In addition, signed documentation indicating the student's ability to meet our essential requirements (with or without reasonable accommodations) for graduation, as well as authorization for a criminal background check (necessitated by Washington state law) is required.

All supplemental materials must be submitted by January 15, 1997. Early submission of application and supplemental materials is encouraged.

Candidates who wish to be considered for the M.D.-Ph.D. program must submit the Medical Scientist Training Program application. This application is sent to all eligible candidates along with the acknowledgment of receipt of the medical school application. All candidates considered eligible for this program after initial review of the MSTP application will be requested to send further supplementary materials.

## SELECTION FACTORS

Candidates for admission are considered comparatively on the basis of academic performance, motivation, maturity, personal integrity, and demonstrated humanitarian qualities. A knowledge of and exposure to the needs of individuals and society and an awareness of health care delivery systems are essential. Extenuating circumstances in an applicant's background are evaluated as they relate to these selection factors.

Students entering in the fall of 1995 had a mean GPA of 3.58. Mean scores on the MCAT were as follows: *VR*-9.9, *PS*-10.2, *BS*-10.3, *WS*-P.

Residents of the states of Washington, Alaska, Montana, or Idaho are eligible to apply. MSTP applicants are considered regardless of residency, as are applicants from underrepresented ethnic minority backgrounds (African American, Mexican American, Native American, and Mainland Puerto Rican). Foreign applicants, in addition to the above requirements, must also have a permanent resident visa.

After the completed applications are screened, applicants considered to be competitive will be invited to Seattle for an interview.

## FINANCIAL AID

Financial status has no bearing on chances for admission. All applicants for aid must submit data for an analysis of need through the FAFSA (see Part 1). The application receipt deadline of February 28 must be met, regardless of admission date, in order to receive highest priority for aid; applicants should mail this form mid-February or earlier. Approximately eighty percent of the student body receive some form of aid, most of which is in the form of loans. Financial aid applications are available in January. Contact the School of Medicine's Financial Aid Office at (206) 685-2520.

## INFORMATION FOR UNDERREPRESENTED MINORITY OR DISADVANTAGED STUDENTS

The Minority Affairs Program is actively involved in the identification, recruitment, retention, and professional development of students from underrepresented ethnic minority and/or disadvantaged backgrounds, who are interested in pursuing M.D. or M.D.-Ph.D. degrees. The program offers the Minority Medical Education Program (MMEP) for pre-med students and the Summer Prematriculation Program for entering medical students. It also provides a range of student services and faculty development programs through its Native American Center of Excellence. Tutoring, counseling, and a variety of other student support services are also available. For more information, please call (206) 685-2489, or visit our MMEP home page at http://weber.u.washington.edu/~dolson/mmep.html.

Public Institution

## APPLICATION AND ACCEPTANCE POLICIES FOR 1997–98 FIRST-YEAR CLASS

*School participates in AMCAS. See Chapter 4.*

Filing of AMCAS application
Earliest date: June 1, 1996
Latest date: Nov. 1, 1996
School application fee to all applicants: $35
Oldest MCAT scores considered: 1994
Does not have Early Decision Program (EDP)
Acceptance notice to regular applicants
Earliest date: Nov. 1, 1996
Latest date: May 5, 1997
Applicant's response to acceptance offer
Maximum time: 2 weeks
Requests for deferred entrance considered: Yes
Deposit to hold place in class (applied to tuition):
$100, due with response to acceptance offer;
nonrefundable
Estimated number of new entrants: 166
Starting date: Sept. 1997

## TUITION AND STUDENT FEES PER YEAR FOR 1995–96 FIRST-YEAR CLASS

Tuition and student fees:
Resident: $7,752
Nonresident: $19,686

## INFORMATION ON 1995–96 FIRST-YEAR CLASS

| Number of | In-State* | Out-of-State | Total |
|---|---|---|---|
| Applicants | 975 | 2,948 | 3,923 |
| Applicants Interviewed | 681 | 75 | 756 |
| New Entrants† | 111 | 9 | 120 |

*In-state figures include Washington, Alaska, Montana, and Idaho residents.

†All took the MCAT and had baccalaureate degrees.

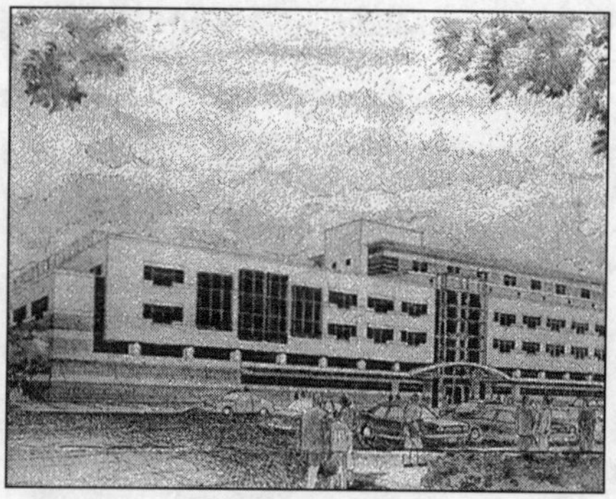

# Marshall University School of Medicine

## Huntington, West Virginia

Dr. Charles H. McKown, Jr., *Vice President and Dean*
Cynthia A. Warren, *Director of Admissions*
Dr. Jack L. Toney, *Director of Student Financial Assistance*

## ADDRESS INQUIRIES TO:

Admissions Office
Marshall University
School of Medicine
1542 Spring Valley Drive
Huntington, West Virginia 25704
(304) 696-7312; (800) 544-8514

## GENERAL INFORMATION

The Marshall University School of Medicine was developed under the Veterans Administration Medical Assistance and Health Training Act passed by Congress in 1972. The School of Medicine was granted full accreditation and graduated its first class in 1981.

The School of Medicine is a community-based program with emphasis on the education of primary care physicians. The teaching affiliates of the School of Medicine include hospitals in Huntington and other communities in West Virginia.

## CURRICULUM

In the first year, the basic sciences courses of anatomy, physiology, neurosciences, medical cell and molecular biology, and biochemistry are supplemented by a clinical interdepartmental course entitled introduction to patient care, which covers early physical diagnosis and behavioral medicine. The second year includes pharmacology, pathology, microbiology, genetics, psychopathology, community medicine, physical diagnosis, immunology, and introduction to clinical medicine. During the third and fourth years, students are rotated through clerkships at participating community hospitals and other locations in the clinical fields of medicine, surgery, pediatrics, psychiatry, family practice, obstetrics-gynecology, and emergency medicine. Several rural health care programs are available for students who demonstrate special interest in primary care medicine. Twenty-three weeks are devoted to electives in the senior year. A standard letter grading system (A, B, C, D, F) is utilized.

## REQUIREMENTS FOR ENTRANCE

The MCAT is required. The baccalaureate degree is preferred. However, exceptionally well qualified students with three years of college education or the equivalent may be considered for admission. Minimum course requirements are:

|  | Sem. hrs. |
| --- | --- |
| General biology or zoology (with lab) | 8 |
| Inorganic chemistry (with lab) | 8 |
| Organic chemistry (with lab) | 8 |
| Physics (with lab) | 8 |
| English composition and rhetoric | 6 |
| Behavioral or social sciences | 6 |

With the exception of these specific courses, applicants are encouraged to pursue their personal educational interests. Quality of course work rather than the field in which it is taken is the more important consideration.

It is urged that applicants take the MCAT in the spring of the year of application but no later than the fall of that year.

## SELECTION FACTORS

There is no discrimination because of race, sex, religion, age, handicap, sexual orientation, or national origin. Qualified members of minority groups are encouraged to apply.

Applicants are evaluated on the basis of their academic records, MCAT scores, recommendations from instructors, and personal qualifications as judged through interviews. Interviews are arranged only by invitation of the Admissions Committee.

Academic achievement alone is not a sufficient foundation for success in the profession of medicine. Applicants must exhibit excellence in character, motivation, and ideals. Behavioral qualities deemed essential for a career in medicine include, but are not limited to, good judgment, integrity, responsibility, and sensitivity.

As a state-assisted institution, the School of Medicine gives preference in selection of students to West Virginia residents. A limited number of positions will be available to well qualified nonresidents from states contiguous to West Virginia or to nonresidents who have strong ties to West Virginia. Other nonresidents are not considered. Only applicants who are U.S. citizens or who have permanent resident visas are eligible for admission.

The August 1995 entering class had the following profile: *resident,* 94 percent West Virginia residents; *mean overall GPA,* 3.4; *gender,* 24 percent women; *undergraduate major,* 80 percent in biological sciences, chemistry or preprofessional curriculum; *degrees,* 43 bachelor's degrees, 1 master's degree, 2 doctoral degrees and 3 students without baccalaureate degrees; *undergraduate schools,* 28 students attended West Virginia schools.

The School of Medicine considers for transfer admissions those applicants who are currently in good standing at an allopathic medical school. Positions are limited by attrition and are rarely available. The residency policy for regular admissions also applies to transfer admissions.

## FINANCIAL AID

The financial needs of the applicant are not a consideration in the admissions process. There is a variety of resources for financial assistance available to medical students. Currently 90 percent of the students are receiving financial assistance. Further information and applications for financial aid may be obtained from Marshall at the following address: Office of Financial Assistance, Marshall University, Huntington, West Virginia 25755.

Because of the rigorous nature of the medical program, students are advised not to attempt outside employment during the academic year.

The supplemental application fee will be waived for individuals who have been granted an AMCAS fee waiver.

Public Institution

## APPLICATION AND ACCEPTANCE POLICIES FOR 1997–98 FIRST-YEAR CLASS

*School participates in AMCAS. See Chapter 4.*

Filing of AMCAS application
    Earliest date: June 1, 1996
    Latest date: Nov. 15, 1996
School application fee to all applicants:
    Residents: $30
    Nonresidents: $50
Oldest MCAT scores considered: 1994
Does have Early Decision Program (EDP)
    For West Virginia residents only
    EDP application period: June 1–Aug. 1, 1996
    EDP applicants notified by: Oct. 1, 1996
Acceptance notice to regular applicants
    Earliest date: Oct. 15, 1996
    Latest date: Until class is filled
Applicant's response to acceptance offer
    Maximum time: 2 weeks
Requests for deferred entrance considered: Yes
Deposit to hold place in class: None
Estimated number of new entrants: 48 (10 EDP)
Starting date: Aug. 1997

## TUITION AND STUDENT FEES PER YEAR FOR 1995–96 FIRST-YEAR CLASS

Tuition                  Student fees: $450
    Resident: $7,784
    Nonresident: $18,210

## INFORMATION ON 1995–96 FIRST-YEAR CLASS

| Number of | In-State | Out-of-State | Total |
|---|---|---|---|
| Applicants | 305 | 1,159 | 1,464 |
| Applicants Interviewed | 253 | 20 | 273 |
| New Entrants* | 46 | 3 | 49 |

*All took the MCAT; 94% had baccalaureate degrees.

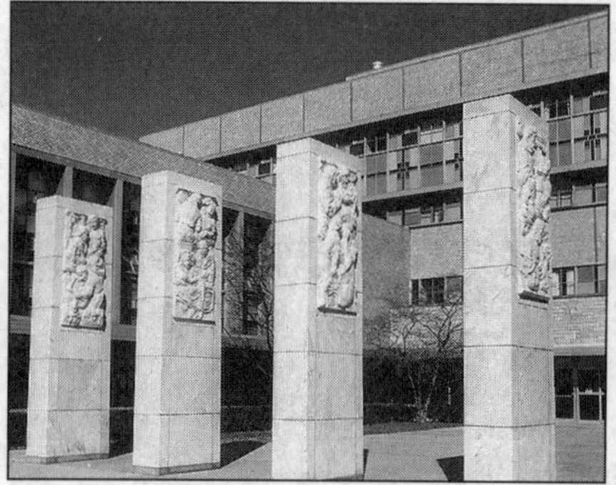

# West Virginia University School of Medicine

## Morgantown, West Virginia

Dr. Robert D'Alessandri, *Dean*
Dr. John W. Traubert, *Associate Dean for Student Affairs*
Kenneth Sears, *Financial Aid Officer*

## ADDRESS INQUIRIES TO:

Office of Admissions and Records
West Virginia University
Health Sciences Center
P.O. Box 9815
Morgantown, West Virginia 26506
(304) 293-3521; 293-7968 (FAX)
E-Mail: dhall@wvuhsc1.hsc.wvu.edu

## GENERAL INFORMATION

West Virginia University, a public institution, has offered the first two years of the medical curriculum continuously since 1902. Three decades ago the Health Sciences Center was established, including the School of Medicine and the schools of dentistry, nursing, and pharmacy. A modern physical plant provides facilities for the schools, including three hospitals— the 400-bed Ruby Memorial Hospital, the 80-bed Chestnut Ridge Psychiatric Hospital, and the 80-bed Mountainview Rehabilitation Hospital—and a cancer center. Clinical instruction is also provided in the Charleston Division of the Health Sciences Center.

Some university housing is available for both married and unmarried students.

## CURRICULUM

The educational program of the School of Medicine is designed to provide students with a foundation upon which they can base further preparation for any branch of medicine, specifically primary care, other specialty practice, teaching, research, or a combination of these career objectives.

In the first and second years the plan of study is directed toward the principles and methodology of the basic medical sciences. However, the basic courses are designed so that the student begins to synthesize concepts of patient care. The first-year basic science courses are integrated through common test methods and through problem-based learning clinical applications. Clinical experiences are introduced the second semester of the first year through behavioral medicine and psychiatry. Summer externships are available in all primary care fields. Additional early exposure to patient-oriented instruction is through the introduction to clinical medicine, community medicine, and other behavioral medicine courses during the second basic science year.

A traditional third-year curriculum gives the student a foundation in history-taking, examination, patient relations, laboratory aids, diagnosis, treatment, and use of medical literature in the major clinical disciplines.

The fourth year is composed of requirements (50 percent) and electives (50 percent). Requirements include critical care medicine, primary care ambulatory medicine, surgical subspecialties, and medicine, family practice, or pediatrics subinternship.

Students with exceptional interest and promise will be considered for the Medical Scientist M.D.-Ph.D. program. The Ph.D. is offered in nine disciplines.

An honors/satisfactory/unsatisfactory grading system is used in the School of Medicine.

## REQUIREMENTS FOR ENTRANCE

The MCAT and a minimum of three years of college (minimum of 90 semester hours or equivalent) are required. All required courses must be passed with a grade of C or better. College work must include:

|  | Sem. hrs. |
|---|---|
| Biology (with lab) | 8 |
| Inorganic chemistry (with lab) | 8 |
| Organic chemistry (with lab) | 8 |
| General physics (with lab) | 8 |
| English | 6 |
| Behavioral or social sciences | 6 |

The best prepared applicants will have completed a course in biochemistry and in cell/molecular biology. Fundamental competence in communication skills is emphasized as a great need. Additional course work should be designed to provide breadth leading toward a bachelor's degree in a major field of the applicant's own choosing, not necessarily in the natural sciences nor in a premedical curriculum.

Applicants are strongly encouraged to take the MCAT in April of the year before they hope to enter medical school. Applicants may apply as early as June 15 and normally should apply no later than mid-August. Interviews are held on site only beginning in September. No applicant is admitted without an interview. Acceptances will be issued periodically throughout the interview period.

Transfer applications are accepted from medical students who are in good academic and professional standing. Students from other doctoral-level programs (dental, podiatric, graduate, etc.) are ineligible. With the exception of West Virginia residents, advanced standing applicants must transfer from LCME-accredited medical schools.

## SELECTION FACTORS

There is no discrimination because of race, creed, sex, or age. Qualified members of minority groups are encouraged to apply. The Health Careers Opportunity Program is available for minority students. Choice of students is based upon scholarship, MCAT scores, and personal qualifications as judged by interviews and recommendations from qualified persons.

As a state-supported school, the School of Medicine gives preference in selection of students to West Virginia residents, but places may be available each year to well qualified non-residents. Although most students present a bachelor's degree at matriculation, a small number of carefully selected individuals are admitted at the end of three years of college work.

A select number of students will be required to spend their clinical years at the Charleston Division of the West Virginia University School of Medicine.

The 1995 entering class had the following profile: *residence,* 97 percent West Virginia residents; *mean overall GPA,* 3.61; *mean MCAT scores, VR*-9.2, *PS*-8.9, *WS*-O, *BS*-9.1; *sex,* 36 percent women; *undergraduate major,* 74 percent in biological sciences, chemistry, or preprofessional curriculum; *degrees,* 80 bachelor's degrees, 8 graduate degrees; *undergraduate schools,* 55 students attended West Virginia schools.

## FINANCIAL AID

A limited number of scholarship awards are available to well qualified students based on financial need. In addition, multiple loan funds are also available. Students' spouses with reasonable training and experience ordinarily have no difficulty in finding work near the medical school, the university, or Morgantown.

---

Public Institution

## APPLICATION AND ACCEPTANCE POLICIES FOR 1997–98 FIRST-YEAR CLASS

*School participates in AMCAS. See Chapter 4.*

Filing of AMCAS application
    Earliest date: June 1, 1996
    Latest date: Nov. 15, 1996
School application fee to all applicants: $30
Oldest MCAT scores considered: 1994
Does have Early Decision Program (EDP)
    For West Virginia residents only
    EDP application period: June 1–Aug. 1, 1996
    EDP applitants notified by: Oct. 1, 1996
Acceptance notice to regular applicants
    Earliest date: Oct. 15, 1996
    Latest date: Until class is filled
Applicant's response to acceptance offer
    Maximum time: 2 weeks
Requests for deferred entrance considered: Yes
Deposit to hold place in class (applied to tuition):
    $100, due with response to acceptance offer
Deposit refundable prior to: May 15, 1997
Estimated number of new entrants: 88 (8 EDP)
Starting date: Aug. 1997

## TUITION AND STUDENT FEES PER YEAR FOR 1995–96 FIRST-YEAR CLASS

| Tuition | Student fees: |
|---|---|
| Resident: $1,640 | Resident: $6,340 |
| Nonresident: $4,550 | Nonresident: $15,164 |

## INFORMATION ON 1995–96 FIRST-YEAR CLASS

| Number of | In-State | Out-of-State | Total |
|---|---|---|---|
| Applicants | 278 | 1,514 | 1,792 |
| Applicants Interviewed | 236 | 48 | 284 |
| New Entrants* | 85 | 3 | 88 |

*All took the MCAT and had baccalaureate degrees.

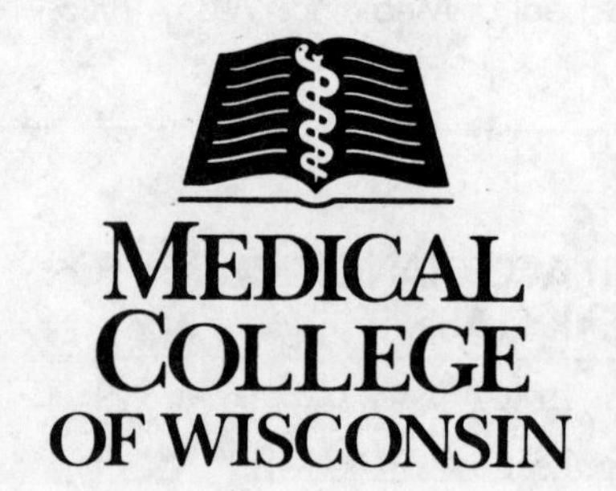

# Medical College of Wisconsin

## Milwaukee, Wisconsin

Dr. Michael J. Dunn, *Dean and Executive Vice President*
Lesley A. Mack, *Director of Admissions and Registrar*
Ruth K. Goldberg, *Director of Student Financial Services*

## ADDRESS INQUIRIES TO:

Office of Admissions and Registrar
Medical College of Wisconsin
8701 Watertown Plank Road
Milwaukee, Wisconsin 53226
(414) 456-8246

## GENERAL INFORMATION

With roots going back to the last century, the Medical College of Wisconsin became an independent, freestanding school of medicine in 1967. Located on the campus of the Milwaukee Regional Medical Center, it is a private medical school with a public mission of education, research, patient care, and community service. Strong relationships and special educational programs are maintained with other educational institutions throughout Wisconsin. Major affiliated teaching hospitals include the Froedtert Memorial Lutheran Hospital, Clement J. Zablocki Veterans Affairs Medical Center, and the Children's Hospital of Wisconsin. Additional affiliations with both private and community hospitals bring the number of teaching beds available for clinical education to over 7,000.

## CURRICULUM

The curriculum is designed to provide a solid foundation for a career in any discipline of medicine. In the first two years, students acquire a thorough knowledge of the basic medical sciences. Courses in anatomy, neuroscience, biochemistry, physiology, biostatistics, and psychiatry comprise the first year. The second-year courses include microbiology, pathology, pharmacology, and psychiatry. The clinical continuum provides first- and second-year students with integrated early generalist experiences, the fundamental skills and attitudes of professional development, and knowledge in the following disciplines: human behavior, bioethics and care of the terminally ill, information management, physical diagnosis, and health care systems.

The third year consists of a brief introduction to clinical skills course, followed by two-month clerkships in medicine, surgery, obstetrics-gynecology, pediatrics, and a combination of psychiatry and anesthesiology. In addition, students have a four-week clerkship in ambulatory medicine, with continuing longitudinal experience in the same clinic setting. Students may also select a two- to four-week elective experience.

During the fourth year, students complete one-month rotations in ward medicine, surgery, a medical selective, and six one-month electives.

Students with a particular interest in research can pursue a variety of options, including the Honors in Research program or joint M.S.-M.D. or M.D.-Ph.D. degree programs. Two students are selected annually for the Medical Scientist Training Program, which culminates with the awarding of both the M.D. and Ph.D. degrees at the end of a seven-year period of study. A five-year extended curriculum is available to students who wish to carry out their studies in the M.D. program over a longer period of time.

## REQUIREMENTS FOR ENTRANCE

All applicants must take the MCAT, usually in the spring or summer of the year in which they apply. A minimum of three years of undergraduate work (90 semester hours) is required; however, almost all students entering the Medical College of Wisconsin have completed a baccalaureate degree. Because the school accepts students from a variety of major fields of study, students are encouraged to determine their fields of major study according to their personal interest. Each prospective medical student must take the following courses for graded credit at an accredited college or university in the United States or Canada:

*Semester Hours*

Biology (with lab) . . . . . . . . . . . . . . . . . . . . . . . . . . . . . . . . 8
General chemistry (with lab) . . . . . . . . . . . . . . . . . . . . . . . 8
Organic chemistry (with lab) . . . . . . . . . . . . . . . . . . . . . . . 8
Physics . . . . . . . . . . . . . . . . . . . . . . . . . . . . . . . . . . . . . . . . 8
English . . . . . . . . . . . . . . . . . . . . . . . . . . . . . . . . . . . . . . . . 6
 Should stress composition
Mathematics
 Completion of a course in algebra in high
 school or college.

Students must be capable of expressing themselves effectively, both orally and in writing.

## SELECTION FACTORS

The college seeks students who are well suited to a competent and ethical practice of medicine. Successful applicants will have a mature sense of values, sound motivation, demonstrated academic achievement, and the willingness and ability to assume responsibility.

The selection of students is based on a careful analysis of each candidate's suitability for the profession of medicine. Undergraduate achievement and MCAT scores are carefully evaluated, but academic excellence alone does not assure acceptance. Subjective factors, including the candidate's statement in the AMCAS application, academic recommendations, and personal interviews are also important.

Interviews are an integral part of the admissions process, and all applicants being seriously considered are interviewed before being offered an acceptance. Interviews are scheduled only at the request of the Admissions Committee, following a review of the application.

The Medical College of Wisconsin accepts about half of its entering class from Wisconsin, with the remainder coming from other states. Women comprised 35 percent of the 1995 entering class. The Medical College of Wisconsin does not discriminate on the basis of race, gender, creed, disability, age, national origin, or sexual orientation.

## FINANCIAL AID

Most financial assistance available through the college, including federal and institutional scholarships and loans, is awarded solely on the basis of need. The Financial Aid Office develops a financial aid package for each student, based upon individual needs. The office helps direct students to additional sources of support. Applicants are strongly encouraged to initiate their financial aid application as soon as they have been interviewed. Because of restrictions placed on loan and scholarship funds, foreign citizens are not eligible for financial aid. All foreign applicants must file proof of financial support before they are eligible for acceptance.

## INFORMATION FOR MINORITIES

The Medical College of Wisconsin actively seeks applications from talented minority students, particularly those who are Wisconsin residents. In addition to academic achievement, MCAT scores, letters of recommendation, and personal interviews, the Admissions Committee carefully considers the student's motivation, cultural, and educational background. Through the Office of Minority Affairs, a variety of programs exist to assist minority students, demonstrating the college's strong commitment to the recruitment, retention, and graduation of underrepresented and disadvantaged minority students. Further information concerning programs for minority students may be obtained from the associate dean for minority student affairs.

Private Institution

## APPLICATION AND ACCEPTANCE POLICIES FOR 1997–98 FIRST-YEAR CLASS

*School participates in AMCAS. See Chapter 4.*

Filing of AMCAS application
    Earliest date: June 1, 1996
    Latest date: Nov. 1, 1996
School application fee to all applicants: $60
Oldest MCAT scores considered: 1994
Does have Early Decision Program (EDP)
    EDP application period: June 1–Aug. 1, 1996
    EDP applicants notified by: Oct. 1, 1996
Acceptance notice to regular applicants
    Earliest date: Oct. 15, 1996
    Latest date: Until class is filled
Applicant's response to acceptance offer
    Maximum time: 2 weeks
Requests for deferred entrance considered: Yes
Deposit to hold place in class (applied to tuition):
    $100, due with response to acceptance offer
Deposit refundable prior to: May 15, 1997
Estimated number of new entrants: 204 (40 EDP)
Starting date: Aug. 1997

## TUITION AND STUDENT FEES PER YEAR FOR 1995–96 FIRST-YEAR CLASS

Tuition                              Student fees: $35
    Resident: $12,894
    Nonresident: $22,985

## INFORMATION ON 1995–96 FIRST-YEAR CLASS

| Number of | In-State | Out-of-State | Total |
|---|---|---|---|
| Applicants | 525 | 7,247 | 7,772 |
| Applicants Interviewed | 176 | 331 | 507 |
| New Entrants* | 94 | 110 | 204 |

*All took the MCAT; 96% had baccalaureate degrees.

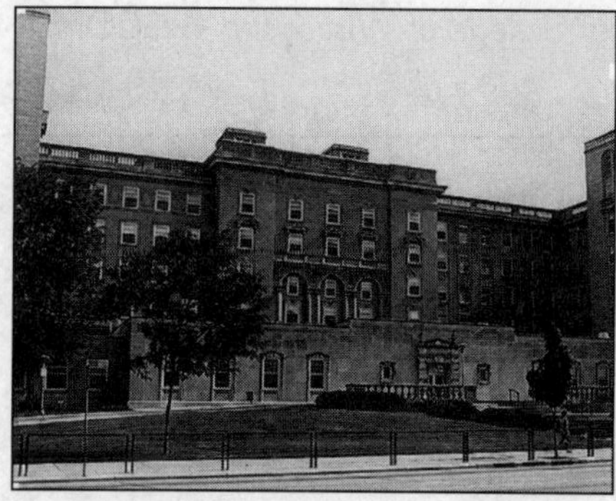

# University of Wisconsin Medical School

## Madison, Wisconsin

Dr. Philip Farrell, *Dean*
Janice Waisman, *Director of Admissions*
John Selbo, *Student Financial Aid*

## ADDRESS INQUIRIES TO:

Admissions Committee
Medical Sciences Center, Room 1250
University of Wisconsin Medical School
1300 University Avenue
Madison, Wisconsin 53706
(608) 263-4925; 262-2327 (FAX)
E-Mail: Janice.Waisman@mail.admin.wisc.edu

## GENERAL INFORMATION

The University of Wisconsin Medical School initiated a two-year program in 1907 and expanded to a full four-year program in 1924. The present University of Wisconsin Center for Health Sciences—which includes the Medical School, University Hospital and Clinics, Psychiatric Research Institute, the schools of nursing, pharmacy, and allied health sciences, and State Hygiene Laboratory—is located on the university campus. The Medical School basic science departments, first- and second-year teaching facilities, and administrative offices are located in the Medical Sciences Center. The Clinical Science Center houses the Medical School clinical departments, University Hospital and Clinics, School of Nursing, and Wisconsin Clinical Cancer Center. In addition to the University Hospital and Clinics, other hospitals in Madison and in Wisconsin are utilized in the educational program.

## CURRICULUM

The educational and research programs have been developed to educate students to become qualified to undertake any career in medicine. Our new curriculum emphasizes the following: active learning; interdisciplinary teaching by the basic science and clinical faculty throughout the first and second years; a four-year generalist curriculum with a focus on health risk assessment, prevention, common illnesses and outcomes; clinical clerkships around the state, including inner city and rural sites with an eight-week, community-based, outpatient primary care clerkship in Year 3, and an eight-week preceptorship with an experienced clinician in Year 4. The senior year provides extensive elective opportunities for study at other institutions and abroad.

Opportunities for research are available to medical students in individually arranged programs leading to the M.S. and Ph.D. degrees or by nondegree arrangements.

Competitive support is being offered to resident and nonresident students entering as M.D.-Ph.D. candidates. Fellowships in the form of tuition and a stipend will be awarded to a select group of applicants who exhibit high academic achievement and interest in medical research.

## REQUIREMENTS FOR ENTRANCE

The MCAT is required. Applicants are strongly encouraged to take the MCAT in the spring before application. Consideration of applicants who indicate they are taking the fall MCAT will be delayed, without detriment, until receipt of those scores.

Applicants must have a minimum of three years (90 semester hours) of college work by the time of matriculation. However, applicants are encouraged to obtain a baccalaureate degree before matriculation. Courses in English, biochemistry, quantitative analysis, and calculus and electives in the humanities and social sciences are recommended. U.S. citizens, as well as foreign nationals, are required to take their prerequisite course work at an undergraduate institution in the United States or Canada. College work must include:

|  | Semesters |
| --- | --- |
| General zoology or biology (with lab) | 1 |
| Advanced zoology or biology (with lab) | 1 |
| Inorganic chemistry (with lab) | 2 |
| Organic chemistry (with lab) | 2 |
| General physics (with lab) | 2 |
| Mathematics | 2 |
| Minimum requirement of college algebra and trigonometry. | |

## SELECTION FACTORS

Intellectual ability, breadth of academic and nonacademic interests and experiences, ability to communicate with others, motivation for medicine, and personal characteristics are some of the factors considered by the Admissions Committee. A preprofessional committee evaluation or three academic letters of recommendation plus one nonacademic letter of recommendation are required and must be submitted no later than December 15. Applicants may or may not be invited for personal interviews to complete the application process, depending upon the selection procedures being used. Applicants are encouraged to make their written applications as complete as possible.

The University of Wisconsin Medical School does not discriminate on the basis of race, sex, creed, national origin, age, or handicap. Women, minorities and/or disadvantaged students, and students from rural areas are encouraged to apply since these groups are presently underrepresented in both the applicant pool and the medical profession. Preference is given to residents of Wisconsin. Non-resident applicants are competing for relatively few places. Only highly qualified nonresidents are encouraged to apply. Applications are accepted from foreign nationals who have a permanent resident visa in the United States.

## FINANCIAL AID

All financial aid allocated by the University of Wisconsin Medical School is awarded on the basis of proven need. Need is calculated as the necessary expenses incurred while attending medical school minus the resources provided to the student by outside agencies, personal resources, and available parental resources. Priority for financial aid, especially grant awards, will be given to students with the greatest need. The major proportion of total financial aid is available in the form of loans.

## INFORMATION FOR MINORITIES

The University of Wisconsin Medical School is committed to increasing the number of physicians from presently underrepresented ethnic groups and providing educational opportunity to individuals who have confronted socioeconomically and educationally disadvantaged conditions. Applications are encouraged from resident and nonresident black Americans, mainland Puerto Ricans, Mexican Americans, American Indians, and all socioeconomically disadvantaged persons, regardless of ethnic identity.

Every effort is made to reach a fair and well informed assessment of intellectual capacity, motivation for medicine, ability to communicate with others, determination to help others, and character. The accomplishments of all applicants will be assessed with due consideration of their backgrounds. Also considered is the diversity of interests which is of value in the training of professionals for good health care delivery.

Public Institution

## APPLICATION AND ACCEPTANCE POLICIES FOR 1997–98 FIRST-YEAR CLASS

*School participates in AMCAS. See Chapter 4.*

Filing of AMCAS application
    Earliest date: June 1, 1996
    Latest date: Nov. 1, 1996
School application fee to all applicants: $38
Oldest MCAT scores considered: 1993
Does have Early Decision Program (EDP)
    For Wisconsin residents only
    EDP application period: June 1–Aug. 1, 1996
    EDP applicants notified by: Oct. 1, 1996
Acceptance notice to regular applicants
    Earliest date: Nov. 15, 1996
    Latest date: Varies
Applicant's response to acceptance offer
    Maximum time: 2 weeks
Requests for deferred entrance considered: Yes
    (for Wisconsin residents only)
Deposit to hold place in class: None
Estimated number of new entrants: 143 (25 EDP)
Starting date: Aug. 1997

## TUITION AND STUDENT FEES PER YEAR FOR 1995–96 FIRST-YEAR CLASS

Tuition and student fees:
    Resident: $13,041
    Nonresident: $18,895

## INFORMATION ON 1995–96 FIRST-YEAR CLASS

| Number of | In-State | Out-of-State | Total |
|---|---|---|---|
| Applicants | 635 | 2,399 | 3,034 |
| Applicants Interviewed | 169 | 57 | 226 |
| New Entrants* | 118 | 25 | 143 |

*All had baccalaureate degrees; 80% took the MCAT.

# Information About Canadian Medical Schools

## Accredited by the LCME and by the CACMS

The 16 medical schools in Canada are affiliate institutional members of the Association of American Medical Colleges (AAMC) and participate in the Association's activities. The Canadian medical schools are accredited jointly by the Liaison Committee on Medical Education (LCME) and the Committee on Accreditation of Canadian Medical Schools (CACMS) of the Association of Canadian Medical Colleges. All are M.D. degree-granting schools with high quality educational programs.

Admission policies and procedures of the Canadian schools are in many respects similar to policies and procedures followed in U.S. schools. Thus, many of the suggestions in chapters 1 through 7 are applicable also to students applying to these schools. Differences exist, however, in the relative importance given by the schools to various factors considered relevant in the selection process. Reference should be made to the individual school entries for details on these differences.

Fourteen Canadian medical schools have four-year programs. McMaster and Calgary have three-year programs. In 1992, the University of Montreal changed from a five-year to a new four-year curriculum. With the introduction of the four-year curriculum some students are now admitted into a one-year preparatory program prior to commencing the four-year M.D. curriculum. Laval University allows students, after admission, to opt to extend the four-year program over five years. Thus there is some variation in the duration of medical curricula in different Canadian faculties of medicine.

## SELECTION CRITERIA

Pre-university education differs in Canada from the straight elementary-secondary 12-year system in the United States. There are also significant differences from province to province within Canada. As reflected in the individual entries, these differences affect the number of years of college/university instruction required of applicants to medical schools located in the different provinces. Individual schools also impose their own requirements independent of the differences that arise out of the educational system itself. Table 11-A shows that biology, organic and inorganic chemistry, physics, humanities, and English are the most common subjects required in undergraduate education by the Canadian schools. Medical schools are drifting away from rigid course prerequisites.

## Language of Instruction

Three Canadian medical schools require fluency in French as all instruction is given in French. These schools are Laval, Montreal, and Sherbrooke—all located in the province of Quebec. Instruction in the other 13 schools is given in English. Students at the University of Ottawa have the option to write their examinations in French and instruction in French is gradually being introduced into the curriculum.

## Residence Requirements

Most medical schools give preference to citizens and landed immigrants residing in the province in which the medical school is located, because universities are a provincial responsibility in Canada. Individual schools within a province may prefer to select students from specific regions within the province. Prospective applicants should be aware of these preferences to maximize their chances of success.

A number of foreign students is accepted into Canadian medical schools each year. In this context, "foreign" refers to persons who are neither citizens of Canada nor landed immigrants in Canada at the time of application.

Some medical schools have a specific quota of places for applicants from the United States. In particular, students from the United States who are contemplating enrollment in Canada should study the admission requirements of Memorial University in St. John's, Newfoundland and McGill University in Montreal, Quebec. Other faculties of medicine in Canada are also currently considering the introduction of such U.S.-specific quotas.

Foreign students, including U.S. students, pay substantially higher tuition fees.

Applicants from outside Canada should check with the particular school in which they are interested to ascertain whether that school considers applications from non-Canadian citizens or nonimmigrants.

## Academic Record/Suitability

Although it is probably fair to state that an excellent academic record is a very important factor in gaining admission to a Canadian medical school, a great deal of effort goes into devising means of assessing suitability for a medical career based on factors other than academic ability. Personal suitability is assessed in a variety of ways by the schools, and so applicants able to demonstrate the qualities considered important in

## TABLE 11-A

### Subjects Required by Three or More Canadian Medical Schools 1997–98 Entering Class

| Required Subject | No. of Schools (n = 13) |
| --- | --- |
| Organic chemistry | 10 |
| Biology/biology or zoology | 9 |
| English | 8 |
| Inorganic (general) chemistry | 8 |
| Physics | 7 |
| Calculus | 4 |
| Humanities | 4 |
| Behavioral and/or social sciences | 3 |
| Biochemistry | 3 |
| College Algebra | 3 |

NOTE: Figures based on data provided fall 1995. Three of the 16 medical schools (Calgary, Dalhousie, and McMaster) did not indicate specific course requirements and are not included in the tabulations. Two schools (Laval and Montreal) require French.

the practice of medicine may occasionally gain access to medical school even if their academic record is not outstanding. Also, applicants with outstanding records who fail to demonstrate the personal qualities considered important may not gain a place in medical school.

Most successful applicants to Canadian medical schools are interviewed prior to acceptance. The discussion of the interview in Chapter 6 also applies in the context of admission to Canadian schools.

### Enrollment Reductions

A comparison of the proportion of applicants who are successful in gaining admission to medical school in Canada with those in the United States indicates that for many years it has been more difficult to gain admission to a Canadian medical school. During the past few years, medical schools in some Canadian provinces reduced the number of available first-year places. The reductions are substantial in some jurisdictions. A consequence is severe competition for the available places.

### MCAT

Eleven Canadian medical schools require applicants to take the Medical College Admission Test (MCAT). These schools are Alberta, British Columbia, Calgary, Dalhousie, Manitoba, McGill, Memorial, Ottawa, Queen's, Toronto, and Western Ontario.

## Other Considerations

Applicants and entrants to Canadian schools today are often older than their counterparts of the past.

Most medical schools no longer have admissions policies related to age, although older applicants are not quite as successful in gaining admission as younger ones. Prospective candidates who are concerned about this should check the statistics of the schools to which they wish to apply.

Canadian faculties of medicine do not use race, religion, and sex as criteria in selection. The admission and enrollment of native Indian and Inuit students are encouraged in several Canadian medical schools. The number of female applicants has risen dramatically in recent years, and correspondingly larger proportions of the entering classes have been made up of women. Women comprised 50 percent of the 1995–96 applicant pool. Overall, 22 percent of the applicants received at least one offer of admission. The success rate of women was higher than that of men. The entering class at Canadian medical schools was 52.2 percent female in 1995–96.

## EXPENSES/FINANCIAL AID

Tuition and student fees for Canadian and non-Canadian students in the 1995–96 entering class are given in Table 11-B and in the individual school entries. Expenses will vary from school to school and from individual to individual. It should be noted that tuition in several Canadian schools is slightly higher for successive years than for the first year. Tuition and fees at all Canadian universities are expected to increase substantially in the next few years.

Some information about financial aid is given in the individual school entries. Eligible Canadian students may apply for a Canadian student loan, or they may apply to the Department of Education of their own province for a provincial student loan.

## ONTARIO MEDICAL SCHOOL APPLICATION SERVICE (OMSAS)

The Ontario Medical School Application Service (OMSAS) is a nonprofit centralized application service for applicants to the five medical schools in the province of Ontario. OMSAS provides only the application processing service; each medical school is completely autonomous in reaching its own admission decisions. *All applications to the Ontario medical schools must be made through OMSAS.*

OMSAS application materials are available July 1. Completed application materials and official transcripts must be received by OMSAS no later than November 1. However, applicants are advised to submit their application materials in advance of the deadline. An instruction booklet, containing information about application procedures, admission requirements, the undergraduate academic record form, and the OMSAS application may be obtained from:

**TABLE 11-B**

**Tuition and Student Fees for 1995–96 First-Year Students<br>at Canadian Medical Schools<br>(In Canadian Dollars)**

| Categories of Students | Range | Median | Average |
|---|---|---|---|
| Canadian | 2,164–5,012 | 3,838 | 3,673* |
| Non-Canadian | 2,929–32,512 | 9,531 | 11,949* |

NOTE: Figures based on data provided fall 1995.
*Average residents were derived from all 16 Canadian schools reporting. Average nonresidents were derived from 14 Canadian schools reporting. Two schools do not accept nonresidents.

OMSAS
Ontario Universities' Application Centre
P.O. Box 1328
650 Woodlawn Road West
Guelph, Ontario N1H 7P4
Canada
Telephone: (519) 823-1940
E-mail: omsas@netserv.ouac.on.ca

## SOURCES OF FURTHER INFORMATION

Further information about admission requirements, curricula of Canadian medical schools, and medical education in Canada is in the catalogs available from each school and in *Admission Requirements to Canadian Faculties of Medicine and Their Selection Policies* (edited in 1996 for admission in 1997–98 or 1998–99). Prices for this publication are $25 in Canada, $30 (U.S.) for requests from the United States, and $35 (U.S.) for requests from overseas and may be ordered from:

Association of Canadian Medical Colleges
774 Echo Drive
Ottawa, Ontario K1S 5P2
Canada

## ABBREVIATIONS

Listed below are the abbreviations used in the school entries in this chapter.

GPA—Grade-point average
MCAT—Medical College Admission Test
  VR—Verbal Reasoning
  PS—Physical Sciences
  WS—Writing Sample
  BS—Biological Sciences
OMSAS—Ontario Medical School Application Service

# Canadian Medical Schools
## School Entries

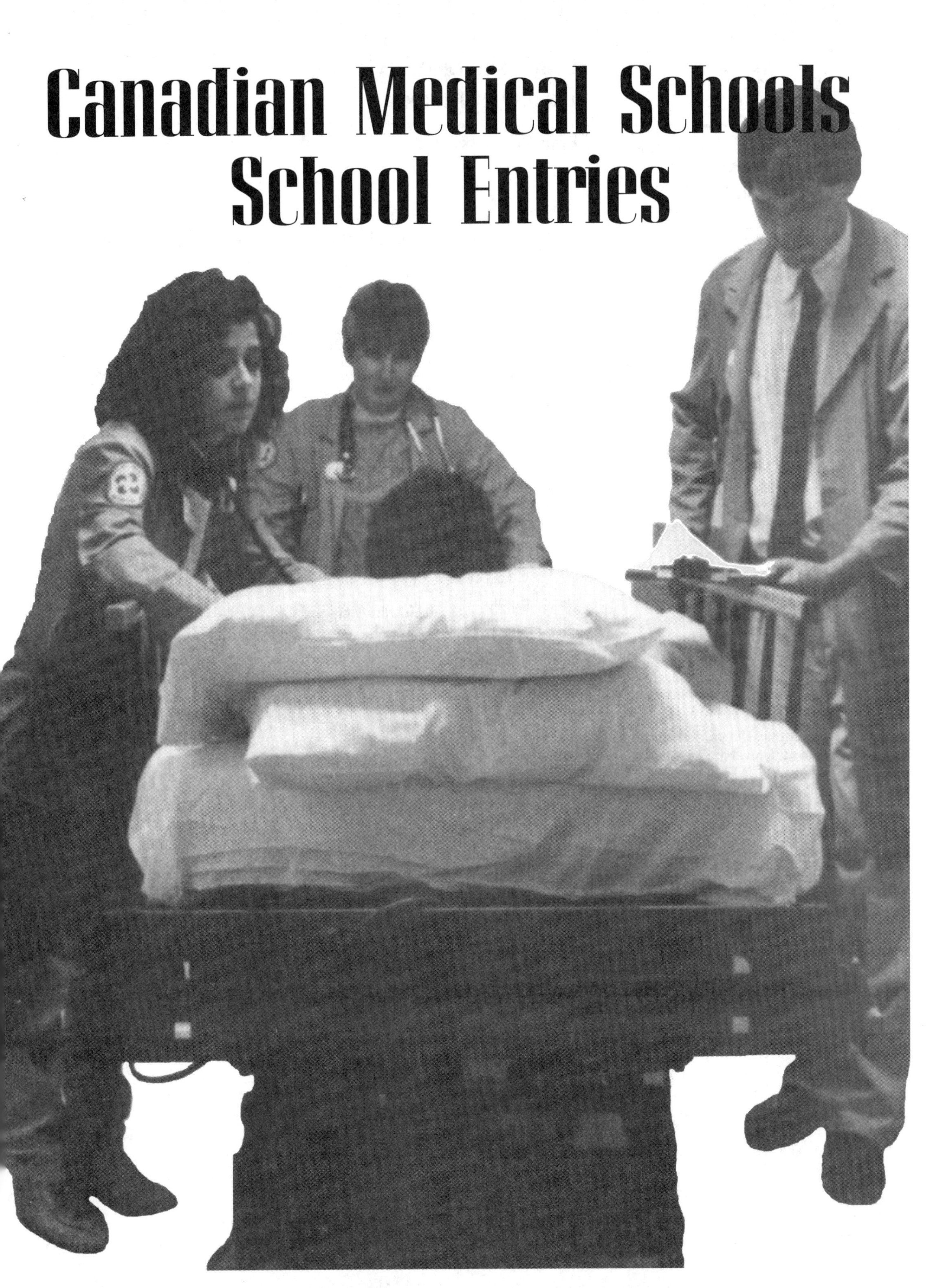

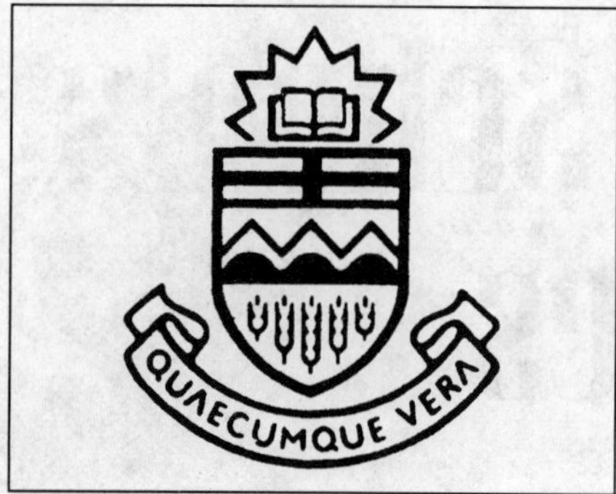

# University of Alberta
# Faculty of Medicine

## Edmonton, Alberta

Dr. D. L. J. Tyrrell, *Dean*
Dr. C. I. Cheeseman, *Assistant Dean, Admissions and Student Affairs*
S. Franklin, *Program Director, Admissions and Student Affairs*

## ADDRESS INQUIRIES TO:

Admissions Officer
2-45 Medical Sciences Building
University of Alberta
Faculty of Medicine
Edmonton, Alberta
Canada, T6G 2H7
(403) 492-6350; 492-9531 (FAX)

## GENERAL INFORMATION

The Faculty of Medicine at the University of Alberta was founded in 1913.

The Medical Sciences Building, the Clinical Sciences Building, the Walter C. Mackenzie Health Sciences Centre, and the University of Alberta Hospitals are located on the university campus. Clinical instruction is also given at the Royal Alexandra Hospital, Edmonton General Hospital, Misericordia Hospital, Alberta Hospital, Glenrose Hospital, Cross Cancer Institute, Grey Nun's Hospital, and Charles Camsell Hospital.

A student counseling service and student health services are available to all University of Alberta students.

## CURRICULUM

The Faculty of Medicine conducts a fully accredited, four-year program leading to the degree of doctor of medicine. Each of the first two years consists of 33 weeks of instruction, from early September until mid-May. The final two years are conducted as a continuum, during which each student has a four-week holiday period.

The first year of the program includes a study of the principles of the basic medical sciences and an introduction to clinical medicine. The second year is a study of the basic and clinical sciences in relation to the mechanisms of disease in a clinical setting on a systems basis. The last two years are composed of a student internship of at least 56 weeks, during which the student is assigned to hospitals affiliated with the Faculty of Medicine for clinical study and experience, a selective program of geriatrics and rural family medicine, and an elective program which allows students to develop their own curriculum and spend a minimum of 10 weeks in one or more subject areas of their choice.

Throughout the program, emphasis is on self-education; much instruction is on a small group basis.

A graduate training program leading to eligibility for specialist qualifications by the Royal College of Physicians and Surgeons of Canada is offered in most clinical specialties. Programs leading to the degree of master of science or doctor of philosophy in any of the basic medical sciences and in most of the clinical medical sciences are conducted under the direction of the Faculty of Graduate Studies and Research of the university.

Opportunity for research in the basic medical sciences is available to those students interested in spending a year or more in this type of work and obtaining a bachelor of science in medicine degree.

## REQUIREMENTS FOR ENTRANCE

The MCAT is compulsory. All students considering medicine must register in a degree program and maintain good standing in that program. Irrespective of the degree program, the student must take courses in the following subjects:

*Biological sciences:* General biology.
*Chemistry:* Inorganic and organic chemistry.
*General physics*
*Statistics*
*English*

These courses must be full-year courses (equivalent to six-credit courses at the University of Alberta) or two single-term courses (equivalent to three-credit courses at the University of Alberta) with the exception of statistics, in which a single three-credit course is acceptable.

Students are encouraged to obtain a baccalaureate degree prior to admission but may apply after two or three years in a degree program. To be considered for early selection, a student must have all the prerequisites as well as exceptional academic (minimum GPA of 8.0 on a 9.0 scale) and personal qualifications. Mature applicants may be given special consideration.

## SELECTION FACTORS

Selection is based upon quality of scholastic achievement, personal suitability, and performance on the MCAT. Alberta residents are preferred, although each year out-of-province applicants are considered for 10 percent of first-year places. An interview, autobiographical essay, and letter(s) of reference may be requested. All information on each candidate is considered by the Admissions Committee, and the quota is filled by the best candidates available.

## FINANCIAL AID

Loans are available under the Canada Student Loan Plan or the Province of Alberta Loan Plan to Canadian citizens or permanent residents who have been in Canada and in Alberta for 12 months prior to the beginning of the academic term.

---

Public Institution

## APPLICATION AND ACCEPTANCE POLICIES FOR 1997–98 FIRST-YEAR CLASS

*Fees and expenses are in Canadian dollars.*

Filing of application
Earliest date: July 1, 1996
Latest date: Nov. 1, 1996
School application fee to all applicants: $60
Oldest MCAT scores considered: 1991
Does have Early Decision Program (EDP)
EDP application period: July 1–Nov. 1, 1996
EDP applications notified by: May 1997
Acceptance notice to regular applicants
Earliest date: July 1, 1997
Latest date: Sept. 1, 1997
Applicant's response to acceptance offer
Maximum time: 14 days
Requests for deferred entrance considered: Yes
Deposit to hold place in class (applied to tuition):
$200, due with response to acceptance offer;
nonrefundable
Estimated number of new entrants: 102 (80 EDP)
Starting date: Aug. 1997

## TUITION AND STUDENT FEES PER YEAR FOR 1995–1996 FIRST-YEAR CLASS

| Tuition | Student fees |
|---|---|
| Canadian: $3,885 | Canadian: $350 |
| Non-Canadian: $7,770 | Non-Canadian: $650 |

## INFORMATION ON 1995–96 FIRST-YEAR CLASS

| Number of | In-Province | Out-of-Province | Total |
|---|---|---|---|
| Applicants | 431 | 393 | 824 |
| Applicants Interviewed | 249 | 110 | 359 |
| New Entrants* | 94 | 9 | 103 |

*All took the MCAT; 80% had baccalaureate degrees.

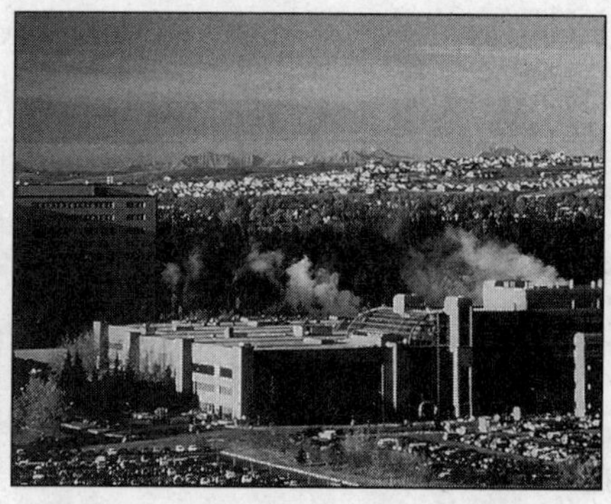

# University of Calgary Faculty of Medicine

## Calgary, Alberta


Dr. Eldon Smith, *Dean of Medicine*
Dr. Wanda Lester, Director, *Office of Admissons and Student Affairs*
Adele Meyers, Coordinator, *Office of Admissions and Student Affairs*


## ADDRESS INQUIRIES TO:

Office of Admissions
University of Calgary
Faculty of Medicine
3330 Hospital Drive, N.W.
Calgary, Alberta
Canada T2N 4N1
(403) 220-4262
E-Mail: meyers@asc.ucalgary.ca
Web Site: http://www.med.ucalgary.ca/ume/infoda.html

## GENERAL INFORMATION

The Faculty of Medicine at the University of Calgary accepted its first students in September 1970. In 1972 the Faculty of Medicine moved into its permanent facilities in the Calgary Health Sciences Centre. The centre has been designed to complement the objectives of the faculty's integrated teaching program.

## CURRICULUM

The curriculum is based on clinical presentations the way patients present to physicians. One hundred twenty clinical presentations have been defined ranging from simple to complex and are grouped by body system and human development. The first course offered is principles for medicine, which serves to introduce the different modes of solving clinical problems and the basic concepts essential to an understanding of human structure, function and growth as well as provision of comprehensive medical care to the individual, the family, and society. Introductory clinical skills of communication and physical examination also commence in the first weeks of the curriculum. Following principles of medicine is the first of the interdisciplinary body systems courses. Approximately two-thirds of the student's time is allocated to these regularly scheduled courses. The remaining period is available for elective study and the independent study or tutorial program. Each academic year lasts about 11 months. The problem-solving approach, combined with the curriculum design, is intended to facilitate the integration between the conventional basic and clinical sciences. As well, students have the opportunity to reinforce in a clinical setting what they have learned in the body systems as they progress through

each of the systems. The curriculum also focuses on the relevance of the family and the community in health and disease.

At the end of the three years, students will be granted the M.D. degree. The school's philosophy is to produce generalist physicians who can proceed to further training in specialty, family medicine, or research.

## REQUIREMENTS FOR ENTRANCE

All students are required to take the new MCAT by the fall of the year before anticipated enrollment. Most students have a B.A. or B.Sc. degree before entering the Faculty of Medicine, although a few extremely well qualified students have been admitted after two years in an arts or science program. There is some advantage to majoring in a science area, but the student who has excelled in behavioral science or any other undergraduate area may be accepted.

The following undergraduate courses are recommended: general biology, cell biology, mammalian physiology, organic and inorganic chemistry, biochemistry, English, physics, calculus, and one course of psychology, sociology, or anthropology.

## SELECTION FACTORS

The Admissions Committee selects applicants without discrimination to gender or race and attempts to apply five criteria: undergraduate academic achievement; an interview; an essay; letters of recommendation; and the MCAT. Final applicants will be required to attend an interview at the University of Calgary at their own expense. Final applicants will also be required to write an on-site essay on a topic assigned by the Admissions Committee. Preference is given to Alberta residents. One position is generally available for international applicants. Rejected applicants are given the opportunity to reapply for admission. Applicants who have been asked to withdraw or who have been suspended or expelled from any medical school will not normally be considered.

## FINANCIAL AID

The majority of students obtain financial aid through student loans. Because the students attend school 11 months each year, summer employment is unlikely, and, therefore, financial support must be sufficient to meet their requirements over the subsequent three years. The student awards officer will provide information about student loans, bursaries, and awards. The financial status of the applicant does not affect acceptance into the program.

Students receive a total stipend of $3,600 for the third (final) year.

Public Institution

## APPLICATION AND ACCEPTANCE POLICIES FOR 1997–98 FIRST-YEAR CLASS

*Fees and expenses are in Canadian dollars.*

Filing of application
 Earliest date: July 15, 1996
 Latest date: Nov. 30, 1996
School application fee to all applicants: $60
Oldest MCAT scores considered: 1991
Does not have Early Decision Program
Acceptance notice to regular applicants
 Earliest date: May 15, 1997
 Latest date: Varies
Applicant's response to acceptance offer
 Maximum time: 15 days
Requests for deferred entrance considered: No
Deposit to hold place in class (applied to tuition):
 $100, due with response to acceptance offer
Deposit refundable prior to: June 15, 1997
Estimated number of new entrants: 69
Starting date: Aug. 1997

## TUITION AND STUDENT FEES PER YEAR FOR 1995–96 FIRST-YEAR CLASS

Tuition                    Student fees: $323
 Canadian: $4,512
 Non-Canadian: $9,024

## INFORMATION ON 1995–96 FIRST-YEAR CLASS

| *Number of* | *In-Province* | *Out-of-Province* | *Total* |
|---|---|---|---|
| Applicants | 402 | 485 | 887 |
| Applicants Interviewed | 99 | 92 | 191 |
| New Entrants* | 43 | 26 | 69 |

*All took the MCAT; 84% had baccalaureate degrees.

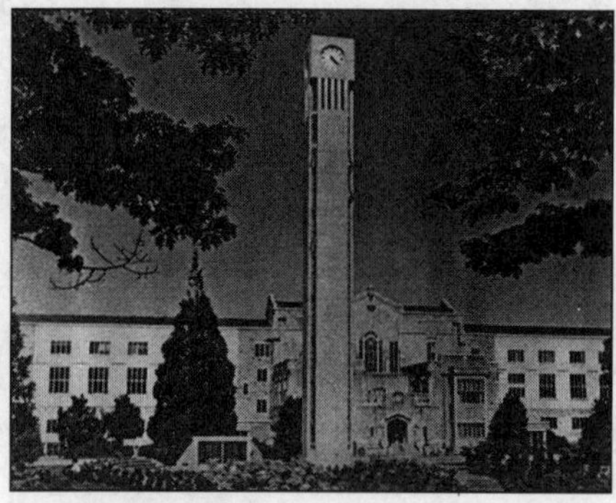

# University of British Columbia Faculty of Medicine

## Vancouver, British Columbia

Dr. M.J. Hollenberg, *Dean*
Dr. J.E. Carter, *Associate Dean, Admissions*
Carol Gibson, *Director, Awards and Financial Aid*

## ADDRESS INQUIRIES TO:

Office of the Dean, Faculty of Medicine
Admissions Office
University of British Columbia
317-2194 Health Sciences Mall
Vancouver, British Columbia
Canada V6T 1Z3
(604) 822-4482; 822-6061 (FAX)

## GENERAL INFORMATION

The Faculty of Medicine of the University of British Columbia received its first students in 1950 and graduated its first class in 1954. It is an integral part of a large provincial university comprising a variety of faculties and schools with a total enrollment of over 30,000 students.

Teaching in the preclinical subject areas is based in the basic medical science departments. Clinical teaching is currently carried out at the Vancouver Hospital and Health Sciences Center, St. Paul's and Children's hospitals, BC Women's Hospital and Health Centre, and a number of other institutions.

The health sciences complex on the university campus comprises a large Instructional Resources Center providing lecture theaters, small group seminar rooms, audiovisual facilities, and student lounge and snack bar areas; a 60-bed psychiatric hospital with additional day care facilities; a 300-bed extended care unit; and a 240-bed acute care hospital. New off-campus hospital facilities at Children's Hospital and an adjoining obstetrical and gynecological unit at BC Women's Hospital and Health Centre were opened in 1982.

## CURRICULUM

The four years of instruction are broadly divided into three phases: an initial 18-month period with emphasis on the basic medical sciences, a second 9-month period of detailed clinical instruction, and a final 12-month clinical clerkship. Teaching in the first year is carried out largely on campus, but during the second year it is transferred in part to the teaching hospitals; in the third and fourth years it is largely hospital-based. The fourth year comprises a 52-week clinical clerkship (including two weeks vacation) with blocks of time assigned exclusively to clerkship experience in each of the major clinical disciplines. The clerkship also provides a six-week elective block.

The elective block can be carried out in the academic departments on campus, in the affiliated teaching hospitals, in a large number of community hospitals throughout British Columbia, or in other medical centers or institutions in Canada or abroad.

Earlier introduction of students to patients in a clinical setting, the integration and coordination of learning experiences in the basic medical sciences and clinical practice, provision of increased elective and self-study time, and the development of more effective measures for evaluation of students and of the educational program are among the major objectives of the Faculty of Medicine.

## REQUIREMENTS FOR ENTRANCE

The MCAT, a minimum of three years (90 semester hours) of accredited college course work, and a minimum of a B average or second class standing (70 percent) are required. Some background in the humanities and behavioral sciences is recommended. A baccalaureate degree is not a prerequisite.

The minimum subject requirements are:

|  | *Years* |
| --- | --- |
| General biology | 1 |
| General biochemistry | 1 |
| General chemistry | 1 |
| Organic chemistry | 1 |
| English literature and composition | 1 |

## SELECTION FACTORS

Selection is not contingent upon applicants' sex, age, race, religion, or national origin. Those accepted are generally within the age range of 19 to 30 years. Preference is given to well qualified British Columbia residents; small numbers of candidates with superior qualifications from other Canadian provinces may be admitted. No applicant is considered who has been required to withdraw from another medical school.

Admission is based on intellectual achievement and potential, as demonstrated by overall academic records and MCAT scores, and on qualities of personality, character, and motivation, evaluated by interviews, preprofessional committee reports, letters of reference, and an autobiographical statement submitted with the application. Applicants will be advised if personal interviews are required.

## FINANCIAL AID

Scholarships are awarded to students showing proficiency and promise in their medical school studies. Generally they are available to only those students who have been in attendance in a university in British Columbia for at least one year. These scholarships are provided through the generosity of various medical and other organizations in British Columbia. Bursaries and loans may be applied for in any academic year.

It is recommended that students devote themselves entirely to the full-time demands of the medical course. Students' spouses may find employment through the university's personnel office.

Public Institution

## APPLICATION AND ACCEPTANCE POLICIES FOR 1997–98 FIRST-YEAR CLASS

*Fees and expenses are in Canadian dollars.*

Filing of application
  Earliest date: Aug. 15, 1996
  Latest date: Dec. 15, 1996
School application fee: $105 British Columbia
  applicants; $155 out-of-province applicants;
  additional $30 to evaluate out-of-province transcripts
Oldest MCAT scores considered: 1991
Does not have Early Decision Program
Acceptance notice to regular applicants
  Earliest date: end of March, 1997
  Latest date: Until class is filled
Applicant's response to acceptance offer
  Maximum time: 4 weeks
Requests for deferred entrance considered: Yes
Deposit to hold place in class (applied to tuition):
  $300, due with response to acceptance offer;
  nonrefundable
Estimated number of new entrants: 120
Starting date: Aug. 1997

## TUITION AND STUDENT FEES PER YEAR FOR 1995–96 FIRST-YEAR CLASS

Tuition                              Student fees: $243
  Canadian: $3,937

## INFORMATION ON 1995–96 FIRST-YEAR CLASS

| Number of | In-Province | Out-of-Province | Total |
|---|---|---|---|
| Applicants | 515 | 191 | 706 |
| Applicants Interviewed | 366 | 3 | 369 |
| New Entrants* | 118 | 2 | 120 |

*All took the MCAT; 93% had baccalaureate degrees.

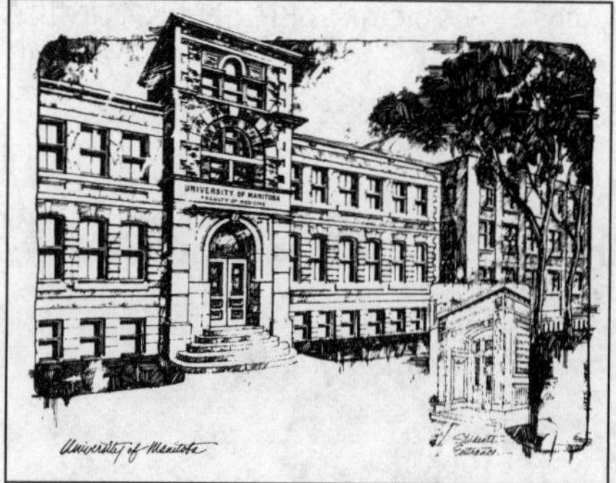

# University of Manitoba
# Faculty of Medicine

## Winnipeg, Manitoba


Dr. N. R. Anthonisen, *Dean*
Dr. P. Mirwaldt, *Associate Dean, Admissions and Student Affairs*
C. K. Paragg, *Registrar*


## ADDRESS INQUIRIES TO:

Chair, Admissions Committee
University of Manitoba
Faculty of Medicine
753 McDermot Avenue
Winnipeg, Manitoba
Canada R3E 0W3
(204) 789-3569; 774-8941 (FAX)
E-Mail: paragg@bldghsc.lanl.umanitoba.ca

## GENERAL INFORMATION

The Manitoba Medical College was established in 1883 and from its beginning was affiliated with the University of Manitoba. The first class of six graduated in 1886. In 1918 the Manitoba Medical College became the Faculty of Medicine of the University of Manitoba. In 1924 it received approval as a Class A medical school. The medical buildings are adjacent to the Health Sciences Centre in Winnipeg, which is some distance from the main university campus.

Teaching hospitals affiliated with the Faculty of Medicine are the Health Sciences Centre (Children's, Adult's, Women's, and Respiratory and Rehabilitation hospitals—1,064 beds); St. Boniface General Hospital (900 beds); Deer Lodge Veterans Hospital (500 beds); Grace Hospital (306 beds); Seven Oaks Hospital (336 beds); Victoria Hospital (254 beds); and Misericordia Hospital (409 beds).

## CURRICULUM

Medicine is a four-year course at the University of Manitoba. In the first and second years there are, on the average, 30 hours of formal instruction per week for 39 weeks. In the first year 14 weeks are devoted to normal human biology, 13 weeks to integration of structure and function of individual organ systems, and the final 12 weeks to general mechanisms of disease. The second year is devoted to clinical sciences and acquisition of basic clinical skills. The third and fourth years are devoted to preclerkship (9 weeks); clerkship (eight clerkships of 7 weeks duration each); elective (13 weeks); and basic science review. A pass/fail system of evaluating student performance has been adopted, and, consequently, no rank in class or grades is given.

## REQUIREMENTS FOR ENTRANCE

The MCAT and a bachelor's degree are mandatory. The academic requirements for admission are clear senior matriculation (comparable with sophomore matriculation in U.S. colleges) and the completion of three premedical years of 32 weeks each (15 full courses) in the Faculty of Arts and Science of the University of Manitoba or its equivalent.

The following subjects must be included in the course of study:

|  | *Credit hrs.* |
|---|---|
| Biochemistry | 6 |
| English | 6 |

In other respects, the content of the course work must satisfy either the university's B.A. or B.Sc. degree requirements, with a minimum of 18 hours in the social sciences/ humanities and 18 hours in the natural/physical sciences.

## SELECTION FACTORS

Selection by the Committee on Admissions is made primarily on the basis of a composite score, calculated as follows: (i) adjusted grade-point score: maximum, 10 percent; (ii) MCAT score: maximum, 50 percent; and (iii) personal assessment score: maximum, 40 percent. The personal assessment score is based on an autobiographical essay of approximately 800 words, the MCAT writing sample, a standardized questionnaire sent to references named by the applicant, and the results of an interview with a panel of three interviewers. Ninety percent of the 70 places available in the entering class normally are filled in this way. However, about 10 percent of successful applicants with acceptable but noncompetitive undergraduate performance may be selected on the basis of special premedical experience (educational or occupational) of relevance to the study and practice of medicine. Preference is given to undergraduates and graduates of the universities in Manitoba who are Canadian citizens or permanent residents of Canada. At the discretion of the committee, a limited number of places may be made available to undergraduates of other universities. The school does not discriminate on the basis of race, sex, creed, or national origin.

Applicants for the 1995 entering class with a minimum GPA of 3.6 were interviewed, and 43 percent of those interviewed were enrolled.

Advanced standing consideration is given to candidates in Medicine I and II attending schools formally accredited by the joint LCME/CACMS accreditation committee to bring a class up to its first-year enrollment limit.

## FINANCIAL AID

Under the Canadian Students Loan Act, Canadians can obtain interest-free loans during their undergraduate course in medicine. Bursaries from the university and from the provincial government are available to deserving students. Students may also obtain assistance from the W. K. Kellogg Student Loan Program and from the Gordon Bell College of Physicians and Surgeons (Manitoba) Loan Fund. A few scholarships of smaller amounts are also available.

## OTHER PROGRAMS

Most graduates of the University of Manitoba, Faculty of Medicine gain licensure by completing the two part Medical Council of Canada Qualifying Examination (MCCQE), plus certification by either the Royal College of Physicians and Surgeons of Canada or the College of Family Physicians of Canada.

Specialty training is approved by the Royal College of Physicians and Surgeons of Canada and is conducted in the Affiliated Teaching Hospitals of the University of Manitoba. The University of Manitoba currently holds Royal College approval for 45 specialty training programs.

The Family Medicine Program is a two-year integrated training program leading to certification by the College of Family Physicians of Canada. The program is conducted in the affiliated teaching hospitals as well as in rural settings.

Continuing Medical Education is provided for practising physicians. The Faculty of Medicine also provides opportunities for graduate studies in all the basic science departments as well as in selected clinical departments. Vibrant research activities are conducted by dedicated basic science and clinical staff.

A formal bachelor of science in the Medicine Research Program is offered to selected medical students in the summers following first- and second-year medicine. Summer opportunities are also available for rural medicine placements as well as placements with the Northern Medical Unit.

---

Public Institution

## APPLICATION AND ACCEPTANCE POLICIES FOR 1997–98 FIRST-YEAR CLASS

*Fees and expenses are in Canadian dollars.*

Filing of application
  Earliest date: Aug. 15, 1996
  Latest date: Nov. 15, 1996
School application fee to all applicants: $45
Oldest MCAT scores considered: 1994
Does not have Early Decision Program
Acceptance notice to regular applicants
  Earliest date: June 1, 1997
  Latest date: Until class is filled
Applicant's response to acceptance offer
  Maximum time: 10 days
Requests for deferred entrance considered: No
Deposit to hold place in class (applied to tuition):
  $100, due with response to acceptance offer
Deposit refundable prior to: Aug. 15, 1997
Estimated number of new entrants: 70
Starting date: Aug. 1997

## TUITION AND STUDENT FEES PER YEAR FOR 1995–96 FIRST-YEAR CLASS

Tuition: $4,197          Student fees: $41

## INFORMATION ON 1995–96 FIRST-YEAR CLASS

| *Number of* | *In-Province* | *Out-of-Province* | *Total* |
|---|---|---|---|
| Applicants | 182 | 202 | 384 |
| Applicants Interviewed | 148 | 12 | 160 |
| New Entrants* | 68 | 1 | 69 |

*All took the MCAT and had baccalaureate degrees.

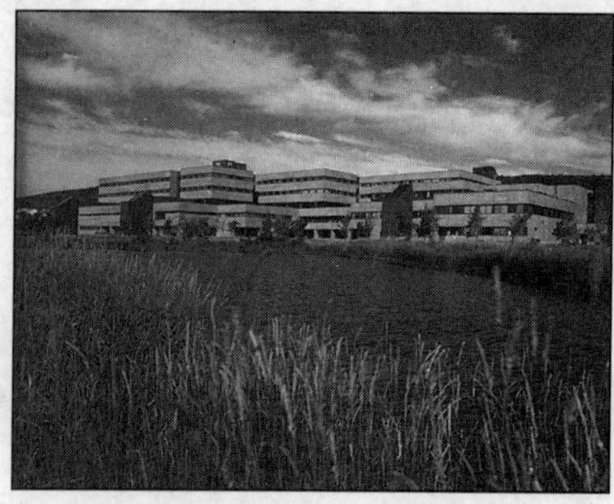

# Memorial University of Newfoundland Faculty of Medicine

## St. John's, Newfoundland

Dr. M.I. Bowmer, *Dean of Medicine*
Dr. W.L. Parsons, *Assistant Dean for Admissions*

## ADDRESS INQUIRIES TO:

Janet McHugh, *Director for Admissions*
Memorial University of Newfoundland
Faculty of Medicine
St. John's, Newfoundland
Canada A1B 3V6
(709) 737-6615; 737-5186 (FAX)
E-Mail: munmed@kean.ucs.mun.ca
Web Site: http://www.aorta.library.mun.ca/med/admissio/

## GENERAL INFORMATION

Memorial is the only university in the province of Newfoundland. The university was established as Memorial College in 1925 and incorporated as a university in 1949. In 1959 campus buildings were erected on a 1,000-acre site. There are some 12,000 undergraduates and a faculty of about 1,000 (including visiting professors) working on the campus, which is situated on the periphery of St. John's. The medical school is one of the four most recently established in Canada. It is housed in the Health Sciences Centre with General Hospital (531 beds) and a biomedical library.

Approved teaching programs for interns and residents are under the direction of the medical school. These programs are based at associate hospitals in St. John's and other provincial centers with a total bed complement of 3,116 covering inpatient and outpatient services in virtually all branches of medicine. Research work is being conducted both in the hospitals and in the Health Sciences Centre.

Residences for single and married students are provided on the campus, and the university maintains a list of approved off-campus accommodations. A health service is open to all students.

## CURRICULUM

The curriculum, the physical structure, and the administrative organization of the school were planned to allow for maximum cooperation among the various basic science and clinical disciplines. The M.D. degree is granted on completion of the fourth year, at which time Medical Council of Canada Examinations may be taken. The fourth year is a clinical clerkship similar to the traditional internship.

During the first year of the medical program, students take introductory courses in cell structure and function, biochemistry, physiology of excitable tissues, pathology, immunology, systems physiology, molecular genetics, pharmacology, microbiology, anatomy, behavioral science, ethics, interviewing skills, and community medicine. They are introduced to patients in the hospital and in the community, and these opportunities are provided in a wide range of medical settings—family practice, general hospital, rural hospital, and public health programs.

Teaching in subsequent years has a systems approach; material from anatomy, physiology, pathology, and clinical medicine is presented in an integrated manner. A considerable portion of time is given for electives in the first, third, and fourth years. These electives take the form either of projects in which the student will investigate research problems or of a more formal in-depth study of a particular subject.

The first academic year of medicine comprises approximately 38 weeks. The second and third years consist of approximately 66 weeks (five semesters). The fourth year (clinical clerkship) has three semesters with 64 weeks.

## REQUIREMENTS FOR ENTRANCE

A bachelor's degree is required. In exceptional circumstances, an application may be considered from someone who does not hold a bachelor's degree; such an applicant will have completed at least 20 one-semester courses and be a student who has work-related or other experience acceptable to the admissions committee. The course of study must include two courses in English. All applicants must take the new MCAT (revised in 1991) prior to the application deadline.

## SELECTION FACTORS

The school admits students on the basis of residency priority as follows: bona fide residents of Newfoundland and Labrador, the rest of Canada, and non-Canadian applicants. In every case a high academic standard is required. Memorial University does not discriminate on the basis of race, sex, creed, national origin, or handicap. Age by itself is not used as a basis for selection or rejection. However, both age and length of time away from full-time academic studies may be taken into consideration.

Public Institution

## APPLICATION AND ACCEPTANCE POLICIES FOR 1997–98 FIRST-YEAR CLASS

*Fees and expenses are in Canadian dollars.*

Filing of application
  Earliest date: Aug. 12, 1996
  Latest date: Nov. 15, 1996
School application fee to all applicants: $50
Oldest MCAT scores considered: 1993
Does not have Early Decision Program
Acceptance notice to regular applicants
  Earliest date: April 1, 1997
  Latest date: Until class is filled
Applicant's response to acceptance offer
  Maximum time: 14 days
Requests for deferred entrance considered: Yes
Deposit to hold place in class (applied to tuition):
  $100, due with response to acceptance offer;
  nonrefundable
Estimated number of new entrants: 60
Starting date: Sept. 1997

## TUITION AND STUDENT FEES PER YEAR FOR 1995–96 FIRST-YEAR CLASS

Tuition                          Student fees: $200
  Resident: $2,312
  Nonresident: $30,000

## INFORMATION ON 1995–96 FIRST-YEAR CLASS

| Number of | In-Province | Out-of-Province | Total |
|---|---|---|---|
| Applicants | 135 | 424 | 559 |
| Applicants Interviewed | 107 | 88 | 195 |
| New Entrants* | 48 | 12 | 60 |

*All took the MCAT and had baccalaureate degrees.

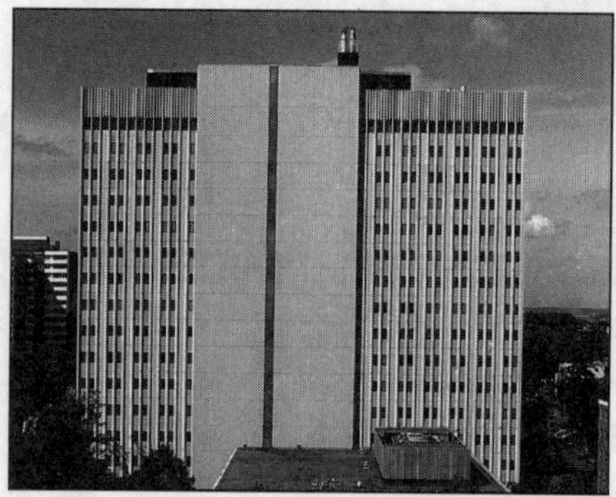

# Dalhousie University Faculty of Medicine

**Halifax, Nova Scotia**

Dr. John Ruedy, *Dean*
Dr. Margaret Casey, *Director of Admissions*
Brian MacDougall, *Finance and Administration*

## ADDRESS INQUIRIES TO:

Brenda L. Detienne, *Admissions Coordinator*
Room C-23, Lower Level, Clinical Research Centre
5849 University Avenue
Dalhousie University
Halifax, Nova Scotia
Canada B3H 4H7
(902) 494-1874; 494-8884 (FAX)

## GENERAL INFORMATION

Dalhousie University, a privately endowed institution founded in 1838, established a Faculty of Medicine in 1868. The main responsibility of the Faculty of Medicine is to the three Maritime Provinces of Canada (Nova Scotia, New Brunswick, and Prince Edward Island), which have a population of some 1.7 million.

The teaching hospitals located in the immediate vicinity of the medical school have a total of 2,300 beds covering inpatient and outpatient services in all branches of medicine.

University housing and comprehensive Student Health Service are available.

## CURRICULUM

The aim of the four-year course of study in medicine is to provide a basic education that would permit a graduate to enter any branch of postgraduate training.

The academic year for Medicine One and Medicine Two begins in early September and extends to the end of May. Medicine Three begins in late August/early September and ends in March. Medicine Four begins in March and extends until May of the following year. The M.D. degree is granted upon successful completion of the fourth year.

During the first two years of the curriculum, students will learn predominantly in small groups, working with a tutor. The curriculum is organized around clinical problems to provide an integrated context for students to learn both basic and clinical science, and to begin the development of clinical reasoning skills. The third and fourth years are predominantly clinical, with the years being broken into a series of rotations within the various clinical disciplines. Starting in the first year, Dalhousie students have extensive patient contact hours, as the school places great emphasis on the development of clinical skills. In addition to small-group teaching, which emphasizes independent learning, teaching methods include lectures, laboratories, and bedside teaching.

In addition to the basic M.D. program, Dalhousie offers a bachelor of science in medicine program and an M.D.-Ph.D. program.

Dalhousie University through its Faculty of Medicine offers university-arranged and university-supervised clinical training, which meets national accreditation standards, for postgraduate medical trainees.

In all provinces with the exception of Quebec, the basis for licensure for the majority of trainees in a postgraduate training program affiliated with a CACMS/LCME medical school is successful completion of the two-part Medical Council of Canada Qualifying Examination of the (MCCQE), plus certification by either the College of Family Physicians of Canada or the Royal College of Physicians and Surgeons of Canada. There is great competition for entry into all programs.

The family medicine program at Dalhousie is a two-year integrated training experience following the M.D. leading to certification by the College of Family Physicians of Canada.

Specialty training is approved by the Royal College of Physicians and Surgeons of Canada and is conducted in affiliated teaching hospitals in both Halifax and Saint John. Dalhousie University currently holds Royal College approval for 41 specialty training programs.

The Faculty of Medicine maintains an active program of continuing medical education for practicing physicians in the Maritime Provinces. Research and graduate education are in all the basic science departments and in most of the clinical departments.

## REQUIREMENTS FOR ENTRANCE

A university degree and the writing of the MCAT are absolute requirements. Students applying in the fall of 1996 for admission in September 1997 must have written either the April 1994 or subsequent MCAT. There are no absolute prerequisite courses required. The major objective is that premedical education emcompasses broad study in the physical, life, and social sciences and the humanities. The minimum requirement for entry, however, is a baccalaureate degree.

Background in the physical and life sciences will help a student to deal with the considerable load of scientific information involved in undergraduate medical study. Courses in the social sciences and humanities will be helpful in understanding human behavior in health and illness. The ability to communicate effectively, both orally and in writing, is essential. The committee believes that attracting students with a rich variety of educational backgrounds is in the interest of all students. Such preparation supports the training of outstanding physicians.

The medical undergraduate student has to deal with a great deal more information per unit of time than is usually the case in university undergraduate programs in arts and science. Therefore, the Admissions Committee will consider not only the academic grades of applicants but the type and degree of difficulty of university courses completed.

Applications from very well qualified students from other provinces and countries will be considered for up to 10 percent of the entering places in each class. Unless such non-resident applicants have reasonable prospects of being accepted at their local medical school, they should not expect to be accepted at Dalhousie and would be well advised not to apply.

## SELECTION FACTORS

Sources of information and factors considered by the Admissions Committee include academic requirements, ability as judged on university records and on the MCAT, confidential assessments received from referees of the applicant's choice and from any others the committee may wish to consult, interviews (selected applicants only), and place of residence. Detailed comments and explanations on these selection factors may be obtained in the Faculty of Medicine Calendar.

Dalhousie does not discriminate on the basis of race, sex, creed, national origin, age, or handicap.

## FINANCIAL AID

A few entrance scholarships and entrance bursaries are awarded to students in the first year who are residents of the Maritime Provinces. The Dalhousie Medical Alumni Association Entrance Scholarship, the Dr. E. James Gordon Scholarship, and the Halifax Medical Society Entrance Scholarship are available to anyone regardless of residency. A number of bursaries and prizes are available in each year. The university maintains a loan fund which is interest-free until graduation. Applicants are advised not to plan to earn money in time-consuming work which may jeopardize their academic standing.

## INFORMATION FOR MINORITIES

Students from minority groups will be considered on their individual merits.

---

Public Institution

## APPLICATION AND ACCEPTANCE POLICIES FOR 1997–98 FIRST-YEAR CLASS

*Fees and expenses are in Canadian dollars.*

Filing of application
    Earliest date: Oct. 1, 1996
    Latest date: Nov. 15, 1996
School application fee to all applicants: $55
Oldest MCAT scores considered: 1994
Does not have Early Decision Program
Acceptance notice to regular applicants
    Earliest date: Feb. 1, 1997
    Latest date: Until class is filled
Applicant's response to acceptance offer
    Maximum time: 3 weeks
Requests for deferred entrance considered: Yes
Deposit to hold place in class (applied to tuition):
    $200, due with response to acceptance offer;
    nonrefundable
Estimated number of new entrants: 82
Starting date: Aug. 1997

## TUITION AND STUDENT FEES PER YEAR FOR 1995–96 FIRST-YEAR CLASS

Tuition                    Student fees: $229
    Canadian: $4,725
    Non-Canadian: $7,425

## INFORMATION ON 1995–96 FIRST-YEAR CLASS

| Number of | In-Province | Out-of-Province | Total |
|---|---|---|---|
| Applicants | 216 | 368 | 584 |
| Applicants Interviewed | 168 | 35 | 203 |
| New Entrants* | 77 | 9 | 86 |

*All took the MCAT and had baccalaureate degrees.

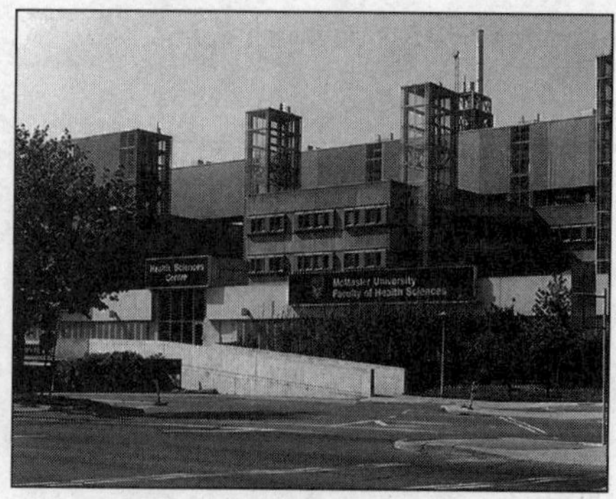

# McMaster University
# Undergraduate Medical Programme
# School of Medicine

**Hamilton, Ontario**

Dr. John Bienenstock, *Dean (Health Sciences)*
Dr. Michael L. Marrin, *Chairman, Admissions Committee*
R. Wakefield, *Student Affairs Office*

## ADDRESS INQUIRIES TO:

Admissions and Records
HSC 1B7-Health Sciences Center
McMaster University
1200 Main Street West
Hamilton, Ontario
Canada L8N 3Z5
(905) 525-9140, Ext. 22235

## GENERAL INFORMATION

The Faculty of Health Sciences at McMaster University offers programs in health sciences education, including undergraduate and postgraduate medical education, and in health sciences research. The clinical programs use the teaching hospital and extensive ambulatory facilities of the McMaster University Health Sciences Centre but also involve clinical teaching units at the major Hamilton hospitals and Community health care centers. The Undergraduate Medical Programme was initiated in 1969, and the first class of students graduated in May 1972.

## CURRICULUM

The three-year program (130 weeks of instruction) in medicine at McMaster uses an approach to learning that will apply throughout the physician's career. The components have been organized in a relevant and logical manner with early exposure to patients. Flexibility is ensured to allow for the variety of student backgrounds and career goals.

The graduates of McMaster's Undergraduate Medical Programme will have developed the knowledge, ability, and attitudes necessary to qualify for further education in any medical career. The general goals for students in the program include the following: the development of competency in problem-based learning and in problem solving, the development of the personal characteristics and attitudes compatible with effective health care, the development of clinical and communication skills, and development of the skills to be a life-long, self-directed learner.

To achieve the objectives of the Undergraduate Medical Programme, students are introduced to patients and their problems with the first unit. They are presented with a series of health care problems and questions requiring the understanding of principles and data collection. Much of the student's

learning occurs within the setting of the small group tutorial. Faculty members serve as tutors/ facilitators or as sources of expert knowledge.

Throughout the course, students are evaluated in a variety of ways, especially by day-today assessment of performance.

The Undergraduate Medical Programme is arranged as a five-unit preclerkship sequence followed by a clerkship; there are additional elective opportunities, both in block periods (totaling 26 weeks) and horizontal electives taken concurrently with ongoing units. Unit I is a 15-week introduction to the determinants of health and illness—environmental, biologic, and behavioral. Units 2, 3, and 4 are 12-week units organized on the basis of organ systems, where biomedical and health care problems are analyzed in depth. Unit 5 is a 12-week integration unit, where case studies are considered on a conception-to-death continuum. The clerkship emphasizes the clinical application of concepts learned in the earlier units and consists of experience in inpatient and ambulatory settings. These include internal medicine, family medicine, surgery psychiatry, obstetrics-gynecology, and pediatrics.

## REQUIREMENTS FOR ENTRANCE

Completion of a minimum of three years at an accredited university with at least an overall second class (B) average is required. There are no course prerequisites. The MCAT is not required.

Applicants who are not Canadian citizens or landed immigrants in Canada will be accepted only when they are considered to be clearly more suitable on all criteria than Canadian candidates.

Both academic achievement and personal qualities are considered. Academic achievement is assessed on the basis of course grades. Personal qualities and attributes are assessed on the basis of a submission written by the applicant, an autobiographical sketch, three references, a personal interview, and the performance in a simulated tutorial.

## SELECTION FACTORS

Students and members of the community and faculty are involved in the assessment of applicants. The aim is to select students who not only have the necessary academic standards but also display characteristics which are deemed to be important for the study and practice of medicine. These include characteristics that suggest sensitivity to the needs of the community; sensitivity to the emotional, psychological, and physical aspects of patients; the ability to detect and solve problems; the ability to learn independently; the ability to function as a member of a small group; and the ability to plan one's career in a way that reflects the needs of the community.

Applicants rating highest in academic achievement and in personal qualities will be invited for an interview. Some weighting according to bona fide residence may be applied according to the following priorities: Hamilton Health Region and Northwestern Ontario, other areas of Ontario, other Canadian provinces, and other countries. From these applicants, 100 students will be selected to fill the entering class.

## FINANCIAL AID

Medical students at McMaster, in addition to facing the general scarcity of financial assistance, are unable to rely on summer employment as a source of funds. In this situation, it is incumbent on students admitted to the Undergraduate Medical Programme to clarify immediately their fiscal situations and to secure or identify sufficient support to meet their financial obligations over the subsequent three years.

There are some government programs (available only to Canadians) and private agencies which offer financial assistance to medical students. The School of Medicine administers a very small loan and bursaries program with a view to supplementing financial resources of some students enrolled in the Undergraduate Medical Programme.

---

Public Institution

## APPLICATION AND ACCEPTANCE POLICIES FOR 1997–98 FIRST-YEAR CLASS

*Fees and expenses are in Canadian dollars.*
*School participates in OMSAS. See Chapter 11.*

Application must be made through Ontario Medical
    School Application Service (OMSAS),
    Ontario Universities' Application Centre,
    P.O. Box 1328, Guelph, Ontario
    Canada N1H 7P4
Filing of OMSAS application
    Earliest date: July 1, 1996
    Latest date: Nov. 1, 1996 (12 p.m. E.S.T.)
OMSAS fee: $150 for one school applied to in
    Ontario; $75 for each additional school
School application fee: None
Oldest MCAT scores considered: 1994
Does not have Early Decision Program
Acceptance notice to regular applicants
    Earliest date: May 31, 1997
    Latest date: Varies
Applicant's response to acceptance offer
    Maximum time: 2 weeks
Requests for deferred entrance considered
Deposit to hold place in class: None
Estimated number of new entrants: 100
Starting date: Aug. 1997

## TUITION AND STUDENT FEES PER YEAR FOR 1995–96 FIRST-YEAR CLASS

Tuition and Student Fees
    Canadian: $5,012
    Non-Canadian: $22,936

## INFORMATION ON 1995–96 FIRST-YEAR CLASS

| Number of | In-Province | Out-of-Province | Total |
|---|---|---|---|
| Applicants | 1,725 | 538 | 2,263 |
| Applicants Interviewed | 360 | 40 | 400 |
| New Entrants* | 94 | 6 | 100 |

*84% had baccalaureate degrees.

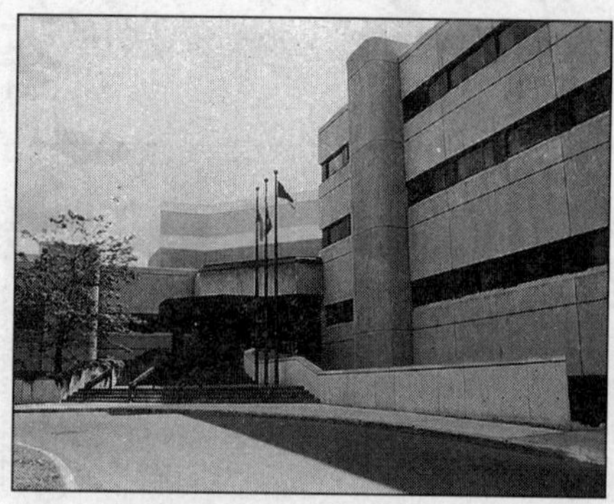

# University of Ottawa Faculty of Medicine

## Ottawa, Ontario

Dr. Peter Walker, *Dean*
Dr. Nadia Z. Mikhael, *Assistant Dean, Admissions*
Nicole Racine, *Admissions Advisor*

## ADDRESS INQUIRIES TO:

Admissions
University of Ottawa
Faculty of Medicine
451 Smyth Road
Ottawa, Ontario
Canada K1H 8M5
(613) 562-5409; 562-5457 (FAX)

## GENERAL INFORMATION

The University of Ottawa received its charter from the province of Ontario in 1866. It was founded by the Missionary Oblates of Mary Immaculate, who were its administrators until 1965, when important structural reforms were introduced through an act of the legislative assembly of the province of Ontario. The management of the university is now under the Board of Governors consisting of members from various sectors of the community. The management, discipline, and control of the university are free from the restrictions and control of any outside body, whether lay or religious. The Faculty of Medicine was established in 1945. In 1978 the health sciences were regrouped into the Faculty of Health Sciences comprising the School of Medicine, the School of Nursing, and the School of Human Kinetics. In 1989, however, the Faculty of Medicine regained its status as a separate academic unit.

## CURRICULUM

During their undergraduate training students acquire the knowledge, skills, and attitudes necessary to recognize, understand, and apply effective, efficient strategies for the prevention and treatment of common and important health problems. The program integrates the basic and clinical sciences throughout the four years of study. Emphasis is placed on self-learning principles, and facts are assimilated in a multidisciplinary fashion, within the context of clinical problems. Lectures and seminars are used to discuss basic concepts, explore new developments, and provide overviews of the biomedical sciences fundamental to the practice of medicine. Training occurs in ambulatory, primary, secondary, and tertiary settings, with students functioning as members of the medical team in collaboration with other health professionals. The program emphasizes health promotion and disease prevention and is responsive to individual needs and abilities and to the changes occurring in society and the health care system.

The program fosters the qualities of trust and compassion, communication skills, ethical professional conduct and patient advocacy.

The program is scheduled over four calendar years and is divided into two stages. The first stage includes 70 weeks of study of essential biomedical principles and consists of thirteen multidisciplinary blocks. The students learn communication and clinical skills in an integrated fashion with the study of body systems. The second stage, of two years duration, is devoted to clinical clerkships; an extended period of sixteen weeks is available for elective study.

## REQUIREMENTS FOR ENTRANCE

The MCAT is compulsory for admission. Results for tests completed prior to 1991 are not accepted.

Students in the following categories are eligible to apply for admission to the first year of the four-year program in the Faculty of Medicine.

(1) Students who have completed successfully in a university the first three years of a bachelor's degree program. Required course work must include:

|  | *Years* |
|---|---|
| Biochemistry* (without laboratory) | 1 |
| General chemistry* (without laboratory) | 1 |
| Organic chemistry* (without laboratory) | 1 |
| General biology or zoology (without laboratory) | 1 |
| Humanities | 1 |

*Two of the three chemistries are required.*

(2) Students of other universities who have completed studies equivalent to those listed above. (Equivalence is determined by the University of Ottawa Faculty of Medicine.)

## SELECTION FACTORS

Academic excellence and interview rating are the main selection criterion used by the Admissions Committee. Academics are measured by an assessment of marks and by a comparison of the applicant's academic record in relationship with those of the other applicants.

Consideration for admission will be given primarily to those eligible candidates who have maintained an overall academic average during the university years of at least B + (or the equivalent GPA). Due to the limited class size, it is to be noted that meeting the above minimum standard does not guarantee admission. No preference is given to academic achievement in one program over another as long as the prerequisites for eligibility have been met. Furthermore, in selecting the students, the Admissions Committee reserves the right to assess, in the applicant's program, the level of difficulty of the courses and/or their pertinence for future medical studies at the University of Ottawa and the performance achieved by the candidate in these courses. No quota is predetermined before the selection is made; each file meeting the requirements is studied individually.

No candidate will be admitted without an interview, and the rating of the interview and of other nonacademic data will be taken into account in the admission process.

Chances of being admitted are greatly reduced for candidates with a score below 8 in any of the MCAT subtests. The MCAT must be written prior to the application deadline.

It is highly desirable that the candidate who has a broad exposure to biology and physical sciences also have a broad exposure to the arts, humanities, and social sciences.

In view of the limited number of places available, a candidate whose GPA is below 3.4 (scale of 4.0) has considerably less chance of being admitted, depending on the year's competition.

Sex, race, age, religion, and socioeconomic status play no part in the selection process. Only applications from Canadian citizens or permanent residents or applications from children of alumni of the University of Ottawa can be considered.

The courses are given in English. Problem-based tutorials and introduction to clinical skills are also offered in French. Knowledge of both official languages of the university will be an asset (but not a prerequisite).

Applicants who are in the third year of a program at the time they apply must, before June 1, submit an official transcript, or no offer of admission will be made.

## FINANCIAL AID

Students who are Canadian citizens may apply to the Student Financial Aid Office of the university and to their respective provincial governments for grant or loan assistance. The Ontario Medical Association Bursaries and Loan Fund, the Kellogg Foundation Loan Fund, and a special bursaries fund are administered by the Awards Committee of the Faculty of Medicine. The Association of Professors of the University also provides a limited number of bursaries. Most of these awards are made on the basis of demonstrable financial need and good academic standing.

Public Institution

## APPLICATION AND ACCEPTANCE POLICIES FOR 1997–98 FIRST-YEAR CLASS

*Fees and expenses are in Canadian dollars.*
*School participates in OMSAS. See Chapter 11.*

Application must be made through Ontario Medical
  School Application Service (OMSAS),
  Ontario Universities' Application Centre,
  P.O. Box 1328, Guelph, Ontario
  Canada N1H 7P4
Filing of OMSAS application
  Earliest date: July 1, 1996
  Latest date: Nov. 1, 1996
OMSAS fee: $150 for one school applied to in
  Ontario; $75 for each additional school
School application fee: $75
Oldest MCAT scores considered: 1991
Does not have Early Decision Program
Acceptance notice to regular applicants
  Earliest date: End of May 1997
  Latest date: Until class is filled
Applicant's response to acceptance offer
  Maximum time: 2 weeks
Requests for deferred entrance considered: Yes
Deposit to hold place in class (applied to tuition)
  $100; nonrefundable
Estimated number of new entrants: 84
Starting date: Sept. 1997

## TUITION AND STUDENT FEES PER YEAR FOR 1995–96 FIRST-YEAR CLASS

Tuition                 Student fees: $239
  Canadian: $3,116
  Non-Canadian: $14,670

## INFORMATION ON 1995–96 FIRST-YEAR CLASS

| Number of | In-Province | Out-of-Province | Total |
| --- | --- | --- | --- |
| Applicants | 1,147 | 513 | 1,660 |
| Applicants Interviewed | * | * | 557 |
| New Entrants† | 75 | 9 | 84 |

*Data not available.
†All took the MCAT; 76.2% had baccalaureate degrees.

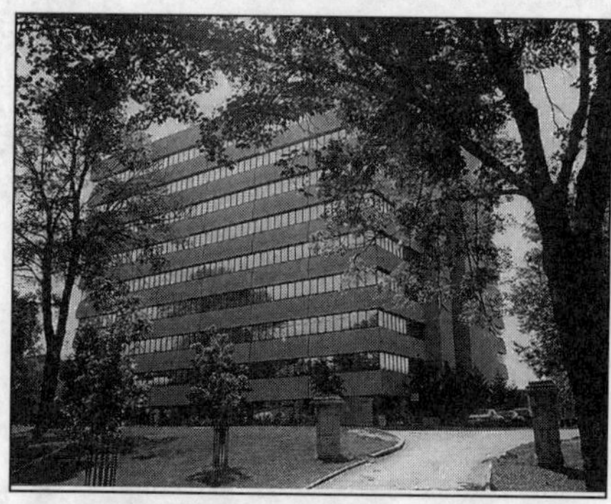

# Queen's University
# Faculty of Medicine

**Kingston, Ontario**

Thelma C. Rikley, *Manager, Undergraduate Medical Education*

## ADDRESS INQUIRIES TO:

Admissions Office
Queen's University
Faculty of Medicine
Kingston, Ontario
Canada K7L 3N6
(613) 545-2542; 545-6884 (FAX)

## GENERAL INFORMATION

Queen's University Faculty of Medicine, established in 1854, is an integral part of a university of more than 10,000 full-time students. The campus is situated within the city of Kingston, which is located on Lake Ontario at the origin of the St. Lawrence River and has an urban and suburban population of 98,000.

Preclinical instruction is given in buildings on the campus. Clinical instruction is conducted in the Kingston General Hospital, immediately adjacent to the campus, the Hotel Dieu Hospital, and a number of specialized hospitals.

## CURRICULUM

The overall goal of the medical curriculum is to produce an undifferentiated or multipotential physician who has the knowledge, skills, and attitudes for further study in the postgraduate training program. Not the least of these skills is the life-long ability to acquire and sustain the new knowledge that will continue to emerge long after graduation. In keeping with this goal, changes in the emphasis and structure of the M.D. program have been made and were implemented in 1991 for students entering the program that year.

The curriculum emphasizes a greater degree of independent student learning and the promotion of the art and the science of medicine, in order to prepare students for a changing health care system. A systems-based approach integrating biomedical and clinical sciences is used to emphasize relevance and avoid undue repetition.

The curriculum is comprised of four phases. Phase I emphasizes selected principles and concepts in the sciences basic to medicine, both for an understanding of these sciences and for their relevance and importance to clinical medicine. A short orientation period and the Horizontal Phase complement Phase I. Phase II uses clinical-based learning, i.e., selected clinical topics that provide a framework for integrating basic and clinical sciences. Instruction in clinical skills is integrated with each systems-based component of Phase II. Phase III, the clinical clerkship, is an integral part of the M.D. program, with structured elements that build upon Phase I, Phase II, and the Horizontal Phase, as well as specific elements and clinical experiences unique to Phase III. The Horizontal Phase introduces broad themes and specific topics and integrate these where appropriate into phases I, II, and III.

The structure of the curriculum, especially the Horizontal Phase, is designed to permit a flexible approach to the introduction and integration of new concepts and topics into the curriculum and to provide students with opportunities to pursue special areas of interest.

## REQUIREMENTS FOR ENTRANCE

The minimum academic requirement for admission is three full years of study in any university program (a minimum of 15 full courses).

Candidates are required to successfully complete the equivalent of a university-level course in each of the following:

|  | *Years* |
| --- | --- |
| Biological sciences | 1 |
| Physical sciences | 1 |
| Humanities or social sciences | 1 |

All applicants are required to write the revised (1991) MCAT prior to the deadline date for submission of applications to OMSAS.

To be eligible for admission, candidates must be Canadian citizens, Canadian permanent residents (landed immigrants) by February 1 following submission of the OMSAS application, or the children of Queen's University alumni who are residents outside Canada. Verification must be sent to the Admissions Office at the time of application.

## SELECTION FACTORS

Seventy-five students are admitted annually into the first medical year and are selected on the basis of a strong academic record and assessment of personal characteristics considered to be most appropriate for the study of medicine at Queen's University and for the subsequent practice of medicine. The following steps are used to identify the group to be invited for interview and for assessment of personal qualities; the cumulative converted GPA based on all years of undergraduate study; and the results of the MCAT. Applications of those below the cutoff will be reviewed by members of the Admissions Committee who will utilize specific guidelines to identify any unusual circumstances.

Candidates who do not make the academic cut based on their undergraduate grade point average but who have completed graduate work are considered in this group. The cutoff is based on the median grade point average of all candidates for the given year.

Given that it is practicable to interview approximately 400 candidates for 75 positions, the Admissions Committee attempts to include as many highly qualified candidates as it can while taking into consideration as many anomalous situations as possible in attempting to give maximum benefit to the applicant population without discriminating against any sector. Unfortunately, it is not possible to interview all of the many highly qualified candidates that apply to our program.

The personal assessment score for those candidates who meet the criteria for steps 1 and 2 is determined from the assessment of the confidential letters of reference, the personal information form, and the autobiographic sketch (50 percent), and the personal interview (50 percent), from which candidates will be ranked for offers and placement on the waiting list.

The Admissions Committee does not give preference to applicants who have studied in any particular university program. Applicants are encouraged to consider all of the undergraduate programs available to them and to embark on the course of studies in which they have the greatest interest and that would prepare them for an alternate career should they not gain a place in medicine.

No preference is shown to applicants at any particular level of training.

Place of residence and location of the university where studies have been undertaken are not criteria in selection. Age, gender, race, and religion are not factors considered in the selection process.

Because of the unique structure of the medical curriculum, candidates are not normally considered for admission with advanced standing or transfer.

Students entering in 1995 presented the following MCAT profile (mean score and range): *BS*-10.84 (9-13), *PS*-11.02 (8-14), *VR*-10.44 (8-13), *WS(M-S)*.

Public Institution

## APPLICATION AND ACCEPTANCE POLICIES FOR 1997–98 FIRST-YEAR CLASS

*Fees and expenses are in Canadian dollars.*
*School participates in OMSAS. See Chapter 11.*

Application must be made through Ontario Medical
  School Application Service (OMSAS),
  Ontario Universities' Application Centre,
  P.O. Box 1328, Guelph, Ontario
  Canada N1H 7P4
Filing of OMSAS application
  Earliest date: July 1, 1996
  Latest date: Nov. 1, 1996
OMSAS fee: $150 plus an institutional levy of $75 for
  each medical school selection
Oldest MCAT scores considered: 1991
Does not have Early Decision Program
Acceptance notice to regular applicants
  Earliest date: May 31, 1997
  Latest date: Until class is filled
Applicant's response to acceptance offer
  Maximum time: 2 weeks
Requests for deferred entrance considered: Yes
Deposit to hold place in class: None
Estimated number of new entrants: 75
Starting date: Sept. 1997

## TUITION AND STUDENT FEES PER YEAR FOR 1995–96 FIRST-YEAR CLASS

Tuition                              Student fees: $539
  Canadian: $3,118
  Non-Canadian: $14,402

## INFORMATION ON 1995–96 FIRST-YEAR CLASS

| Number of | In-Province | Out-of-Province | Total |
|---|---|---|---|
| Applicants | 933 | 489 | 1,422 |
| Applicants Interviewed | 239 | 171 | 410 |
| New Entrants* | 60 | 15 | 75 |

*All took the MCAT; 69% had baccalaureate degrees.

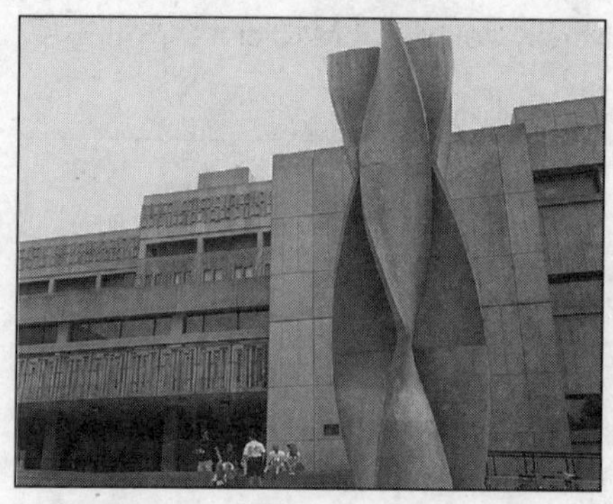

# University of Toronto
# Faculty of Medicine

**Toronto, Ontario**

Dr. A. Aberman, *Dean*
Dr. M. Rossi, *Associate Dean, Student Affairs*
Judy Irvine, *Coordinator, Admissions, Awards and Registrarial Affairs*

## ADDRESS INQUIRIES TO:

University of Toronto
Faculty of Medicine
Toronto, Ontario
Canada M5S 1A8
(416) 978-2717; 971-2163 (FAX)

## GENERAL INFORMATION

The medical school was founded in 1843 as part of King's College, which later became the University of Toronto. The school is a faculty of the university and, as such, receives support from the government of Ontario.

## CURRICULUM

The four-year curriculum is focused on student-centered learning. The pre-clerkship phase (approximately 82 weeks) consists of six multidisciplinary courses, each of which is built upon a series of patient-based cases. Selected lectures, seminars, and laboratory exercises will complement small-group, problem-based learning sessions. Themes for the courses will include the following: the determinants of health; structure and function; the brain, behavior and communication; metabolism and nutrition; pathobiology of disease; and the foundations of medical practice. Students are required to fulfill specific learning objectives for each course and will be assessed both within and at the completion of each course. In addition, longitudinal clinical and community experiences—beginning in Year I— are intended to provide students with the opportunity to acquire knowledge and skills through direct interaction with patients.

Following the pre-clerkship, students spend approximately 78 weeks as clinical clerks. This phase of medical education enables the student to participate in the study and care of patients as a member of a clinical team, which includes interns, residents, and the attending staff physician or surgeon. As clerks, medical students rotate for defined periods through hospital services, including medicine, surgery, obstetrics, paediatrics, family medicine, and psychiatry. Each rotation includes community experiences as well as elements of problem-based learning and basic sicence.

As part of the clerkship, students spend a total of 18 weeks in elective rotations to allow them to explore areas of medicine of particular interest. Clerks may choose to participate in the most technically sophisticated medical units or medical research, work with family physicians in rural setting, or spend part of their elective working in another country.

During the clerkship, students apply to the Canadian Resident Matching Service to select the program in which they wish to do their postgraduate training. Applications must be submitted in the fall, and students are notified in March as to the program to which they have been matched.

A joint M.D.-Ph.D. program is offered in the Faculty of Medicine and the School of Graduate Studies for individuals wishing to make a commitment to research in addition to the practice of clinical medicine. Students accepted into the combined program may pursue the dual degrees via either a sequential or an integrated route. Interested individuals must apply to the M.D. program at the Faculty of Medicine in the normal manner and request an application from the coordinator of the M.D.-Ph.D. program. Entry into the M.D.-Ph.D. program is dependent upon acceptance into the M.D. program.

## REQUIREMENTS FOR ENTRANCE

All applicants are required to write the revised (1991) MCAT prior to the deadline date for submission of applications to OMSAS. A minimum of three years in a degree program at a Canadian university or, for applicants enrolled at a non-Canadian university, a bachelor's degree is required. The faculty does not accept applications for transfer into the program.

Enrollment in the first-year class is currently 177 students.

All applicants are required to have satisfactorily completed the following courses: two full course equivalents in life sciences plus one full course equivalent in social sciences or humanities or languages.

It is recommended, although not required, that applicants complete a university-level course in biometrics or statistics.

## SELECTION FACTORS

Applicants are judged initially upon their academic and non-academic records. In addition, attention is paid to the results of the MCAT, statements of referees, and an autobiographical essay. Applicants are also required to appear for an interview in Toronto. Definite preference is given to Ontario residents. No more than 35 places will be offered to outstanding nonresidents, and of these, a maximum of 9 places will be offered to applicants with student visas. Sex, race, and religion are not considered in determining those applicants to whom places are offered.

Successful candidates must be deemed by the Admissions Committee to be acceptable in all aspects of the admissions process. This may include cumulative grade point average, MCAT scores, published papers, supervisor's letters, non-academic factors, English proficiency performance on interview, and any other criteria put forward by the Admissions Committee.

## FINANCIAL AID

Financial aid is available under the Province of Ontario Student Assistance Program and the Canada Student Loan Program. Applicants are referred to the publications of the Department of University Affairs for details of the regulations governing these awards. Applicants are advised not to plan to earn money in time-consuming work which may jeopardize their standing during the academic year.

Public Institution

## APPLICATION AND ACCEPTANCE POLICIES FOR 1997–98 FIRST-YEAR CLASS

*Fees and expenses are in Canadian dollars.*
*School participates in OMSAS. See Chapter 11.*

Application must be made through Ontario Medical
   School Application Service (OMSAS),
   Ontario Universities' Application Centre,
   P.O. Box 1328, Guelph, Ontario
   Canada N1H 7P4
Filing of OMSAS application
   Earliest date: July 1, 1996
   Latest date: Nov. 1, 1996 12 noon E.S.T.
OMSAS fee: $150 for one school applied to in
   Ontario; $75 for each additional school
School application fee to all applicants: $50
Oldest MCAT scores considered: 1991
Does not have Early Decision Program
Acceptance notice to regular applicants
   Earliest date: May 1997
   Latest date: Until class is filled
Applicant's response to acceptance offer
   Maximum time: 2 weeks
Requests for deferred entrance considered
Deposit to hold place in class: None
Estimated number of new entrants: 177
Starting date: Sept. 1997

## TUITION AND STUDENT FEES PER YEAR FOR 1995–96 FIRST-YEAR CLASS

Tuition
   Canadian: $3,118
   Non-Canadian: $15,069

Student fees:
   Canadian: $764.66
   Non-Canadian: $1,300

## INFORMATION ON 1995–96 FIRST-YEAR CLASS

| Number of | In-Province | Out-of-Province | Total |
|---|---|---|---|
| Applicants | 1,171 | 396 | 1,567 |
| Applicants Interviewed | * | * | 392 |
| New Entrants† | 142 | 30 | 172 |

*Data not available.
†All took the MCAT; 70% had baccalaureate degrees.

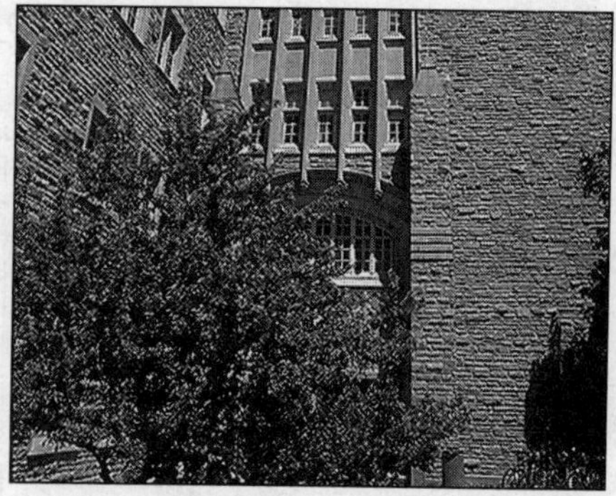

# University of Western Ontario
# Faculty of Medicine

### London, Ontario

Dr. R. Y. McMurtry, *Dean*
Dr. J.A. Silcox, *Associate Dean, Undergraduate Medical Education*
Belle Potts, *Administrative Officer, Admissions Office*

## ADDRESS INQUIRIES TO:

Admissions Office
Room H-104, Health Sciences Centre
University of Western Ontario
London, Ontario
Canada N6A 5C1
(519) 661-3744; 661-3797 (FAX)
E-Mail: Admissions@do.med.uwo.ca

## GENERAL INFORMATION

The Faculty of Medicine of the University of Western Ontario had its origin in 1882 and came under the direct control of the university in 1912. The University of Western Ontario is a private university but in receipt of government grants in common with other universities of Ontario having faculties of medicine.

Students are free to choose any approved residency program. The teaching hospitals, incorporating the clinical science departments, are approved for the graduate training leading to certification in the Royal College of Physicians and Surgeons of Canada.

## CURRICULUM

The undergraduate medical curriculum provided by the Faculty of Medicine is designed to permit the acquisition of a core of fundamental knowledge and basic technical skills, and to assist in developing attitudes that will form a basis for further postgraduate study. The curriculum aims to produce doctors who are life-long learners, caring in their practice of medicine, and in touch with the local community problems that contribute to health care.

The first two years of the curriculum are designed to provide the student with a solid grounding in the basic and clinical sciences. The content of this phase is organized into a series of systems and uses a variety of teaching methods, including lectures, small group tutorials, problem-based learning, self-instructional materials, and laboratories. Students participate in early patient contact and an emphasis is placed on community involvement.

The third and fourth years of medicine are comprised of a 52-week integrated clerkship, 16 weeks of clinical electives, and 6 weeks of basic science electives. During the clerkship, the student becomes an active member of a clinical care team taking major rotations in the following: family medicine, medicine, obstetrics and gynecology, pediatrics, psychiatry, and surgery. The clerkship provides students with an opportunity to participate in patient care in the hospital, clinic, and office setting. Under the supervision of faculty and more senior housestaff, clerks are given graded responsibility in the diagnosis, investigation, and management of patients. Following the clerkship, 16 weeks of clinical electives are arranged entirely by the student in any area of medicine, at UWO or in other centres. After completion of the clinical electives, students return to UWO for 6 weeks of basic science electives. This permits students to further integrate the basic and clinical aspects of medicine in light of their clinical experience.

## REQUIREMENTS FOR ENTRANCE

All applicants must submit results of the revised MCAT (April 1991 or later). The MCAT must be written prior to the application deadline of Nov. 1.

Individuals in the third year of study or those who have successfully completed three full years of study (15 full or equivalent courses) in any degree program at a recognized university are eligible to apply. Five full or equivalent courses must be included in the final undergraduate year and in one other year. In addition, three full or equivalent honors level courses (level 200 or higher) must be included in each of two years (one being the final undergraduate year.)

Individuals who have earned a degree from a recognized university may elect to continue in full-time undergraduate studies for the purpose of improving academic standing for application to medical school for a one-year period only. The special year must contain five full or equivalent courses with a minimum of four full or equivalent honors courses.

Graduate students will be expected to have completed all requirements (including submission of the thesis, if one is required) for their graduate degree prior to registration in the Faculty of Medicine.

Prior to being permitted to register in the Faculty of Medicine, all applicants granted admission will be required to have successfully completed one full or equivalent laboratory course in biology and organic chemistry plus one other full or equivalent science course from a science discipline unrelated to biology and organic chemistry. In addition, three full or equivalent nonscience courses are required; two of these courses must be from different disciplines, one of which must be at the first-year level (one of these courses must be literature (English) or history, if the applicant does not have OAC English or equivalent from secondary school); and one other full or equivalent nonscience course must be at the honors level from one of the nonscience disciplines chosen above.

## SELECTION FACTORS

Enrollment is limited. Admission to the Faculty of Medicine is competitive, and the possession of the minimum requirements does not assure acceptance. Admission consideration is based on academic achievement, MCAT scores, and a personal interview score. Only those applicants deemed competitive will be selected for an interview.

Applications will not be accepted from individuals who are not Canadian citizens or landed immigrants.

## FINANCIAL AID

Financial aid information may be obtained by contacting the Financial Aid Office, Somerville House, the University of Western Ontario at (519) 661-3775.

Public Institution

## APPLICATION AND ACCEPTANCE POLICIES FOR 1997–98 FIRST-YEAR CLASS

*Fees and expenses are in Canadian dollars.*
*School participates in OMSAS. See Chapter 11.*

Application must be made through Ontario Medical
  School Application Service (OMSAS),
  Ontario Universities' Application Centre,
  P.O. Box 1328, Guelph, Ontario
  Canada N1H 7P4
Filing of OMSAS application
  Earliest date: July 1, 1996
  Latest date: Nov. 1, 1996
OMSAS fee: $150 for one school applied to in Ontario,
  $75 for each additional school
School application fee: $50 (subject to change)
Oldest MCAT scores considered: 1991
Does not have Early Decision Program
Acceptance notice to regular applicants
  Earliest date: early July 1996
  Latest date: Until class is filled
Applicant's response to acceptance offer
  Maximum time: 2 weeks
Requests for deferred entrance considered: No
Deposit to hold place in class: None
Estimated number of new entrants: 96
Starting date: Sept. 1997

## TUITION AND STUDENT FEES PER YEAR FOR 1995–96 FIRST-YEAR CLASS

Tuition and student fees: $3,496

## INFORMATION ON 1995–96 FIRST-YEAR CLASS

| Number of | In-Province | Out-of-Province | Total |
|---|---|---|---|
| Applicants | 1,181 | 587 | 1,768 |
| Applicants Interviewed | * | * | 417 |
| New Entrants† | 78 | 18 | 96 |

*Data not available.
†All took the MCAT; 70% had baccalaureate degrees.

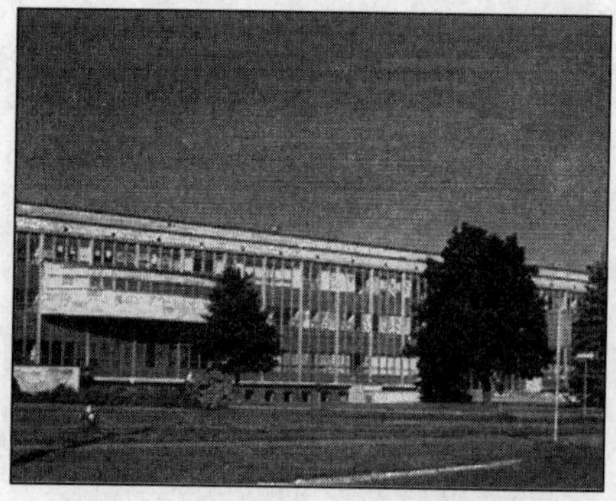

# Université Laval
# Faculty of Medicine

**Ste-Foy, Quebec**

Dr. Louis Larochelle, *Dean*
Dr. Guy Pomerleau, *Chairman, Admission Committee*
Dr. Guy Belanger, *Admission Officer*

## ADDRESS INQUIRIES TO:

Secretary, Admissions Committee
Université Laval
Faculty of Medicine
Ste-Foy, Quebec
Canada G1K 7P4
(418) 656-2492; 656-2733 (FAX)
E-Mail: admission@fmed.ulaval.ca
Web Site: http://www.fmed.ulaval.ca/fmed/fmed.html

## GENERAL INFORMATION

Université Laval, a private institution, was established in 1852 by a Royal Charter granted by Queen Victoria. It was named after Monsignor de Laval, first bishop of Quebec.

Research opportunities are provided in all the basic sciences and in many fields of clinical investigations. The clinical teaching is provided through a network of six major affiliated hospitals and five minor affiliated hospitals. Residence accommodations are provided for many students. There is a University Health Service for students as well as vocational guidance and counseling services.

## CURRICULUM

The curriculum aims to prepare students to undertake any career in medicine. During the first two years, the program provides early introduction to clinical problems and interdepartmental teaching by both basic science and clinical faculty. This part of the curriculum is designed to be flexible and can be spread over three calendar years. The basic clinical clerkships are given in the third and fourth years and provide a basic exposure to each major clinical discipline, including family medicine. The curriculum is monitored by both faculty and students.

## REQUIREMENTS FOR ENTRANCE

Since all instruction is in French, fluency in the French language is an essential prerequisite.

Under the present Quebec educational system, the minimum requirements are two years of college (Health Sciences Program) and the diploma of collegial studies of the Ministry of Education (D.E.C.).

For other applicants, the college curriculum should provide a wide cultural background, including behavioral and social sciences.

Specific course requirements are:

| | *Sem. hrs* |
|---|---|
| General biology (with lab) | 8 |
| General or inorganic chemistry (with lab) | 8 |
| Organic chemistry | 8 |
| General physics (with lab) | 2 |
| Mathematics through calculus | 2 |

Must include analytical geometry, college algebra, and trigonometry.

French
Humanities
Behavioral and social sciences

The MCAT is not required, although the scores are considered when available.

## SELECTION FACTORS

Preference is given to applicants from the province of Quebec. Admission requirements for application from Quebec College (CEGEP) and universities include a standardized C.V. and a three-hour group session called Assessment by Simulation (ABS). This test evaluates different behavioral characteristics of the candidates. A few outstanding French-speaking candidates are admitted from other Canadian provinces and the United States. These candidates are selected on the basis of different parameters: scholastic achievement, interview, curriculum vitae, and letters of recommendation. Sex, race, religion, age, and socioeconomic status are not considered in the selection process.

## FINANCIAL AID

Financial aid is available to Quebec residents through the Bursaries Division of the Provincial Ministry of Education. Summer scholarships of $2,000 are also available to students who wish to devote their vacation period to research.

Public Institution

## APPLICATION AND ACCEPTANCE POLICIES FOR 1997–98 FIRST-YEAR CLASS

*Fees and expenses are in Canadian dollars.*

Filing of application
Earliest date: Jan. 1, 1997
Latest date: March 1, 1997 (for Canadians)
Feb. 1, 1997 (for non-Canadians)

School application fee to all applicants: $55
Oldest MCAT scores considered: 1992
Does not have Early Decision Program
Acceptance notice to regular applicants
   Earliest date: May 15, 1997
   Latest date: Until class is filled
Applicant's response to acceptance offer
   Maximum time: 10 days
Requests for deferred entrance considered: No
Deposit to hold place in class: None
Estimated number of new entrants: 120
Starting date: Sept. 1997

## TUITION AND STUDENT FEES PER YEAR FOR 1995–96 FIRST-YEAR CLASS

Tuition                Student fees: $200
  Resident: $1,964
  Nonresident: $7,696

## INFORMATION ON 1995–96 FIRST-YEAR CLASS

| Number of | In-Province | Out-of-Province | Total |
| --- | --- | --- | --- |
| Applicants | 1,857 | 161 | 1,908 |
| Applicants Interviewed | 360 | 45 | 405 |
| New Entrants | 126 | 11 | 137 |

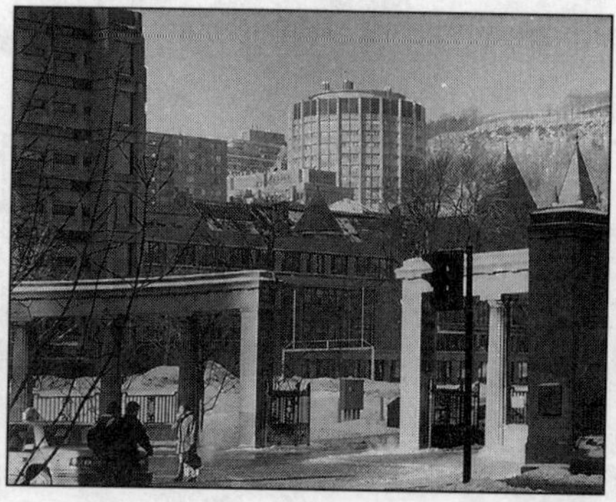

# McGill University
# Faculty of Medicine

**Montreal, Quebec**

Dr. Abraham Fuks, *Dean*
Dr. Nelson Mitchell, *Associate Dean, Admissions*
Judy Stymest, *Director of Student Aid*

## ADDRESS INQUIRIES TO:

Admissions Office
McGill University
Faculty of Medicine
3655 Drummond Street
Montreal, Quebec
Canada H3G 1Y6
(514) 398-3517; 398-3595 (FAX)

## GENERAL INFORMATION

The Faculty of Medicine was established as the original faculty of McGill University in 1829. It seeks to retain its character as an integral part of a diverse university with an international constituency by selecting students from a variety of academic backgrounds and providing them with a medical education which places emphasis upon both basic medical sciences and clinical medicine. There are five university teaching hospitals, three specialty teaching hospitals, and 14 special research centers and units. Research opportunities, available at the undergraduate and graduate levels, are provided in all of the basic medical sciences and in many fields of clinical medicine. The university offers residential facilities and provides student services, including a health service.

The language of instruction is English.

The Faculty of Medicine is identical to a U.S. medical school from the point of view of accreditation, internship and residency training, and licensing, including USMLE eligibility. U.S. students usually choose to return to the U.S. for their residency training and are very competitive in obtaining positions.

## CURRICULUM

McGill University introduced a new curriculum for undergraduate medical education in August 1994. The new curriculum recognizes the importance of a solid data base and a multidisciplinary approach to medical education with interdigitation (integration) of clinical and basic science experience. It is designed to permit a variety of teaching and evaluation methods, recognizing the importance of small-group teaching and the clinical relevance of teaching. It also focuses on the strengths of teaching available in basis science departments and the close cooperation and coordination between the basic and clinical scientists at McGill University.

The new curriculum is composed of four components entitled basis of medicine (BOM), introduction to clinical medicine (ICM), practice of medicine (POM) and back to basics (BTB). The BOM component occupies the first 18 months of medical school, ICM occurs in the second half of the second year and POM is given in the third year and half of the fourth year. The BTB component occupies the remainder of the fourth year. Each component is composed of individual units of interdisciplinary basic science and clinical teaching.

## REQUIREMENTS FOR ENTRANCE

Applicants to the four-year program must have received, or be in the final year of a course of study leading to, a bachelor's degree. The course of study, whether in the natural or social sciences or the humanities, should be selected because it appeals to the intending applicant and offers a broad education and intellectual training. Specific requirements include the MCAT and university level courses in each of the following:

*Credit hrs.*

| | |
|---|---|
| General biology (with lab) | 6 |
| Cellular biology | 3 |
| Molecular biology | 3 |
| General chemistry (with lab) | 6 |
| Organic chemistry (with lab) | 6 |
| Physics (with lab) | 6 |

A university level course in biochemistry (6 credit hrs.) may be substituted for the cellular and molecular biology requirements.

A five-year program is restricted to residents of the province of Quebec who are attending the provincial colleges of general and professional education. Successful applicants take a medical preparatory year in the Faculty of Science before entering the four-year program.

No places for transfer are available.

## SELECTION FACTORS

Selection of students by the admissions committee is based upon academic achievement at the time of application and an assessment of personal characteristics and accomplishments. Academic achievement is determined from the academic record in unergraduate studies and the result of the Medical College Admission Test. Factors taken into account include the subject matter, academic level, and relative difficulty of the program of studies in addition to the actual grades. Completed graduate degrees add additional weight to the application. Applicants to the four-year program should have undergraduate CGPA's of 3.5 or better and a total of 30 or more in the MCAT scores.

The initial assessment of personal qualities and achievements is made from a study of the autobiographical letter and the confirmatory statements and amplifications contained in the letters of reference. A number of those applicants who are deemed the most competitive will be invited for interviews. The decision to offer an interview, however, is not affected by academic performance above the minimums described above. The files of candidates who are not invited for interviews are not considered further.

Once the interviews have been completed, all the components of the application process are considered including GPA's, MCAT scores, and scores assigned to the autobiographical letter. The interview performance and letters of reference are aggregated. Places in the entering class are offered to those whose assembled scores are the most competitive.

The decisions described above are final and are not subject to appeal.

Students accepted into the 1995 entering class had the following academic profile: *mean GPA, 3.5; mean MCAT scores (new test) VR-9.82, PS-10.59, BS-11.04.*

## FINANCIAL AID

A limited amount of financial aid in the form of scholarships, bursaries, and loans is available to students in all years. Information is available from: Student Aid Office, McGill University, 3637 Peel Street, Montreal, Quebec H3A 1X1.

Public Institution

## APPLICATION AND ACCEPTANCE POLICIES FOR 1997–98 FIRST-YEAR CLASS

*Fees and expenses are in Canadian dollars.*

Filing of application
   Earliest date: Sept. 1, 1996
   Latest date: Nov. 15, 1996 (out-of-province applicants); Feb. 1, 1997 (Quebec resident applicants to 4-year program); March 1, 1997 (Quebec resident applicants to 5-year program)
School application fee to all applicants: $60
Oldest MCAT scores considered: 1993
Does not have Early Decision Program
Acceptance notice to regular applicants
   Earliest date: March 31, 1997
   Latest date: Varies
Applicant's response to acceptance offer
   Maximum time: 2 weeks
Requests for deferred entrance considered: Yes
Deposit to hold place in class (applied to tuition):
   $500, due with response to acceptance offer
Deposit refundable prior to: July 1, 1997
Estimated number of new entrants: 130
Starting date: Aug. 1997

## TUITION AND STUDENT FEES PER YEAR FOR 1995–96 FIRST-YEAR CLASS

Tuition                                Student fees: $823
   Resident: $1,845
   Nonresident: $7,635

## INFORMATION ON 1995–96 FIRST-YEAR CLASS

| Number of | In-Province | Out-of-Province | Total |
|---|---|---|---|
| Applicants | 773 | 233 | 1,006 |
| Applicants Interviewed | 250 | 101 | 351 |
| New Entrants* | 94 | 25† | 119 |

*All new entrants into four-year programs took the MCAT and had baccalaureate degrees.

†Of this total, 16 entrants were U.S. citizens, and 9 were citizens of foreign countries.

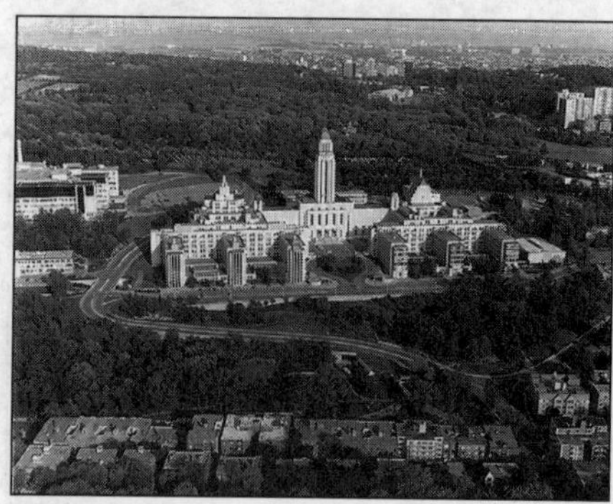

# Université de Montréal
# School of Medicine

**Montreal, Quebec**

Dr. Patrick Vinay, *Dean*
Dr. Michel Gagnon, *Committee on Admissions*

## ADDRESS INQUIRIES TO:

Committee on Admission
Université de Montréal
Faculty of Medicine
P.O. Box 6128, Station Centre-Ville
Montreal, Quebec
Canada H3C 3J7
(514) 343-6265; 343-6629 (FAX)
E-Mail: admmed@ere.umontreal.ca

## GENERAL INFORMATION

The Faculty of Medicine of the University of Montreal can be traced back to a school first established in Montreal in 1843 and incorporated in 1845 under the name of Ecole de Médecine et de Chirurgie de Montréal. In 1891 the school merged with the Faculty of Medicine of the Montreal Branch of Laval University, which had been founded in 1877. In 1920, by an act of the Quebec legislature, the Montreal Branch of Laval University was granted its independence, and the school of medicine became known by its present name.

All instruction is in French, and clinical instruction is carried out at 14 affiliated teaching hospitals and research centers.

## CURRICULUM

In September 1993 a new four- year curriculum came into effect. The first year is devoted to basic biological and behavioral sciences. Clinical exposure begins with Year 1. It consists of two years (70 weeks) of problem-based learning during which students are exposed to biomedical and psychosocial sciences basic to medicine. Courses are interdisciplinary and system-based. Introduction to clinical skills takes place in a continuous fashion throughout those two preclinical years. Ninety hours of electives are mandatory during the first two years. The third and fourth years consist of an 80-week clerkship.

In the new curriculum, formal lecturing is reduced to a minimum and replaced by active methods, especially problem-based learning and small-group discussion.

A premedical year is restricted to students having just graduated from the provincial colleges of general and professional education. Students who have completed one to three years at the university level in humanities are also eligible for the pre-

medical year. Opportunities exist to pursue a combined M.D.-M.Sc. and M.D.-Ph.D. curriculum.

Residency training in the teaching hospitals is under the responsibility of the Faculty of Medicine. Various courses and symposia are organized by the continuing medical education division.

## REQUIREMENTS FOR ENTRANCE

A thorough knowledge of the French language is a prerequisite. Under the present Quebec educational system, the minimum requirement is two years of college (Health Sciences Program) and the diploma of collegial studies of the Department of Education (D.E.C.).

The college curriculum should provide a wide cultural background. Course work must include: philosophy, behavioral and social sciences, French, English, mathematics (analytical geometry, calculus, college algebra, and trigonometry), and sciences (biology, inorganic and organic chemistry, and physics).

## SELECTION FACTORS

Candidates accepted must be either Canadian citizens or landed immigrants, but due consideration will be given to French-speaking applicants from other provinces of Canada and from the United States. Selection of candidates is competitive and based on a global score derived from scholastic records and an interview. Interviews, conducted on the site of the medical school, are granted to about one quarter of the applicants selected from their scholastic records. This interview can be eliminatory. For candidates holding a Ph.D. degree, performance in research may constitute an important selection factor. No consideration is given to race, sex, creed, or age.

## FINANCIAL AID

Financial aid is available to students through the Bursaries Division of the Department of Education, the Kellogg Foundation Loan Fund, the Scholarships and Loan Committee of the university, and the Jean Frappier Fund. Summer scholarships are also available.

Public Institution

## APPLICATION AND ACCEPTANCE POLICIES FOR 1997–98 FIRST-YEAR CLASS

*Fees and expenses are in Canadian dollars.*

Filing of application
   Latest date: March 1, 1997
School application fee to all applicants: $55
Does not have Early Decision Program
Acceptance notice to regular applicants
   Earliest date: May 15, 1997
   Latest date: Until class is filled
Applicant's response to acceptance offer
   Maximum time: 14 days
Requests for deferred entrance considered: No
Deposit to hold place in class: None
Estimated number of new entrants: 145
Starting date: Sept. 1997

## TUITION AND STUDENT FEES PER YEAR FOR 1995–96 FIRST-YEAR CLASS

Tuition                Student fees: $30
   Resident: $2,260
   Nonresident: $7,455

## INFORMATION ON 1995–96 FIRST-YEAR CLASS

| Number of | In-Province | Out-of-Province | Total |
|---|---|---|---|
| Applicants | 2,059 | 143 | 2,202 |
| Applicants Interviewed | 457 | 37 | 494 |
| New Entrants* | 152 | 9 | 161 |

*44% had baccalaureate degrees.

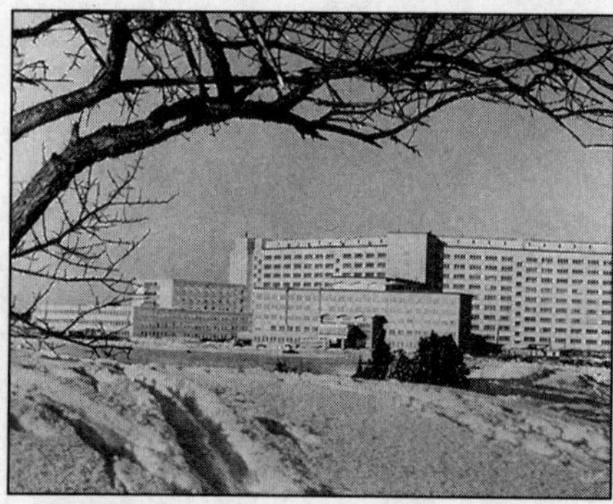

# University of Sherbrooke
# Faculty of Medicine

### Sherbrooke, Quebec

Dr. Michael Baron, *Dean*
Dr. Carolle Bernier, *Chair, Admission, Committee*
Robert Rouleau, *Financial Aid Officer*

## ADDRESS INQUIRIES TO:

Admission Office
University of Sherbrooke
Faculty of Medicine
Sherbrooke, Quebec
Canada J1H 5N4
(819) 564-5208; 564-5378 (FAX)
E-Mail: mmoreau@courrier.usherb.ca
Web Site: http://www.usherb.ca

## GENERAL INFORMATION

Officially founded in February 1961, the Faculty of Medicine at the University of Sherbrooke is a French-speaking institution. It admitted its first students in September 1966.

As required by modern medical teaching, the Faculty of Medicine is integrated into a developing Health Sciences Center to serve all members of the health team. This center includes a modern 400-bed teaching hospital. A Department of Nursing offers several programs of study at university level. The Faculty of Medicine offers residential facilities on campus. Twelve hospitals, many health centers, and CLSC are affiliated with the Faculty of Medicine.

## CURRICULUM

Since 1987, a new four-year curriculum has begun. The form of teaching is now a problem-based learning program. Formal lecturing has been reduced to a minimum. Audiovisual facilities, seminars, small group discussions, panels, field work, and case studies are used extensively. Most learning sessions integrate many disciplines representing various departments.

The M.D. degree is granted after successful completion of a four-year course. Students work in the hospital from the beginning of their first year. The fourth year is a 16-month clerkship starting immediately after the end of the third year.

Postgraduate programs are available in most departments leading to the M.Sc. or Ph.D. degree, and a diploma can be obtained in community health. Residency training is offered in all major specialties.

## REQUIREMENTS FOR ENTRANCE

The minimum requirement for admission is two years of college under the present Quebec educational system—College d'enseignement general et professionel (C.E.G.E.P.). B.A. or B.Sc. degrees are fully acceptable. The minimum science curriculum is as follows:
Candidates with a B.A. or B.Sc. degree:

|  | *Semesters* |
|---|---|
| General biology (with lab) | 2 |
| General chemistry (with lab) | 2 |
| Organic chemistry (with lab) | 2 |
| General physics (with lab) | 3 |
| Mathematics through calculus | 3 |

Must include analytical geometry, college algebra, and trigonometry.

C.E.G.E.P. candidates:

College diploma (D.E.C.) with major in sciences.

The college curriculum should also provide a wide cultural background in the humanities (including philosophy and literature) and in the social and behavioral sciences (including history, psychology, and sociology). Since all instruction is in French, fluency and reading ability in the French language are essential prerequisites.

The MCAT is not required.

## SELECTION FACTORS

Admission to the Faculty of Medicine is based primarily on ability and premedical achievement, as demonstrated by scholastic records. Actually, the selection procedures are being revised due to our new curriculum of medical studies.

Eighty-six places are reserved for applicants from the province of Quebec. Seven additional places are reserved for applicants from New Brunswick. Two places are available for qualified foreign applicants with visas. Applicants must have a very good knowledge of the French language.

## FINANCIAL AID

Financial aid is available to resident students through the Bursaries Division of the Provincial Ministry of Education, the Scholarships and Loans Committee of the university, and a few private foundations.

Public Institution

## APPLICATION AND ACCEPTANCE POLICIES FOR 1997–98 FIRST-YEAR CLASS

*Fees and expenses are in Canadian dollars.*

Filing of application
 Earliest date: Nov. 1996
 Latest date: March 1, 1997
School application fee to all applicants: $30
Oldest MCAT scores considered: 1994
Does not have Early Decision Program
Acceptance notice to regular applicants
 Earliest date: May 1997
 Latest date: Aug. 1997
Applicant's response to acceptance offer
 Maximum time: 15 days
Requests for deferred entrance considered: No
Deposit to hold place in class (applied to tuition):
 $200, due Aug. 1, 1997
Deposit refundable prior to: Aug. 1, 1997
Estimated number of new entrants: 88
Starting date: Aug. 1997

## TUITION AND STUDENT FEES PER YEAR FOR 1995–96 FIRST-YEAR CLASS

Tuition and student fees:
 Canadian: $2,942
 Non-Canadian: $11,624

## INFORMATION ON 1995–96 FIRST-YEAR CLASS

| *Number of* | *In-Province* | *Out-of-Province* | *Total* |
|---|---|---|---|
| Applicants | 1,540 | 191 | 1,731 |
| New Entrants* | 82 | 9 | 91 |

*5% had baccalaureate degrees.

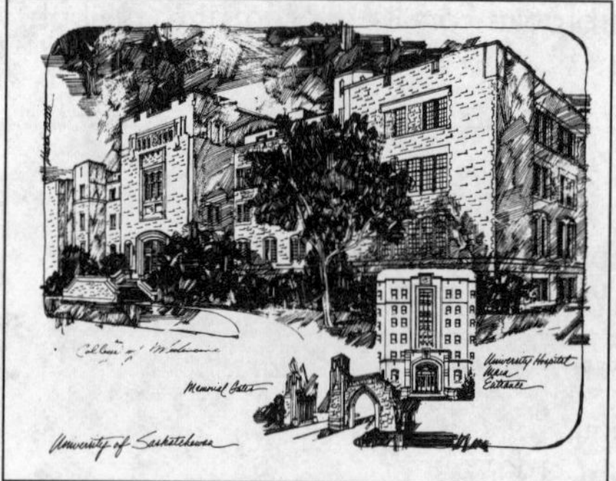

# University of Saskatchewan College of Medicine

## Saskatoon, Saskatchewan

Dr. D. R. Popkin, *Dean of Medicine*
M.D. Evered, *Director of Admissions and Student Affairs*
J. R. Pitzel, *Administrative Assistant, Admissions*

## ADDRESS INQUIRIES TO:

Secretary, Admissions
University of Saskatchewan
College of Medicine
B103 Health Sciences Building
Saskatoon, Saskatchewan
Canada S7N 0W0
(306) 966-8554; 966-6164 (FAX)

## GENERAL INFORMATION

The University of Saskatchewan began teaching medical students in a two-year medical sciences program in 1926. The present college was introduced in 1953 with a four-year curriculum leading to the M.D. degree. In 1968 the curriculum changed to five years with a one-year premedical university requirement. The curriculum reverted to a four-year program in 1988 with a minimum two-year premedical requirement.

Clinical teaching is based at the Royal University Hospital, St. Paul's and Saskatoon City hospitals in Saskatoon, and the Plains Health Centre and General Hospital in Regina.

The maximum size of each entering class is 55 students.

## CURRICULUM

The College of Medicine provides a curriculum leading to the general professional education of the physician; graduates may select careers in family medicine, specialty practice, public health, research, or teaching. During the course of the undergraduate M.D. curriculum, students may obtain a B.Sc. (Med.) degree in the basic medical sciences.

The curriculum consists of at least two years of premedical study followed by four medical years. The four years are divided into five phases: Phase 1 (8 weeks) provides students with an overview of the basic science disciplines appropriate to the understanding of medicine; Phase 2 (25 weeks) enables students to acquire specific knowledge in basic sciences; Phase 3 (14 weeks) enables students to acquire specific knowledge in those subjects bridging the basic and clinical sciences and to learn basic clinical skills; Phase 4 (47 weeks) enables learning of the principles, methods, and core clinical knowledge; Phase 5 (52 weeks of clinical clerkships) provides students with an opportunity to apply the knowledge, skills, and attitudes they have acquired to the management of patients.

Learning in the basic and clinical sciences has been organized by body systems with a problem-solving emphasis. Significant time blocks have been reserved in phases 1-4 for independent study. Provision is made for clinical electives.

## REQUIREMENTS FOR ENTRANCE

Two full years of university study are required after graduation from secondary school. The following courses or their equivalent are required:

| | Credit hrs. |
|---|---:|
| General biology (with lab) | 6 |
| General chemistry (with lab) | 3 |
| General physics (with lab) | 6 |
| Organic chemistry | 3 |
| English (lit. and comp.) | 6 |
| Social sciences or humanities (full course) | 6 |

The MCAT is not required.

The applicant must be a Canadian citizen or landed immigrant.

## SELECTION FACTORS

The Admissions Committee considers academic ability and personal qualities assessed through scholastic records, letters of recommendation, and results of a personal interview by a team of four persons. All eligible candidates are interviewed during a weekend in March. At the time of selection, academic ability and personal qualities are weighted approximately 3 to 1. For the 1995 entering class, the average GPA was 85.8 percent, and the average interview score was 21 of a possible 24 points.

## FINANCIAL AID

Various loan funds and scholarships are available. A limited number of bursaries enable students to engage in research between the end of one academic year and the beginning of another.

## INFORMATION FOR MINORITIES

There is an Aboriginal Access Program for Saskatchewan Residents.

Public Institution

## APPLICATION AND ACCEPTANCE POLICIES FOR 1997–98 FIRST-YEAR CLASS

*Fees and expenses are in Canadian dollars.*

Filing of application
  Earliest date: Sept. 1, 1996
  Latest dates
    In-province: Jan. 15, 1997
    Out-of-province: Dec. 1, 1996
School application fee:
  In-province: $40
  Out-of-province: $75 plus transcript fee*
Does not have Early Decision Program
Acceptance notice to regular applicants
  Earliest date: June 25, 1997
  Latest date: Varies
Applicant's response to acceptance offer
  Maximum time: 2 weeks
Requests for deferred entrance considered: Yes
Deposit to hold place in class (applied to tuition):
  $100, due with response to acceptance offer;
  nonrefundable
Estimated number of new entrants: 55
Starting date: Aug. 1997

## TUITION AND STUDENT FEES PER YEAR FOR 1995–96 FIRST-YEAR CLASS

Tuition: $5,000                    Student fees: $105

## INFORMATION ON 1995–96 FIRST-YEAR CLASS

| Number of | In-Province | Out-of-Province | Total |
|---|---|---|---|
| Applicants | 240 | 198 | 438 |
| Applicants Interviewed | 205 | 17 | 222 |
| New Entrants† | 54 | 1 | 55 |

*Transcript fees are $25 for Canadian universities and $50 for non-Canadian universities.

†32% had baccalaureate degrees.